How to Pass the
FRACP Written
Examination

How to Pass the FRACP Written Examination

Jonathan Gleadle
Professor of Medicine and Consultant Nephrologist
College of Medicine and Public Health
Flinders University, South Australia;
Division of Medicine, Critical and Cardiac Care
Flinders Medical Centre, South Australia, Australia

Jordan Li
Associate Professor of Medicine and Consultant Nephrologist
College of Medicine and Public Health
Flinders University, South Australia;
Department of Renal Medicine
Flinders Medical Centre, South Australia, Australia

Danielle Wu
Consultant Nephrologist and General Medicine Physician, Adjunct Senior Lecturer
Department of Medicine
Mackay Base Hospital, Queensland;
College of Medicine and Dentistry
James Cook University, Queensland, Australia

Paul Kleinig
Consultant in General Medicine, Palliative Care and Care of the Elderly, Senior Lecturer
Division of Rehabilitation, Aged Care and Palliative Care
Flinders Medical Centre, South Australia;
College of Medicine and Public Health
Flinders University, South Australia, Australia

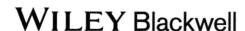

Registered Offices

John Wiley & Sons, Inc., 111 River Street, Hoboken, NJ 07030, USA
John Wiley & Sons Ltd, The Atrium, Southern Gate, Chichester, West Sussex, PO19 8SQ, UK

Editorial Office
9600 Garsington Road, Oxford, OX4 2DQ, UK

For details of our global editorial offices, customer services, and more information about Wiley products visit us at www.wiley.com.

Wiley also publishes its books in a variety of electronic formats and by print-on-demand. Some content that appears in standard print versions of this book may not be available in other formats.

Library of Congress Cataloging-in-Publication Data

Names: Gleadle, Jonathan, author. | Li, Jordan, author. | Wu, Danielle,
    author. | Kleinig, Paul, author.
Title: How to pass the FRACP written examination / Jonathan Gleadle, Jordan
    Li, Danielle Wu, Paul Kleinig.
Description: Hoboken, NJ : Wiley-Blackwell, 2022. | Includes
    bibliographical references and index.
Identifiers: LCCN 2021028006 (print) | LCCN 2021028007 (ebook) | ISBN
    9781119599500 (paperback) | ISBN 9781119599494 (Adobe PDF) | ISBN
    9781119599548 (epub)
Subjects: MESH: Internal Medicine | Australia | New Zealand | Examination
    Questions
Classification: LCC RC58 (print) | LCC RC58 (ebook) | NLM WB 18.2 | DDC
    616.0076–dc23
LC record available at https://lccn.loc.gov/2021028006
LC ebook record available at https://lccn.loc.gov/2021028007

Cover Design: Wiley
Cover Images: © magicmine/getty images

Set in size of 8.5/11pt FrutigerLTStd by Straive, Chennai, India

10 9 8 7 6 5 4 3 2 1

Contents

Introduction, vii

Acknowledgements, ix

Abbreviations, xiii

Features contained in your study aid, xvii

1. **Cardiology,** 1
   Answers, 13

2. **Critical Care Medicine,** 34
   Answers, 43

3. **Dermatology,** 57
   Answers, 63

4. **Endocrinology,** 71
   Answers, 79

5. **Epidemiology, Statistics, and Research,** 97
   Answers, 100

6. **Gastroenterology,** 107
   Answers, 118

7. **General and Geriatric Medicine,** 141
   Answers, 151

8. **Genetic Medicine,** 170
   Answers, 175

9. **Haematology,** 184
   Answers, 199

10. **Immunology and Allergy,** 223
    Answers, 228

11. **Infectious Disease,** 237
    Answers, 244

12. **Medical Obstetrics,** 262
    Answers, 264

13. **Medical Oncology,** 269
    Answers, 274

14. **Mental Health,** 289
    Answers, 293

15. **Nephrology,** 302
    Answers, 312

16. **Neurology,** 334
    Answers, 342

17. **Palliative Medicine,** 360
    Answers, 363

18. **Pharmacology, Toxicology and Addiction Medicine,** 368
Answers, 376

19. **Respiratory and Sleep Medicine,** 393
Answers, 409

20. **Rheumatology,** 430
Answers, 442

21. **Basic Science,** 458
Answers, 461

Index 471

Introduction

This book follows on from the successful 'Passing the FRACP Written Examination. Questions and Answers'. We were encouraged by the responses of readers and trainees to generate this completely new text. It is similar in style to the first book in providing an array of multiple choice and extended matching questions which follow the current format of the FRACP written examination. Every question is chosen to reflect the RACP core training curriculum. However, this is not just a practice exam paper; it also provides an explanation of the answer with a mini review of the topic with referenced QR code links to the best recent review or relevant article in the area.

We have endeavoured to ground many of the questions in clinically relevant cases recalling Osler '*He who studies medicine without books sails an uncharted sea, but he who studies medicine without patients does not go to sea at all*' and we have sought to provide coverage of areas of medicine that are new, contemporary, or evolving. We hope that readers will use the book to help them define areas of their own medical knowledge that are incomplete and would benefit from focussed learning and revision. Whilst many of the questions are designed to be similar in level to those in the actual examination, some are specialised or difficult, designed to 'teach' particularly important issues, stretch the reader's knowledge or to draw attention to contemporary topics. Furthermore, these questions often require clinical reasoning with many being two step questions where simple recall of knowledge is insufficient.

Whilst the main audience for the book is intended to be Trainees undertaking the FRACP written examination, we hope that it may be useful to physicians seeking to update their knowledge or to undertake other postgraduate examinations.

Questions in the written examination are based on the curriculum and all candidates should familiarise themselves with the RACP curriculum for Basic Physician training, which is available electronically from the College website (https://www.racp.edu.au/docs/default-source/default-document-library/knowledge-guides-for-basic-trainees-in-adult-internal-medicine.pdf?sfvrsn=38dc0d1a_4). It is vital to carefully read the most updated examination instructions in any past questions provided by the RACP.

In undertaking the written examination:

- **Read the question carefully!**
- **Read the possible answers carefully!**
- **Answer all of the questions! (make an informed guess if you are uncertain)**
- If you are uncertain about the correct response, look at which options you think are definitely incorrect. Think about why the question is being asked; what is the question 'getting at?'; what are the important 'teaching points' that are being tested? If you still are uncertain, move to the other questions and then come back to those you are not certain of.

We hope that this book will improve your medical knowledge and thereby help you to pass the FRACP examination. Good luck! Clinical practice and biomedical sciences are constantly changing and today's incontrovertible facts can quickly become outdated when a new trial is published or a new scientific discovery made. Therefore, trainees are strongly encouraged to keep up-to-date with their reading and learning, and to check appropriate drug selection, dosage and route of administration. If you have any questions or suggestions, please write to us care of the publisher.

Jonathan Gleadle
Professor of Medicine
College of Medicine and Public Health
Flinders University and Consultant Nephrologist
Flinders Medical Centre
Adelaide, Australia

Jordan Li
Associate Professor of Medicine
College of Medicine and Public Health
Flinders University and Consultant Nephrologist
Flinders Medical Centre
Adelaide, Australia

Danielle Wu
Adjunct Senior Lecturer
College of Medicine and Dentistry, James Cook University and
Consultant Nephrologist and General Physician
Mackay Base Hospital
Queensland, Australia

Paul Kleinig
Clinical Associate Lecturer
College of Medicine and Public Health
Flinders University and Consultant in General Medicine
Palliative Care and Care of the Elderly
Flinders Medical Centre
Adelaide, Australia

Acknowledgements

We would like to thank many of our colleagues who have made major contributions to this book. We would particularly like to acknowledge Dr Katherine Punshon, Dr Sonia Huang, Dr Naukhez Asif, and Dr Telena Kerkham for contributing questions and review.

We would like to thank Oliver Mountain, Justine Li, our student reviewers, and Jasmin Shuen who all provided meticulous review, editing of the manuscript, references and QR codes. Your contributions were essential in the generation of this book.

Finally, a special thanks to Anne Hunt, Anupama Sreekanth, James Watson, and Mary Malin at Wiley for your support in making this book possible.

We would like to acknowledge the following specialists and advanced trainees for their expertise, comments and reviews of the relevant chapters.

Cardiology
Professor Bill Heddle
Consultant Cardiologist
Department of Cardiology
Flinders Medical Centre and College of Medicine and Public Health, Flinders University

Critical Care Medicine
Dr Hanmo Li
Senior Registrar, Advanced Trainee in Critical Care Medicine
Intensive and Critical Care Unit
Flinders Medical Centre

Dermatology
Dr Alain Tran
Senior Registrar, Advanced Trainee in Dermatology, Associate Lecturer
Department of Dermatology
Flinders Medical Centre and College of Medicine and Public Health, Flinders University

Endocrinology
Dr Angela Chen
Consultant Endocrinologist
Department Endocrinology
Flinders Medical Centre

Epidemiology, Statistics and Research
Paul Hakendorf
Manager, Clinical Epidemiology Unit
Flinders Medical Centre

Chris Horwood
Senior Epidemiologist and Data Analyst
Clinical Epidemiology Unit
Flinders Medical Centre

Gastroenterology
Dr Alex Barnes
Consultant Gastroenterologist, Associate Lecturer
Department of Gastroenterology
Flinders Medical Centre and College of Medicine and Public Health, Flinders University

General and Geriatric Medicine
Dr Pravin Shetty
Consultant General Physician and Senior Lecturer
Department of General Medicine
Flinders Medical Centre and College of Medicine and Public Health, Flinders University

Genetic Medicine
Associate Professor Karen Lower
Department of Molecular Medicine and Genetics
College of Medicine and Public Health, Flinders University

Haematology
Dr Angelina Yong
Consultant Haematologist
Department of Haematology
Lyell McEwin Hospital

Immunology
Dr Claire Reynolds
Senior Registrar, Advanced Trainee in Immunology
Department of Immunology
Flinders Medical Centre

Infectious Disease
Dr Nicholas Anagnostou
Consultant Infectious Disease Physician
Department of Infectious Disease
Flinders Medical Centre

Medical Obstetrics
Dr Jessica Gehlert
Consultant Endocrinologist, Clinical Pharmacologist and Obstetric Medicine
Department of Clinical Pharmacology
Flinders Medical Centre

Medical Oncology
Dr Anna Mislang
Consultant Medical Oncologist
Department of Medical Oncology
Flinders Medical Centre

Mental Health
Professor Michael Baigent
Consultant Psychiatrist
Centre for Anxiety and Related Disorders
Flinders Medical Centre and College of Medicine and Public Health, Flinders University

Nephrology
Dr Sarah Tan
Senior Registrar, Advanced Trainee in Nephrology, Associate Lecturer
Department of Renal Medicine
Flinders Medical Centre and College of Medicine and Public Health, Flinders University

Neurology

Associate Professor Tim Kleinig
Consultant Neurologist and Stroke Physician
The Central Adelaide Neurology Service
Royal Adelaide Hospital

Pharmacology, Toxicology and Addiction Medicine

Dr Jessica Gehlert
Consultant Endocrinologist, Clinical Pharmacologist and Obstetric Medicine
Department of Clinical Pharmacology
Flinders Medical Centre

Radiology

Dr Ramon Pathi
Consultant Radiologist
Medical Imaging Services
Flinders Medical Centre

Respiratory and Sleep Medicine

Dr Brendan Dougherty
Consultant Respiratory Physician
Department of Respiratory & Sleep Medicine
Flinders Medical Centre

Dr Teng Yuan Kang
Senior Registrar, Advanced Trainee in Respiratory & Sleep Medicine, Associate Lecturer
Department of Respiratory & Sleep Medicine
Flinders Medical Centre and College of Medicine and Public Health, Flinders University

Rheumatology

Associate Professor Mihir Wechalekar
Consultant Rheumatologist
Department of Rheumatology
Flinders Medical Centre and College of Medicine and Public Health, Flinders University

Dr Anthea Gist
Senior Registrar, Advanced Trainee in Rheumatology
Canberra Hospital, ACT

Abbreviations

AAA	Abdominal aortic aneurysm
ABG	Arterial blood gas
ACE	Angiotensin-converting enzyme
ACS	Acute coronary syndrome
ADH	Antidiuretic hormone
AF	Atrial fibrillation
AFP	Alpha-fetoprotein
AIDS	Acquired immune deficiency syndrome
AKI	Acute kidney injury
ALP	Alkaline phosphatase
ALT	Alanine aminotransferase
ANA	Antinuclear antibody
ANCA	Anti-neutrophil cytoplasmic antibody
Anti-CCP	Anti-cyclic citrullinated peptide
APTT	Activated partial thromboplastin time
ARB	Angiotensin II receptor blocker
ARDS	Acute respiratory distress syndrome
AST	Aspartate aminotransferase
ATSI	Aboriginal and Torres Strait Islander
AUC	Area under the curve
AXR	Abdominal X-ray
BCC	Basal cell carcinoma
Beta-HCG	Beta human chorionic gonadotropin
BGL	Blood glucose level
BMI	Body mass index
BP	Blood pressure
bpm	Beat per minute
CABG	Coronary artery bypass grafting
CCF	Congestive cardiac failure
CFTR	Cystic fibrosis transmembrane conductance regulator
CK	Creatine kinase
CKD	Chronic kidney disease
CMV	Cytomegalovirus
CNS	Central nervous system
CPAP	Continuous positive airway pressure
CPR	Cardiopulmonary resuscitation
COPD	Chronic obstructive pulmonary disease
COVID-19	Coronavirus disease 2019
CRP	C-reactive protein
CSF	Cerebrospinal fluid
CT	Computed tomography
CTPA	Computed tomography pulmonary angiography
CVA	Cerebrovascular accident
CVP	Central venous pressure
CXR	Chest X-ray
DIC	Disseminated intravascular coagulation
DKA	Diabetic ketoacidosis
DMARDs	Disease-modifying anti-rheumatic drugs
DNA	Deoxyribonucleic acid

ds-DNA	Double-stranded DNA
DVT	Deep vein thrombosis
eGFR	Estimated glomerular filtration rate
EBV	Epstein-Barr virus
ECG	Electrocardiogram
ECT	Electroconvulsive therapy
EEG	Electroencephalogram
EGFR	Epidermal growth factor receptor
ELISA	Enzyme-linked immunosorbent assay
EMG	Electromyography
ENA	Extractable nuclear antigens antibodies
ERCP	Endoscopic retrograde cholangiopancreatography
ESKD	End stage kidney disease
ESR	Erythrocyte sedimentation rate
EUC	Electrolyte, urea, creatinine
FBE	Full blood examination
FDA	The United States Food and Drug Administration
FEV1	Forced expiratory volume in one second
FFP	Fresh frozen plasma
FNA	Fine needle aspiration
FOBT	Faecal occult blood test
G-CSF	Granulocyte colony stimulating factor
GCS	Glasgow Coma Scale
GGT	Gamma-glutamyl transferase
GI	Gastrointestinal
GORD	Gastro-oesophageal reflux disease
GP	General practitioner
Hb	Haemoglobin
HBV	Hepatitis B virus
HCV	Hepatitis C virus
HDL	High-density lipoprotein
HIV	Human Immunodeficiency virus
HLA	Human leukocyte antigen
HPV	Human papillomavirus
HR	Heart rate
HRCT	High-resolution computed tomography
HSV	Herpes simplex virus
HUS	Haemolytic uremic syndrome
IBD	Inflammatory bowel disease
IBS	Irritable bowel syndrome
ICD	Implantable cardioverter-defibrillator
ICU	Intensive care unit
IDC	indwelling catheter
IgA	Immunoglobulin A
IHD	Ischaemic heart disease
INR	International normalised ratio
IV	Intravenous
IVIG	Intravenous immunoglobulin
JVP	Jugular venous pressure
LDH	Lactate dehydrogenase
LDL	Low-density lipoproteins

LFTs	Liver function tests
MAP	Mean arterial pressure
MCV	Mean corpuscular volume
MGUS	Monoclonal gammopathy of undetermined significance
MHC	Major histocompatibility complex
MI	Myocardial infarction
MPO	Myeloperoxidase
MRCP	Magnetic resonance cholangiopancreatography
MRI	Magnetic resonance imaging
MRSA	Methicillin-resistant *Staphylococcus aureus*
NSAIDs	Nonsteroidal anti-inflammatory drugs
NT-proBNP	N-terminal pro B-type natriuretic peptide
OSA	Obstructive sleep apnoea
PBS	Pharmaceutical Benefits Scheme
PCR	Polymerase chain reaction
PE	Pulmonary embolism
PET	Positron emission tomography
PFTs	Pulmonary function tests
PPI	Proton pump inhibitor
PSA	Prostate specific antigen
PTH	Parathyroid hormone
PVD	Peripheral vascular disease
RBC	Red blood cell
RCT	Randomised, controlled trial
RF	Rheumatoid factor
SGLT2	Sodium-glucose co-transporter 2
SIADH	Syndrome of inappropriate antidiuretic hormone secretion
SLE	Systemic lupus erythematosus
SSRI	Selective serotonin reuptake inhibitor
STD	Sexually transmitted disease
STEMI	ST-elevation myocardial infarction
TB	Tuberculosis
TFTs	Thyroid function tests
TIA	Transient ischaemic attack
TNF	Tumour necrosis factor
TOE	Transoesophageal echocardiogram
TSH	Thyroid stimulating hormone
TTE	Transthoracic echocardiogram
TTP	Thrombotic thrombocytopenic purpura
USS	Ultrasound scan
UTI	Urinary tract infection
VBG	Venous blood gas
VEGF	Vascular endothelial growth factor
VF	Ventricular fibrillation
V/Q	Ventilation/Perfusion scan
VRE	Vancomycin-resistant Enterococci
VT	Ventricular tachycardia
VTE	Venous thromboembolism
VZV	Varicella zoster virus
WBC	White blood cells
WHO	World Health Organization

Features contained in your study aid

Question and answer sections are clearly indicated for quick reference.

Question sections:

> ## 1 Cardiology
>
> ## Questions
> **BASIC SCIENCE**
>
> Answers can be found in the Cardiology Answers section at the end of this chapter.
>
> 1. Beta-blockers are recommended as first-line therapy for stable angina by both the American College of Cardiology/American Heart Association (ACC/AHA) and the European Society of Cardiology. Their mechanism of action in this condition is explained by:
>   A. Plaque stabilisation
>   B. Increased coronary blood flow
>   C. Reduction in blood pressure
>   D. Reduction in myocardial oxygen demand
>   E. Reduction in systemic vasodilatation

> **CLINICAL**
>
> 9. A 47-year-old man presents with chest pain. He reports moderately severe central chest pain of 24 h duration. The pain is worse with inspiration and is alleviated by maintaining an upright position. He also reports having had a fever recently. His medical history and physical examination are unremarkable. His ECG is shown below. What is the most likely diagnosis and the most appropriate treatment approach for this patient?

Answer sections:

> 16 Cardiology
>
> ## Answers
> **BASIC SCIENCE**
>
> **1. Answer D**
> The beneficial effects of beta-blockers in stable angina are secondary to reduction in myocardial oxygen demand. Myocardial oxygen demand varies directly according to the heart rate, contractility and left ventricular wall stress, each of which is decreased by beta-blockers.

> **CLINICAL**
>
> **9. Answer B**
> The clinical diagnosis of acute pericarditis rests primarily on the findings of chest pain, pericardial friction rub and ECG changes (Imazio et al., 2010). The chest pain of acute pericarditis typically develops suddenly and is severe and constant over the anterior chest. In acute pericarditis, the pain worsens with inspiration – a response that helps to distinguish acute pericarditis from myocardial infarction.

Answers are linked to an authoritative reference to supplement your study. Scan the QR code on your mobile device to be taken directly to the reference.

> Phan, T.T., Shivu, G.N., Choudhury, A., et al. (2009). Multi-centre experience on the use of perhexiline in chronic heart failure and refractory angina: old drug, new hope. *Eur J Heart Failure* 11, 881–886. http://eurjhf.oxfordjournals.org/content/11/9/881.long

1 Cardiology

Questions

Answers can be found in the Cardiology Answers section at the end of this chapter.

1. A 65-year-old accountant undergoes an abdominal ultrasound because of mildly abnormal liver function tests. The ultrasound reveals a few mobile gallstones and a 5 cm abdominal aortic aneurysm. He drinks three to four standard drinks of alcohol every day and is an ex-smoker. He is known to have hypertension and is taking irbesartan 150 mg daily. Blood pressure control is satisfactory with mean systolic BP of 130 mmHg.

What is your most appropriate course of action?

   A. Abdominal CT with contrast immediately and suspension of driver's license.
   B. Endovascular aneurysm repair immediately.
   C. Follow up ultrasound in 6 months and continue driving.
   D. Open surgical aneurysm repair immediately.

2. A 39-year-old man with a known atrial septal defect presents to emergency department with a 6-hour history of palpitations. His ECG is shown below:

Which one of the following signs is **UNLIKELY** to be present?

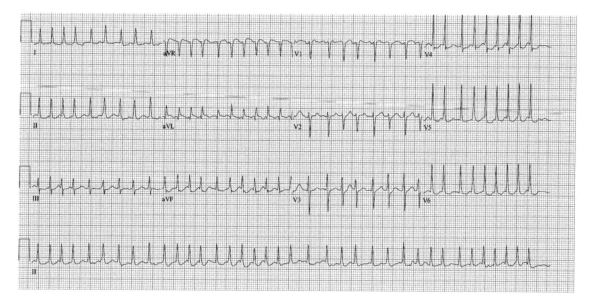

   A. Fixed splitting of second heart sound.
   B. Fourth heart sound.
   C. Loud first heart sound.
   D. Third heart sound.

How to Pass the FRACP Written Examination, First Edition. Jonathan Gleadle, Jordan Li, Danielle Wu, and Paul Kleinig.
© 2022 John Wiley & Sons Ltd. Published 2022 by John Wiley & Sons Ltd.

3. Which of the following patient characteristics is **LEAST LIKELY** to increase an individual's susceptibility to anthracycline cardiomyopathy?
  A. Age of 70 years.
  B. Male sex.
  C. Mediastinal radiotherapy.
  D. Positive carrier status for *C282Y HFE* gene.

4. A 65-year-old-man presents with a three-month history of exertional dyspnoea. He is found to have aortic stenosis with a valve area of 0.9 cm^2 and a mean transvalvular pressure gradient of 15 mmHg. His left ventricle ejection fraction (LVEF) is 35%. A Dobutamine Stress Echocardiography (DSE) has been arranged which will provide all of the following information, **EXCEPT**:
  A. Confirming the suitability for valve replacement.
  B. Deciding the need for cardiac resynchronisation therapy.
  C. Predicting prognosis post valve replacement.
  D. Diagnosing low-flow, low-gradient aortic stenosis.

5. An 84-year-old man with severe aortic stenosis complains of shortness of breath after walking for 20 metres and a couple of episodes of unexplained collapse. He is independent with activities of daily living. His medical history includes hypertension, hyperlipidaemia, cholecystectomy, and hernia repair.
  What is the most appropriate management approach?
  A. Aortic valve balloon valvuloplasty.
  B. Implantable cardioverter–defibrillator (ICD).
  C. Surgical aortic valve replacement (SAVR).
  D. Transcatheter aortic valve implantation (TAVI).

6. You see a 75-year-old woman with a new diagnosis of atrial fibrillation. Her CHA$_2$DS$_2$-VASc score is 4. She has a history of myocardial infarction four years ago, treated with percutaneous coronary intervention and a bare-metal stent inserted in the right coronary artery, and is currently on aspirin.
  Which of the following options is the most appropriate regarding ongoing anti-thrombotic therapy?
  A. Coronary angiogram to guide further therapy.
  B. Rivaroxaban and clopidogrel.
  C. Rivaroxaban and aspirin.
  D. Rivaroxaban monotherapy.

7. Beta-blockers are recommended as first line therapy for stable angina. Their main mechanism of action is explained by:
  A. Increased coronary artery blood flow.
  B. Plaque stabilisation.
  C. Reduction in blood pressure.
  D. Reduction in myocardial oxygen demand.

8. What is the management strategy for a patient with the following ECG?

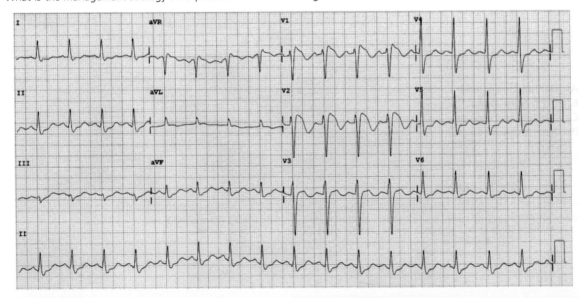

A. Amiodarone.
B. Beta-blocker.
C. Implantable cardioverter–defibrillator (ICD).
D. Pacemaker.

9. A 54-year-old man is admitted to hospital because of syncope. This is his third presentation with syncope due to severe postural hypotension over the past six months. He has developed chronic diarrhoea and lost 6 kg of body weight in the past six months. He has no significant past medical history. On examination, BP is 90/50 mmHg. HR is 86 bpm. There are no murmurs. Urinary analysis shows ++++ protein but no RBCs nor RBC casts. His investigation results are shown below. ECG shows sinus rhythm and low voltage in all leads. Echocardiogram reports moderate left ventricular hypertrophy, biatrial dilatation and grade 2 diastolic dysfunction.

Tests	Results	Normal values
Haemoglobin	108 g/L	135–175
White blood cell	5.48 x 10^9/L	4.0–11.0
Platelet	206 x 10^9/L	150–450
Sodium	133 mmol/L	135–145
Potassium	4.3 mmol/L	3.5–5.2
Creatinine	156 µmol/L	60–110
Albumin	22 g/L	34–48
Globulin	42 g/L	21–41
Liver function tests	normal	
Troponin	<29 ng/L	0–29
N-terminal pro b-type Natriuretic Peptide (NT-proBNP)	1800 ng/L	0–124

What would you consider the most appropriate next investigation?
A. Cardiac MRI.
B. Coronary artery angiogram.
C. Holter monitor.
D. Implantable loop recorder.

10. Which one of the following increases cardiac output?
A. Atropine.
B. Acidosis.
C. Beta-blockers.
D. Hypertension.

11. A 72-year-old woman presents to emergency department after an episode of loss of consciousness. Which of the following clinical features, if present, **DO NOT** increase the likelihood that her loss of consciousness was due to cardiac syncope?
A. Breathlessness prior to the episode.
B. Cyanosis during the episode.
C. History of atrial fibrillation.
D. Significant injury as a result of loss of consciousness.

12. An 80-year-old man presents to emergency department with sudden onset of left-sided weakness two hours ago. His medical history includes hypertension, hypercholesterolaemia, and atrial fibrillation for which he is taking aspirin only. CT head shows acute right middle cerebral artery territory infarction. He is treated with thrombolysis followed by bridging low molecular weight heparin then a direct thrombin inhibitor. Two weeks later while in rehabilitation, he develops low grade fever, myalgia, painful feet (shown below), anaemia, and AKI.

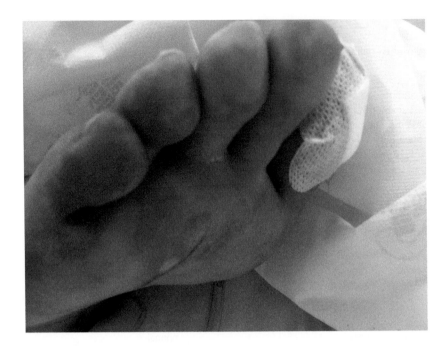

The most likely diagnosis is:
   A. Acute allergic reaction to direct thrombin inhibitor.
   B. Antiphospholipid syndrome.
   C. Cholesterol embolisation.
   D. Multiple emboli due to inappropriate use of an oral direct thrombin inhibitor.

13. Which one of the following patients can be investigated appropriately with a computed tomography coronary angiography (CTCA)?
   A. An asymptomatic patient with history of type 2 diabetes and normal renal function.
   B. A patient with previous coronary stents presenting with chest pain and possible in-stent restenosis.
   C. A patient presenting with central chest pain and rapid atrial fibrillation.
   D. A patient with chest pain but with a low pre-test probability of coronary artery disease.

14. A 75-year-old man presents with transient weakness of his left arm. He is diagnosed with a transient ischaemic attack. He is known to have hypertension, type 2 diabetes, alcohol dependence, recent weight loss, and a low-grade fever. He undergoes a transthoracic echocardiogram which reveals a 12 mm mitral-valve vegetation.
   Which one of the following statements is true?
   A. Blood culture is negative in over 20% of cases of infectious endocarditis.
   B. Cerebral complications are the most frequent extracardiac complications.
   C. Majority (80%) of cases of infectious endocarditis develop in patients with known valvular disease.
   D. Streptococci in the most common pathogen isolated.

15. A 75-year-old man presents with increasing dyspnoea. You note that he had four admissions in the past year due to decompensated CCF. He is known to have ischaemic heart disease with a drug eluting stent in two coronary arteries, insulin dependent type 2 diabetes, hypertension, stage 4 CKD with an eGFR of 26 ml/min/1.73 m^2 and severe smoking related COPD. His medications include aspirin, clopidogrel, perindopril, gliclazide, frusemide, digoxin, spironolactone, atorvastatin, formoterol/,budesonide inhaler, and tiotropium inhaler. Physical examination findings are consistent with decompensated CCF. His ECG is shown below. A dobutamine stress echocardiogram demonstrates no reversible ischaemic change but a large antero-apical area of akinesia. The ejection fraction is 30%.

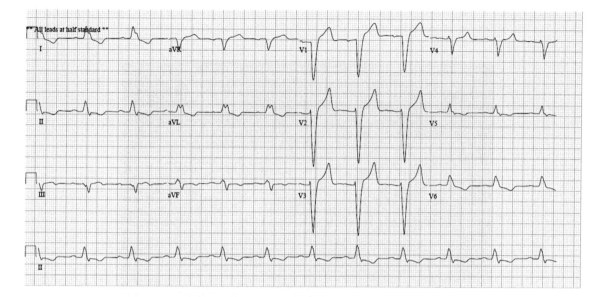

The most effective treatment to reduce the frequency of readmissions and improve survival is:
- **A.** Add a SGLT2 inhibitor.
- **B.** Commence a beta-blocker.
- **C.** Insert a biventricular pacemaker and defibrillator.
- **D.** Insert a dual-chamber pacemaker.

16. Which one of the following medications is recommended in patients with type 2 diabetes with cardiovascular disease and inadequate glycaemic control despite metformin, to reduce the risk of cardiovascular events and hospitalisation for heart failure?
- **A.** Dipeptidyl peptidase-4 (DPP-4) inhibitors.
- **B.** Glucagon-like peptide-1 (GLP-1) analogues.
- **C.** Sodium-glucose co-transporter-2 (SGLT2) inhibitors.
- **D.** Thiazolidinediones.

17. A 70-year-old woman presents with a 2-month history of exertional dyspnoea for evaluation. Her medical history includes longstanding hypertension, obesity, OSA, and permanent AF. On examination, there are clinical signs consistent with CCF. Her troponin level is normal, but NT-pro BNP level is elevated. Her echocardiogram demonstrates a left ventricular ejection fraction of 55%, left ventricular end-diastolic volume index (LVEDI) <97 mL/m^2 and the ratio of mitral early diastolic inflow velocity to mitral early annular lengthening velocity (E/e′)>15.
  Which one of the following treatments will reduce mortality for this patient?
- **A.** Angiotensin-converting enzyme inhibitor.
- **B.** No pharmacological treatment proven to reduce mortality.
- **C.** Phosphodiesterase-5 inhibitor.
- **D.** Selective sinus node I_f sodium channel inhibitor.

18. In a 28-year-old man with known hypertrophic cardiomyopathy (HOCM) who has had one episode of syncope at work, which one of the following treatments should be instituted?
- **A.** Amiodarone.
- **B.** Anticoagulation.
- **C.** Atenolol.
- **D.** Implantable cardioverter–defibrillator.

19. A 56-year-old man presents to emergency department with severe headaches and blurred vision. He is known to have IgA nephropathy but has no regular follow up for this. His BP is 210/110 mmHg. You have performed a fundoscopic examination which is shown below:

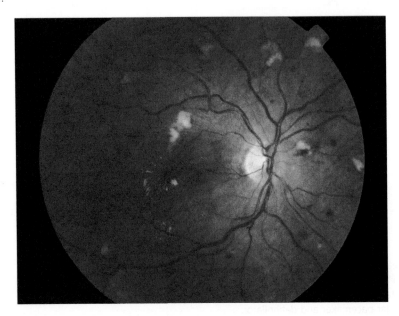

What does the fundoscopy show?
- **A.** Keith-Wagener (KG) grade 3 hypertensive retinopathy.
- **B.** Keith-Wagener (KG) grade 4 hypertensive retinopathy.
- **C.** Retinal artery occlusion.
- **D.** Retinal vein occlusion.

20. Which one of the following patients **DOES NOT** have an indication for an implantable cardioverter defibrillator (ICD) implantation?
- **A.** A 20-year-old man with congenital long QT syndrome with recurrent syncope who cannot tolerate beta-blockers.
- **B.** A 65-year-old woman with haemodynamically unstable ventricular tachycardia not due to reversible causes.
- **C.** A 59-year-old man with ischaemic cardiomyopathy with a myocardial infarction two weeks ago with left ventricular ejection fraction of 30%.
- **D.** A 22-year-old asymptomatic female with hypertrophic cardiomyopathy, unexplained syncope but no family history of sudden cardiac death.

21. A 56-year-old man with a background history of type 2 diabetes, hypertension, and hyperlipidaemia presents with unexplained syncope and palpitations that happen around 6-monthly. His previous cardiac investigations, including repeated 12-lead ECG and 24-hour Holter monitoring, are normal.
What is the appropriate next step to investigate palpitations?
- **A.** Three-day Holter monitoring.
- **B.** Seven-day Holter monitoring.
- **C.** Wearable device.
- **D.** Implantable loop recorder.

22. Which one of the following lipid-lowering agents acts by blocking the inhibition of lysosomal degradation of low-density lipoprotein (LDL) receptors, thereby increasing the body's ability to sequester LDL?
- **A.** Evolocumab.
- **B.** Ezetimibe.
- **C.** Mipomersen.
- **D.** Rosuvastatin.

23. A 65-year-old man presents with dizziness and syncope. His ECG shows a QTc interval of 520 ms. Review of medical history, family history, medications, electrolytes, and echocardiogram did not find a reversible cause of the condition.

What is the first-line treatment for this patient?
A. Amiodarone.
B. Beta-blockers.
C. Implantable cardioverter defibrillator (ICD).
D. Left cardiac sympathetic denervation (LCSD).

24. A 25-year-old Aboriginal and Torres Strait Islander woman presents with a 3-month history of exertional dyspnoea. She has had an unproductive cough but no fevers, chest pain or other illnesses. She takes no medication. On examination, BP is 120/70 mmHg, HR 90/min and regular, there is a 2/6 diastolic murmur and a 3/6 systolic murmur, chest is clear, there is pitting oedema of both ankles. Echocardiogram reveals mitral stenosis with a mean transvalvular gradient of 14 mmHg and moderate mitral regurgitation. The left atrium is enlarged. There is normal biventricular size and function, as well as pulmonary hypertension with a pulmonary arterial pressure of 50 mmHg.

Which of the following is the most appropriate management?
A. Balloon mitral valvuloplasty.
B. Commence ACE inhibitor and repeat echocardiogram in 6 months.
C. Mitral valve open commissurotomy.
D. Mitral valve replacement.

25. A 65-year-old man suffers from ischaemic heart disease, chronic AF, insulin-dependent type 2 diabetes, stage 3 CKD, peripheral vascular disease with chronic claudication. He is taking multiple medications and is asking your advice about taking omega-3 fish oil supplements.

Which one of the following pieces of advice regarding omega-3 fish oil supplements for this patient is correct?
A. It is associated with a statistically significant reduction on all-cause mortality.
B. It has a beneficial effect on glycaemic control and increased fasting insulin levels.
C. It can improve walking distance, ankle brachial pressure index, and angiographic findings.
D. It can reduce serum triglycerides and raise HDL and LDL levels.

26. A 55-year-old man presents with repeated clinic blood pressure measurements of around 150/90 mmHg, after six months of therapy with perindopril, amlodipine, and hydrochlorothiazide at maximal doses. He is compliant with his medications and is engaging actively with lifestyle modifications.

Which one of the following additional agents is most likely to be beneficial?
A. Atenolol.
B. Doxazosin.
C. Hydralazine.
D. Spironolactone.

27. A 50-year-old woman with haemochromatosis presents with dyspnoea. She undergoes an echocardiogram. Which of the echocardiogram findings is most commonly seen in patients with early-stage restrictive cardiomyopathy?
A. Left ventricular dilatation with reduced left ventricular ejection fraction <45%.
B. Left ventricular outflow tract obstruction.
C. Normal ventricular size and systolic function with a restrictive ventricular filling pattern.
D. Regional wall motion abnormality in a non-coronary distribution.

28. Which of the following statements is correct regarding acute rheumatic fever (ARF) in Aboriginal and Torres Strait Islander (ATSI)?
A. It is usually associated with Group B streptococcal infection.
B. Secondary prophylaxis following rheumatic fever should be oral doxycycline.
C. The highest rates of ARF in ATSI are between the ages 34 to 45.
D. The major manifestations of ARF include carditis and chorea.

29. A 60-year-old woman presents with epigastric pain, nausea, vomiting, and shortness of breath. She has a HR of 58 bpm and a BP of 90/60 mmHg. Her ECG is shown below:

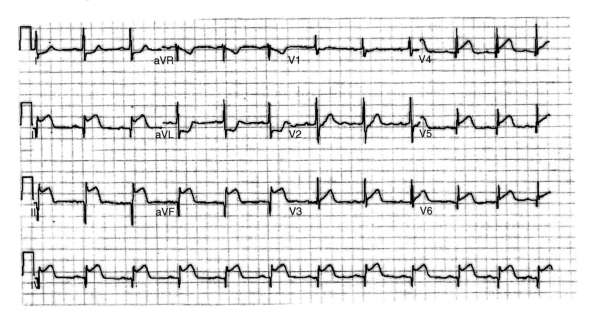

The occlusion of which coronary artery is likely to have produced this presentation.
  A. Circumflex.
  B. Left anterior descending.
  C. Left marginal.
  D. Right.

30. A 55-year-old man is referred by his GP because of bradycardia with a heart rate as low as 45 bpm at night. He has hypertension for which he is taking amlodipine 5 mg daily. An ECG performed today shows a sinus bradycardia 55/min and he is asymptomatic.
  Which one of the following statements is correct?
  A. Nocturnal bradycardia is an indication for permanent pacing.
  B. Sinus node dysfunction is most likely due to ischaemic heart disease.
  C. Sleep apnoea is not associated with nocturnal bradycardia.
  D. There is no minimum heart rate or pause duration for which permanent pacing is recommended in sinus node dysfunction.

31. A 38-year-old woman is admitted to intensive care unit because of septic shock due to meningococcal septicaemia. She complains of increased dyspnoea on day 3 when she is discharged to the ward. She has a medical history of asthma and chronic back pain. She has been experiencing depressive symptoms since her husband passed away one year ago. Her ECG shows ST depression in the lateral leads. Initial Troponin I level is 54 ng/L [<29], N-terminal pro-B-type brain natriuretic peptide (NT-proBNP) level is 5400 ng/L [0–124]. Her echocardiogram shows ballooning of the left ventricular apex.
  Which of the following medications will improve her survival at one year?
  A. Angiotensin-receptor blockers.
  B. Beta-blockers.
  C. Calcium channel blockers.
  D. Digitalis glycosides.

32. Which of the following statements is correct regarding transcatheter aortic valve implantation (TAVI) in inoperable and high-risk elderly patients?
  A. Patients should be anticoagulated with a novel oral anticoagulant (NOAC) for 3 months post implantation.
  B. Patients should be anticoagulated with dual antiplatelet therapy for 3 months post implantation.
  C. Patients with asymptomatic severe aortic stenosis at intermediate surgical risk should be offered TAVI.
  D. The need for permanent pacemaker insertion due to bradyarrhythmias post TAVI is about 30%.

33. A 62-year-old man presents with vague chest discomfort for 6 hours. He is known to have insulin-dependent type 2 diabetes, hypertension, hyperlipidaemia, stage 3A CKD with serum creatinine 150 µmol/L [60–110] and psoriatic arthritis treated with adalimumab. His ECG is shown below. His coronary artery angiography shows 50% stenosis of the left main, 75% stenosis of the left circumflex, 70% stenosis of the proximal left anterior descending artery, and 50% stenosis of the right coronary artery. Left ventricular systolic function is reduced with an ejection fraction of 40%.

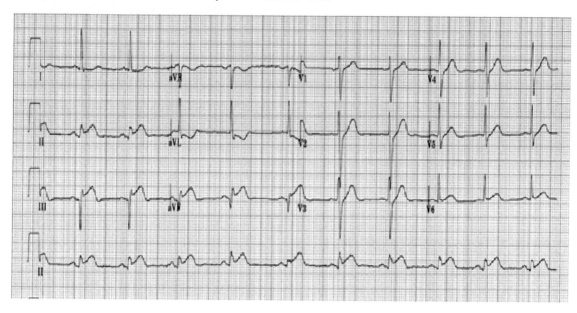

Which one of the following is the best management option?
A. Coronary artery bypass graft surgery (CABG).
B. Infarct-related artery (IRA)-only revascularisation in primary PCI.
C. PCI plus biventricular pacemaker–defibrillator.
D. Percutaneous coronary intervention (PCI).

34. A 51-year-old woman presents to the emergency department with cellulitis of her left lower leg and epigastric discomfort after being on oral antibiotics for three days. She is otherwise well and has no other symptoms and ECG is normal. She is known to have autosomal dominant polycystic kidney disease with a serum creatinine of 86 µmol/L [60–110]. A serum high-sensitivity troponin (hs-cTn) is requested and the result is 40 ng/L [<29].
What is the best interpretation of this result in terms of the likelihood of acute coronary syndrome?
A. Likely because the specificity of hs-cTn is high.
B. Likely because the pre-test probability is high.
C. Unlikely because the specificity of hs-cTn is low.
D. Unlikely because the pre-test probability is low.

35. A 78-year-old woman is admitted to the Acute Medical Unit with severe community acquired pneumonia. Her BP is 90/60 mmHg and oxygen saturation is 90% on 4 L of oxygen. Her other medical history includes type 2 diabetes, stage 3B CKD, and hypertension. A central venous line is inserted because of difficult venous access. She complains of increased dyspnoea. A bedside ECG is taken and shown below. Troponin level is 289 ng/L [<29].

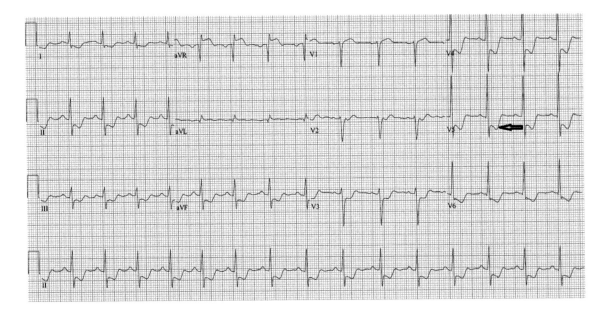

Which one of the following is the most likely diagnosis?
   A. Type 1 myocardial infarction.
   B. Type 2 myocardial infarction.
   C. Type 3 myocardial infarction.
   D. Type 4 myocardial infarction.

36. A 55-year-man presents with a 2-hour history of palpitations and chest discomfort. He had a similar episode one year ago. He is known to have ankylosing spondylitis, diet-controlled type 2 diabetes, and asthma. He uses a salbutamol inhaler two to three times a week. On examination, he is alert and orientated, BP is 110/60 mmHg, pulse rate is 150 bpm, SaO2 on room air is 95%. There is scattered expiratory wheeze. There is no heart murmur. His current ECG is shown in Figure 1.1A, while Figure 1.1B shows

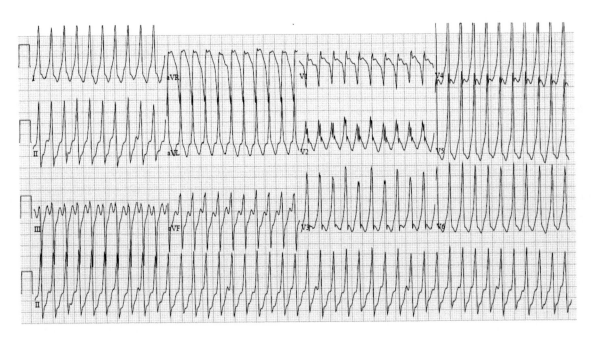

Figure 1.1A

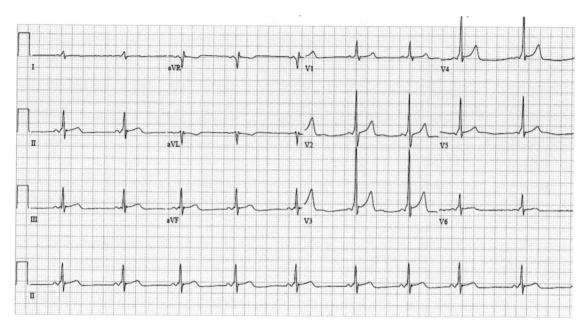

Figure 1.1B

an ECG taken 1-year ago during an infective exacerbation of asthma. His biochemistry results and troponin T are within normal reference range.

The most appropriate treatment for rate control is:
A. Intravenous adenosine.
B. Intravenous digoxin.
C. Intravenous flecainide.
D. Intravenous verapamil.

QUESTIONS (37–43) REFER TO THE FOLLOWING INFORMATION
Match the following blood pressure lowering agents to their mechanism of action.
A. Decreased renin secretion and decreased heart rate.
B. Decreased central synthesis of catecholamines.
C. Decreasing degradation of circulating natriuretic peptides.
D. Relaxation of smooth muscle through opening K_{ATP} channels.
E. Blocking the angiotensin I binding site on angiotensin converting enzyme (ACE).
F. Interfering with Ca^{2+} release on the sarcoplasmic reticulum.
G. Increased guanylyl cyclase activity.

37. Minoxidil

38. Sacubitril

39. Moxonidine

40. Captopril

41. Glyceryl trinitrate

42. Nebivolol

43. Hydralazine.

QUESTIONS (44–51) REFER TO THE FOLLOWING INFORMATION

Match the clinical features listed below to the most likely type of congenital heart disease or clinical syndrome found in patients.

A. Atrial septal defect (ASD).
B. Ventricular septal defect (VSD).
C. Patent ductus arteriosus (PDA).
D. Coarctation of the aorta (CoA).
E. Eisenmenger's syndrome.
F. Marfan's syndrome.
G. Tetralogy of Fallot.
H. Transposition of the great arteries.

44. Cyanosis, clubbing, polycythaemia, an elevated JVP with a dominant *a* wave pattern, right ventricular heave, palpable pulmonary component of the second heart sound (P2), loud P2, fourth heart sound, pulmonary ejection click, and pulmonary regurgitation on auscultation.

45. Cyanosis, clubbing, polycythaemia, right ventricular heave, a thrill at the left sternal edge, a single second heart sound (A2) and short pulmonary ejection murmur on auscultation, a boot shape heart, right ventricular enlargement, and decreased vascularity of lung vessels on CXR.

46. A better developed upper body in comparison with the lower limbs, radiofemoral delay, and hypertension in the upper limbs only, midsystolic murmur over the precordium and back, hypertensive changes in the fundi, a small aortic knuckle and rib notching on CXR.

47. Fixed splitting of the second heart sound (S2), pulmonary systolic ejection murmur (increasing on inspiration), signs of pulmonary hypertension.

48. A thrill and a harsh pansystolic murmur to the left sternal edge, mitral regurgitation.

49. Arachnodactyly, joint hypermobility, long, thin limbs, a long and narrow face, lens dislocation, blue sclerae, a high-arched palate, pectus excavatum, aortic regurgitation, mitral valve prolapse, kyphoscoliosis, and arm span exceeding overall height.

50. A continuous murmur along the left sternal border, ECG shows left ventricular hypertrophy, CXR shows increased pulmonary vasculature.

Answers

1. Answer: C

An aneurysm is an artery that has enlarged to greater than 1.5 times the expected diameter. In the infrarenal aorta, the threshold diameter is accepted as 3.0 cm. Abdominal aortic aneurysm (AAA) affects approximately 4–7% of men and 1–2% of women over the age of 65 years.

Medical therapy options remain limited and no aneurysm-specific pharmacotherapy is currently available. Medical management of AAA generally involves cardiovascular risk reduction, including antiplatelet, statin, and antihypertensive therapy. The best medical management is generally not intended to limit expansion or reduce the size of the AAA. However, managing cardiovascular risk factors is crucial for improving the overall survival of patients and the outcomes of future AAA repair.

Australian national driving regulations stipulate that untreated atherosclerotic aortic aneurysms >5.5 cm disqualify patients from an unconditional driver's licence, except with the approval of a treating vascular surgeon.

Patients with large aneurysms (men >5.5 cm; women >5.0 cm) should be considered for elective aneurysm repair. The optimal management of small AAAs (4.0–5.5 cm) has been clarified by several large, randomised control trials which demonstrate no long-term survival benefit with open or endovascular repair.

Most AAAs detected with screening or as an incidental finding are below the threshold for elective repair. The risk of AAA rupture increases with AAA diameter (Table 1.1). The surveillance interval for asymptomatic AAA also depends on AAA diameter (Table 1.2).

Table 1.1 Annual AAA rupture risk by diameter.

AAA diameter (cm)	Rupture risk (%/year)
3.0–3.9	0%
4.0–4.9	1%
5.0–5.9	1–10%
6.0–6.9	10–22%
>7.0	30–50%

Source: Based on Chuen J. Abdominal aortic aneurysm: An update AJGP 2018;47:252–56

Table 1.2 AAA surveillance intervals by diameter.

AAA diameter (cm)	Surveillance interval (months)
3.0–3.9	24
4.0–4.5	12
4.6–5.0	6
>5.0	3

Chuen J. Abdominal aortic aneurysm: An update AJGP 2018;47:252–56.
https://www1.racgp.org.au/ajgp/2018/may/aaa-an-update/

2. Answer: B

The ECG shows Atrial Fibrillation (AF) with a rapid ventricular response. A fourth heart sound (S4) is a late diastolic sound due to a high pressure atrial wave reflected back from a poorly compliant ventricle. It does not occur in patients with AF because S4 depends on effective atrial contraction. In patients with an atrial septal defect, there is fixed splitting of the second heart sound because there is equalisation of volume loads between the two atria occurring through the defect. A loud S1 can occur in AF due to reduced diastolic filling time so the mitral valve remains widely open at the end of diastole. S3 is a mid-diastolic sound. It can occur in children and young people due to rapid diastolic filling. A pathologic S3 is present in patient with congestive heart failure (CCF) and other heart disorders due to reduced ventricular compliance and rapid diastolic filling.

Voin V, Oskouian R, Loukas M, Tubbs R. Auscultation of the heart. Clinical Anatomy. 2016;30(1):58–60.
https://www.ncbi.nlm.nih.gov/pubmed/27576554

3. Answer: B

Anthracyclines such as doxorubicin and idarubicin exhibit an anti-cancer action through inhibition of topoisomerase (Top) 2α in cancer cells, and their toxicity is largely through inhibition of Top 2β in cardiac myocytes. Topoisomerases are highly expressed in proliferating eukaryotic cells and are involved in detangling and relegating aberrant DNA coils. By binding Top 2α in cancer cells' DNA, anthracyclines facilitate the cleavage function of topoisomerase, but not the religation, which leads to accumulation of double stranded DNA breaks and initiates programmed cell death pathways. Anthracyclines also cause mitochondrial dysfunction and excessive intracellular reactive oxygen species, which results in increased apoptosis. This process is promoted by high intracellular iron availability. Both of these pathways are thought to contribute to the death of cardiac myocytes, and result in cardiomyopathy.

Patient factors predictive of higher risk for anthracycline cardiomyopathy include lifetime cumulative dose, age less than 18 or over 65, female gender, renal failure, radiotherapy involving the heart, pre-existing cardiac disease, carbonyl reductase gene polymorphisms, and carrier status for haemochromatosis genes. Exposure to anthracycline chemotherapy also increases risk of cardiotoxicity with trastuzumab. Trials evaluating the pharmaceutical prevention of anthracycline related cardiomyopathy have found small but statistically significant differences in deterioration of left ventricular function for ACE inhibitors, beta-blockers, aldosterone antagonists and angiotensin 2 receptor blockers in predominantly low-exposure and low-risk patients. These results may or may not be clinically significant.

Trials that target those at highest risk of cardiomyopathy are most likely to yield more meaningful clinical results. For example, in one trial patients receiving high dose chemotherapy were randomised to receive placebo or ramipril should they have a troponin rise after their first cycle of chemotherapy. The results of the study found that the treatment arm had a roughly stable left ventricular ejection fraction over the trial period, but the placebo arm decreased by around 14%, which could translate to meaningful patient-centred outcomes. Dexrazoxane competitively binds Top 2β, preventing anthracycline binding, and very effectively prevents anthracycline cardiomyopathy. Previous concerns regarding increased risk of secondary cancers with dexrazoxane are being re-evaluated as the result of multiple influential trials, and it is now available for use in a number of settings.

Henriksen P. Anthracycline cardiotoxicity: an update on mechanisms, monitoring and prevention.
Heart. 2017;104(12):971–977.
https://heart.bmj.com/content/104/12/971.long

4. Answer: B

Most patients with symptomatic severe aortic stenosis (AS) have a valve area <1.0 cm² and/or a mean transvalvular pressure gradient >40 mmHg. Low gradient AS is defined as severe AS (valve area <1.0 cm²) with a transvalvular pressure gradient <30 mmHg. Low gradient AS is seen in patients with left ventricular (LV) systolic dysfunction with reduced left ventricular ejection fraction (LVEF). A challenging clinical task in those with low gradient AS is differentiating who will survive and improve after aortic valve replacement surgery and those who will not. There is a subset of patients with AS and low transvalvular gradients who do not benefit from aortic valve replacement and are at considerable risk of operative death. These patients have a significant degree of LV dysfunction but only mild to moderate AS. They are considered to have pseudo-stenosis because their symptoms are primarily due to poor LV function, not significant valvular disease.

Dobutamine Stress Echocardiography (DSE) is useful to differentiate true aortic stenosis from pseudo-aortic stenosis. Patients with severe AS and secondary LV dysfunction that leads to a low transvalvular pressure gradient are considered to have true stenosis. In this setting, the severe stenotic lesion results in excessive afterload and a reduced LVEF, thereby producing both a markedly decreased stroke volume and low transvalvular pressure gradient. It is logical to assume that aortic valve replacement will be beneficial in these patients. In pseudostenosis, patients have a low transvalvular pressure gradient because of the combination of moderate AS and low cardiac output. The low output reduces the valve opening forces, resulting in limited mobility of a valve that is not severely diseased. The calculated valve area may mistakenly suggest severe stenosis because of valve area equation limitations when applied to low flow rate conditions. In contrast to true stenosis, surgical correction in these patients is unlikely to be beneficial.

There are no other clinical or haemodynamic variables that are helpful to stratify risk in such patients and determine the appropriate therapy. The aortic valve calcium score (determined by CT) has been associated with AS haemodynamic severity, progression rate, and clinical outcomes but not validated in patients with low ejection fraction. Patients with contractile reserve have a much better outcome after surgery.

 Annabi M, Touboul E, Dahou A, et al. Dobutamine Stress Echocardiography for Management of Low-Flow, Low-Gradient Aortic Stenosis. Journal of the American College of Cardiology. 2018;71(5):475–485. https://www.sciencedirect.com/science/article/pii/S0735109717417785?via%3Dihub

5. Answer: D
There is an increased prevalence of AS in an ageing population. Severe AS is defined on transthoracic echocardiogram as a reduced aortic valve area (AVA) of < 1.0 cm², peak velocity of > 4 m/s and a mean gradient of greater than 40 mmHg across the valve. Patients with less severe aortic stenosis may remain asymptomatic for years. Once the symptoms of syncope, angina, or heart failure develop, average survival reduces rapidly, with an increased risk of sudden cardiac death. Until transcatheter aortic valve implantation (TAVI) became available, the options to treat severe AS include medical (palliative management), surgical aortic valve replacement (SAVR), or a Ross procedure (where a diseased aortic valve is replaced by a patient's own pulmonary valve). SAVR involves a midline sternotomy, general anaesthetic, cardiopulmonary bypass, typically requires 24 to 48 hours stay in an intensive care unit (ICU) and 10 to 14 days as an inpatient for post-op recovery and mobilisation, and an even longer hospital stay for rehabilitation in the frail and elderly. Patients who are greater than 75 years old have an increased morbidity and mortality associated with SAVR.

Since the advent of TAVI in 2002, elderly patients who were not suitable candidates for SAVR, can now be considered for TAVI if appropriate, provided they do not have severe COPD, debilitating stroke, active malignancy, and dementia indicating a survival of < 1 year.

The majority of TAVI procedures are performed with local anaesthetic and conscious sedation. In uncomplicated TAVI cases, patients can be mobilised 4 hours post-procedure and do not require ICU admission and likely to be discharged within 48 hours after telemetry monitoring to rule out conduction disturbance. Patients usually require dual-antiplatelets (aspirin and clopidogrel) for at least 3–6 months, with aspirin continued lifelong.

 Adams H, Ashokkumar S, Newcomb A, et al. Contemporary review of severe aortic stenosis. Internal Medicine Journal. 2019;49(3):297–305. https://www.ncbi.nlm.nih.gov/pubmed/30091235

6. Answer: D
A randomised non-inferiority trial was terminated early due to safety concerns around the combination of rivaroxaban and antiplatelets in patients with coronary artery disease (CAD) and intervention (percutaneous coronary intervention or bypass grafting) more than one-year prior – or medically treated CAD. The primary efficacy measure of cardiovascular events or death from any cause was significantly lower in patients taking rivaroxaban alone compared to rivaroxaban plus aspirin. Bleeding was significantly lower in the monotherapy group, and the secondary outcome measure of death from any cause was significantly lower in the monotherapy group.

 Yasuda S, Kaikita K, Akao M, Ako J, Matoba T, Nakamura M et al. Antithrombotic Therapy for Atrial Fibrillation with Stable Coronary Disease. New England Journal of Medicine. 2019;381(12):1103–1113. https://www.nejm.org/doi/full/10.1056/NEJMoa1904143

7. Answer: D
The anti-anginal action of β-blockers is predominantly through reduced heart rate, which results in a relative decrease in myocardial oxygen demand. This leads to decrease in angina symptoms. β-blockade also results in decreased heart contractility, decreased atrioventricular conduction and nodal refractiveness, and competitive catecholamine inhibition to prevent cardiac remodelling.

Angina results from myocardial ischemia, due to a mismatch between myocardial oxygen demand and supply. Heart rate is the major determinant of oxygen consumption, and increased heart rate precedes most episodes of angina. Other determinants of myocardial oxygen demand include BP, myocardial wall tension, cardiac hypertrophy, and myocardial contractility. Coronary blood flow is the major determinant of myocardial oxygen supply, which is dependent on the pressure gradient across the coronary circuit, integrity of the coronary arteries, and oxygen carrying capacity of the blood. Typically, angina results from exercise or emotional stress precipitating further reduced coronary blood flow in patients with obstructive coronary artery disease (CAD). In a minority of patients, angina is secondary to functional alterations of coronary vessels, where coronary arteries can be angiographically normal, so called non-obstructive CAD.

Treatment for stable angina includes lifestyle changes such as weight loss, exercise, smoking cessation, aspirin, moderate to high intensity statin therapy, and antianginal therapy as listed below. Heart rate should be targeted <70/min and BP <120/85 mmHg, with β-blockers, calcium channel blockers, and/or nitrates, before considering newer agents.

1. Medications which reduce heart rate (reduce myocardial demand): β-blockers, ivabradine, non-dihydropyridine calcium antagonists.
2. Medications which induce coronary and vascular artery relaxation (increase myocardial supply): Dihydropyridine calcium channel blockers, nitrates, and nicorandil.
3. Medications which induce cellular tolerance to ischemia: Piperazine derivatives including trimetazidine, ranolazine.

 Ohman E. Chronic Stable Angina. New England Journal of Medicine. 2016;374(12):1167–1176. https://www.nejm.org/doi/full/10.1056/NEJMcp1502240

8. Answer: C

Brugada syndrome (BS) is a rare inherited disease with ECG findings of coved type ST-segment elevation (≥ 2mm) followed by a negative T wave in (≥ 1) the right precordial leads in V1 to V3 in patients with a structurally normal heart in patients with Type I BS.

ECG of Type II BS: The ST segments also have a high take-off but the J amplitude of ≥ 2mV gives rise to a gradually descending ST elevation remaining ≥ 1mV above the baseline followed by a positive or biphasic T wave that results in a saddle back configuration. Type III BS ECG: Right precordial ST elevation of saddle-back type or coved type.

BS is genetically transmitted as an autosomal dominant syndrome with incomplete penetrance and has a male predominance. Mutations of several genes have been reported to be linked to BS, with mutations of SCN5A gene the most common.

Presenting clinical symptoms include syncope, seizures, agonal breathing at night due to polymorphic ventricular tachycardia (PVTs), ventricular fibrillation and sudden cardiac death (SCD). Lethal arrhythmias are mainly observed during the night or at rest during the day suggesting a likely association with bradycardia or vagal events. Clinical manifestations are also noted in patients with fever, which requires prompt management with antipyretics to minimise the risks of arrhythmias.

The mainstay of management currently is to prevent SCD associated with arrhythmias with an implantable cardioverter defibrillator (ICD). More recently, radiofrequency epicardial catheter ablation has been suggested as to be a new therapeutic option for patients with BS.

 Larkin D. Brugada Syndrome • LITFL • ECG Library Diagnosis [Internet]. Life in the Fast Lane • LITFL • Medical Blog. 2019 [cited 8 September 2019]. Available from: https://litfl.com/brugada-syndrome-ecg-library/

 Brugada J, Campuzano O, Arbelo E, Sarquella-Brugada G, Brugada R.et al. Present Status of Brugada Syndrome. Journal of the American College of Cardiology [Internet]. 2018 [cited 16 November 2020];72(9):1046–1059. Available from: https://www.sciencedirect.com/science/article/pii/S0735109718353622?via%3Dihub

9. Answer: A

This presentation is highly suspicious for cardiac amyloidosis (CA). His echocardiogram suggests cardiac involvement especially left ventricular hypertrophy in the context of hypotension and low voltage ECG, which could be further investigated with cardiac MRI.

Amyloidosis is a collection of diseases in which a protein-based infiltrate deposits in tissues as beta-pleated sheets. In >95% of CA, the main protein being deposited is light chain [termed light chain amyloidosis (AL)] and less commonly transthyretin [termed transthyretin amyloidosis (ATTR)].

AL is a plasma cell dyscrasia, where misfolded antibody light chain fragments can deposit systemically in any organ. The typical presentation is heart failure with preserved ejection fraction, with pathognomonic but infrequent presentations with macroglossia and/or periorbital purpura, and other symptoms dependent on organ involvement, commonly kidneys (proteinuria, especially nephrotic range) gastrointestinal tract (diarrhoea, weight loss), and nervous system (peripheral neuropathy, carpal tunnel syndrome, orthostatic hypotension). AL presents in adults, with a median age of diagnosis of 63, and median untreated survival of 6 months if the initial presentation is heart failure. It is rare for patients to have clinical involvement of all of these organ systems. The diagnosis is often delayed. Physician should have a heightened clinical suspicion for amyloidosis in appropriate clinical context and should consider it until proven otherwise.

ATTR is due to monomerization and misfolding of the protein transthyretin, which is produced by the liver and functions as a transporter of thyroxine and retinol. There are two main subtypes of ATTR amyloidosis: (i) acquired wild type ATTR (ATTRwt, previously senile CA) which typically presents as heart failure or hypertrophic restrictive cardiomyopathy in a male >60, often preceded by carpal tunnel syndrome and/or spinal stenosis, and (ii) hereditary mutant variant (ATTRm) which can be due to >100 point mutations, and subsequently presents heterogeneously as polyneuropathy, cardiomyopathy, or mixed. ATTR prognosis is better than AL, with median survival of 4 years for ATTRwt and variable for ATTRm.

Echocardiogram is the first step in the CA diagnostic workup to identify patients likely to have the disease and prompting further workup. Typical features of CA on echocardiogram include:
- Left ventricular hypertrophy in the absence of secondary causes
- Mismatch between ECG finding of low voltage and echocardiogram finding of left ventricular hypertrophy
- Granular sparking appearance of left ventricular wall
- Apical sparing
- Diastolic dysfunction
- Biatrial dilatation and reduced left ventricular cavity dimensions

ECG hallmarks are low voltages. Further investigations include:
- sFLC ratio and serum/urine immunofixation (to investigate for AL).
- Cardiac imaging (non-invasive diagnosis)
  - Longitudinal strain imaging using 2D speckle tracking for 'apical sparing' pattern
  - Cardiac MRI for diffuse and subendocardial 'late gadolinium enhancement' pattern that does not respect coronary distributions (93% sensitive, 70% specific)
  - 99mTcPYP scintigraphy for grade 2 or 3 myocardial radiotracer uptake (100% specificity and positive predictive value, in absence of monoclonal gammopathy)
- Endomyocardial biopsy (diagnostic gold standard, 100% sensitive for CA).

Definitive diagnosis of amyloidosis requires biopsy (Table 1.3).

Table 1.3 Sensitivity of different organ biopsy in diagnosis of amyloidosis.

Organ	Sensitivity
Abdominal fat pad	70%
Bone marrow	50% to 60%
Clinically involved organ	99% to 100%
Rectum	70% to 85%

Donnelly J, Hanna M. Cardiac amyloidosis: An update on diagnosis and treatment. Cleveland Clinic Journal of Medicine. 2017;84(12 suppl 3):12–26.
https://www.ccjm.org/content/84/12_suppl_3/12.long

10. Answer: A

Cardiac output is defined by the amount of blood ejected by each ventricle in one minute. Cardiac output (litres/min) is the product of the stroke volume (litres/beat) and the heart rate (beats/min). There are four determinants of cardiac output, including heart rate, preload, afterload, and contractility.

Heart rate is affected by chronotropic factors. Sympathetic stimulation by noradrenaline, adrenaline, and medications such as atropine can increase heart rate. Activation of the parasympathetic system and chemicals, such as acetylcholine and adenosine, slows down the heart rate.

Preload is the amount of blood entering the ventricle during diastole, also known as the end-diastolic volume. It is influenced by blood volume, venous return, and atrial contraction.

Afterload occurs during systole when ventricle contracts and ejects blood out of the aorta and into the pulmonary trunk. Atherosclerosis, peripheral vasoconstriction, and hypertension increase afterload due to increased resistance.

Inotropic factors affect the contractility of the heart. Positive inotropes such as sympathetic stimulation by noradrenaline and dobutamine increases cardiac output. The parasympathetic system, acetylcholine, beta blockers, acidosis, and calcium channel blockers can have negative inotropic effect on the heart and reduce cardiac contractility.

Atropine increases heart rate, causing a higher cardiac output. Adenosine slows down heart rate hence reduces cardiac output. Hypertension increases the force against which the ventricles must pump in order to eject blood, hence reducing cardiac output. Beta blockers have negative inotrope effect and also slow down the heart rate, resulting in decreased cardiac output.

Acidosis reduces left ventricle contractility. However, this is compensated for by an increased heart rate and a reduced systemic vascular resistance, resulting in an increased cardiac output.

Vincent J. Understanding cardiac output. Critical Care. 2008;12(4):174.
https://www.ncbi.nlm.nih.gov/pmc/articles/PMC2575587/

11. Answer D

Episodic loss of consciousness is most commonly caused by cardiac syncope, reflex syncope, orthostatic syncope, and less commonly seizure. Clinical features present on history, examination and basic investigation findings can be useful in determining the likelihood of various causes, although no individual feature is diagnostic for a particular cause.

Patient features that increase the likelihood of cardiac syncope are increasing patient age, history of atrial fibrillation or flutter, history of cardiac failure, and history of severe structural heart disease. Some precipitating factors can decrease the likelihood of cardiac syncope, such as syncope in a warm place, during a medical procedure, or after using the toilet. Dyspnoea or chest pain prior to syncope are associated with higher likelihood of cardiac syncope, whereas cold sensitivity, headache, mood change, and abdominal discomfort decrease the likelihood of cardiac syncope. Witnessed cyanosis is associated with higher likelihood of cardiac syncope, whereas inability to remember details prior to the episode and mood changes after the episode are associated with lower likelihood of cardiac syncope. A combination of normal ECG and no history of cardiac disease is associated with a lower likelihood of cardiac syncope. Contrary to popular teaching, the presence or absence of injury does not predict for or against cardiac syncope.

Two clinical scores, Evaluation of Guidelines in SYncope Study (EGSYS) and vasovagal score), assign scores on the basis of a combination of clinical factors and have some predictive value over and above individual patient characteristics. EGSYS uses six patient variables and a score less than three has a likelihood ratio of cardiac syncope of 0.12–0.17. The vasovagal score has only been prospectively evaluated in one study but a cut-off score of less than −2 has likelihood ratio of over 8 for cardiac syncope and equal to or more than −2 has a likelihood ratio of 0.10, making this score a potentially good discriminator, if results can be duplicated.

Biomarkers are not yet utilised in widespread practice for the evaluation of syncope, but there is some evidence that high-sensitivity troponin and N-terminal pro-B-type natriuretic peptide may become useful in ruling out cardiac syncope.

Several clinical features have high specificity, but low sensitivity for the diagnosis of seizure. These include head turning during the event, unusual posturing during the event, urinary incontinence, tongue trauma, and the patient having no recall of witnessed unusual behaviours.

Albassam O, Redelmeier R, Shadowitz S, et al. Did This Patient Have Cardiac Syncope? JAMA. 2019;321(24):2448.
https://jamanetwork.com/journals/jama/article-abstract/2736568

12. Answer: C

This patient's clinical features, unexplained fever, myalgia, sudden appearance of several small, cool, cyanotic and painful areas of the toe, and AKI are consistent with cholesterol embolisation. Cholesterol embolism is caused by showers of cholesterol crystals from an atherosclerotic plaque that occludes small arteries. Embolisation can occur spontaneously or as an iatrogenic complication from an invasive vascular procedure (angiography or vascular surgery) and after anticoagulant therapy as a result of interference with the protective clot over ulcerative atheromatous plaques and thrombolytic therapy may lyse thrombi, including those covering atherosclerotic plaques.

Once in the circulation, cholesterol crystal emboli lodge in small arteries (150–200 um in diameter); which then cause an inflammatory reaction, intimal proliferation, and intravascular fibrosis leading to the narrowing or obliteration of the lumen and ischaemic changes. Peak incidence is usually two to four weeks after a procedure.

The true incidence of cholesterol embolisation is difficult to estimate. Retrospective autopsy (incidence 10–27%) or biopsy (incidence 1%) studies may include subclinical cases. The hallmark of the condition is the presence of needle-shaped empty spaces in histological sections as the lipids are dissolved by the techniques used to prepare the tissue for histological examination (See below).

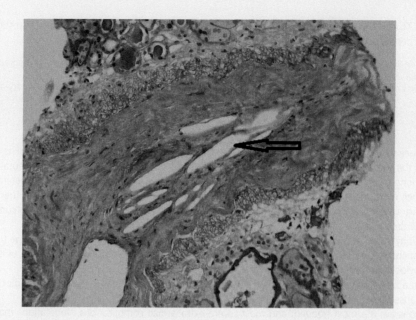

Patients can be asymptomatic, or they can present with a distinct clinical syndrome, ranging from a cyanotic toe to a multiorgan systemic disease that can mimic other systemic diseases such as vasculitis. The distribution of end-organ damage depends on the anatomical location of the original atherosclerotic plaques and the extent of organ involvement. Laboratory investigations are non-specific. Eosinophilia appears to be the most common finding up to 80% of cases.

The presence of a triad of a precipitating event, AKI, and peripheral embolisation strongly suggests the diagnosis. The presence of other complications of atheroembolism, such as gastrointestinal bleeding and neurological involvement, should raise the suspicion level. To confirm diagnosis, a biopsy of the target organs is needed.

There is no effective treatment apart from symptomatic and supportive measures, including dialysis. Anticoagulants should be avoided if possible because they can potentiate the problem. Disagreement exists concerning steroid treatment. Recently, statins have been found to be associated with better renal outcome likely due to statin-induced plaque stabilisation and regression. Patients with cholesterol embolisation have a poor prognosis with one-year mortality rate ranging from 64–87%.

 Kronzon I, Saric M. Cholesterol Embolization Syndrome. Circulation. 2010;122(6):631–641.
https://www.ncbi.nlm.nih.gov/pubmed/21993354

 Scolari F, Ravani P. Atheroembolic renal disease. The Lancet. 2010;375(9726):1650–1660.
https://www.ncbi.nlm.nih.gov/pubmed/20381857

13. Answer: D

Computed tomography coronary angiography (CTCA) is an imaging test that has been shown in meta-analyses to have excellent sensitivity (98%) and good specificity (88%) for significant coronary artery disease (CAD) with stenosis >50%. Its high negative predictive values (96–100%) suggest CTCA is an excellent test for ruling out significant disease in patients with low-to-intermediate pretest probability of CAD. Current data does not support the use of CTCA in asymptomatic patients.

CTCA is not recommended in patients with previous coronary stents as the stents may produce artefact and make the results uninterpretable. Stent diameter <3 mm is thought to be unevaluable. However, very selective cases can be evaluated using CTCA, including large stents and simple left main stents. CTCA is not appropriate for patients with STEMI given the need for invasive coronary angiogram without any delay.

To avoid artefacts which may hamper interpretation of the results, the patient should be in sinus rhythm with a heart rate <65 beats/min, able to hold their breath for 10 seconds, able to tolerate beta blockers and nitrates (nitrates are given to dilate the coronary arteries by most centres), and able to hold their arms above the head during the scan. Previous contrast allergy must be ruled out prior to CTCA. If the patient has significant renal impairment, CTCA may not be the best investigation for CAD due to the risk of contrast nephropathy.

 Liew G, Feneley M, Worthley S. Appropriate indications for computed tomography coronary angiography. Medical Journal of Australia. 2012;196(4):246–249.
https://www.mja.com.au/journal/2012/196/4/appropriate-indications-computed-tomography-coronary-angiography

14. Answer: B

This patient has evidence of native mitralvalve infective endocarditis (IE) complicated by cerebral emboli. IE is the infection of the endocardial surface of the heart and may involve one or more heart valves, the mural endocardium, or a septal defect. The highest rates are observed among patients with prosthetic valves, intracardiac devices, unrepaired cyanotic congenital heart diseases, or a history of IE. However, more than 50% of cases are not associated with underlying valvular disease. Other risk factors include chronic rheumatic heart disease, age related degenerative valvular lesions, haemodialysis, and co-existing conditions such as diabetes, and intravenous drug use.

Streptococci and staphylococci account for 80% of cases of IE, with proportions varying according to valve (native vs prosthetic), source of infection, patient age, and coexisting conditions. Staphylococci are now the most common cause of IE and approximately 35%–60.5% of staphylococcal bacteraemia are complicated by IE.

Cases of IE in which a blood culture is negative (10% of cases) may be due to patients exposed to antibiotic agents before the diagnosis of IE or IE caused by fastidious microorganisms.

Cerebral complications are the most frequent and most severe extracardiac complications. Vegetations that are large, mobile, or in the mitral position and IE due to Staphylococcus aureus are associated with an increased risk of symptomatic embolism.

IE remains a diagnostic and therapeutic challenge. Identifying the causative microorganism is central to diagnosis and appropriate treatment; two or three blood cultures should routinely be drawn before antibiotic therapy is initiated. When IE is suspected, echocardiogram should be performed as soon as possible. However, the diagnosis of IE can never be excluded on the basis of negative echocardiogram findings, either from transthoracic echocardiogram or transesophageal echocardiogram.

Appropriate antibiotic treatment of IE is guided by Australian Therapeutic Antibiotic Guidelines. Approximately 15%–25% of patients with IE eventually require surgery. Indications for surgical intervention in patients with native valve IE are as follows:
- Congestive heart failure that is refractory to standard medical therapy
- Fungal infective endocarditis
- Persistent sepsis after 72 hours of appropriate antibiotic treatment
- Recurrent septic emboli, especially after 2 weeks of antibiotic treatment
- Rupture of an aneurysm of the sinus of Valsalva
- Conduction disturbances caused by a septal abscess
- Kissing infection of the anterior mitral leaflet in patients with IE of the aortic valve.

 Hoen B, Duval X. Infective Endocarditis. New England Journal of Medicine. 2013;368(15):1425–1433.
https://www.ncbi.nlm.nih.gov/pubmed/23574121

15. Answer: C

According to the ACC/AHA guideline, a biventricular pacemaker and defibrillator should be offered to patients with NYHA class III or IV heart failure, an ejection fraction <35% and a QRS complex >0.12 second. Approximately 70% of patients' symptoms improve due to resynchronisation of the timing of the left and right ventricular contraction. Device treatment has been shown to improve mortality, ejection fraction, quality of life, and functional status, as well as reduce readmission.

A dual-chamber pacemaker does not provide symptomatic relief or protect patients from ventricular arrhythmias and sudden cardiac death. Recent clinical trials have demonstrated SGLT2 inhibitors reduces mortality and hospitalisation in patients with type 2 diabetes and established cardiovascular disease. However, it is currently contraindicated in patients with eGFR <30 ml/min/1.73 m². Adding a beta blocker in an elderly patient with severe airway disease and insulin dependent diabetes may need careful consideration and is not the most effective treatment for this patient.

 Normand C, Linde C, Singh J, Dickstein K.Ref: Indications for Cardiac Resynchronization Therapy. A Comparison of the Major International Guidelines JACC: Heart Failure. 2018;6(Issue 4):308-316., April 2018
https://www.sciencedirect.com/science/article/pii/S2213177918301203

16. Answer: C

SGLT2 inhibitor (SGLT2i) works by inhibiting SGLT2 in the proximal convoluted tubule, to prevent reabsorption of glucose and facilitate its excretion in urine. As glucose is excreted in urine, its plasma levels fall leading to an improvement in glycaemic parameters. This mechanism of action of SGLT2i is dependent on blood glucose levels and has minimal potential for hypoglycaemia. SGLT2i's mode of action depends upon normal renal glomerular–tubular function and their efficacy is reduced in persons with renal impairment. SGLT2i are not prescribed on their own but can be used in combination with other diabetes medications. SGLT2i may also cause modest weight loss and reduce systolic blood pressure, which are beneficial for patients with heart failure.

Thiazolidinediones may cause water retention, weight gain, or worsen heart failure and are contraindicated in patients with New York Heart Association (NYHA) class II–IV heart failure. They should be used cautiously in patients with NYHA class I heart failure.

Atherton J, Sindone A, De Pasquale C, et al. National Heart Foundation of Australia and Cardiac Society of Australia and New Zealand: Australian clinical guidelines for the management of heart failure 2018. Medical Journal of Australia. 2018;209(8):363–369.
https://onlinelibrary.wiley.com/doi/abs/10.5694/mja18.00647?sid=nlm%3Apubmed

17. Answer: B

This patient's clinical presentation, risk factors, and echocardiogram findings are consistent with heart failure with preserved ejection fraction (HFpEF). No therapy has been proven to reduce mortality in patients with HFpEF.

HFpEF predominantly affects elderly (>65 years) hypertensive women. Other risk factors include obesity, coronary artery disease, diabetes, atrial fibrillation, and hyperlipidaemia. It is established that the prevalence of HFpEF among patients with heart failure averages 47% and its prevalence in the community is estimated to be 1.1% to 5.5% of the general population. The prevalence of HFpEF has increased over the last two decades, due to ageing population, increasing prevalence of risk factors, such as hypertension, diabetes, and increased survival.

The diagnosis of HFpEF can be challenging because the symptoms and signs are non-specific, hence it is a strictly clinical diagnosis. For patients presenting with heart failure and relatively normal LV ejection fraction (LVEF), valvular heart disease, infiltrative cardiomyopathies, pericardial disease, high-output heart failure, chronic pulmonary disease, and pulmonary arterial hypertension should be excluded. An elevated BNP or NT-proBNP on its own is insufficient for the diagnosis or exclusion of HFpEF.

Echocardiogram is the imaging modality of choice to establish the diagnosis of HFpEF by criteria; exclude valvular, right-sided, or pericardial disease; and assess for other differential diagnoses. The following are the echocardiographic criteria recommended by the European Society of Cardiology for the diagnosis of HFpEF:

- LVEF ≥50%
- LV end-diastolic volume index (LVEDI) <97 mL/m²
- Raised LV filling pressure is indicated by a ratio of mitral early diastolic inflow velocity to mitral early annular lengthening velocity (E/e')>15.

Cardiac catheterisation is the gold standard for the diagnosis of HFpEF. Criteria for raised LV filling pressure include LV end-diastolic pressure >16 mmHg or a mean pulmonary capillary wedge pressure >12 mmHg.

In contrast to heart failure with reduced ejection fraction, there is limited clinical trial evidence guiding the treatment of HFpEF. At present, no therapy including ACE inhibitors, angiotensin receptor blockers, β-blockers and aldosterone antagonists has demonstrated mortality benefit in patients with HFpEF.

Managing comorbidities including hypertension, obesity, OSA, rate control for AF, and diabetes, are the mainstay of HFpEF treatment strategies. Diuretics can be used to reduce congestion and improve symptoms. Low-dose spironolactone is recommended to reduce hospital admission on the basis of the TOPCAT trial results. Sildenafil is an inhibitor of phosphodiesterase-5 that increases cGMP levels by blocking catabolism. Increased availability of cGMP could provide benefits for both vascular and myocardial remodelling, including attenuating hypertrophy, fibrosis, and impaired cardiac relaxation. In the RELAX trial, sildenafil did not improve 6 min walk distance or quality of life. Ivabradine is a selective sinus node If sodium channel inhibitor that reduces HR without affecting contractility. It can increase peak VO₂ and reduced exercise mitral early diastolic velocity/mitral annular velocity (E/e') ratio.

Harper A, Patel H, Lyon A.AR. Heart failure with preserved ejection fraction. Clinical Medicine.Clin Med (Lond). 2018;18(Suppl 2): s24–s29.
https://pubmed.ncbi.nlm.nih.gov/29700089/

18. Answer: D

Hypertrophic cardiomyopathy (HOCM) is a common monogenic cardiovascular disorder with a prevalence of 1 in 500. It is diagnosed with echocardiogram and MRI which shows a hypertrophic left ventricule without dilatation and it is not associated with another cardiac, systemic, metabolic, or syndromic disease. HOCM is diverse in clinical, phenotypic expression, and natural history. It is often underdiagnosed.

HOCM is inherited in an autosomal dominant pattern. It is associated with mutations (nucleotide sequence variants) in 11 or more genes encoding proteins of thick and thin myofilament contractile components of the cardiac sarcomere (Z-disk), with beta-myosin heavy chain and myosin-binding protein C genes most commonly involved.

HOCM is predominantly an obstructive disease, with 70% of patients having mechanical impedance to left ventricular outflow (gradients ≥30 mm Hg) at rest or with exertion. Left ventricular outflow obstruction is usually produced by mitral-valve systolic anterior motion and septal contact due to flow drag, causing complications such as mitral regurgitation, diastolic dysfunction, atrial fibrillation, congestive heart failure, and ventricular tachyarrhythmias.

HOCM is associated with increased sudden cardiac death associated with ventricular tachyarrhythmias, disorganised myocardial architecture, interstitial collagen deposition, and replacement scarring after myocyte death as a consequence of coronary microvascular mediated flow dysfunction and ischemia. Patients with a diagnosis of HOCM are often disqualified from participating in intensive competitive sports due to high risks of sudden cardiac death.

The American College of Cardiology and the American Heart Association (ACC–AHA) have developed an algorithm for risk stratification in patients with HOCM who would benefit from primary prevention of sudden cardiac death with implantable cardioverter–defibrillators (ICDs). ICDs should be considered in young and middle-aged patients whose clinical profiles include one or more major risk factors, include family history of HOCM-related sudden death, unexplained syncope, multiple, repetitive non-sustained VT, massive LVH (≥30 mm), left ventricle apical aneurysm, and extensive late gadolinium enhancement. If the level of risk remains uncertain, other clinical features such as left ventricular outflow obstruction, hypotensive response to exercise, can serve as mediating factors.

Management strategies for variable clinical manifestation of HOCM include ICDs to reduce the risk of sudden cardiac death, surgical myectomy (with alcohol septal ablation as a selective alternative) for permanent reversal of heart failure in patients with outflow obstruction, heart transplantation for patients with non-obstructive end-stage disease, and anticoagulant therapy to prevent embolic stroke caused by atrial fibrillation.

Maron B. Clinical Course and Management of Hypertrophic Cardiomyopathy. New England Journal of Medicine. 2018;379(7):655–668.
https://www.ncbi.nlm.nih.gov/pubmed/30110588

19. Answer: B

This patient has papilloedema with almost complete obliteration of the margins of the optic disc and several hypertensive haemorrhages. Changes in hypertensive retinopathy include: Focal arteriolar narrowing and arterial venous nicking, flame or blot haemorrhages, microaneurysm, hard exudates, cotton wool spots, and papilloedema.

The Keith-Wagner grade is used to classify the severity of hypertensive retinopathy:

Grade 1: Isolated narrowing of the arterioles.

Grade 2: There is moderate to marked narrowing of retinal arterioles associated with a copper wire appearance or arteriovenous nicking.

Grade 3: Hypertensive retinal haemorrhage or exudates are present.

Grade 4: Papilloedema is present.

Modi P, Arsiwalla T. Hypertensive Retinopathy [Internet]. Statpearls.com. 2020 [cited 16 November 2020]. Available from: https://www.statpearls.com/articlelibrary/viewarticle/35600/

20. Answer: C

All of the above patients have a Class I indication for an ICD implantation except in the patient who just had a myocardial infarction two weeks ago. There is no survival benefit of early ICD implantation in patients with ischaemic cardiomyopathy. Evaluation of patients for ICD implantation should wait at least 40 days post-myocardial infarction and an ICD is then indicated in patients with left ventricular ejection fraction less than or equal to 35% and at least 90 days post revascularisation, with NYHA class II/III symptoms despite guideline directed medical therapy.

The current indications for ICD to prevent sudden cardiac death (SCD) are summarised in Table 1 in the following full text article based on the 2017 American Heart Association/American College of Cardiology/Heart Rhythm Society (AHA/ACC/HRS) guidelines for management of patients with ventricular arrhythmias and the 2015 European Society of Cardiology (ESC) guidelines for management of patients with ventricular arrhythmias.

Chieng D, Paul V, Denman R. Current Device Therapies for Sudden Cardiac Death Prevention – the ICD, Subcutaneous ICD and Wearable ICD. Heart, Lung and Circulation. 2019;28(1):65-75.
https://www.heartlungcirc.org/article/S1443-9506(18)31920-6/fulltext

21. Answer: D

This patient has infrequent palpitations which happen around once every 6 months. Three- or seven-day Holter monitoring may not capture arrythmias due to the infrequent events.

It is important to know the frequency of palpitations or syncopal events to decide what the best way is to investigate potential underlying arrhythmias.

The next preferred step of investigation for this patient is an implantable loop recorder due to the infrequent symptoms and the long duration between events.

It will be important to investigate underlying coronary artery disease in this patient with significant risk factors for cardiovascular disease due to his past medical history, which may contribute to his symptoms.

In patients with infrequent unexplained syncopal episodes, implantable loop recorders have high rates of diagnosing arrythmias compared to external loop recorders or physician follow-up. Implantable loop recorders are pen drive sized device inserted under the skin under local anaesthetic and are capable of recording cardiac events for up to three years. Implantable loop recorders can be considered in patients with cryptogenic stroke to detect paroxysmal or infrequent atrial fibrillation if the initial in-hospital or Holter monitoring are unable to detect atrial fibrillation, which is a risk factor for embolic stroke.

Wearable devices are gaining popularity in the recent years and may aid in detection of arrythmias such as atrial fibrillation and supraventricular tachycardia. However, in patients with syncopal episodes, they are unable to record these events due to potential loss of consciousness with syncope. More studies are required to see how to integrate smart devices to improve patient care.

Khalil C, Haddad F, Al Suwaidi J. Investigating palpitations: the role of Holter monitoring and loop recorders. BMJ. 2017; 358: j3123.
https://www.bmj.com/content/358/bmj.j3123.long

22. Answer: A

Evolocumab and alirocumab are monoclonal antibodies inhibiting Proprotein Convertase Sublitisin/Kexin Type-9 (PCSK9). PCSK9 inhibits low-density lipoproteins (LDL) receptor recycling, which in turn limits the ability for tissue to sequester LDL from the extracellular space. Individuals with activating mutations of the PCSK9 gene have high LDL and poor cardiac outcomes; conversely individuals with inactivating mutations of the PCSK9 gene have low LDL levels and relatively good cardiac outcomes. PCSK9 inhibitor therapy is administered by subcutaneous injection and is indicated where statin/combination therapy has failed to reach LDL targets. PCKS9 inhibitors have shown small but meaningful reductions in cardiovascular risk and mortality and have a greater protective effect for individuals with higher baseline LDL.

The primary action of statins (eg. rosuvastatin) is to decrease hepatocyte production of cholesterol by inhibition of HMG-CoA (3-hydroxy-3-methylglutaryl-coenzyme A) reductase, thereby increasing LDL receptor synthesis, and increasing LDL clearance. Ezetimibe is an azetidinone cholesterol absorption inhibitor, which acts by blocking NPC1L1 (Niemann-Pick C1-Like 1) a key brush-border transport protein. Mipomersen is an example of a newer advance in lipid-lowering therapy, which inhibits synthesis of apoB-100 and LDL, and can be considered for use in homozygous familial hypercholesterolaemia but hepatotoxicity is a significant potential adverse effect.

Burnett J, Hooper A. PCSK9 — A Journey to Cardiovascular Outcomes. New England Journal of Medicine. 2018;379(22):2161–2162.
https://www.nejm.org/doi/full/10.1056/NEJMe1813758

23. Answer: B

Long QT syndrome (LQT) is diagnosed by QT prolongation and T-wave abnormalities on an ECG. A QT interval is measured from the onset of the QRS complex to the end of the T wave. The corrected QT interval (QTc, corrected for heart rate) can be calculated as QTc = QT interval + square root of the RR interval. The latest European Society of Cardiology guideline suggests upper limits of the QT interval of 480 ms on the ECG strip, regardless of gender. Presenting symptoms of LQT include dizziness, syncope, seizures, and in some cases cardiac arrest due to the presence of Torsades-de-Pointes which can degenerate to ventricular fibrillation causing sudden cardiac death. LQT can be congenital or acquired. LQT is associated with multiple risk factors, including a family history of LQT, ion channel abnormalities, structural heart disease, heart failure, advanced age, hypokalaemia, subarachnoid bleed, medications, diabetes, epilepsy, emotional stress, and physical stress, etc.

The aim of the treatment of LQT is to ensure patients are symptom free. The mainstay of management of LQT is beta blockers in both asymptomatic and symptomatic patients with LQT. Medication compliance is important to avoid life-threatening consequences. Unfortunately, cardiac events cannot be completely prevented by taking beta blockers.

Life-style modification such as avoiding strenuous exercises, emotional stress, physical stress, sleep disturbance, and medications that prolong the QT interval, should be implemented as much as possible.

ICD should be considered in symptomatic patients with syncope who are already on beta blockers, high risk patients with a very long QTc interval (> 550 ms), patients with T-wave alternans, or in patients who cannot tolerate beta blocker therapy. If there are reversible causes of LQT, an ICD is not indicated.

Left cardiac sympathetic denervation (LCSD) is a rarely performed but effective procedure for management of LQT in patients who cannot have beta blockers or ICD. LCSD procedure involves high thoracic left sympathectomy and ablation of the lower half of the stellate ganglion along with T2 to T4. It reduces noradrenaline release at the ventricles and increase the threshold for ventricular fibrillation.

 Shah S, Park K, Alweis R. Long QT Syndrome: A Comprehensive Review of the Literature and Current Evidence. Current Problems in Cardiology. 2019;44(3):92–106.
https://www.sciencedirect.com/science/article/abs/pii/S0146280618300513?via%3Dihub

24. Answer: D

This patient is likely to have a history of rheumatic fever leading to mixed mitral valve disease. She is symptomatic with pulmonary hypertension which is the indication for intervention. The mortality for untreated symptomatic severe mitral stenosis is 85% over 10 years. Complications for untreated severe mitral stenosis include endocarditis, atrial fibrillation, stroke, pulmonary hypertension, and right heart failure. The clinical features of severe mitral stenosis are:

- Transmitral mean gradient >10 mmHg
- Enlarged left atrium
- Mitral valvular area <1.5cm^2
- Pulmonary hypertension.

In terms of intervention, percutaneous valvuloplasty should be considered if valve anatomy is amenable. Percutaneous valvuloplasty is less invasive and avoids anticoagulation which is an important consideration in an Aboriginal and Torres Strait Islander patient. Percutaneous valvuloplasty should not be performed in patient with moderate mitral regurgitation as the procedure will worsen mitral regurgitation. Recent emphasis on mitral valve conservation may lead to increased use of mitral valve open commissurotomy, wherein the surgeon, under direct vision, may be able to provide relief of obstruction in patients not suitable for balloon mitral valvuloplasty because of poor valve morphology. However, the percentage of patients that would likely have a bad outcome with balloon mitral valvuloplasty yet a good outcome with open commissurotomy is unknown but is probably small. When the valve can be conserved, it avoids the risks inherent to prosthetic valves and also avoids the need for anticoagulation for patients in sinus rhythm.

Putting these together, this patient has symptomatic, severe mitral stenosis with moderate mitral regurgitation and no other comorbidities therefore she should be considered for mitral valve replacement.

 Carabello B. Modern Management of Mitral Stenosis. Circulation. 2005;112(3):432–437.
https://www.ahajournals.org/doi/10.1161/CIRCULATIONAHA.104.532498

25. Answer: D

Polyunsaturated fatty acids (PUFAs), such as omega-3 and omega-6 fatty acids, have multiple roles in membrane structure, lipid metabolism, coagulation, blood pressure, and inflammation. It has been suggested that regular supplementation of omega-3 fatty acids is linked to a reduction in cardiovascular disease and other beneficial effects.

According to a recent Cochrane review, increasing PUFA intake may slightly reduce the risk of cardiovascular events but has no effect on all-cause or cardiovascular disease mortality based on an extensive systematic review of RCTs conducted to date. The number need to treat to prevent one cardiovascular event is 63. The mechanism may be via serum triglycerides reduction.

Omega-3 PUFA supplementation in type 2 diabetes lowers triglycerides and VLDL cholesterol, but may raise LDL cholesterol (although results were nonsignificant in subgroups) and has no statistically significant effect on glycaemic control or fasting insulin levels.

Omega-3 fatty acids appear to have limited benefit in blood viscosity reduction in patients with intermittent claudication. However, there is no evidence of consistent improved clinical outcomes including quality of life, walking distance, ankle brachial pressure index, or angiographic findings. Supplementation may also cause adverse effects such as increased total and LDL cholesterol levels.

Direct evidence on the effect of omega-3 PUFA on incident dementia is lacking. The available trials showed no benefit of omega-3 PUFA supplementation on cognitive function in cognitively healthy older people.

Abdelhamid A, Martin N, Bridges C, et al. Polyunsaturated fatty acids for the primary and secondary prevention of cardiovascular disease. Cochrane Database of Systematic Reviews. 2018.
https://www.cochranelibrary.com/cdsr/doi/10.1002/14651858.CD012345.pub3/full

26. Answer: D

Treatment resistant hypertension is defined as persistent hypertension despite adherent and optimal therapy with three different classes of antihypertensive medication including a diuretic, or any four agents. Cardiovascular and renal risk for such patients is two- to six fold higher than for patients with controlled hypertension. Medication compliance is an important factor in evaluating this patient. In addition to screening for secondary causes, which should be guided by history, examination, and laboratory findings, guidelines now suggest addition of a mineralocorticoid receptor antagonist (MRA) for this patient group. This is a result of multiple studies showing significant benefit for MRAs in this patient population. It is suggested that this may be due to high levels of undiagnosed hyperaldosteronism, but the benefits of MRA therapy, while predicted by presence of hyperaldosteronism, are not limited to this sub-population, and suggests of resistant hypertension is often indicative of a salt-retaining state.

Carey M, Whelton PK. Prevention, detection, evaluation and management of high blood pressure in adults: Synopsis of the 2017 American College of Cardiology/American Heart Association hypertension guideline. Ann Intern Med. 2018;168(5):351–8.
https://www.acc.org//media/Non-Clinical/Files-PDFs-Excel-MS-Word-etc/Guidelines/2017/Guidelines_Made_Simple_2017_HBP.pdf

27. Answer: C

Restrictive cardiomyopathy (RCM) is a heterogeneous group of diseases with variable pathogenesis, clinical features, diagnostic criteria, management strategies and prognosis. It is the least common of the cardiomyopathies and is often underdiagnosed.

In patients with RCM, a restrictive ventricular filling pattern is noted secondary to ventricular stiffness. Biventricular size and normal or near-normal ventricular systolic function are usual in the early stages of the disease. Depending on the ventricle involved, patients may have signs of right or left heart failure, conduction disturbance or arrhythmias. Diagnosis of RCM is based on echocardiogram, cardiac MRI and in some cases endomyocardial biopsy.

RCM is categorised as infiltrative (amyloidosis, sarcoidosis, primary hyperoxaluria), storage disease (Fabry disease, Gaucher disease, hereditary haemochromatosis, glycogen storage disease, mucopolysaccharidosis type I and type II, Niemann-Pick disease), noninfiltrative (idiopathic, diabetic, scleroderma, myofibrillar myopathies, pseuxanthoma elasticum, sarcomeric protein disorders, Werner's syndrome), and endomyocardial (carcinoid heart disease, endomyocardial fibrosis including idiopathic, hypereosinophilic syndrome, chronic eosinophilic leukaemia, drug-induced secondary to serotonin, methysergide, ergotamine, mercurial agents, busulfan, anthracyclines), endocardial fibroelastosis, metastatic cancer, and radiation, etc.

Left ventricular outflow tract obstruction is often seen in patients with subaortic stenosis, bicuspid aortic valve, supravalvular aortic stenosis, coarctation of the aorta, and hypertrophic cardiomyopathy. Option C is often seen in patients with sarcoidosis and RCM. Option D is seen in patients with dilated cardiomyopathy, which is the most common cause of cardiomyopathy.

Treatment should be of the underlying cause(s) of RCM if possible. Diuretics should be used with caution for patients with fluid overload, as some patients with RCM rely on high filling pressure to maintain cardiac output. Excessive diuresis may cause reduced cardiac tissue perfusion. β-blockers and calcium channel blockers could be used to manage arrhythmias or increase filling time. However, careful monitoring of the response is required as some patients may be intolerant. Angiotensin-converting enzyme (ACE) inhibitors and angiotensin receptor blockers should be considered. However, currently there is no evidence that these agents may be beneficial, and they may not be well tolerated by patients with RCM. Anticoagulation is required in patients with atrial fibrillation, mural thrombus, or evidence of systemic embolisation to prevent strokes. Left ventricular assist device may be beneficial in patients with advanced heart failure as a definitive therapy or as a bridge to cardiac transplant.

 Muchtar E, Blauwet L, Gertz M. Restrictive Cardiomyopathy: Genetics, Pathogenesis, Clinical Manifestations, Diagnosis, and Therapy. Circulation Research. 2017;121(7):819–837.
https://www.ncbi.nlm.nih.gov/pubmed/28912185

28. Answer: D

Acute rheumatic fever (ARF) and rheumatic heart disease (RHD) remain a significant cause of cardiovascular morbidity and mortality worldwide. In Australia, ARF and RHD disproportionately affect the ATSI population, with up to ×10 higher incidence, ×8 higher ARF hospitalisation rates, and ×20 higher mortality. The highest rates of ARF are in children aged 5–14 years old, and highest rates of RHD in adults aged 35–39, with an all-age RHD incidence up to 2% in ATSI populations in the Northern Territory.

All patients with suspected ARF should be hospitalised to enable appropriate diagnostic investigations including echocardiogram. In high risk groups there should be a lower threshold for diagnosis as listed below and high-risk groups are populations with an incidence of ARF >30/100 000 per year in 5–14 years old or incidence of RHD >2/1000 in all age groups.

ARF diagnosis requires evidence of a preceding group A streptococcus infection, and two major manifestations or one major manifestation and two minor manifestations listed below in low risk populations:

- Major manifestations:
  - Carditis (including subclinical evidence of rheumatic valve disease on echocardiograms)
  - Polyarthritis or aseptic monoarthritis or polyarthralgia
  - Chorea
  - Subcutaneous nodules
  - Erythema marginatum.
- Minor manifestations:
  - Fever
  - Polyarthralgia or aseptic monoarthritis
  - ESR ≥30 mm/hr or CRP ≥30 mg/L
  - Prolonged PR interval on ECG.

Treatment of ARF is benzathine penicillin G every four week, or every three week for high risk patients, for a minimum of 10 years after the last episode of ARF, or until aged 21 if no RHD or 35–40 if moderate–severe RHD.

 ARF RHD Guideline [Internet]. Rheumatic Heart Disease Australia. 2019 [cited 19 August 2019]. Available from: https://www.rhdaustralia.org.au/arf-rhd-guideline

29. Answer: D

This patient's presentation and ECG changes are consistent with inferior and right ventricular (RV) myocardial infarction (MI). RV ischaemia complicates 30% to 50% of inferior MIs. Isolated RV myocardial infarction (RVMI) is rare. The coronary artery involved is usually an occluded right coronary artery (RCA). The proximal segment of the RCA supplies the sinoatrial (SA) node and the right atrial wall; the middle segment supplies the lateral and inferior right ventricle (RV); and the posterior portion of the left ventricle, the inferior septum, inferior left ventricular wall and atrioventricular (AV) node are perfused by the distal segment of the RCA. A few patients (10%) may have a right ventricle that is supplied by the circumflex artery.

Although the RVMI often shows good long-term recovery, in the short term RVMI has a worse prognosis to uncomplicated inferior MI, with haemodynamic and electrophysiologic complications increasing in-hospital morbidity and mortality. Acute RV shock has an equally high mortality to left ventricular (LV) shock.

Clinically, the triad of hypotension, elevated jugular venous pressure (JVP), and clear lung fields should raise the possibility of RVMI in patients with acute inferior MI. The classic 12 lead ECG provides information on the LV, but limited information on the electrical activity of the RV. Only lead V1 provides a partial view of the RV free wall. Right precordial leads are obtained by placing the precordial electrodes over the right chest in positions mirroring their usual arrangement. The presence of acute ST segment elevation, Q waves or both in the right precordial leads (V3R to V6R), is highly reliable in the diagnosis of RVMI. ST segment elevation 0.1 mV in the right precordial leads, especially V4R, is observed in 60–90% of patients with acute RVMI. ST elevation from the RV free wall may also be detected by ST elevation in lead III being more than that in lead II or by reciprocal ST depression in leads I and aVL. Echocardiogram should be performed in patient with or suspected RVMI. It may show RV dysfunction.

Additional features of RV involvement include paradoxical septal motion due to increased RV end diastolic pressure, tricuspid regurgitation, and increased right heart pressure.

Cardiac MRI (CMR) can directly evaluate RV size, mass, morphology, and function in an accurate and reproducible manner. CMR is now considered the gold standard for non-invasive assessment of RV function, particularly as it provides additional information on RV anatomy and myocardial mass.

It is important to recognise and diagnose RVMI, as the treatment is different to LVMI and inferior MI. Please see the following principles of the RVMI management.

1. Reperfusion therapy
   - Primary percutaneous coronary intervention preferable to thrombolysis, this should be performed as early as possible to preserve right heart function.
2. Optimise RV preload
   - Avoid morphine, diuretics, β-blockers, nitrates, ACE inhibitor
   - Trial of judicious fluid administration in the absence of pulmonary oedema
   - Consider intravenous fluid therapy to increase right sided preload in the absence of pulmonary oedema.
3. Reduce RV afterload
   - Inotropes, pulmonary vasodilators (nitric oxide, prostacycline)
   - Intra-aortic balloon pump.
4. Maintain chronotropic competence and atrioventricular synchrony
   - Avoid β-blockers in patients with proximal right coronary artery occlusion
   - Consider dual-chamber temporary pacing.

 Kakouros N, Cokkinos D. Right ventricular myocardial infarction: pathophysiology, diagnosis, and management. Postgraduate Medical Journal. 2010;86(1022):719–728. https://www.ncbi.nlm.nih.gov/pubmed/20956396

30. Answer: D

Permanent pacing for sinus node dysfunction is only indicated in patients with symptoms directly attributable to bradycardia, irrespective of minimum heart rate or pause duration.

Sinus node dysfunction is most often related to age-dependent progressive fibrosis of the sinus nodal tissue and surrounding atrial myocardium. It may lead to abnormalities of the sinus node, and atrial impulse formation and propagation, which will therefore result in various bradycardic or pause-related syndromes. Less common causes include acute myocardial ischemia, atrial tachyarrhythmias, electrolyte abnormalities, hypothyroidism, medications, infections, and metabolic abnormalities. Evaluation for these potentially treatable or reversible causes can be performed non-urgently in most cases.

Nocturnal bradycardias should prompt consideration of screening for sleep apnoea. Nocturnal bradycardias are common in patient with sleep apnoea. Treatment of sleep apnoea not only reduces the frequency of nocturnal bradycardias but also might offer cardiovascular benefits. The presence of nocturnal bradycardia is not in itself an indication for permanent pacing.

 Kusumoto F, Schoenfeld M, Barrett C, et al. 2018 ACC/AHA/HRS Guideline on the Evaluation and Management of Patients with Bradycardia and Cardiac Conduction Delay. Circulation. 2018. https://www.ahajournals.org/doi/abs/10.1161/CIR.0000000000000628

31. Answer: A

This patient has classical clinical features of Takotsubo (stress) cardiomyopathy which was first described in 1990. Its characteristic finding is the left ventricular apex ballooning. Presenting symptoms include chest pain, dyspnoea, and syncope and can be similar to those in patients with acute coronary syndrome (ACS). 80% of patients have elevated troponin levels and 80% of patients have ischaemic changes on ECG and most have elevated levels of NT-pro BNP.

Diagnosis of Takotsubo cardiomyopathy does not preclude the diagnosis of ACS. Up to 15% of patients with Takotsubo cardiomyopathy have concurrent coronary artery disease on coronary angiography. Diagnostic criteria for Takotsubo cardiomyopathy includes the presence of a transient abnormality in left ventricular wall motion beyond a single epicardial coronary artery perfusion territory, the absence of obstructive coronary artery disease or angiographic evidence of acute plaque rupture, the presence of new ECG abnormalities or elevation in cardiac troponin levels, and the absence of pheochromocytoma and myocarditis. There are four types of Takotsubo cardiomyopathy: apical type (in most patients) followed by the midventricular type, the basal type, and the focal type.

Takotsubo cardiomyopathy has a higher incidence in patients with a past medical history of neurological and psychiatric disorders, such as epilepsy, stroke, subarachnoid haemorrhage, electroconvulsive therapy, anxiety, and depression. Previous studies suggest Takotsubo cardiomyopathy is associated with emotional triggers. Subsequent studies have found the condition may also occur with physical triggers or even without preceding triggers. Takotsubo cardiomyopathy has a female predominance.

Takotsubo cardiomyopathy was once thought a benign disease with transient systolic and diastolic left ventricular dysfunction with a variety of wall-motion abnormalities. However, rates of in-hospital shock and death were similar in patients with Takotsubo cardiomyopathy and ACS. Other complications such as ventricular tachycardia, ventricular aneurysm, and ventricular rupture have been reported. The rate of major adverse cardiac and cerebrovascular events is 10% per patient-year, and the rate of death is 5.6% per patient-year, during long-term follow-up.

Angiotensin-converting enzyme (ACE) inhibitors or angiotensin-receptor blockers have been shown to improve survival at one year. Beta-blockers showed no survival benefits at one year following diagnosis of Takotsubo cardiomyopathy.

Templin C, Ghadri J, Diekmann J, et al Clinical Features and Outcomes of Takotsubo (Stress) Cardiomyopathy.
New England Journal of Medicine. 2015;373(10):929–938.
https://www.ncbi.nlm.nih.gov/pubmed/26332547

32. Answer: B
TAVI valves are bioprosthetic, so the recommendation is for dual antiplatelet therapy with aspirin and clopidogrel for 3–6 months, with aspirin continued lifelong.

Severe aortic stenosis (AS) is the most common form of valvular heart disease in the developed world, affecting 7% of adults older than 65 years. Most patients with early AS are asymptomatic. Currently, there is no evidence to support surgical aortic valve replacement (SAVR) or TAVI in asymptomatic patients, even with severe AS. However, once symptoms of angina, syncope, or heart failure develop, there is significantly increased mortality if untreated. SAVR remains the preferred treatment for low risk patients. For intermediate and high- risk patients, TAVI in suitable candidates is at least non-inferior.

According to the largest trial comparing TAVI to SAVR, major complications include:
- Major vascular complication rate (7.9% TAVI vs 5% SAVR).
- Major stroke rate (3.2% TAVI vs 4.3% SAVR).
- Heart block (secondary to direct compression of the bioprosthetic valve on the conduction tissue) requiring pacemaker insertion (8.5% TAVI vs 6.9% SAVR).
- Acute kidney injury (1.3% TAVI vs 3% SAVR).
- Other: Paravalvular aortic regurgitation (<5%), infectiveInfective endocarditis, catastrophic complications: coronary obstruction, aortic dissection, cardiac perforation (0.2–1.1%).

Adams H, Ashokkumar S, Newcomb A, et al. Contemporary review of severe aortic stenosis. Internal Medicine Journal.
2019;49(3):297–305.
https://onlinelibrary.wiley.com/doi/abs/10.1111/imj.14071

33. Answer: A
This patient has an inferolateral STEMI due to multivessel coronary disease. CABG is indicated in patients with severe left main coronary artery disease or triple vessel disease. CABG offers improved survival and quality of life for patients with more extensive coronary disease with reduced left ventricular systolic dysfunction and remodelling. Furthermore, patients with diabetes and multivessel disease have been shown to benefit from CABG.

Percutaneous coronary intervention (PCI) may be considered for patients with multivessel coronary artery disease who are not a candidate for open heart surgery due to comorbidities and poor functional status. PCI even with biventricular pacemaker–defibrillator is not the best option for this patient. He is young; stage 3A CKD and treatment with adalimumab are not contraindications for CABG.

Infarct-related artery (IRA) or culprit-only revascularisation in primary PCI is associated with higher rate of long-term major adverse cardiac events (MACE) compared with multivessel treatment. Patients scheduled for staged revascularisation experienced a similar rate of MACE to patients undergoing complete simultaneous treatment of non-IRA.

Pineda AM, Carvalho N, Gowani SA, Desouza KA, Santana O, Mihos CG, Stone GW, Beohar N. Managing Multivessel
Coronary Artery Disease in Patients With ST-Elevation Myocardial Infarction: A Comprehensive Review. Cardiol Rev.
2017 Jul/Aug;25(4):179–188.
https://pubmed.ncbi.nlm.nih.gov/27124268/

34. Answer: D

Troponin is a protein complex of three subunits (T, I, and C) that are involved in the contractile process of skeletal and cardiac muscle. Both cardiac and skeletal muscle express troponin C; whereas troponin T and I are cardiac-specific. Cardiac troponin (cTn) is integral to the diagnosis of acute coronary syndrome (ACS), but is elevated in many patients without ACS.

Conditions associated with non-ACS cTn elevations include:

- Tachyarrhythmias
- Congestive heart failure
- Malignant hypertension
- Sepsis
- Myocarditis
- Valvular heart disease (aortic stenosis)
- Aortic dissection
- Pulmonary embolism, pulmonary hypertension
- Chronic kidney disease
- Acute ischaemic or haemorrhagic stroke
- Cardiac contusion or cardiac procedures (CABG, PCI, ablation, pacing, cardioversion, or endomyocardial biopsy)
- Infiltrative diseases (amyloidosis, hemochromatosis, sarcoidosis)
- Myocardial drug toxicity or poisoning (doxorubicin, trastuzumab, snake venoms)
- Rhabdomyolysis.

As cTn can be detected among healthy adults, there are guidelines regarding what is considered an 'elevated' level. The joint European/American College of Cardiology guidelines define a clinically relevant increase in cTn levels as a level that exceeds the 99th percentile of a normal reference population. However, using a statistical cut-off means that some normal individuals will have a value above this cut-off, and because other clinical causes can cause an elevation, cTn should be interpreted in the context of pre-test probability of ACS. cTn concentrations are elevated in one in eight patients in the emergency department (ED).

High-sensitivity assays can accurately detect cTn at lower levels than older-generation assays, giving them higher sensitivity for the detection of ACS at presentation, which means that the time interval to the second measurement of high-sensitivity cTn (hs-cTn) can be significantly shortened, thereby reducing the time to diagnosis and improving efficiency in the ED. There is concern that hs-cTn may have lower diagnostic accuracy in patients with low pre-test probability for ACS. Concern of misinterpretation of these hs-cTn elevations as ACS and patient harm associated with potential unnecessary therapies such as anticoagulation and coronary angiography has led some experts to recommend withholding hs-cTn testing in patients with a low pre-test probability for ACS.

However, practice guidelines also highlight that ACS frequently presents with atypical symptoms especially in the elderly and patients with diabetes. It recommends scrutiny for ACS with ECG and hs-cTn. These divergent recommendations result in uncertainty in clinical practice regarding hs-cTn testing in patients with low pre-test probability for ACS. A recent retrospective analysis reported low specificity for hs-cTn to diagnose MI when grouping ED patients with suspected MI together with patients with acute heart failure and patients with documented PE. Hence, it is very important to highlight that diagnostic testing with hs-cTn should be applied to the correct population, at the optimal time and in the appropriate clinical context. This patient has very low pretest probability because her epigastric discomfort is nonspecific; her renal function is normal, and there are no other cardiovascular risk factors.

Twerenbold R, Boeddinghaus J, Nestelberger T, Wildi K, Rubini Gimenez M, Badertscher P et al. Ref: JACC 70(8):996–1012. Clinical Use of High-Sensitivity Cardiac Troponin in Patients With Suspected Myocardial Infarction. Twerenbold et al. 2017;70(8):996–1012.
https://pubmed.ncbi.nlm.nih.gov/28818210/

35. Answer: B

This elderly woman is septic due to severe pneumonia. She has multiple cardiovascular risk factors. Her ECG shows ischaemic change, and the troponin level is elevated. This is a typical case of type 2 myocardial infarction (MI).

MI can be classified into various types, based on pathological, clinical, and prognostic differences, along with different treatment strategies:

Type 1: Spontaneous myocardial infarction

Spontaneous MI related to atherosclerotic plaque rupture, ulceration, erosion, or dissection with resulting intraluminal thrombus in one or more of the coronary arteries leading to decreased myocardial blood flow or distal platelet emboli with ensuing myocyte necrosis. The patient may have underlying severe coronary artery disease (CAD) but on occasion non-obstructive or no CAD.

Type 2: Myocardial infarction secondary to an ischemic imbalance

In instances of myocardial injury with necrosis where a condition other than CAD contributes to an imbalance between myocardial oxygen supply and/or demand, e.g. coronary endothelial dysfunction, coronary artery spasm, coronary embolism, tachy-/brady-arrhythmias, anaemia, respiratory failure, hypotension.

Type 3: Myocardial infarction resulting in death when biomarker values are unavailable.

Type 4a: Myocardial infarction related to percutaneous coronary intervention (PCI).

Type 4b: Myocardial infarction related to stent thrombosis.

Type 5: Myocardial infarction related to coronary artery bypass grafting (CABG).

Patients with type 2 MI are frequently encountered in clinical practice and may be more common than type 1 MI. Diagnostic criteria for type 2 MI include:

Detection of a rise and/or fall of troponin values with at least one value above the 99th percentile, and evidence of an imbalance between myocardial oxygen supply and demand unrelated to acute coronary atherothrombosis, requiring at least one of the following:

- Symptoms of acute myocardial ischaemia
- New ischaemic ECG changes
- Development of pathological Q waves
- Imaging evidence of new loss of viable myocardium or new regional wall motion abnormality in a pattern consistent with an ischaemic aetiology.

The diagnosis of type 2 MI is associated with a poor prognosis: less than 40% of patients will live 5 years past their diagnosis. In contrast, 65% of patients with type 1 MI will survive for 5 years. This is because type 2 MI typically occurs among older patients with multiple comorbidities and is identified in the context of hemodynamic instability, including shock, tachycardia, respiratory failure, gastrointestinal bleeding, decompensated heart failure, or recent surgery. Moreover, in contrast to type 1 MI that has a clear set of guideline-based recommendations for treatment, management of type 2 MI remains uncertain.

Although the benefits of antiplatelet agents, β-blockers, and statins have been demonstrated among patients with type 1 MI, the utility of these medications among patients with type 2 MI remains uncertain. Currently, patients with type 2 MI are less likely to be discharged while taking these cardioprotective agents.

Reported prevalence of CAD among patients with type 2 MI varies with study design, ranging from 36% to 78%. About 30% of patients with type 2 MI experiencing major adverse cardiovascular events at 5 years, it is plausible that coronary revascularisation could be beneficial in those with obstructive CAD.

Thygesen K, Alpert J, Jaffe A, et al. Fourth universal definition of myocardial infarction (2018). European Heart Journal. 2018;40(3):237–269.
https://academic.oup.com/eurheartj/article/40/3/237/5079081

36. Answer: C

This patient's ECG, while in sinus rhythm 1-year ago shows classic pattern of pre-excitation – Wolff-Parkinson-White (WPW) syndrome. The ECG features a short PR interval; a slurred, thickened initial upstroke of the QRS complex, which is termed a delta wave; and a slight widening of the QRS deflexion with increased ventricular activation time. He presents with symptomatic pre-excited atrial fibrillation (AF) with a rapid ventricular response requiring urgent treatment.

AF is a medical emergency when rapid antegrade conduction over an accessory pathway occurs in WPW syndrome. This is because the normal rate-limiting effects of the atrioventricular (AV) node are bypassed, and the resultant excessive ventricular rates may lead to ventricular fibrillation and sudden death. The incidence of paroxysmal AF is between 10% and 38% in patients with WPW syndrome.

Urgent treatment for patients with WPW syndrome presenting with a tachydysrhythmia who are haemodynamically unstable, regardless of the QRS duration or regularity is direct current cardioversion. The electrical shock depolarises all excitable myocardium, lengthens refractoriness, interrupts re-entrant circuits, discharges foci, and establishes electrical homogeneity that terminates re-entry. Embolic episodes occur in 1–3% of the patients converted from AF to sinus rhythm if the episodes are longer than 48 hours. In those patients, anticoagulation must be addressed prior to cardioversion, with consideration of a transesophageal echocardiogram to exclude left atrial thrombus.

The acute treatment of pre-excited AF WPW syndrome in a haemodynamically stable patient requires a rapid acting drug that can be given intravenously and can lengthen antegrade refractoriness and slow conduction in both the AV node/His-Purkinje system and the accessory pathway. The class IC antiarrhythmic drugs such as flecainide which prolong the refractory period of the accessory connection are effective in this setting. Amiodarone, a class III antiarrhythmic drug, may also be used. AV node blockers (β-blockers, non-dihydropyridine calcium channel blockers and digoxin) are contraindicated for pre-excited AF because inhibition of AV node conduction can increase pre-excitation and lead to an increase in the ventricular rate and ventricular fibrillation. Intravenous adenosine is also contraindicated because it causes an effect similar to verapamil and can precipitate ventricular fibrillation. Catheter ablation is the recommended treatment for the long-term therapy of pre-excited AF.

Svendsen J, Dagres N, Dobreanu D, et al. Current strategy for treatment of patients with Wolff-Parkinson-White syndrome and asymptomatic preexcitation in Europe: European Heart Rhythm Association survey. Europace. 2013;15(5):750–753.
https://academic.oup.com/europace/article/15/5/750/675642

37. Answer: D
Minoxidil is metabolised to an active sulfate metabolite, which antagonises the effect of ATP on K_{ATP} channels. The cell is thus hyperpolarised, which deactivates voltage-dependant calcium channels. The net effect of this action is smooth muscle relaxation. Undesirable side effects of K_{ATP} channel blockade include hirsutism and marked salt and water retention. Therefore, minoxidil is usually co-administered with a loop diuretic.

38. Answer: C
Sacubitril (through its active metabolite sacubitilat) inhibits neprolysin, which in turn increases circulating levels of natriuretic peptides, thus decreasing extracellular volume through induction of renal sodium excretion. In combination with valsartan, sacubitril shows efficacy in treating symptomatic patients with heart failure with reduced ejection fraction. Neprolysin is involved in the degradation of other peptides including bradykinin which elicited adverse effects of renal failure, angioedema, and hyperkalaemia in the randomised controlled trial.

39. Answer: B
Moxonidine antagonises the central control of sympathetically mediated vasoconstriction by stimulating the imidazoline (I_1) receptor present in the brainstem, which in turn decreases central catecholamine synthesis. Moxonidine and clonidine act at α_2 receptors as well, however moxonidine has much higher affinity for the I_1 receptor.

40. Answer: E
Captopril is the archetypal ACE inhibitor that decreases the production of angiotensin II by competitively adhering to the binding site for angiotensin I on ACE. ACE is a membrane bound enzyme predominantly present on vascular endothelium which is most extensively, but not exclusively, expressed in the lung. Angiotensin I undergoes conformational change when interacting with ACE to produce angiotensin II. Angiotensin II has multiple effects which increase blood pressure including proximal tubular absorption of sodium, increased secretion of aldosterone, increased noradrenaline release, and growth of cardiac and vascular cells. ACE is also involved in the degradation of bradykinin, consequently angioedema is a well-known side effect.

41. Answer: G
Some drugs induce relaxation of vascular smooth muscle by increasing cellular concentration of either cyclic adenosine monophosphate (cAMP) or cyclic guanine monophosphate (cGMP). Nitrates are reduced to nitric oxide by a variety of mechanisms. Nitric oxide activates guanylyl cyclase, which in turn increases cGMP production from guanosine triphosphate, which stimulates dephosphorylation of myosin, leading to vasodilation.

42. Answer: A
Beta receptor blockers decrease blood pressure by two main mechanisms. The first is by decreasing cardiac output by blockade of cardiac β_1-receptors, the second is by blocking renal β_1-receptors, resulting in decreased renin secretion.

43. Answer: F
Hydralazine is an arterial and arteriolar vasodilator that directly causes a fall in systemic vascular resistance by interfering with inositol triphosphate's effects on the sarcoplasmic reticulum, which decreases calcium release, resulting in less smooth muscle contraction. The fall in blood pressure is usually accompanied by reflex tachycardia and increased cardiac output. Hydralazine causes drug-induced lupus, which can limit its use in the medium to long term.

Rang H, Ritter J, Flower R, et al. Rang and Dale's pharmacology. 9th ed. Edinburgh: Elsevier; 2019.
https://www.elsevierhealth.com.au/rang-dales-pharmacology-9780702074486.html

44. Answer: E

All of the signs suggest pulmonary hypertension, pointing to Eisenmenger's syndrome, which may be found in older adults who have had a reversal of shunt from right-to-left before open-heart surgery is available. It is the most advanced form of pulmonary arterial hypertension due to elevated pulmonary vascular resistance causing right-to-left intracardiac shunt or great artery shunting, leading to systemic arterial desaturation.

45. Answer: G

Tetralogy of Fallot is associated with a combination of four clinical features:
1. VSD
2. Right ventricular outflow obstruction
3. Overriding aorta
4. Right ventricular hypertrophy

Although the long-term survival has improved for patients with repaired tetralogy of Fallot, residual haemodynamic and electrophysiological sequalae are common in adults. These groups of patients may have symptoms of arrythmias, heart failure, exercise intolerance, and death in early adulthood. Implantable cardioverter–defibrillators (ICDs) as a primary intervention should be considered in patients who meet standard qualifying criteria (i.e. LV ejection fraction ≤35% with NYHA class II or III symptoms).

46. Answer: D

The most common site for coarctation (CoA) is just distal to the origin of the left subclavian artery. An ECG may show signs of systolic overload, including left ventricular hypertrophy.

Sometimes the diagnosis can be easily missed if the lower limb blood pressure is not routinely measured. The long-term complications of CoA are generally related to chronic upper body systemic hypertension. Complications in patients with repaired CoA include recoarctation of the aorta, aneurysm, pseudoaneurysm, and dissection; thus, patients will require ongoing monitoring after operation. CoA is also known to be associated with Turner's syndrome.

47. Answer: A

There are two common types of ASD in adults: ostium secundum (most common) and ostium primum. These patients characteristically exhibit a left-to-right intracardiac shunt which may lead to right heart enlargement and, in a minority of the patients, pulmonary arterial hypertension (PAH). ECG findings may demonstrate right-axis deviation, right bundle branch block pattern, right ventricular hypertrophy from systolic overload and CXR findings may show an enlarged right atrium and ventricle, increased pulmonary vasculature, a dilated main pulmonary artery, and a small aortic knob. Almost all ASDs need to be closed surgically or, if the patient is suitable, with a percutaneous closure device when a pulmonary-to-systemic blood flow (shunt) ratio (Qp/Qs) >1.5:1. It is important to evaluate severe PAH prior to operation since closure of ASDs is contraindicated in this group of patients.

ASD due to ostium primum is caused by an endocardial cushion defect adjacent to the atrioventricular valves. In addition to the aforementioned signs in patients with ostium secundum, there is also associated mitral regurgitation, tricuspid regurgitation or VSD. ECG findings should show left-axis deviation, right bundle branch block and sometimes a prolonged PR interval. The condition is associated with Down's syndrome and Holt-Oram syndrome.

48. Answer: B

VSD in adults are usually small or large with Eisermenger's syndrome. Small restrictive defects may be monitored conservatively without the need for operation. ECG and CXR findings may demonstrate left ventricular hypertrophy. Closure of the VSD is indicated when the left-to-right shunt is moderate to large when the pulmonary-to-systemic flow is >1.5 to 1. Eisermenger's syndrome and severe PAH are contraindications to operative intervention due to significantly increased surgical risks. VSD is associated with Down syndrome.

49. Answer: F

A Marfanoid habitus is suggestive of a diagnosis of Marfan's syndrome. Patients with Marfan's syndrome are at an increased risk of experiencing progressive aortic root dilatation and aortic dissection. Serial echocardiograms are required to monitor the size of the aortic root over time. A slit-lamp examination may be required to diagnose lens dislocation. Patients with lens dislocation may have had lens replacement surgery in the past.

50. Answer: C

The ductus arteriosus usually closes shortly after birth. Failure of the ductus to close in the early weeks of life results in a PDA, which allows blood to flow between the aorta and the pulmonary artery, increasing blood flow in the pulmonary circulation.

Patients with a large PDA can exhibit signs and symptoms of pulmonary hypertension and heart failure. Patients with a small PDA are often asymptomatic but may develop infective endocarditis. PDAs are most commonly closed using catheter-based or surgical intervention. An enlarged left ventricle and calcification of the duct may be evidenced on CXR.

Stout K, Daniels C, Aboulhosn J, et al. 2018 AHA/ACC Guideline for the Management of Adults With Congenital Heart Disease: A Report of the American College of Cardiology/American Heart Association Task Force on Clinical Practice Guidelines. Circulation. 2019;139(14).
https://ahajournals.org/doi/pdf/10.1161/CIR.0000000000000603

2 Critical Care Medicine

Questions

Answers can be found in the Critical Care Medicine Answers section at the end of this chapter.

1. Which of the following treatment options reduces the mortality of acute respiratory distress syndrome (ARDS)?
   A. Aggressive intravenous fluid administration for reversal of shock.
   B. Intravenous albumin administration.
   C. Intravenous hydrocortisone administration.
   D. Lung-protective invasive mechanical ventilation with lower tidal volumes and airway pressures.

2. A 70-year-old man returns to the cardiology ward from the operating theatre after a pacemaker implantation for complete heart block. He complains of shortness of breath and chest pain. On examination, his HR is 120/min, BP is 90/70 mmHg and his respiratory rate is 30/min. His JVP is markedly elevated and his heart sounds are quiet. Air entry is symmetrical on lung auscultation. Oxygen saturation is 90% on room air. An ECG shows sinus tachycardia but is otherwise within normal limits.
   What is the next most appropriate investigation?
   A. CXR.
   B. CT of the chest.
   C. Echocardiogram.
   D. Serial troponin levels.

3. Which of the following clinical findings would be **UNUSUAL** in severe acute carbon monoxide poisoning?
   A. Chest pain.
   B. Headache.
   C. Loss of consciousness.
   D. Low oxygen saturation on pulse oximetry.

4. A 42-year-old man is admitted to the intensive care unit with severe sepsis. Regarding the diagnosis of disseminated intravascular coagulation (DIC), which of the following statements is most correct?
   A. Abnormal prothrombin time is required to diagnose DIC.
   B. A low fibrinogen level (<100 g/mL) is present in about 30% of septic patients with DIC.
   C. DIC affects less than 20% of patients with septic shock.
   D. The most frequent clinical manifestation of DIC in sepsis is haemorrhage.

5. Which type of circulatory shock is the most common in patients in the intensive care unit?
   A. Cardiogenic shock.
   B. Distributive shock.
   C. Hypovolaemic shock.
   D. Obstructive shock.

How to Pass the FRACP Written Examination, First Edition. Jonathan Gleadle, Jordan Li, Danielle Wu, and Paul Kleinig.
© 2022 John Wiley & Sons Ltd. Published 2022 by John Wiley & Sons Ltd.

6. A 48-year-old man presents to the Acute Medical Unit because he experienced chest discomfort three hours ago and generalised weakness in the last two days. He is known to have IgA nephropathy and hypertension, but he does not have regular follow up. His BP is 90/60 mmHg. His rapid troponin level is 1320 ng/L [<29]. His previous ECG was normal 1 year ago when he was admitted for a kidney biopsy.

Which one of the following ECGs would make you call the on-call cardiology registrar immediately and prepare the patient to go to the cardiac catheter laboratory?

(A)

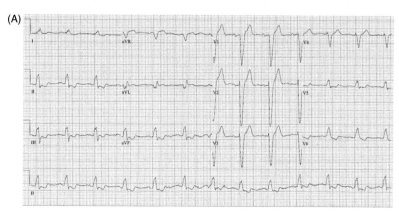

(B)

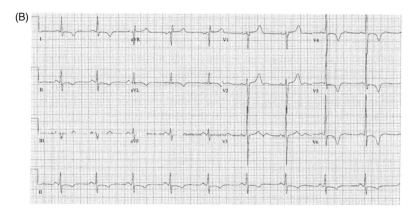

(C)

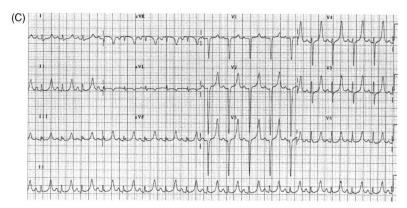

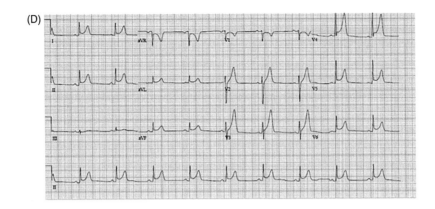

(D)

7. Which one of the following is **NOT** an indication for extracorporeal membrane oxygenation (ECMO) treatment?
- **A.** Acute myocardial infarction with cardiogenic shock.
- **B.** Cardiac failure due to intractable arrhythmias.
- **C.** Postcardiac arrest as part of advanced life support.
- **D.** Refractory septic shock in adults with preserved left ventricular function.

8. You are reviewing a 78-year-old woman who was admitted yesterday with an infective exacerbation of COPD, with a baseline FEV_1 of 40% of the predicted value. She has become progressively drowsier throughout the day, as her GCS is now 12. She is confused and responds to voice on review, is moving all four limbs spontaneously and eyes open to voice. On examination, she is saturating 92% on 4 L of oxygen via nasal cannulae, her respiratory rate is 20/min, and other observations are normal. Her neurological examination shows normal power, tone reflexes and sensation, pupils are normal, but there is slowed thinking and lack of interest in the world, and she is not oriented to place or time. She takes 20 mg of slow release morphine for relief of breathlessness daily and is not on long-term oxygen therapy at home. There is no obvious tremor or myoclonus at rest, but asterixis is present.
   Which of the following is likely the biggest contributor to her drowsiness?
- **A.** Hypercarbia.
- **B.** Hypoxia.
- **C.** Infection.
- **D.** Opiates.

9. A 65-year-old has an anterior myocardial infarction. He has cardiogenic shock despite successful revascularisation. An intra-aortic balloon pump (IABP) is inserted, which will:
- **A.** Decrease diastolic blood pressure.
- **B.** Increase the afterload of left ventricle.
- **C.** Increase coronary blood flow.
- **D.** Increase systolic blood pressure.

10. Which of the following outcomes has the **LEAST** evidence for being improved by advance care planning?
- **A.** Comfort at the end of life.
- **B.** Decreased use of hospital resources.
- **C.** Enhanced surrogate decision making.
- **D.** Patient and family satisfaction.

11. A 62-year-old man is admitted to intensive care unit because of necrotising fasciitis of the left leg after sustaining an injury while changing a flat tyre. He is known to have type 2 diabetes and hypertension.
   Which one of the following complications is **LEAST** likely in this patient?
- **A.** Capillary leak syndrome.
- **B.** Intravascular haemolysis.
- **C.** Posterior reversible encephalopathy syndrome.
- **D.** Systolic heart failure.

12. A 25-year-old woman is brought in by ambulance to the emergency department. Her partner has found a few empty packets of immediate-release paracetamol (~40 gm paracetamol ingestion) at home. Her family thinks she might have taken an overdose of paracetamol within the last 6 hours after she was last seen well. Past medical history includes depression, borderline personality disorder, and previous suicide attempts. On examination, her temperature is 37 °C, BP is 85/50 mmHg, HR is 110 bpm, and respiratory rate is 12/min. Her investigation results are shown below:

Tests	Results	Normal values
Urea	6 mmol/L	2.7–8.0
Creatinine	170 umol/L	45–90
Haemoglobin	129 g/L	115–155
Platelet count	170 x 10⁹/L	150–450
Glucose level	4.0 mmol/L	3.2–5.5
Phosphate level	0.80 mmol/L	0.75–1.50
Alanine aminotransferase (ALT)	150 U/L	0–55
INR	1.3	0.9–1.3
pH on ABG	7.34	7.35–7.45
Arterial lactate	3.5 mmol/L	0.2–2.0

Which one of the following is the appropriate next step of management?
  A. Commence activated charcoal.
  B. Commence 'two-bag' N-acetylcysteine infusion regimen.
  C. Commence 'three-bag' N-acetylcysteine infusion regimen.
  D. Urgent referral to the liver transplant unit.

13. You attend a Medical Emergency Teams (MET) call. The patient is a 64-year-old man who was admitted one hour ago because of an infective exacerbation of COPD and dehydration. His past medical history includes congestive heart failure and hypertension. ECG shows pulseless electrical activity (PEA) with no features of acute myocardial infarction. His troponin is normal on admission. PEA in this patient when compared with ventricular tachycardia (VT) or ventricular fibrillation (VF) cardiac arrest:
  A. Has a good prognosis as it is not likely caused by acute myocardial infarction.
  B. Is more common in patients with congestive heart failure.
  C. Is more common in patients with respiratory failure.
  D. Is not due to hypoxia or tension pneumothorax.

14. A 37-year-old woman has been admitted to intensive care unit (ICU) with pneumococcal pneumonia. She has a history of alcohol induced liver cirrhosis and has required intubation and ventilation.
  Which of the following is correct regarding prophylaxis with proton-pump inhibitors (PPIs) or histamine H_2–receptor antagonists against gastrointestinal bleeding?
  A. Clinically important gastrointestinal bleeding occurs in 30% of ICU patients.
  B. Patients with mechanical ventilation but no enteral feeding are at higher risk of bleeding.
  C. PPIs are clearly superior to ranitidine in reducing bleeding and ICU mortality.
  D. Prophylaxis reduces ICU mortality.

15. In patients with AKI due to septic shock who are admitted to the intensive care unit, which of the following statements regarding dialysis treatment is correct?
  A. AKI is not associated with worsening mortality.
  B. Delayed dialysis compared to early dialysis has a lower mortality rate.
  C. Early dialysis compared to delayed dialysis has a lower mortality rate.
  D. There is no difference in mortality rate in early vs. delayed dialysis.

16. A 70-year-old woman presents to the emergency department following a 3-day history of chills and dysuria. She reports dizziness and light-headedness. She has a temperature of 38.6°C, heart rate of 125 bpm and her BP is 85/55 mmHg. Physical examination reveals dry mucous membranes, undetectable JVP. She is tachycardic with no adventitious sounds and her chest is clear. There is suprapubic tenderness. Her investigations reveal the following:

Tests	Results	Normal values
Serum creatinine	159 µmol/L	45–90
Urea	27 mmol/L	2.7–8.0
Lactate	5.0 mmol/L	0.2–2.0
Anion gap	25 mmol	7–17
WCC	20 x 10^9/L	4–11
Haemoglobin	90 g/L	115–155
Urine microscopy	>100 WBC/HPF, abundant bacteria	

Which of the following is most appropriate regarding management of this patient?
  A. Placement of central venous catheter and administration of intravenous fluid guided by central venous pressure.
  B. Intravenous fluid administration of 60ml/kg body weight.
  C. Intravenous fluid administration of 30ml/kg body weight.
  D. Intravenous fluid administration to achieve mean arterial pressure 85 mmHg.

17. A 43-year-old woman is admitted to a high dependency unit because of exacerbation of asthma. This is her third admission within 12 months. She is diagnosed with severe asthma. Which one of the following considerations in this case is **INCORRECT**?
  A. Approximately 50% of patients with severe asthma have type 2 inflammation.
  B. Exhaled nitric oxide should be monitored in patients with severe asthma and used to guide therapy.
  C. Mepolizumab is indicated for use as an add-on treatment for patients with an eosinophilic phenotype of severe asthma.
  D. Recurrent exacerbations of severe asthma are often associated with gastroesophageal reflux.

18. A 72-year-old man is day 7 in ICU because of severe biliary sepsis. He has been on piperacillin/tazobactam for 7 days and develops severe diarrhoea. He is diagnosed with severe *Clostridium difficile* colitis. His repeat abdominal CT shows large intestine distension, colonic wall thickening, and fat stranding.
  What is your first line treatment of choice in this case?
  A. Faecal microbiota transplantation.
  B. Intravenous metronidazole.
  C. Oral fidaxomicin.
  D. Oral vancomycin.

19. Which one of the following measures is **NOT** in the Hour-1 Bundle of care elements in the initial resuscitation for sepsis and septic shock?
  A. Administer broad-spectrum antibiotics.
  B. Apply vasopressors if hypotensive during or after fluid resuscitation to maintain mean arterial pressure (MAP) ≥80 mmHg.
  C. Begin rapid administration of 30 mL/kg crystalloid for hypotension or lactate level ≥ 4 mmol/L.
  D. Measure lactate level.

20. A 76-year-old man has had an inferior myocardial infarction 4 days ago. Today he is feeling lightheaded. On examination his blood pressure is 85/65 mmHg. An ECG is done immediately. Which one of the following findings is an indication for temporary pacing?

(A)

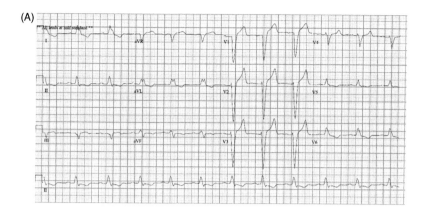

(B)

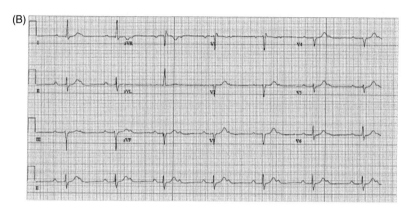

(C)

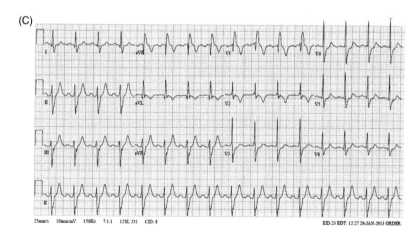

25mm/s   10mm/mV   150Hz   7.1.1   12SL 231   CID: 8   EID:23 EDT: 12:27 29-JAN-2013 ORDER.

(D)

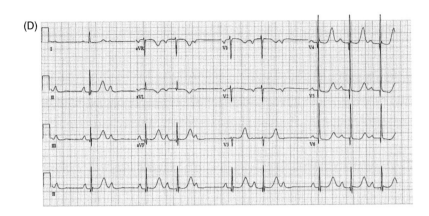

21. A 25-year-old man is brought into the emergency department by ambulance after a motor bike injury 40 min ago. On examination, his GCS is 9, he is unable to move his right hand due to pain. Both pupils are reactive to light. He does not take regular medications. X-ray shows a right-sided distal radius fracture. CT brain shows intra-cranial haemorrhage in the right hemisphere with no mass effect and no major extracranial bleeding.

Which one of the following medications has been shown to reduce head injury related death compared to placebo when given within 3 hours of injury?
- **A.** Desmopressin.
- **B.** Fresh frozen plasma.
- **C.** Prothrombinex.
- **D.** Tranexamic acid.

22. Which of the following measurements in the VBG **DOES NOT** correlate with the readings in ABG in critically ill patients?
- **A.** Bicarbonate.
- **B.** Lactate.
- **C.** pH.
- **D.** The partial pressure of Oxygen (PaO2).

23. A 72-year-old man is admitted with pneumonia and treated with intravenous penicillin and azithromycin. He is known to have CCF, smoking related COPD and AF for which he is taking sotalol. He has a cardiac arrest in the medical ward. After 3 cycles of CPR, 3 boluses of 1mg epinephrine and 3 defibrillator shocks, he remains unconscious with the below ECG trace.

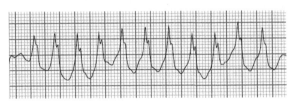

What is the next most appropriate step?
- **A.** 5 mg epinephrine intravenously.
- **B.** 10 mls of 10% calcium gluconate intravenously.
- **C.** 10 mls of magnesium sulphate intravenously.
- **D.** 300 mg amiodarone intravenously.

24. An 80-year-old woman presents to emergency department following a 2-day history of fever and dysuria. She reports dizziness and light-headedness. She has a temperature of 39.6°C, HR of 120 bpm and her BP is 80/55 mmHg. Physical examination reveals dry mucous membranes and undetectable JVP. Her chest is clear on auscultation. There is renal angle tenderness. Her investigations reveal the following:

Tests	Results	Normal values
Serum creatinine	178 μmol/L	45–90
Urea	28 mmol/L	2.7–8.0
Lactate	3.0 mmol/L	0.2–2.0
Anion gap	25 mmol	7–17
WCC	26 x 10⁹/L	4–11
Haemoglobin	90 g/L	115–155
Urinalysis	3+ leukocyte esterase, nitrate positive	

After taking blood cultures and commencing fluid resuscitation and intravenous antibiotics, her BP improves to 100/60 mmHg and HR is 98/min.

Which of the following strategies is most appropriate in further managing her haemodynamic state?
- **A.** Placement of central venous catheter with serial central venous pressure and central venous oxygen saturation ($Scvo_2$) measurement.
- **B.** Whole blood transfusion and serial haemoglobin measurement.
- **C.** Administration of inotropic medication.
- **D.** Continued monitoring of blood pressure and urine output.

25. Which one of the following measures is **NOT** recommended in the treatment of severe sepsis or septic shock, according to the latest guidelines from the Surviving Sepsis Campaign?
- **A.** Use antimicrobial treatment for 7 to 10 days for most serious infections associated with sepsis and septic shock.
- **B.** Use combination antimicrobial therapy for the routine treatment of neutropenic sepsis.
- **C.** Use empiric broad-spectrum antimicrobials for patients presenting with sepsis or septic shock to cover all likely pathogens.
- **D.** Use intravenous antimicrobials within one hour after recognition of sepsis or septic shock.

QUESTIONS (26–31) REFER TO THE FOLLOWING INFORMATION

Match each of the following inotropic/vasopressor agents with the best description of their mechanism of action:
- **A.** Dobutamine.
- **B.** Levosimendan.
- **C.** Metaraminol.
- **D.** Milrinone.
- **E.** Noradrenaline.
- **F.** Omecamtiv.
- **G.** Phenylephrine.
- **H.** Vasopressin.

26. A mixed alpha and beta agonist with greater alpha-1 activity than beta activity.

27. Enhancement of troponin C sensitivity to intracellular calcium.

28. Inhibition of the enzyme responsible for breakdown of cyclic adenylate monophosphate (cAMP).

29. Direct stimulation of actin-myosin cross-bridging.

30. A mixed alpha and beta agonist with greater beta activity than alpha activity.

31. Pure alpha-1 receptor agonist.

QUESTIONS (32–35) REFER TO THE FOLLOWING INFORMATION

You are the co-leader for Medical Emergency Response Team. When you attend the following medical emergency, what is the most appropriate immediate management?

    A. intravenous amiodarone.
    B. intravenous appropriate antibiotics.
    C. intravenous calcium chloride.
    D. intravenous calcium gluconate.
    E. intravenous epinephrine.
    F. intravenous fluid.
    G. intravenous dextrose.
    H. intravenous hydrocortisone.
    I. intravenous insulin.
    J. intravenous magnesium.
    K. intravenous naloxone.

32. A 26-year-old woman known to have asthma and type 1 diabetes presents to emergency department with severe dyspnoea and wheeze. She is unable to speak in a full sentence. Her HR is 120 bpm, respiratory rate of 26/min and BP is 90/60 mmHg. Oxygen saturation while breathing 4 L of oxygen is 91%. She is using her accessory muscles; has quiet breath sounds and few wheezes. Her BGL is 26 mmol/L [3.2–5.5]. She has been given three consecutive salbutamol nebulisers.

33. A 59-year-old man who has end stage kidney disease due to diabetic nephropathy presents to haemodialysis centre for dialysis. He has missed his previous dialysis because he is worried about contracting COVID-19 at the dialysis centre. He collapses just before commencing dialysis. CPR is started, ECG shows ventricular tachycardia, and VBG shows a potassium level of 7.9 mmol/L [3.5–5.2].

34. A 53-year-old man known to have cirrhosis due to alcoholic hepatitis is admitted to the Acute Medical Unit after binge drinking. He has been given intravenous thiamine and 5% dextrose infusion. He is found to have an irregular and difficult to palpate pulse with a BP of 110/70 mmHg. His cardiac monitor shows intermittent runs of the following rhythm.

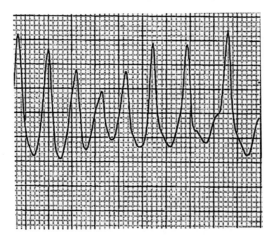

35. An 85-year-old man is transferred from a peripheral hospital due to a fracture of neck of right femur. He has been given analgesia, settled in the ward and is fasting and waiting for surgery. He is a fit farmer apart from stage 3B CKD. However, the nurse finds him unconscious 4 hours later. He is afebrile, BP 120/80 mmHg, HR 76 bpm, respiratory rate 8/min, SaO2 90% on 6 L of oxygen. He has bilateral pin-point pupils.

Answers

1. Answer: D

Acute Respiratory Distress Syndrome (ARDS) is a heterogenous syndrome with symptoms of tachypnea, refractory hypoxemia, and diffuse opacities on CXR or CT chest. More than 85% of patients with ARDS have risk factors such as pneumonia, aspiration of gastric contents, and sepsis. Other risk factors for ARDS include pulmonary contusion, inhalation injury, near drowning, non-thoracic trauma, haemorrhagic shock, pancreatitis, major burns, drug overdose, transfusion of blood products, cardiopulmonary bypass, and reperfusion oedema after lung transplantation or embolectomy.

Direct or indirect insult to the alveolar structure causes alveolar macrophage activation. This leads to the release of pro-inflammatory mediators and chemokines that attract neutrophils and monocytes. Toxic mediators are released by activated neutrophils causing alveolar injury, leading to loss of barrier function, interstitial, and intra-alveolar flooding. Expression of tissue factor mediated by tumor necrosis factor then promotes platelet aggregation, intra-alveolar coagulation, and hyaline-membrane formation.

In patients with severe ARDS, mortality is up to 46%. Long-term sequelae for the survivors of ARDS include depression, skeletal-muscle weakness, post-traumatic stress disorder, and cognitive decline. Identification and treatment of the underlying cause(s) of ARDS is the first priority in the care of the patients with this condition.

The volumes of the aerated lungs are reduced in patients with ARDS. Using lung-protective invasive mechanical ventilation with lower tidal volumes and airway pressure has been reported to reduce ventilator-associated lung injury and mortality. Avoidance of fluid administration following reversal of shock has been shown to reduce mortality in a large randomised trial. IV albumin administration was not associated with reduced mortality in a large randomised trial in patients with ARDS. Currently, no pharmacologic therapy has been shown to reduce short-term or long-term mortality in patients with ARDS. A recent trial shows that infusion of muscle relaxant for 48 hours may improve oxygenation but does not improve mortality. Placing the patient in the prone position for moderate to severe ARDS may reduce mortality. Introducing inhaled nitric oxide therapy improves oxygenation but does not improve mortality.

Distinguishing between initial fluid resuscitation for shock and maintenance fluid therapy is important. Early aggressive resuscitation for associated circulatory shock and its associated remote organ injury are essential. However, several small trials have demonstrated improved outcome for ARDS in patients treated with diuretics or dialysis to promote a negative fluid balance in the first few days. Primary ARDS due to aspiration, pneumonia, or inhalational injury can be treated with fluid restriction. Secondary ARDS due to sepsis or inflammation requires initial fluid and potential vasoactive drug therapy to stabilize the patient.

An ARDS Clinical Trials Network study of a fluid-conservative strategy versus a fluid liberal strategy in the management of patients with ARDS found no statistically significant difference in 60-day mortality between the two groups 72 hours after presentation with ARDS. However, patients treated with the fluid-conservative strategy had an improved oxygenation index and lung injury score and an increase in ventilator-free days, without an increase in non-pulmonary organ failures.

 Thompson B, Chambers R, Liu K. Acute Respiratory Distress Syndrome. New England Journal of Medicine. 2017;377(6):562–572.
https://www.ncbi.nlm.nih.gov/pubmed/28792873

2. Answer: C

This patient's clinical presentation and signs are consistent with cardiac tamponade which is a rare complication after pacemaker insertion. The diagnosis of cardiac tamponade is clinical and requires prompt recognition. Echocardiogram is the best imaging modality to use at the bedside, as it can confirm the presence of a pericardial effusion, determine its size, and whether it is causing compromise of cardiac function such as right ventricular diastolic collapse, right atrial systolic collapse, plethoric inferior vena cava (IVC). The commonest ECG finding of cardiac tamponade is sinus tachycardia. ECG may show low voltages or electrical alternans, which is the classic ECG finding in cardiac tamponade. A CXR may show an enlarged heart and may strongly suggest pericardial effusion if a prior CXR is available for comparison. CT chest can also detect pericardial effusion.

Differential diagnosis includes large pleural effusion, pneumothorax, pulmonary embolism, constrictive pericarditis, CCF, and shock.

Cardiac tamponade is a medical emergency. The urgent treatment of cardiac tamponade is the removal of pericardial fluid/blood to relieve the pressure surrounding the heart. This can be done by performing a needle pericardiocentesis at the bedside, performed either using traditional landmark technique in a sub-xiphoid window or using a point-of-care echocardiogram to guide needle placement in real-time. Surgical options include creating a pericardial window or removing the pericardium.

Complications of pacemaker insertion may occur during the immediate or early post-insertion period and can be related to (ii) venous access (pneumothorax, haemothorax, air embolism, haematoma, arterial puncture, wound healing problems, infection, pain), (ii) the pacemaker lead (cardiac perforation, tamponade, malposition or dislodgement of the lead), (iii) or the generator device. Late complications are related to infections, thrombosis, endocarditis, pulmonary embolism, superior vena cava (SVC) syndrome (due to thrombus formation and/or fibrosis of the pacing wires within the SVC), and pericarditis.

 Mahadevan V, Agrawal H. Cardiac tamponade – Symptoms, diagnosis, and treatment | BMJ Best Practice [Internet]. Newbp.bmj.com. 2019 [cited 22 August 2019]. Available from: https://bestpractice.bmj.com/topics/en-gb/459

3. Answer: D

Carbon monoxide (CO) poisoning causes a large number of deaths due to intentional self-injury and non-intentional injury related to fires. Chronic CO poisoning is more commonly encountered as a result of faulty heating. CO binds to heme products with much greater affinity than oxygen and reduces oxygen delivery to tissues. However, this mechanism only accounts for some of the toxicity of CO, and as a result, carboxyhaemoglobin levels do not necessarily correlate with severity of toxicity. CO poisoning also produces toxicity by binding many intracellular heme products resulting in impaired cellular function. For example, CO inhibits mitochondrial respiration by binding ferrous heme, which is the active site on cytochrome c oxidase complex IV. CO inhibits platelet function, causes inflammation, central demyelination and global brain ischaemic injury, through acidosis and oxidative stress. CO poisoning can be diagnosed by consistent symptoms, history of recent CO exposure, and elevated carboxyhaemoglobin levels. Conventional pulse oximetry cannot distinguish between carboxyhaemoglobin and oxyhaemoglobin, so pulse oximetry usually returns normal values. Treatment focuses on accelerating the dissociation of CO through oxygen therapy. Whilst hyperbaric oxygen has been shown to accelerate this process faster than normobaric oxygen, it has not shown improved clinical outcomes. Long term sequelae of CO poisoning are common, with cardiovascular toxicity and neurological deficits occurring most frequently.

 Rose J, Wang L, Xu Q, McTiernan C, Shiva S, Tejero J et al. Carbon Monoxide Poisoning: Pathogenesis, Management, and Future Directions of Therapy. American Journal of Respiratory and Critical Care Medicine. 2017;195(5):596–606. https://www.atsjournals.org/doi/full/10.1164/rccm.201606-1275CI

4. Answer: B

Disseminated intravascular coagulation (DIC) is an overactivation of the coagulation cascade resulting in consumption of coagulation factors, and disordered haemostasis, manifesting as either coagulation or bleeding. DIC affects about 35% of patients who have sepsis. Depending on the cause, DIC manifests in different ways. This is thought to be due to differential effects of the causative pathology on fibrinolysis and procoagulant factors. For example, DIC caused by trauma or acute promyelocytic leukaemia tends to result in bleeding, whereas sepsis most frequently causes multi-organ dysfunction through microembolic damage. Obviously, the treatment of these differentially manifesting pathologies will differ. The typical laboratory parameters in DIC are decreased platelet count, increased prothrombin time, increased (often dramatically) D-dimer, and decreased fibrinogen. However, the individual components of laboratory diagnosis are not all required and DIC can go undiagnosed if this possibility is not recognised. For example, low fibrinogen is only present in around 30% of DIC associated with sepsis. One of the most thoroughly validated scoring systems for the diagnosis of DIC is that of the International Society of Thrombosis and Haemostasis (ISTH), which gives weight to the above-mentioned laboratory parameters and a score of 5 or more denotes DIC. There is still some controversy surrounding the supportive management of DIC (other than addressing the underlying cause), but treatment strategies in sepsis induced DIC include replacing factors, activated protein-C and systemic anticoagulation.

 Iba T, Levy JH, Warkentin TE et.al. Diagnosis and management of sepsis-induced coagulopathy and disseminated intravascular coagulation. J Thromb Haemost. 2019; 17(11): 1989–1994. https://onlinelibrary.wiley.com/doi/10.1111/jth.14578

5. Answer: B

Septic shock is a type of distributive shock and is the most common cause of circulatory shock among patients in the ICU (62% of the patients). It is followed by cardiogenic (16%), hypovolemic (16%), and obstructive shock (2%). Causes of shock may be obvious from history, clinical examination, and/or investigations. Patients who present with a history of trauma/gastrointestinal bleeding may have hypovolaemic shock; patients with massive pneumothorax/pulmonary emboli/cardiac tamponade are likely to have obstructive shock; patients with fever, symptoms/signs of infection, an elevated WBC count, a high CRP, and an elevated procalcitonin level may have septic shock; patients present after a recent acute coronary syndrome are likely to have cardiogenic shock, etc. Some patients may have mixed types of circulatory shock.

Initial presentations may be similar in patients with different types of shock. Depending on the organ involvement after circulatory shock, the patient may have mental status changes, hypotension, tachycardia, tachypnoea, reduced urine output, coagulation abnormalities, etc. Blood lactate levels are elevated in patients with impaired tissue perfusion.

Further investigations by performing a septic screen, assessing cardiac output by echocardiogram, monitoring mixed venous oxygen saturation (SvO2), monitoring of central venous pressure, or performing a CTPA can help to differentiate the underlying cause(s) of circulatory shocks. If an echocardiogram shows large ventricles and poor contractility, cardiogenic shock is likely. An echocardiogram may help to rule out pericardial effusion, cardiac tamponade, etc. some of the common causes of obstructive shock.

After failing initial intravenous fluid resuscitation, it may be appropriate to provide vasopressor support, intensive blood pressure monitoring via an arterial line, and central venous catheters in the ICU if patients wish to have more intensive monitoring and treatment. Broad spectrum antibiotics administration according to the possible sites of infections should be considered as soon as possible without delay after a septic screen is performed if there is suspicion of septic shock, to minimise morbidity and mortality associated with sepsis.

 Vincent J, De Backer D. Circulatory Shock. New England Journal of Medicine. 2013;369(18):1726–1734.
https://www.nejm.org/doi/10.1056/NEJMra1208943

6. Answer: A

The ECGs show
   A. Left bundle branch block (LBBB)
   B. ST change associated with severe left ventricular hypertrophy (LVH)
   C. ST changes associated 'Tented' T wave in patient with hyperkalaemia
   D. Widespread concave ('saddleback') ST segment elevation in a patient with pericarditis

The key point is that not all ST elevation is due to ST elevation acute myocardial infarction (STEMI). ECG A is typical for LBBB which is new. New LBBB alone is not necessarily an indication for immediate cardiac catheterisation. However, the following criteria are the indications for immediate cardiac catheterisation:
• Unstable patient with hypotension, acute pulmonary oedema or electrical instability
• Sgarbossa Criteria (electrocardiographic findings used to identify myocardial infarction (MI) in the presence of a LBBB)
   o Concordant ST-segment elevation of 1 mm in at least 1 lead
   o Concordant ST-segment depression of at least 1 mm in leads V1 to V3
• Smith-Modified Sgarbossa criteria – any single lead with at least 1 mm of discordant ST elevation that is ≥25% of the preceding S-wave.

In patients with old LBBB, ST–T abnormalities are common, making it difficult to assess the presence of AMI. ST segment and T–waves are usually discordant with the QRS in LBBB, since they are directed in opposite directions. A concordant ST segment shift should always be presumed to be a myocardial lesion and considered as strongly indicative of AMI. On the other hand, a discordant ST segment displacement may be indicative of a myocardial lesion when specific standard criteria are exceeded. For example, discordant elevation of the J point ≥0.5 mV in V1–V2 is strongly suggestive of AMI in the presence of LBBB. Moreover, in LBBB, the QRS/T ratio appears to be more predictive than the amplitude of ST elevation. When this ratio is near to or less than 1, the probability that the repolarisation abnormality is related to an MI is high.

ECG B is typical of LVH with associated concave ST elevation not STEMI. In LVH, the repolarisation pattern is usually discordant to the QRS as in LBBB, The elevation is more commonly observed in leads V2–V3 and is usually <0.3 mV with minor abnormalities in V4–V6. ECG shows high voltage of R waves in antero-lateral leads associated to Q waves in anterior and inferior leads. The T waves, usually being very deep and inverted in V2–V4, may resemble a non-Q AMI.

ECG C has ST changes associated 'Tented' T wave in a patient with hyperkalaemia. Significant variations of potassium levels have dramatic effects on electrical activities and cause arrhythmias. Hyperkalaemia induces an ST elevation in right precordial leads that can resemble an AMI. Other ECG changes in hyperkalaemia include reduction in the amplitude of P waves, prolongation of the PQ interval, enlargement of QRS complex and concave ST segment elevation.

ECG D shows widespread concave ('saddleback') ST segment elevation in a patient with pericarditis. Although pericardium is electrically inactive, its infection and/or inflammation as seen in this case of uraemic pericarditis may affect the external part of epicardium and cause concave ST elevation in almost all leads, as pericarditis generally affects the whole pericardium.

 Smith S, Dodd K, Henry T, Dvorak D, Pearce L. Diagnosis of ST-Elevation Myocardial Infarction in the Presence of Left Bundle Branch Block With the ST-Elevation to S-Wave Ratio in a Modified Sgarbossa Rule. Annals of Emergency Medicine. 2012;60(6):766–776.
https://www.annemergmed.com/article/S0196-0644(12)01368-6/fulltext

7. Answer: D

Extracorporeal membrane oxygenation (ECMO) is an advanced form of temporary life support which helps to maintain respiratory and/or cardiac function. It diverts venous blood through an extracorporeal circuit and returns it to the body after gas exchange through a semi-permeable membrane. ECMO can be used for oxygenation, carbon dioxide removal and haemodynamic support. Additional components allow thermoregulation and haemofiltration. The two most common forms of ECMO are: (i) veno-arterial ECMO (VA-ECMO) to support patients with a reversible cause of cardiogenic shock that is refractory to maximal therapy. VA-ECMO can also be a salvage treatment option in the setting of cardiac arrest with unsuccessful advanced life support. (ii) veno-venous ECMO (VV-ECMO) is indicated for patients with a reversible cause of acute respiratory failure with refractory hypoxaemia or hypercapnia despite optimal ventilation. VV-ECMO allows reduction in the ventilatory insult caused by mechanical ventilation.

The indications and contraindications for ECMO in critically ill patients are listed in Tables 2.1 and 2.2.

Table 2.1 Indications for ECMO.

Indications for VA-ECMO	Indications for VV-ECMO
Acute myocardial infarction	Reversible causes of acute respiratory failure
Fulminant myocarditis	ARDS
Acute exacerbations of chronic CCF	Trauma—extensive pulmonary contusion
Cardiac failure due to intractable arrhythmias	Massive pulmonary embolism with refractory shock and/or cardiac arrest
Primary graft failure following cardiac transplantation	Graft dysfunction following lung transplantation
Acute heart failure secondary to drug toxicity	Inability to provide adequate gas exchange without risk of ventilatory injury
Postcardiac arrest (as part of advanced life support)	Pulmonary haemorrhage

Table 2.2 Contraindications to ECMO.

Chronic respiratory or cardiac disease with no hope of recovery or transplant
Out-of-hospital cardiac arrest with prolonged down time
Severe aortic regurgitation or type A aortic dissection or severe peripheral vascular disease if using VA-ECMO
Refractory septic shock in adults with preserved left ventricular function
ARDS with advanced multiorgan failure
ARDS in patient with advanced age
Prolonged pre-ECMO mechanical ventilation
Therapeutic anticoagulation is a relative contraindication

Ali J, Vuylsteke A. Extracorporeal membrane oxygenation: indications, technique and contemporary outcomes. Heart 2019; 105:1437–43.
https://heart.bmj.com/content/105/18/1437.abstract

8. Answer: A

The most common cause of drowsiness in the admitted patient is a metabolic encephalopathy. Thorough neurological examination is needed, however, to rule out focal central nervous system pathology. Common causes of encephalopathy are infection, medications, decompensated hepatic failure, and hypercania. Less common causes include endocrine causes and electrolyte disturbance. In this case, type 2 respiratory failure is the most likely cause given the findings on history and examination.

Alpert J. Evaluation of the Poorly Responsive Patient. The Neurologic Diagnosis [Internet]. 2018 [cited 30 June 2020]; 163–206. Available from: https://link.springer.com/chapter/10.1007/978-3-319-95951-1_5

9. Answer: C

Intra-aortic balloon pump (IABP) is a percutaneous temporary mechanical circulatory support that creates more favourable balance of myocardial oxygen supply and demand by using systolic unloading and diastolic augmentation.

The IABP, by inflating during diastole, displaces blood volume from the thoracic aorta. In systole, as the balloon rapidly deflates, this creates a vacuum effect, reducing afterload for myocardial ejection and improving forward flow from the left ventricle. The net effect is to decrease systolic aortic pressure by as much as 20% and increase diastolic pressure, but the MAP is usually unchanged. This subsequently results in decreased left ventricle wall stress reducing the myocardial oxygen demand. Overall, these haemodynamic changes indirectly improve the cardiac output by increasing stroke volume, particularly in patients with reduced left ventricular function. The augmentation of diastolic pressure by IABP leads to an increase in myocardial perfusion especially epicardial coronary circulation.

Indication for placement can include:

- Myocardial infarction with decreased left ventricular function leading to cardiogenic shock
- Myocardial infarction with mechanical complications causing cardiogenic shock, i.e., acute mitral regurgitation due to papillary muscle rupture or ventricular septal rupture
- Acute congestive heart failure exacerbation with hypotension
- As prophylaxis or adjunct treatment in high risk percutaneous coronary intervention
- Low cardiac output state after coronary artery bypass grafting surgery
- As a bridge to definitive treatment in patients with any of the following conditions: intractable myocardial ischaemia, refractory heart failure, or intractable ventricular arrhythmias

However, studies have not shown any survival benefits with the use of IABP and there is no convincing randomised data to support the routine use of IABP in infarct-related cardiogenic shock.

 Unverzagt S, Buerke M, de Waha A, Haerting J, Pietzner D, Seyfarth M et al. Intra-aortic balloon pump counterpulsation (IABP) for myocardial infarction complicated by cardiogenic shock. Cochrane Database of Systematic Reviews. 2015. https://www.cochranelibrary.com/cdsr/doi/10.1002/14651858.CD007398.pub3/abstract

10. Answer: A

Advance care planning in a health care context can be described as the process by which an individual sets out their wishes for medical care in the event that they are unable to make decisions themselves. In addition, advance care planning can set out who they would like to assist in medical decision making such as family or close friends. Advance care planning has been shown in multiple studies as being valuable to patients and their families. Additionally, randomised controlled trials have shown significant improvement in several outcomes; decreased utilisation of healthcare and cost, increased satisfaction with care, decreased use of hospital resources, improved concordance with wishes. However, these trials have not been of sufficient rigour and size to evaluate whether advance care planning improves quality of end-of-life care such as by measures of individual comfort.

 Weathers E, O'Caoimh R, Cornally N, Fitzgerald C, Kearns T, Coffey A et al. Advance care planning: A systematic review of randomised controlled trials conducted with older adults. Maturitas. 2016;91: 101–109. https://pubmed.ncbi.nlm.nih.gov/27451328/

11. Answer: C

Necrotising fasciitis is a rapidly progressive infection of the fascia, with secondary widespread necrosis of the subcutaneous tissues. The frequency of necrotising fasciitis has been increasing because of an increase in immunocompromised patients with diabetes, peripheral vascular disease, alcoholism, organ transplants, and neutropenia. The causative bacteria may be aerobic, anaerobic, or mixed flora. The three most important types are as follows:

- Type I, or polymicrobial
- Type II, or group A streptococcal
- Type III gas gangrene, or clostridial myonecrosis

The reported mortality in patients with necrotising fasciitis has ranged from 20% to as high as 80%. Early diagnosis is key and requires a high index of suspicion as the initial lesion is often trivial. In many cases of necrotising fasciitis, antecedent trauma or surgery can be identified. Necrotising fasciitis requires urgent surgical intervention, and the urgent initiation of broad spectrum antibiotics. Admission to the intensive care unit is likely required, as these patients are usually profoundly shocked.

While caring for critically ill patients with necrotising fasciitis the following complications should be close monitored:

- Capillary leak syndrome: Circulating bacterial toxins and host cytokines cause diffuse endothelial damage. Intravenous fluid requirements may be extremely high (10 to 12 litres of normal saline per day). Profound hypoalbuminaemia is also common, and replacement with albumin is needed to maintain oncotic pressure.

- Intravascular haemolysis: Bacterial haemolysins cause striking and rapid reductions in the haematocrit in the absence of DIC. Thus, the haematocrit may be a better indicator of the need for transfusion than the haemoglobin level.
- Stress cardiomyopathy: necrotising fasciitis especially caused by streptococcal infection can cause global hypokinesia, severe systolic heart failure, low cardiac output. This cardiomyopathy is reversible, fully resolving in 3 to 24 months after infection.

Posterior reversible encephalopathy syndrome (PRES) is a clinico-radiological syndrome characterised by headache, visual disturbances, seizures and altered consciousness. It is most commonly associated with accelerated and malignant hypertension. It can also be associated with eclampsia/preeclampsia, HUS, TTP, drug toxicity and very rarely sepsis. CT or/and MRI of the brain commonly show vasogenic oedema within the occipital and parietal regions, The oedema is usually symmetrical. PRES can be found in a non-posterior distribution, mainly in watershed areas, including within the frontal, inferior temporal, cerebellar, and brainstem regions. Both cortical and subcortical locations are affected.

 Stevens D, Bryant A. Necrotizing Soft-Tissue Infections. New England Journal of Medicine. 2017;377(23):2253–2265. https://www.nejm.org/doi/10.1056/NEJMra1600673

12. Answer: B

The updated paracetamol overdose management guidelines in 2019 recommend a two-bag N-acetylcysteine (NAC) infusion regimen (200 mg/kg over 4 hours, then 100 mg/kg over 16 hours) instead of the previous three-bag regimen since they have similar efficacy and the two-bag regimen has less adverse reactions. All patients with risks of hepatotoxicity secondary to paracetamol overdoses should receive NAC treatment. In patients with massive paracetamol overdoses which result in blood paracetamol level more than double the nomogram line should receive increased doses of NAC. In patients whose time of ingestion is unclear, it may be worthwhile to commence NAC infusion regardless given the unlikelihood of harm associated with the treatment.

The nomogram is only validated for a single ingestion of immediate release paracetamol. If extended-release paracetamol is ingested, and or the overdose has occurred over a longer period of time, it is no longer validated. In these cases, NAC infusion should be commenced regardless, given the lack of harm. If there was co-ingestion of opioids or anticholinergics, as they can affect gastric emptying and absorption of paracetamol, NAC should be given.

For patients who present within 2 hours of immediate release paracetamol overdoses or present within 4 hours of immediate release paracetamol ingestions greater than 30 gm, activated charcoal should be given in alert and co-operative patients.

Only a small percentage of patients develop hepatotoxicity following acute paracetamol overdoses with symptoms that can include nausea, vomiting, abdominal pain, and right-upper quadrant tenderness. Of these patients, a small number of patients develop fulminant hepatic failure. Most patients recover after standard treatment.

Liver transplant unit should be consulted if patients meet any of the following criteria:

- INR >3.0 at 48 hours or >4.5 at any time.
- Oliguria or serum creatinine is >200 μmol/L.
- Persistent acidosis (pH <7.3) or arterial lactate >3 mmol/L.
- Systolic blood pressure <80 mmHg, despite fluid resuscitation.
- Hypoglycaemia, severe thrombocytopenia, or encephalopathy.
- Any alteration of consciousness (GCS <15) not associated with concomitant sedative overdoses.

 Chiew A, Reith D, Pomerleau A, Wong A, Isoardi K, Soderstrom J et al. Updated guidelines for the management of paracetamol poisoning in Australia and New Zealand. Medical Journal of Australia. 2019;212(4):175–183. https://onlinelibrary.wiley.com/doi/abs/10.5694/mja2.50428

13. Answer: C

Pulseless electrical activity (PEA), previously known as electromechanical dissociation (EMD) is defined as the absence of a palpable pulse in an unconscious patient with organized electrical activity other than VT on ECG. The proportion of PEA among cases of sudden cardiac arrest increases with age. Females are more likely to develop PEA than males. Patients with PEA are more likely to have one or more co-morbidities than those in the VF/VT group. However, PEA is less likely to occur in those with CCF. In one study, PEA was responsible for 68% of monitored in-hospital deaths and 10% of all in-hospital deaths.

PEA more commonly has an underlying cause of the arrest including the Hs and Ts listed below and the most frequent causes are hypoxemia secondary to respiratory failure and hypovolemia due to internal bleeding or a recent haemodialysis. This patient's PEA is possibly due to hypoxia caused by his infective exacerbation of COPD. Tension pneumothorax also needs to be excluded.

Hs
- Hypoxia
- Hypovolemia
- Hydrogen ion (acidosis)
- Hypokalaemia/ hyperkalaemia, hypoglycaemia
- Hypothermia

Ts
- Toxins
- Tamponade (cardiac)
- Tension pneumothorax
- Thrombosis (massive PE or AMI)
- Trauma

The overall prognosis for patients with PEA arrest is dismal unless a rapidly reversible cause is identified and corrected. Only 11% of patients who have PEA as their first documented rhythm survives to hospital discharge. ECG characteristics are related to the patient's prognosis. The more abnormal the ECG characteristics, the less likely the patient is to recover from PEA; patients with a wider QRS (>0.2 sec) have worse prognosis.

PEA is treated in the same way as asystole. It is not a shockable rhythm. You should continue with CPR, administer epinephrine and begin to consider possible causes. Epinephrine can be given every 3 to 5 min.

Pulseless Electrical Activity: Background, Etiology, Epidemiology [Internet]. Emedicine.medscape.com. 2019 [cited 17 August 2019]. Available from: https://emedicine.medscape.com/article/161080-overview

The Australian Resuscitation Council Guidelines [Internet]. Resus.org.au. 2019 [cited 17 August 2019]. Available from: https://resus.org.au/guidelines/

14. Answer: B

Patients with critical illness are at risk of upper gastrointestinal bleeding, a condition that may be associated with increased mortality. Clinically important gastrointestinal bleeding occurs in 3–5% of ICU patients. Until recently guidelines have recommended preventive therapy with either histamine H_2–receptor antagonists or proton-pump inhibitors (PPIs) for patients in ICU who are at risk for stress ulceration and bleeding. However, any benefit from PPIs might be reduced by harmful events that are associated with the use of these agents, including nosocomial pneumonia, *Clostridium difficile* enteritis, and myocardial ischemia. The use of enteral feeding may also reduce the risk of gastrointestinal bleeding.

In a recent large trial, patients were randomly assigned to daily intravenous pantoprazole (40 mg) or placebo during their ICU admission. The patients were at high risk for gastrointestinal bleeding because of a history of liver disease, coagulopathy, shock, treatment with anticoagulant agents, renal replacement therapy, or mechanical ventilation that was expected to last for more than 24 hours. There was no significant difference between the groups in the rate of the primary outcome of death nor gastrointestinal bleeding, pneumonia, *C. difficile* infection, or myocardial ischemia. A further study of use with PPIs vs histamine H_2–receptor antagonists for stress ulcer prophylaxis among adults requiring mechanical ventilation did not result in a statistically significant difference for in-hospital mortality.

Barkun A, Bardou M. Proton-Pump Inhibitor Prophylaxis in the ICU — Benefits Worth the Risks? New England Journal of Medicine. 2018;379(23):2263–2264.
https://www.nejm.org/doi/full/10.1056/NEJMe1810021

15. Answer: D

AKI is a frequent complication associated with septic shock in patients who require ICU admission. AKI is also associated with an increased mortality rate in these patients.

In a large, multicenter, RCT, patients with early-stage septic shock with severe AKI based on the failure stage of the risk, injury, failure, loss, and end-stage kidney disease (RIFLE) system but without life-threatening complications of AKI were randomised to either receive dialysis within 12 hours after documentation of AKI (early dialysis) or 48 hours after the AKI if no renal recovery was observed (delayed dialysis).

The failure stage of the RIFLE classification system is characterised by a serum creatinine level 3 times the baseline level (or ≥4 mg/dL with a rapid increase of ≥0.5 mg/dL), urine output less than 0.3 ml per kilogram of body weight per hour for 24 hours or longer, or anuria for at least 12 hours.

The trial was stopped early for futility after the second planned interim analysis showed no significant difference in overall mortality at 90 days in the early dialysis vs. delayed dialysis groups.

Barbar S, Clere-Jehl R, Bourredjem A, Hernu R, Montini F, Bruyère R et al. Timing of Renal-Replacement Therapy in Patients with Acute Kidney Injury and Sepsis. New England Journal of Medicine. 2018;379(15):1431–1442. https://www.ncbi.nlm.nih.gov/pubmed/30304656

16. Answer: C

This patient is in septic shock, likely of urinary origin. Sepsis and septic shock are medical emergencies and treatment and resuscitation should begin immediately. Latest guidelines dictate that following initial fluid resuscitation, administration of additional fluids should be guided by frequent assessment of haemodynamic status. This includes thorough clinical examination including blood pressure, heart rate, respiratory rate, temperature, oxygen saturation and urine output.

Previous resuscitation guidelines in septic shock have recommended a protocolised approach, known as early goal-directed therapy (EGDT) which described the use of goals that included central venous monitoring and serial haemoglobin monitoring. Previously, the EGDT dictated that early placement of a central venous catheter (CVC) improved outcomes in patients with septic shock. However, this approach has now been challenged following the results of three large, multicentre RCTs which showed no mortality benefit, as discussed in the Protocolised Resuscitation In Sepsis Meta-Analysis (PRISM). New evidence found that the use of CVP alone to guide fluid resuscitation can no longer be justified given the limited ability of CVP to predict a response to a fluid challenge when the CVP is within a relatively normal range (8–12 mmHg).

Recommended volume of fluid resuscitation starts at 30 mL/kg; however, the balance of additional fluids and the use of vasopressors remains uncertain. Several clinical trials are underway which will evaluate this, however currently the goal of fluid resuscitation should be targeted at a mean arterial pressure (MAP) of 65 mmHg through the use of fluids and vasopressors, while normalising the lactate level. Two clinical trials show the potential for harm with starch-related intravenous fluids, but limited evidence to support the use of colloids over crystalloids. (Starch trial: https://www.nejm.org/doi/full/10.1056/NEJMoa1204242 and ALBIOS trial: https://www.nejm.org/doi/full/10.1056/nejmoa1305727). There is emerging evidence for the use of balanced crystalloid solutions over 0.9% sodium chloride (SMART trial, https://www.nejm.org/doi/full/10.1056/NEJMoa1711584). There is also some emerging evidence for fluids potentially leading to higher mortality (FEAST trial, https://www.nejm.org/doi/full/10.1056/NEJMoa1101549).

In summary:
- Septic shock is a medical emergency and resuscitation should begin immediately.
- Initial fluid volume administered should start at 30 mL/kg.
- Further fluid administration should be based on haemodynamic status as determined by physiologic parameters (BP, HR, urine output, oxygen saturation and temperature).
- A target MAP of 65 mmHg may be used for vasopressor and fluid adjustment.
- Serial measurement of CVP, Scvo$_2$ and haemoglobin using a CVC is no longer recommended.

Berger R, Rivers E, Levy M. Management of Septic Shock. New England Journal of Medicine. 2017;376(23):2282–2285. https://www.nejm.org/doi/full/10.1056/NEJMclde1705277?url_ver=Z39.88-2003&rfr_id=ori:rid:crossref.org&rfr_dat=cr_pub%3dpubmed

Rhodes A, Evans L, Alhazzani W, Levy M, Antonelli M, Ferrer R et al. Surviving Sepsis Campaign: International Guidelines for Management of for Management of Sepsis and Septic Shock: 2016. Critical Care Medicine: 2017; 45: 486–552. https://journals.lww.com/ccmjournal/Fulltext/2017/03000/Surviving_Sepsis_Campaign___International.15.aspx

17. Answer: B

Severe asthma is defined as uncontrolled asthma despite adherence to maximum optimised therapy and treatment of contributing factors or that exacerbates when high-dose treatment is decreased. Patients with severe asthma suffer a substantial burden of symptoms, exacerbations, and side effects from medications. Patients with comorbidities such as severe sinus disease, recurrent respiratory infections, sleep apnoea, and gastroesophageal reflux experience more frequent recurrent exacerbations of severe asthma.

According to Global Initiative for Asthma (GINA) guidelines, approximately 50% of patients with severe asthma have type 2 inflammation which is characterised by eosinophils, increased fractional inhaled nitric oxide (FeNO), and cytokines such as interleukin [IL]-4, IL-5, IL-13. GINA guidelines do not suggest use of exhaled nitric oxide to guide therapy in patients with severe asthma.

Mepolizumab is a humanised immunoglobulin G1 kappa monoclonal antibody specific for IL-5. It binds to IL-5 and stops IL-5 from binding to its receptor on the surface of eosinophils. Therefore, it reduces blood, tissue, and sputum eosinophil levels. It is indicated for add-on maintenance treatment of patients with severe asthma and with an eosinophilic phenotype.

Global Initiative for Asthma – Global Initiative for Asthma – GINA [Internet]. Global Initiative for Asthma – GINA. 2020 [cited 7 July 2020]. Available from: http://www.ginasthma.org

18. Answer: D

This patient has clinical evidence of severe and complicated *Clostridium difficile* infection (CDI). The incidence of CDI continues to rise. Oral vancomycin 125 mg four times daily is recommended as first-line therapy for severe CDI. It can be administrated via nasogastric tube or per rectum. Oral metronidazole 400 mg three times daily for 10 days is recommended as first-line therapy for first episode mild CDI. Fidaxomicin, a first-in-class macrocyclic bactericidal antibiotic, has targeted bactericidal activity against *C. difficile* through inhibiting clostridial RNA polymerase. Fidaxomicin demonstrates minimal impact on normal gut flora and spares *Bacteroides spp.*, a major 'protective' constituent of faecal flora. Fidaxomicin has minimal oral absorption like vancomycin and a prolonged post-antibiotic effect and has been approved by the Therapeutic Drug Administration (TGA) for use in CDI. Oral fidaxomicin 200 mg twice daily is a treatment alternative in recurrent CDI. Faecal microbiota transplantation (FMT) is a treatment option alternative in recurrent CDI for appropriately selected patients.

Trubiano J, Cheng A, Korman T, Roder C, Campbell A, May M et al. Australasian Society of Infectious Diseases updated guidelines for the management of Clostridium difficile infection in adults and children in Australia and New Zealand. Internal Medicine Journal. 2016;46(4):479–493.
https://onlinelibrary.wiley.com/doi/epdf/10.1111/imj.13027

19. Answer: B

Sepsis is life threatening organ dysfunction caused by an infection-induced dysregulated host response, which may be complicated by septic shock. Sepsis and septic shock are major causes of morbidity and mortality worldwide. The Surviving Sepsis Campaign (SSC) has strongly emphasised the importance of speed and appropriateness of therapy in improving outcomes. Since the application of the first SSC guidelines, a substantial reduction in mortality has been reported. Both sepsis and septic shock should be viewed as medical emergencies requiring rapid diagnosis and immediate intervention.

The hour-1 bundle encourages clinicians to act as quickly as possible to obtain blood cultures, administer broad spectrum antibiotics, start appropriate fluid resuscitation, measure lactate, and begin vasopressors if clinically indicated. Ideally these interventions would all begin in the first hour from sepsis recognition but may not necessarily be completed in the first hour.

SSC Hour-1 Bundle of Care Elements:
- Measure lactate level, remeasure lactate if initial lactate is elevated (>2 mmol/L).
- Obtain blood cultures before administering antibiotics.
- Administer broad-spectrum antibiotics.
- Begin rapid administration of 30 mL/kg crystalloid for hypotension or lactate level ≥4 mmol/L.
- Apply vasopressors if hypotensive during or after fluid resuscitation to maintain MAP ≥65 mm Hg.

Rhodes A, Evans L, Alhazzani W, Levy M, Antonelli M, Ferrer R et al. Surviving Sepsis Campaign. Critical Care Medicine [Internet]. 2017 [cited 21 June 2020];45(3):486–552. Available from: https://journals.lww.com/ccmjournal/Fulltext/2017/03000/Surviving_Sepsis_Campaign___International.15.aspx

20. Answer: B

The ECGs show
  A. Left bundle branch block
  B. Mobitz type II 2:1 heart block
  C. Bifascicular block
  D. Mobitz type I (Wenckebach) heart block.

Temporary transvenous pacing is necessary for patients with severe and symptomatic bradyarrhythmias. It should be considered for patients with second-degree or third-degree atrioventricular (AV) block associated with symptoms or hemodynamic compromise. Temporary transvenous pacing is necessary to increase heart rate and improve symptoms.

In summary, temporary transvenous pacing should be considered following an acute myocardial infarction (AMI), if there is:

- Complete (third-degree) heart block.
- Mobitz type II second-degree AV block.
- New or age-indeterminate bifascicular block (RBBB with LAFB or LPFB or LBBB) with PR prolongation.
- Bradycardia-induced tachyarrhythmias.
- Symptomatic bradycardia of any aetiology if hypotension is present and the bradyarrhythmia is not responsive to atropine.

Despite reperfusion treatment, the incidence of intraventricular conduction disturbances post AMI has not changed, whereas the incidence of AV block post AMI has decreased but still remains high. AV block occurs in almost 7% of cases of AMI.

 Kusumoto FM. 2018 ACC/AHA/HRS Guideline on the Evaluation and Management of Patients With Bradycardia and Cardiac Conduction Delay. Journal of the American College of Cardiology. 2018.
https://www.sciencedirect.com/science/article/pii/S073510971838985X?via%3Dihub

21. Answer: D

Tranexamic acid has been shown to reduce surgical bleeding and decrease mortality in patients with mild to moderate traumatic extracranial bleeding. A 7-year large randomised, placebo-controlled, multi-centre trial (CRASH-3) with 12,737 patients in 29 countries has shown that tranexamic acid (loading dose 1 g over 10 min then infusion of 1 g over 8 h) is safe in patients with acute traumatic brain injury. The trial patients had a GCS score of 12 or lower or any intracranial bleeding on CT brain, and no major extracranial haemorrhage. Patients with a GCS score of 3 or bilateral unreactive pupils, severe brain injury, at baseline were excluded. Patients should be started on tranexamic acid as soon as possible after injury, within 3 hours of injury. Early treatment had more effect than later treatment in patients with mild and moderate head injury (p=0.005). There was no difference of the risk of vascular occlusive events and the risk of seizures in the tranexamic acid and placebo groups. It should be noted the benefit is mostly restricted to the moderate head injury group (and done as a subgroup analysis). However, given its low risk of causing harm, it may be beneficial to give to all groups of traumatic head injuries.

 Effects of tranexamic acid on death, disability, vascular occlusive events and other morbidities in patients with acute traumatic brain injury (CRASH-3): a randomised, placebo-controlled trial. The Lancet. 2019;394(10210):1713–1723.
https://www.ncbi.nlm.nih.gov/pmc/articles/PMC6853170/

22. Answer: D

There is an increasing trend of using VBG instead of ABG to assess critically unwell patients in the emergency department, ICU, or when inpatients are acutely unwell. VBG can be obtained from the peripheral veins and is a safer, easier to obtain, and less invasive alternative. VBG blood test results can provide rapid and accurate information on acid-base and CO2 status, along with SpO2, and provide direction on ventilation requirement and the need for ICU or high dependency unit admission. The pH of a VBG and ABG correlates closely and accurately measures the severity of an acidosis. The average VBG pH is 0.03–0.04 less than the ABG pH values. SpO2 values correlate well with PaO2 on ABG analysis as predicted by the standard oxygen–haemoglobin dissociation curve, but PaO2 level does not correlate well between the venous and arterial blood gases. PaO2 readings in VBG can significantly underestimate arterial oxygen level or miss patients with hyperoxia, a state in which oxygen supply is excessive. It is important to also recall that the oxygen-haemoglobin dissociation curve is altered by arterial pH, PaCO2, and temperature. The bicarbonate (HCO3) correlates well between arterial and venous samples, and similar to the pH will closely approximate the arterial values, with a difference of 0.52–1.5 mmol/L. The lactate level correlates well between ABG and VBG, with a mean difference of 0.02–0.08. The venous lactic acid can be used determine trends in lactate during resuscitation.

In patients with a clinical suspicion of ARDS demonstrating signs and symptoms of dyspnoea, tachypnoea, hypoxaemia, and bilateral infiltrates on CXR, PaO2 in ABG results is required as part of the diagnostic criteria. A ratio of partial pressure of arterial oxygen to fraction of inspired oxygen (PaO2/FiO2) of 200 or less, regardless of positive end-expiratory pressure, is supportive of the diagnosis of ARDS.

Please note that peripheral VBG may be skewed by prolonged tourniquet time. Central VBG or mixed VBG may be a useful marker in monitoring a patient's cardiac function.

 Zeserson E, Goodgame B, Hess J, Schultz K, Hoon C, Lamb K et al. Correlation of Venous Blood Gas and Pulse Oximetry With Arterial Blood Gas in the Undifferentiated Critically Ill Patient. Journal of Intensive Care Medicine. 2016;33(3):176–181.
https://www.ncbi.nlm.nih.gov/pmc/articles/PMC5885755/

23. Answer: D

Azithromycin is considered to have minimal cardiotoxicity and is the safest of the macrolide derivatives due to divergent pharmacokinetic properties (e.g. minimal CYP3A4 metabolism/inhibition) and is limited in blockade of the rapid delayed rectifier potassium current (IKr) conducted by hERG-encoded Kv11.1 potassium channel at therapeutic concentrations. There is a small absolute increased risk of ventricular arrhythmia and cardiovascular deaths, which is most pronounced among patients with a high baseline risk of cardiovascular disease and/or concomitant use of other QT-prolonging drugs such as sotalol in this case. Prescribing physicians should carefully assess the risks and benefits of azithromycin use especially in patients with underlying cardiovascular disease and concomitant use of other QT-prolonging drugs.

This patient has ongoing VT despite defibrillation three times. The next line of therapy is amiodarone.

According to the 2018 Australian and New Zealand Council of Resuscitation (ANZCOR) Advanced Life Support Guideline, intravenous amiodarone (300 mg) should be administered after the third failed attempt at defibrillation, at the time of recommencement of CPR. There is no evidence that giving any antiarrhythmic drug routinely during cardiac arrest increases rate of survival to hospital discharge. However, in comparison with placebo and lignocaine the use of amiodarone in shock-refractory VF improves the short-term survival. Despite the lack of long-term outcome data, it is reasonable to continue to use antiarrhythmic drugs on a routine basis.

Magnesium sulphate is indicated only in the treatment of VF or pulseless VT arrest due to drug induced prolonged QT interval associated with torsades de pointes.

There are no placebo-controlled studies that show that the routine use of any vasopressor at any stage during cardiac arrest increases survival to hospital discharge, though they have been demonstrated to increase return of spontaneous circulation. Current evidence is insufficient to support or refute the routine use of any particular drug or sequence of drugs. Despite the lack of human data, it is reasonable to continue to use vasopressors on a routine basis. Adrenaline (1 mg), when indicated, should be administered after rhythm analysis (± shock), at the time of recommencement of CPR.

 Guidelines [Internet]. Resus.org.au. 2019 [cited 24 March 2019]. Available from: https://resus.org.au/guidelines/

24. Answer: D

This patient is in septic shock, likely due to urosepsis. Sepsis and septic shock are medical emergencies and treatment and resuscitation should begin immediately. Latest guidelines dictate that following initial fluid resuscitation, administration of additional fluids should be guided by frequent assessment of haemodynamic status. This includes thorough clinical examination including blood pressure, heart rate, respiratory rate, temperature, oxygen saturation and urine output. This patient is responding to initial fluid resuscitation; therefore, it is appropriate to continue monitor blood pressure and urine output and give additional fluid.

New evidence found that the use of CVP alone to guide fluid resuscitation can no longer be justified given the limited ability of CVP to predict a response to a fluid challenge when the CVP is within a relatively normal range (8–12 mmHg).

Recommended volume of fluid resuscitation starts at 30mL/kg; however, the balance of additional fluids and the use of vasopressors remains uncertain. Several clinical trials are underway which will evaluate this, however currently the goal of fluid resuscitation should be targeted at a mean arterial pressure (MAP) of 65mmHg through the use of fluids and vasopressors, while normalising the lactate level.

In summary:
- Septic shock is a medical emergency and resuscitation should begin immediately.
- Initial fluid volume administered should start at 30 mL/kg.
- Further fluid administration should be based on haemodynamic status as determined by physiologic parameters (blood pressure, heart rate, urine output, oxygen saturation and temperature).
- A target MAP of 65mmHg may be used for vasopressor and fluid adjustment.
- Serial measurement of CVP, $Scvo_2$ and haemoglobin using a CVC is no longer recommended.

 Berger R, Rivers E, Levy M. Management of Septic Shock. New England Journal of Medicine. 2017;376(23):2282–2285. https://www.nejm.org/doi/full/10.1056/NEJMclde1705277

 Rhodes A, Evans L, Alhazzani W, Levy M, Antonelli M, Ferrer R et al. Surviving Sepsis Campaign: International Guidelines for Management of Sepsis and Septic Shock: 2016. Intensive Care Medicine. 2017;43(3):304–377. https://link.springer.com/article/10.1007%2Fs00134-017-4683-6

25. Answer: B

The latest guidelines from the Surviving Sepsis Campaign give detailed recommendations of initial resuscitation, screening and diagnosis of sepsis, antibiotic therapy, fluid administration, source control, administration of vasopressors and steroids, blood products, anticoagulants, immunoglobulins, mechanical ventilation, sedation, analgesia, glucose control, blood purification, renal replacement therapy, bicarbonate, venous thromboembolism and stress ulcer prophylaxis, and nutrition.

Specific recommendations in antimicrobial treatment include:

- Administration of IV antimicrobials be initiated as soon as possible after recognition, and within one hour for both sepsis and septic shock.
- Empiric broad-spectrum therapy with one or more antimicrobials for patients presenting with sepsis or septic shock to cover all likely pathogens (including bacterial and potentially fungal or viral coverage) should be used initially.
- Empiric antimicrobial therapy be narrowed once pathogen identification and sensitivities are established and/or adequate clinical improvement is noted.
- Daily assessment for de-escalation of antimicrobial therapy in patients with sepsis and septic shock should be performed.
- Do not use systemic antimicrobial prophylaxis in patients with severe inflammatory states of non-infectious origin such as severe pancreatitis, burn injury.
- Dosing strategies of antimicrobials should be optimised based on accepted pharmacokinetic/pharmacodynamic principles and specific drug properties in patients with sepsis or septic shock.
- Do not use combination therapy for the routine treatment of neutropenic sepsis/bacteraemia.
- An antimicrobial treatment duration of 7 to 10 days is adequate for most serious infections associated with sepsis and septic shock.

Rhodes A, Evans L, Alhazzani W, Levy M, Antonelli M, Ferrer R et al. Surviving Sepsis Campaign. Critical Care Medicine [Internet]. 2017 [cited 21 June 2020];45(3):486–552. Available from: https://journals.lww.com/ccmjournal/Fulltext/ 2017/03000/Surviving_Sepsis_Campaign___International.15.aspx

26. Answer: E

27. Answer: B

28. Answer: D

29. Answer: F

30. Answer: A

31. Answer: G

Inotropes and vasopressors are used in shock states to improve perfusion by increasing BP. As BP is a function of both cardiac output and systemic vascular resistance, medications can increase BP by either increasing one or both of these parameters. Vasopressors induce vasoconstriction and thereby elevate BP. Inotropes increase cardiac contractility; however, many drugs have both vasopressor and inotropic effects.

One of the key mechanisms by which medications can improve BP is by stimulation of adrenoreceptors. Dobutamine predominantly stimulates beta adrenoreceptors and very short half-life, thus having greater effect on cardiac output than systemic vascular resistance. Noradrenaline has a greater effect on peripheral resistance than cardiac output, through greater alpha than beta action. Phenylephrine has predominantly alpha adrenoreceptor action, resulting in increased BP through increased peripheral resistance. Dopamine is a precursor to both noradrenaline and adrenaline, but also acts independently on the renal arteries, resulting in renal arteriolar dilatation. Vasopressin also acts has vasopressor actions through stimulation of V2 receptors on peripheral vessels. Milrinone is a phosphodiesterase III inhibitor, which has its inotropic effect through decreasing metabolism of cAMP, leading to prolonged cardiac myocyte contraction – cAMP causes vasodilation both in the pulmonary arteries and peripheral arteries, which can be a useful by-effect, for example in pulmonary hypertension. As adrenoreceptor agonists and phosphodiesterase inhibitors increase intracellular calcium, they have an unwanted effect of increasing myocardial oxygen demand and are potentially pro-arrhythmic.

Levosimendan enhances the calcium sensitivity of troponin C, resulting in increased cardiac output, and also causes peripheral vasodilation, through activation of ATP-sensitive potassium channels in peripheral vessels. Omecamtiv is a newer inotrope that acts as a selective cardiac myosin activator, which is currently being studied in relation to therapy for left ventricular dysfunction.

Arrigo M, Mebazaa A. Understanding the differences among inotropes. Intensive Care Medicine. 2015;41(5):912–915. https://link.springer.com/article/10.1007/s00134-015-3659-7

32. Answer: H

This patient has clinical features of life-threating asthma. Please see the following criteria.

Near fatal asthma

Raised PaCO2 and/or requiring mechanical ventilation with raised inflation pressures.

Life-threatening asthma

Any one of the following in a patient with severe asthma:

- Peak expiratory flow (PEF) <33% best or predicted
- SpO2<92%
- PaO2<60mmHg
- Normal PaCO2
- Silent chest
- Cyanosis
- Feeble respiratory effort
- Bradycardia
- Dysrhythmia
- Hypotension
- Exhaustion
- Confusion
- Coma

Acute severe asthma

Any one of:

- PEF 33–50% best or predicted
- Respiratory rate >25/min
- Heart rate >110/min
- Inability to complete sentences in one breath.

Initial management for life-threatening asthma includes:

- Take an ABG.
- Give high concentrations of inspired oxygen aiming to achieve oxygen saturations >92%.
- Give short-acting β2-agonists, salbutamol repeatedly in 5mg doses or by continuous nebulization at 10 mg/h driven by oxygen.
- Add nebulized ipratropium bromide to nebulized salbutamol for all patients with life-threatening asthma as it has been shown to produce significantly greater bronchodilation than β2 agonists alone.
- Give high dose intravenous hydrocortisone to all patients with life-threatening asthma as early as possible in the episode, as this may improve survival.
- Give a single intravenous dose of magnesium sulphate 1.2–2g over 20 min if there is no improvement after performing the above. It has been shown to be safe and effective in acute severe asthma. Magnesium is a smooth muscle relaxant, producing bronchodilation. Rapid administration may be associated with hypotension. As this patient's BP is low, it is better to be given after transfer to ICU.
- Transfer to ICU for consideration of intravenous bronchodilators, epinephrine and mechanical ventilation.

Australian Asthma Handbook [Internet]. Asthmahandbook.org.au. 2020 [cited 7 July 2020]. Available from: http://www.asthmahandbook.org.au/acute-asthma/clinical

33. Answer: C

This patient has collapse and VT due to hyperkalaemia after missing his regular haemodialysis. The best immediate treatment is intravenous administration of 10 ml 10% calcium chloride to stabilise the myocardial cell membrane and lower the risk of VF. Calcium chloride is preferred over calcium gluconate for a patient experiencing a cardiac arrest because the chloride formulation has approximately 3 times the amount of elemental calcium compared with the gluconate formulation. Furthermore, gluconate must be hepatically metabolized before its associated calcium becomes bioavailable, which is unlikely in the setting of hemodynamic instability or poor liver function during cardiac arrest. Calcium chloride is preferably given intravenously via a central or a large peripheral line to avoid any potentially harmful effects should extravasation occur.

Hyperkalaemia raises the resting membrane potential, causing a narrowing between resting membrane potential and threshold potential for action potential generation. Calcium restores this initial narrowing back towards 15 mV by raising the threshold potential to being 'less negative'. Calcium results in improvement in ECG changes within minutes of administration.

Calcium is essential for normal muscle and nerve activity. It transiently increases peripheral resistance, myocardial excitability and contractility. Randomized control trials and observational studies have demonstrated no survival benefits when calcium was given in-hospital or out-of-hospital cardiac arrest patients. In VF, calcium did not restore spontaneous circulation.

 Ahee P. The management of hyperkalaemia in the emergency department. Emergency Medicine Journal. 2000;17(3): 188–191.
https://emj.bmj.com/content/17/3/188

34. Answer: J

This patient's cardiac monitor demonstrates torsade de pointes. It is the result of QTc prolongation which can either be congenital or acquired. Acquired QTc prolongation is most often drug-related. There are many medications that can predispose a person to torsades such as antiarrhythmics, antipsychotics, antiemetics, antifungals, and antimicrobials. Prolonged QTc and Torsades are also associated with hypokalaemia, hypocalcaemia, hypomagnesemia, bradycardia, and heart failure.

Magnesium is an electrolyte essential for membrane stability. Hypomagnesaemia causes myocardial hyperexcitability particularly in the presence of hypokalaemia and digoxin. Electrical cardioversion should be performed for patients with hypotension or in cardiac arrest from torsades de pointes. Intravenous magnesium is the first-line pharmacologic therapy of torsades de pointes. The recommended initial dose of magnesium is a slow 2 g IV push. An infusion of 1g to 4 g/hr should be started to keep the magnesium levels >2 mmol/L. Once the magnesium level is >3 mmol/L, the infusion can be stopped. Severe magnesium toxicity is seen with levels >3.5 mmol/L which can cause confusion, respiratory depression, and cardiac arrest. It is important to remember to correct any hypokalaemia as well. There is insufficient data to recommend for or against its routine use in cardiac arrest.

There are many causes of hypomagnesaemia. Heavy binge alcohol intake can lead to a loss of magnesium from tissues and increased urinary loss. Chronic alcohol abuse has been reported to deplete the total body supply of magnesium. This is the most likely cause in this case.

 Schwartz PJ. Predicting the Unpredictable Drug-Induced QT Prolongation and Torsades de Pointes. J Am Coll Cardiol 2016; 67:1639–50.
https://www.sciencedirect.com/science/article/pii/S0735109716003387

35. Answer: K

This case is a very typical occurrence in hospital. The patient is in pain after the fracture and is waiting for surgery. He receives opioid analgesia regularly. Opiate toxicity should be suspected when the clinical triad of depressed level of consciousness (reduced GCS), respiratory depression, and pupillary miosis are present. It is important to remember opioid exposure/toxicity does not always result in miosis and that respiratory depression is the most specific sign. Respiratory failure and respiratory acidosis is due to hypoventilation.

Airway control and adequate oxygenation is the primary supportive treatment. Intravenous naloxone should be given in patient with reduced level of consciousness and/or respiratory depression. The usual dose is between 0.4 and 2 mg. The onset of effect following intravenous naloxone is 1–2 min; maximal effect is observed within 5–10 min. A repeat dose is indicated for partial response and can be repeated as often as needed. To avoid precipitous withdrawal (nausea, vomiting, agitation) and consequent aspiration, naloxone may be started with low doses such as 0.1 mg and titrated up gradually until reversal of respiratory depression is achieved.

 Boyer E. Management of Opioid Analgesic Overdose. New England Journal of Medicine. 2012;367(2):146–155.
https://pubmed.ncbi.nlm.nih.gov/22784117/

3 Dermatology

Questions

Answers can be found in the Dermatology Answers section at the end of this chapter.

1. A 65-year-old man with a history of type 2 diabetes presents with blistering skin lesions affecting the trunk and upper and lower extremities. Histopathology of a punch biopsy and an excision biopsy of the affected skin and blister confirms a diagnosis of bullous pemphigoid.

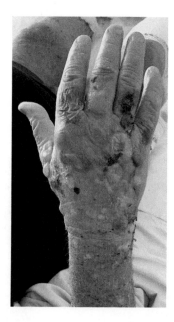

Which one of the following medications may have contributed to the development of bullous pemphigoid?
  A. Gliclazide.
  B. Insulin.
  C. Linagliptin.
  D. Metformin.

2. A 27-year-old woman with an 18-year history of type 1 diabetes and a 5-year history of hypothyroidism now presents with fatigue, bloating, abdominal pain, diarrhoea, and a 4 kg weight loss over the past 6 months. On examination, she has symmetric papulovesicles over the external surface of the extremities and on the trunk.
  What other classic characteristic of her skin lesion would you expect to find?
  A. Absence of any pain.
  B. Firm nodules on the scalp.
  C. Intense pruritus.
  D. Target lesions on the palms.

How to Pass the FRACP Written Examination, First Edition. Jonathan Gleadle, Jordan Li, Danielle Wu, and Paul Kleinig.
© 2022 John Wiley & Sons Ltd. Published 2022 by John Wiley & Sons Ltd.

3. A 34-year-old woman has developed several tender red swellings on her shins and right ankle (picture shown below) over the past 3 weeks. She has been feeling generally unwell and has a low-grade fever. She has not had a recent sore throat, cough, or sputum. Over the past 12 months she has had recurrent aphthous ulcers in her mouth but no genital ulceration. She has also experienced intermittent abdominal pain, diarrhoea, and lost 7 kg of body weight. She is a current heavy smoker and drinks alcohol only occasionally. On examination, she is afebrile, there are no aphthous ulcers, active arthritis, lymphadenopathy, or organomegaly. The initial investigation results and CXR are displayed below.

Tests	Results	Normal values
Sodium	136 mmol/L	135–145
Potassium	3.5 mmol/L	3.5–5.2
Urea	5.9 mmol/L	2.7–8.0
Creatinine	96 μmol/L	60–100
Calcium	2.01 mmol/L	2.10–2.60
Albumin	28 g/L	38–48
Bilirubin	16 mmol/L	2–24
ALP	63 U/L	30–110
GGT	46 U/L	0–60
ALT	52 U/L	0–55
AST	45 U/L	0–45
Hb	92 g/L	135–175
WBC	16.5 x 10⁹/L	4.0–11.0
Platelet	259 x 10⁹/L	150–450
MCV	72 fL	80–98
ESR	82 mm/h	<20

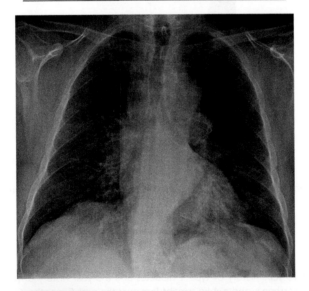

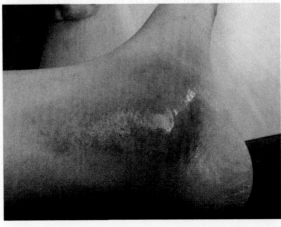

What is your most likely diagnosis?
- **A.** Crohn's disease.
- **B.** Glandular fever.
- **C.** Lymphoma.
- **D.** Sarcoidosis.

4. An 18-year-old man presents to the emergency department with central colicky abdominal pain and arthralgia. He has become unwell with coryzal symptoms since yesterday. He reports smoky coloured urine and reduced oral intake due to sore throat. He does not have a significant past medical history and no history of intravenous drug use. On examination, a palpable rash is present on both legs (see below). He is hypertensive.

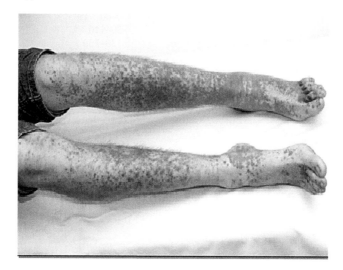

Which of the following statement regarding this condition is correct?
- **A.** 80% of patients will have a negative FOBT.
- **B.** 90% of patients will have high level of serum IgA.
- **C.** 90% of patients will have thrombocytopenia.
- **D.** 90% of patients will have a positive ANCA and MPO.

5. Which of the following gene mutations are frequently detected in melanoma?
- **A.** BRAF and CDKN2A.
- **B.** Epidermal growth factor receptor (EGFR).
- **C.** K-ras and p53.
- **D.** Vascular endothelial growth factor (VEGF).

6. A 58-year-old woman presents to the clinic following an excisional biopsy of an asymmetrical pigmented lesion on her right lower leg with widest diameter measuring 9 mm. The Breslow thickness has been reported at 4 mm. She is known to have poorly controlled type 2 diabetes, which is complicated by nephropathy, retinopathy, and neuropathy. She had several small foot and leg ulcers before which took a long time to heal. There is no documented macrovascular complication so far.
The best management plan is:
- **A.** Require no wider local excision; however require a sentinel node biopsy.
- **B.** Require a wider local excision with a surgical margin of 2 cm and a sentinel node biopsy.
- **C.** Require a wider local excision with a surgical margin of 1 cm and a sentinel node biopsy.
- **D.** Require a wider local excision with a surgical margin of 4 cm without a sentinel node biopsy.

7. A 58-year-old butcher presents with a 4-month history of fatigue. He has noticed a few small blisters developing initially on both hands and since then the rash is getting worse especially when exposed to sun. He is concerned about the scarring marks left on his hands. He drinks two to three standard drinks of alcohol per day. He has no history of previous skin disease or other medical problems. He does not take any medication. His hands are shown below. The full skin examination reveals similar small lesions and scars on his face. The biochemistry results are shown below:

Tests	Results	Normal values
Hb	170 g/L	135–175
Creatinine	139 µmol/L	80–120
ALT	98 U/L	0–55
AST	155 U/L	0–45
GGT	89 U/L	0–60
ALP	169 U/L	30–110
LDH	213 U/L	120–250
Ferritin	547 µg/L	30–300
Transferrin saturation	26 %	10–55

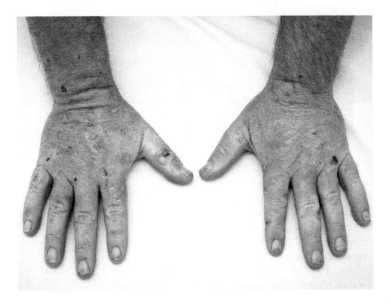

What is the most likely diagnosis?
- **A.** Bullous pemphigoid.
- **B.** Cutaneous lichen planus.
- **C.** Dermatitis herpetiforms.
- **D.** Porphyria cutanea tarda.

8. A 42-year-old woman presents with a 9-month history of repeated facial flushing, often precipitated by sun exposure. She reports that the flushing occurs on the nose, both cheeks, and the central forehead. On examination, she has multiple telangiectasia on both malar surfaces, but no evidence of inflamed papules or pustules. There are no features suggestive of systemic lupus erythematosus.

Which of the following treatments is most likely to be helpful in reducing her symptoms?
- **A.** Oral doxycycline.
- **B.** Oral isotretinoin.
- **C.** Topical brimonidine.
- **D.** Topical metronidazole.

9. An 82-year-old man with vascular dementia is constantly scratching his hands and elbows. There are diffuse scaly rashes on hands, elbows, and scrotum with several vesicles and scratch marks. A clinical diagnosis of scabies is made.

Which of the following statements is true in regard to this patient?

A. A skin biopsy should be performed prior to the treatment.

B. He is at risk of having highly contagious crusted scabies.

C. His pruritus is caused by direct irritation from mites and eggs.

D. The mite can survive on bedding, clothes for more than one week.

10. A 40-year-old woman who received a heart transplant two years ago is seeking your advice regarding sunscreen usage to prevent skin cancers.

Which of the following do you advise her?

A. High-number SPF (Sun Protection Factor) sunscreen allows longer time intervals between application.

B. SPF 30 sunscreen blocks 60% of the sun's UVB rays.

C. SPF 30 sunscreen decrease the skin's production of vitamin D.

D. UVA rays mainly cause sunburn and UVB rays cause skin cancers.

11. A 66-year-old man has a skin lesion on his right shoulder which is suspicious for a BCC. He has a history of ischaemic heart disease with a coronary artery stent and hypertension. His dermatologist excises the lesion without stopping clopidogrel and causes profuse bleeding.

Which layer of the skin has the dermatologist most likely transversed to cause this bleeding?

A. Papillary dermis.

B. Reticular dermis.

C. Stratum basale.

D. Stratum granulosum.

12. A 60-year-old man presents with a 2-week history of flu-like symptoms including malaise, sore throat, and fever. His GP had commenced him on amoxicillin, but he did not respond to this treatment. On examination, he has an erythematous, desquamating rash over his torso with injected conjunctivae.

Which of the following has the most benefit on mortality in this condition?

A. Etanercept.

B. High dose systemic steroids.

C. Intravenous Immunoglobulin (IVIG).

D. Supportive care.

QUESTIONS (13–17) **REFER TO THE FOLLOWING INFORMATION**

Match each of the clinical scenarios with the best fitting dermatological emergency:

A. Drug rash with eosinophilia and systemic symptoms.

B. Meningococcaemia.

C. Necrotising fasciitis.

D. Disseminated candidiasis.

E. Staphylococcal scalded skin syndrome.

F. Stevens-Johnson syndrome.

G. Acute generalised exanthematous pustulosis.

H. Toxic epidermal necrolysis.

13. A 21-year-old woman presents with a 6-hour history of fever and rash over her body. She was started on oral trimethoprim for UTI 7 days ago. She takes no other medication and has no known allergies. On examination, she is febrile and other vital signs are in normal range. There are erythematous, urticarial, targetoid rashes studded with small, tense blisters on the shoulders, back, palms but less than 10% of body surface area involved. There are also small vesicles and crusts on the upper and lower lips, but there are no lesions are present on the soles or genitalia. Nikolsky's sign is positive. Her FBE, LFTs, and renal function are normal.

14. A 25-year-old woman with a history of epilepsy, depression, and diabetes presents with fever (39°C), a morbilliform eruption and facial swelling. Her GP had commenced her on paracetamol, carbamazepine and metformin 6 weeks ago. On examination, the rash has varying morphology with targetoid lesions, pustules and blisters, however she is Nikolsky sign negative. She has WCC of 16×10^9/L, eosinophil of 4×10^9/L, deranged LFTs and a serum creatinine of 300 μmol/L [45-85]. The skin biopsy shows lichenoid infiltrate with focal necrotic keratinocytes.

15. A 58-year-old man presents with fever, malaise, and conjunctivitis progressing to a tender erythematous rash in the face, neck, axilla, and groin with mucous membranes spared. Nikolsky's sign is positive and flaccid bullae develop in areas of erythema.

16. A 42-year-old woman presents with fever and examination showswidespread erythema worse on the skin folds progressing to widespread small coalescing pustules.

17. A 56-year-old man presents with a 3-day history of worsening skin erythema, blistering and pain. He is known to have smoking related COPD. He was started with allopurinol 7 days ago, because of frequent acute gout attack. On examination, he is febrile, HR is 110 bpm, there is confluent erythema of the entire trunk and all extremities with blistering and erosions affecting >30% of the body surface. On palpation, mild pressure causes several non-blistered skins to slough. There is mild neutrophilia, slight elevation in liver aminotransferase levels.

Answers

1. Answer: C

Bullous pemphigoid is a rare autoimmune skin condition with an increasing incidence over the last two decades. It is caused by autoantibody-mediated damage to the epithelial basement membrane of the epidermis. IgG +/- IgE antibody and activated T cells attack the protein BP180 (Type XVII collagen), or less frequently BP230 (a plakin), in the basement membrane.

There are HLA associations to suggest genetic predisposition to the disease. It most commonly affects elderly patients over the age of 70. However, drug-induced bullous pemphigoid is linked to patients who are younger than 70 years of age and has a male predominance. The risk of developing bullous pemphigoid is greater in elderly patients with neurological disease, such as stroke, dementia, Parkinson's disease, unipolar disorder, bipolar disease, and multiple sclerosis. The risk of developing bullous pemphigoid is also increased in patients with psoriasis and in patients treated with phototherapy. A medication, trauma, or skin infection can trigger the onset of bullous pemphigoid. Medications which are associated with bullous pemphigoid include penicillamine, frusemide, spironolactone, captopril, penicillin and its derivative, sulfasalazine, salicylazosulfapyridine, phenacetin, nalidixic acid, topical fluorouracil, neuroleptics, and dipeptidyl-peptidase 4 (DPP-4) inhibitors. Bullous pemphigoid is associated with underlying malignancy and appropriate screening is important.

Schmidt E, Zillikens D. Pemphigoid diseases. The Lancet. 2013;381(9863):320–332.
https://www.ncbi.nlm.nih.gov/pubmed/23237497

2. Answer: C

This patient is likely to have coeliac disease. Classically, patients with coeliac disease present with steatorrhea, weight loss, nutrient deficiency, and resolution of the mucosal lesions (villous atrophy) and symptoms upon withdrawal of gluten-containing foods. The malabsorption may cause weight loss, severe anaemia, neurologic disorders from deficiencies of B vitamins, and osteopenia from deficiency of vitamin D and calcium. Coeliac disease can exist in a very mild form and go largely undetected.

Dermatitis herpetiformis (DH) is a rare but persistent immunobullous disease associated with coeliac disease. It develops in 15 to 25% of patients with coeliac disease. There is a genetic predisposition with an association with HLA, DQ2, and DQ8. Some patients have a personal or family history of other autoimmune diseases including thyroid disease, pernicious anaemia, type 1 diabetes, vitiligo, and Addison disease.

DH is characterised by its intense pruritus. Because of severe itching, intact vesicles are rarely seen. DH has a symmetrical distribution. The location of the lesions aids in the diagnosis. Lesions are most commonly seen on the extensor surfaces of knees, elbows and on buttocks. Lesions are seldom seen on the face, neck, scalp, palms, or soles.

DH diagnosis is based on typical clinical picture and demonstration of IgA deposition in papillary dermis. DH usually has a good prognosis, with the majority of patients responding well to a strict gluten-free diet and medication.

Salmi T. Dermatitis herpetiformis. Clinical and Experimental Dermatology. 2019;44(7):728–731.
https://onlinelibrary.wiley.com/doi/full/10.1111/ced.13992

3. Answer: A

This patient has erythema nodosum which is likely secondary to previously undiagnosed Crohn's disease which can be hypothesised from her history of mouth ulcers, abdominal pain, diarrhoea, and microcytic anaemia. Her serum calcium level is normal and CXR is normal which does not suggest sarcoidosis. There is also no lymphadenopathy or hepatosplenomegaly to suggest lymphoma.

Erythema nodosum is the most common type of panniculitis. Generally, it is idiopathic in 50% of cases, however there are many possible causes (Table 3.1). Erythema nodosum often occurs in association with granulomatous disease including sarcoidosis, tuberculosis, and granulomatous colitis. The hallmark of erythema nodosum is painful, tender, erythematous, subcutaneous nodules that typically are located symmetrically on the anterior surface of the lower extremities and is a nonspecific cutaneous reaction pattern to a variety of antigens.

Evidence supports the involvement of a type IV delayed hypersensitivity response to numerous antigens. Erythema nodosum represents an inflammatory process involving the septa between subcutaneous fat lobules, with an absence of vasculitis and the presence of radial granulomas. These nodules tend to be self-limiting; they do not ulcerate and usually resolve without atrophy or scarring. Pain can be managed with NSAIDs and prednisolone (1 mg/kg) may be used until the erythema nodosum resolves if underlying infection has been excluded. However most importantly, any underlying causes should be treated.

Table 3.1   Common causes of erythema nodosum.

Infection
   Streptococcal pharyngitis
   Mycoplasma
   Tuberculosis
   Syphilis
   Viral infection: HSV, EBV, hepatitis B and C, HIV

Inflammatory bowel disease
   Ulcerative colitis
   Crohn's disease

Sarcoidosis

Drugs
   Antibiotics: sulfonamides, amoxicillin; oral contraceptives

Lymphoma and other malignancies

 Chowaniec M, Starba A, Wiland P. Erythema nodosum – review of the literature. Reumatologia/Rheumatology. 2016;2:79–82. https://www.termedia.pl/Erythema-nodosum-review-of-the-literature,18,27671,1,1.html

4. Answer: A

The combination of palpable purpura, arthritis/arthralgia, abdominal pain. and haematuria in a young person is highly suggestive of Henoch-Schonlein (HSP) or IgA vasculitis. HSP is an immune-mediated vasculitis associated with IgA deposition. Skin biopsy shows leukocytoclastic vasculitis with IgA staining of superficial dermal vessels. Some degree of renal involvement is seen in 35 to 54% of adult patients. Renal biopsy primarily shows IgA deposition in the mesangium in both HSP and IgA nephropathy suggesting similar pathogenesis.

The majority of HSP cases are preceded by an upper respiratory tract infection suggesting a potential infectious trigger. Streptococcus, staphylococcus, and parainfluenza are the most commonly implicated pathogens.

Diagnosis of HSP is based on the presence of purpura (palpable) or petechiae (without thrombocytopaenia) with lower limb predominance (mandatory criterion) plus at least one of the following four features: (i) abdominal pain, (ii) arthritis or arthralgia, (iii) leukocytoclastic vasculitis or proliferative glomerulonephritis with predominant deposition of IgA on histology, (iv) renal involvement (haematuria, red blood cell casts, proteinuria). Laboratory tests focus on assessing renal involvement (urinalysis, urine microscopy, proteinuria, serum creatinine).

There are no blood tests specific for HSP. Although the IgA system plays a central role in the pathophysiology, measurement of serum levels of total IgA is not helpful in confirming the diagnosis or providing prognostic information. Galactose-deficient IgA1 serum levels seem to distinguish patients with HSP nephritis from patients without nephritis.

Gastrointestinal involvement is relatively common with typical colicky abdominal pain. In a recent case series, main clinical manifestations were abdominal pain (100%), nausea and vomiting (14.4%), melaena and/or rectorrhagia (12.9%), and positive FOBT (10.3%). Symptoms are caused by bowel ischemia and oedema. Serious complications include infarction and perforation. Descending duodenum and the terminal ileum are frequently involved, with endoscopic features including diffuse mucosal redness, petechiae, haemorrhagic erosions, and ulcers. CT scan features are commonly bowel wall thickening with engorgement of mesenteric vessels.

Patients with HSP usually do not have thrombocytopenia. It is extremely rare that patients with HSP also have positive ANCA and MPO. If present, patient usually have severe and rapid progressive renal failure. It has been suggested these patients should be treated with high dose steroid and cyclophosphamide.

Management of HSP includes supportive care, symptomatic therapy and, in some cases, immunosuppressive treatment. Immunosuppressive treatment of HSP nephritis is used in patients with severe kidney involvement (nephrotic range proteinuria and/or progressive renal impairment). In these cases, renal biopsy should be considered before treatment. Mild renal involvement (microscopic haematuria or mild proteinuria) does not require biopsy or immunosuppressive treatment.

In patients with rapidly progressive glomerulonephritis or nephrotic syndrome (usually accompanied by crescents on kidney biopsy), pulsed intravenous methylprednisolone followed by 3- to 6-month course of oral steroids is most commonly used. A current KDIGO guideline suggests adding cyclophosphamide to steroid treatment for crescentic IgA glomerulonephritis.

Audemard-Verger A, Pillebout E, Guillevin L, Thervet E, Terrier B. IgA vasculitis (Henoch–Shönlein purpura) in adults: Diagnostic and therapeutic aspects. Autoimmunity Reviews. 2015;14(7):579–585.
https://www.sciencedirect.com/science/article/abs/pii/S1568997215000361?via%3Dihub

5. Answer: A

The malignant transformation of melanocytes into melanoma is due to a complex interaction between exogenous and endogenous triggers as well as tumour-intrinsic and immune-related factors. Cutaneous melanomas carry a particularly high mutational load and harbour a high number of ultraviolet-signature mutations, such as C→T (caused by ultraviolet B) or G→T (caused by ultraviolet A) transitions. Although many pathogenetically relevant mutations in melanoma are assumed to originate from a direct mutagenic effect of ultraviolet B and A, indirect effects such as the production of free radicals resulting from the biochemical interaction of ultraviolet A with melanin also cause mutations and genetic aberrations.

Melanoma is a molecularly heterogenous malignancy. Malignant transformation into melanoma follows a sequential genetic model that results in constitutive activation of oncogenic signal transduction. Systematic genome-wide screening has identified missense mutations in *BRAF*, a component of the mitogen activated protein kinase (MAPK) pathway in 66% of melanomas. BRAFv600 mutation is a typical feature of benign naevus formation. Further progression into intermediate lesions and melanomas in situ requires additional mutations – for example, mutations in the telomerase reverse-transcriptase (TERT) promoter. To gain invasive potential, tertiary mutations in cell-cycle controlling genes (cyclin-dependent kinase-inhibitor 2A [CDKN2A]) or chromatin-remodelling (AT-rich interaction domain [ARID]1A, ARID1B, ARID2) are required. Metastatic melanoma progression is associated with mutations in phosphatase- and-tensin homologue (PTEN) or tumour-protein p53 (TP53).

BRAF inhibitors such as dabrafenib and trametinib are standards of care in patients with stage-3 BRAF mutated melanoma. Several randomised phase 3 clinical trials have shown objective response rates to BRAF inhibitors of approximately 50%, which can be increased to 70% when combined with MEK inhibitors.

Schadendorf D, van Akkooi A, Berking C, Griewank K, Gutzmer R, Hauschild A et al. Melanoma. The Lancet. 2018;392(10151):971–984.
https://www.thelancet.com/journals/lancet/article/PIIS0140-6736(18)31559-9/fulltext

6. Answer: B

This patient has melanoma in the context of diabetic neuropathy which may have impact on the wound healing. However, the Breslow thickness is 4 mm and she will require a wider local excision with margins of 2 cm. The guidelines for surgical margins of melanomas can be seen in the table below.

Sentinel lymph node biopsy (SLNB) is a surgical technique to identify low volume metastatic disease within the draining lymph node basin in patients undergoing treatment for primary melanoma. SLNB is a staging procedure to identify patients with a positive draining nodal basin and thereby minimise the morbidity associated with elective lymph node dissection in patients who may not require this procedure. Moreover, it provides prognostic stratification. Numerous studies have consistently demonstrated that the status of the sentinel lymph node (SLN) reflects the status of the entire draining nodal basin as measured by elective lymph node dissection. The recently revised American Joint Committee on Cancer (AJCC) staging system (8th edition) requires a SLNB for patients with primary melanoma >1 mm in thickness and for some patients with thin melanomas but with high risk factors in order to perform microstaging of the lymph node basin and accurately allocate a pathological disease stage.

SLNB involves pre-operative lymphoscintigraphy to identify the draining nodal basin for the anatomical location of the primary melanoma. This is followed by intraoperative intradermal injection of the melanoma site with patent blue dye. Intraoperative exploration through a small incision allows the identification of SLNs. A node is considered a SLN if it has tracer uptake and/or is stained blue. This dual modality approach allows the successful identification of a SLN in over 95% of patients. SLNs are carefully examined pathologically to identify metastasis.

Breslow thickness	Surgical margin for excision
Melanoma in situ	5 mm
Melanoma <1 mm	1 cm
Melanoma 1–2 mm	1–2 cm
Melanoma 2–4 mm	1–2 cm
Melanoma >4 mm	2 cm

Gyorki D, Barbour A, Mar V, Sandhu S, Hanikeri M. When is a sentinel node biopsy indicated? – Clinical Guidelines Wiki [Internet]. Cancer Council Australia: Clinical Guideline Network. 2020 [cited 15 February 2020]. Available from: https://wiki.cancer.org.au/australia/Clinical_question:When_is_a_sentinel_node_biopsy_indicated%3F

7. Answer: D

Porphyria is a predominantly inherited metabolic disorder resulting from a deficiency of an enzyme in the heme production pathway and overproduction of toxic heme precursors. There are three principal types of porphyria: porphyria cutanea tarda, (PCT), acute intermittent porphyria, and protoporphyria.

This patient's clinical picture is consistent with PCT: the most common porphyria affecting 5–10 persons per 100 000 people. The cause is inhibition of the fifth enzyme in heme biosynthetic pathway: uroporphyrinogen decarboxylase. PCT is associated with several precipitating factors such as haemochromatosis (53%) and uroporphyrinogen decarboxylase mutations (17%), as well as hepatitis C (69%), alcohol (8%), tobacco (81%), oestrogen (6%), and HIV (15%). Typically, patients are >40 year old and male. The clinical picture is of painless blistering lesions in sun exposed areas, typically the back of the hands. Sun exposed skin can be friable, scarred, or develop hypertrichosis. Remission may occur in the winter months, if sunlight exposure is decreased. Urine is brown–reddish, due to excess uroporphyrin. PCT is usually associated with mild abnormal LFTs. Advanced liver disease is uncommon at initial presentation but may be seen in older patients with recurrent disease. Diagnosis is made with an elevated urine or plasma porphyrin with predominantly uroporphyrin and heptacarboxyporphyrin. Erythrocyte porphyrins are usually normal. A total plasma porphyrin measurement may be most useful for initial screening. A skin biopsy reveals subepidermal bullae. Wood's lamp examination of the urine shows orange red fluorescence.

First line treatment for PCT involves addressing modifiable risk factors: treating hepatitis C or HIV if present, and restricting alcohol, tobacco, and oestrogen. These factors, in combination with hepatic iron depletion via phlebotomy or iron chelation to a target ferritin at the low end of the normal range, often produces remission. Hydroxychloroquine is an alternative to iron depletion. Once in remission, patients may relapse, especially if they drink >4 standard drinks/ day or continue smoking, so urine or plasma uroporphyrin should be measured annually.

Acute intermittent porphyria is an autosomal dominant partial deficiency of the third enzyme of heme synthesis: porphobilinogen deaminase (or hydroxymehtlbilane synthase). 90% of patients are females, typically presenting aged 18–45 with a prodrome of days of severe fatigue and lack of concentration, then worsening abdominal pain, nausea, vomiting, afebrile tachycardia, and neurological signs including weakness dysthesia, and seizures (20% of patients). Risk factors include cytochrome P450 inducers, oral contraceptive pill, and severely restricted caloric intake. Abdominal exam is often unremarkable and blood tests usually show mild liver derangement and hyponatremia. Diagnosis requires elevated porphobilinogen in urine and plasma, often up to 10–150x normal. Urine colour can be unremarkable, however if exposed to light can turn dark amber when heme precursors form uroporphyrin-like-pigments. Treatment is primarily supportive: fluids (preferable 10% dextrose in 0.45% saline), antiemetics, analgesics, and anticonvulsants. Of note, many anticonvulsants are not safe in acute porphyria, including phenytoin, valproic acid, carbamazepine, clonazepam. Intravenous heme is the only specific treatment but is not widely available.

Protoporphyria occurs when there is bone marrow overproduction of protoporphyrin. It is typically diagnosed in early childhood, with toddlers develop pain, stinging, oedema, and itching of sun exposed skin often within 10 minutes of being in the sun but can be longer in adults. Total blood porphyrin over five times the upper limit of normal is diagnostic. Urine colour is normal as protoporphyrin is universally excreted into bile. This leads to complications such as gallstones and cholestasis. Treatment with oral beta-carotene is most effective, but only works in <1/3 of cases. Activated charcoal, and colestipol are also trialled but often ineffective. Avoidance of sunlight is the main treatment for most patients, is associated with vitamin D deficiency in 50% of patients.

Bullous pemphigoid is a subepidermal blistering disorder that most commonly occurs in older adults. The classic skin lesions are urticarial plaques and tense bullae on the trunk and extremities. Intense pruritus is common, and lesions typically do not scar. Cutaneous lichen planus is most commonly expressed as an eruption of shiny, flat, polygonal, violaceous papules. Dermatitis herpetiformis is an autoimmune blistering disease associated with coeliac disease and characterised by intensely itchy polymorphous vesicular lesions located over the extensor surfaces, back, and scalp.

Bissell D, Anderson K, Bonkovsky H. Porphyria. New England Journal of Medicine. 2017;377(9):862–872. https://www.nejm.org/doi/full/10.1056/NEJMra1608634

8. Answer: C

Rosacea is an inflammatory facial condition of unknown cause associated with high morbidity due to social avoidance, and mood disorder. Rosacea most commonly manifests in middle age, mostly effects women, and can present with flushing and telangiectasia, inflammatory papules and pustules, or a combination of both. Keratitis is commonly seen in rosacea, but is rarely severe enough to be vision threatening. Long-term sequelae include phymatous changes, most commonly of the nose.

Despite the unclear pathophysiology, several anti-inflammatory, and vasoactive medications have been shown to significantly improve symptoms associated with the condition. Topical medications blockading alpha-receptors significantly reduce vascular symptoms – for example brimonidine and oxymetazoline. For inflammatory symptoms, medications such as metronidazole, ivermectin, azelaic acid have shown significant efficacy. For lesions refractory to topical therapy, combination with low-dose oral doxycycline or tetracycline is indicated, and for cases refractory to this, low-dose isotretinoin is effective. For inflamed phymatous changes, anti-inflammatory treatments can be effective, but for more fibrosed lesions, ablative laser therapies can be effective.

van Zuuren E. Rosacea. New England Journal of Medicine. 2017;377(18):1754–1764. https://www.nejm.org/doi/full/10.1056/NEJMcp1506630?af=R&rss=currentIssue&page=2&sort=newest

9. Answer: B

In developed countries, scabies epidemics occur primarily in nursing homes, prisons and other long-term care facilities. Transmission of scabies is predominantly through direct skin-to-skin contact. Prevalence rates for scabies are higher in sexually active individuals, immunocompromised, and elderly patients. The *S scabiei hominis* mite that infects humans is female and is large enough (0.3–0.4 mm long) to be seen with the naked eye. Its life cycle occurs completely on the human, but the mite is able to live on bedding, clothes, or other surfaces at room temperature for 2–3 days, while remaining capable of infestation and burrowing.

Patients usually present with pruritus, erythematous papules, and vesicles in webbed spaces of the fingers, wrist, elbows, and scrotum. Burrows are a pathognomonic sign and represent the intraepidermal tunnel created by the moving female mite.

There are three types of scabies:

1. Classic scabies: Typically, 10–15 mites live on the host. After 4 weeks of primary infection and with subsequent infections, a delayed type IV hypersensitivity reaction to the mites and eggs occurs, which causes the classic skin eruption and its associated intense pruritus.
2. Crusted scabies is a distinctive and highly contagious form of the disease. In this variant, hundreds to millions of mites infest the patient, who is usually immunocompromised, elderly, or physically or mentally disabled and impaired. It can be confused with severe dermatitis or psoriasis because widespread, crusted lesions appear with thick, hyperkeratotic scales over the elbows, knees, palms, and soles. Serum IgE and IgG levels are high in patients with crusted scabies, but the immune reaction is not protective. Crusted scabies carries a higher mortality rate than the classic form of the disease, because of the frequency of secondary bacterial infections.
3. Nodular scabies occur in 7–10% of patients with scabies, particularly young children.

The diagnosis of scabies can often be made clinically in patients with a pruritic rash and characteristic linear burrows. The diagnosis is confirmed by light microscopic identification of mites, larvae, ova, or scybala (feces) in skin scrapings, and skin biopsy is not required.

Scabies treatment includes administration of a scabicidal agent such as permethrin, lindane, ivermectin. There is no single agent ranked most effective with respect to cure and control of adverse effects from the scabies infection.

Chandlera DJ. A Review of Scabies: An Infestation More than Skin Deep. Dermatology 2019;235:79–90. https://www.karger.com/Article/FullText/495290

10. Answer: C

Organ transplant recipients are at a higher risk (up to a 100-fold higher) for developing skin cancer compared to the general population. Heart and lung transplant patients develop skin cancer more frequently than liver or kidney transplant patients. The common skin cancers after solid organ transplant are squamous cell carcinoma (SCC), basal cell carcinoma (BCC), melanoma, and Merkel cell carcinoma (MCC). This higher risk is due to immunosuppression. Many centres advise transplant patients to check their skin monthly for worrisome lesions and have yearly dermatological review. Patients should practise adequate sun protection measures, including using sunscreen and wearing protective clothing and be aware of the significant UV exposure that can occur in all seasons.

Sunlight consists of two types of harmful rays that reach the earth: UVA and UVB rays. Overexposure to either can lead to skin cancer. In addition to causing skin cancer, UVA rays can cause age spots or solar lentigines, UVB rays are the primary cause of sunburn.

It is recommended to use a broad-spectrum sunscreen with a Sun Protection Factor (SPF) of at least 30, which blocks 97% of the sun's UVB rays. Broad spectrum sunscreen can protect skin from both harmful UVA rays and the UVB rays. Higher-number SPFs block slightly more of the sun's UVB rays, but no sunscreen can block 100% of the sun's UVB rays. High-number SPFs last the same amount of time as low-number SPFs and high-number SPF does not allow you to spend additional time outdoors without reapplication. Sunscreens should be reapplied approximately every two hours when outdoors.

There are two types of sunscreen: (i) Chemical sunscreens, which work by absorbing the sun's rays. They contain one or more of the following active ingredients, oxybenzone, avobenzone, octisalate, octocrylene, homosalate, or octinoxate, (ii) Physical or mineral sunscreens act like a shield deflecting the sun's rays. They contain the active ingredients titanium dioxide, zinc oxide, or both, which are safe for sensitive skin. Using sunscreen can decrease skin's production of vitamin D.

 Iannacone MR. Effects of sunscreen on skin cancer and photoaging. Photodermatol Photoimmunol Photomed 2014; 30: 55–61. https://onlinelibrary.wiley.com/doi/full/10.1111/phpp.12109

11. Answer: B

The skin is made up of three layers, the most superficial layer is the epidermis and the layer below is the dermis, followed by the third layer of subcutaneous tissue. The epidermis is further divided into five layers in areas of thick skin, such as the palms and soles: stratum basale, stratum spinosum, stratum granulosum, stratum lucidum, and stratum corneum. While in areas of thinner skin, the epidermis has four layers, without the stratum lucidum.

The dermis is further divided into two layers, the papillary dermis (the upper layer) and the reticular dermis (the lower layer) which contains the vasculature. The skin is highly vascularised; there is an extensive network of larger blood vessels and capillaries that extend from regional branches of the systemic circulation to local sites throughout subcutaneous tissue and dermis, respectively. Therefore, it is likely that the excision has traversed the reticular dermis to cause profuse bleeding. In addition, there is an extensive lymphatic network that runs alongside many of the skin's blood vessels, particularly those attached to the venous end of the capillary networks.

12. Answer: D

Stevens Johnson Syndrome (SJS)/Toxic Epidermal Necrolysis (TEN) are severe skin disorders characterised by mucosal involvement, extensive skin necrosis and epidermal detachment. SJS is classified by <10% body surface area (BSA) involvement, Overlap syndrome 10–20% BSA and TEN >30% BSA. It is usually caused by antibiotics, anticonvulsants, allopurinol, and anti-inflammatory medications commenced 2–3 weeks prior to presentation.

Supportive care has been shown to be the most important treatment for patients with SJS/TEN. It should consist of managing skin wounds, haemodynamic stability, electrolyte balance, maintenance of airway and pain control. Guidelines suggest that covering the denuded skin can improve skin barrier function, reduce water and protein loss, limit microbial colonisation and promote reepithelialisation.

Systemic steroids were considered to be the primary treatment option for many years, however recent studies have reported a lack of efficacy and in some cases worsened mortality from increased risk of infection, delayed healing and prolonged hospitalisation. The use of IVIG has had controversial conflicting results. A recent meta-analysis showed no difference in mortality when comparing patients who received IVIG compared to those who received supportive care. Although some studies have showed that higher dosages of IVIG may lower mortality.

There have also been several case reports with positive results for TNFα inhibitors such as Etanercept in the treatment of SJS/TEN. There is one published case series of 10 patients who responded well with complete reepithelialisation, however it will need further studies to validate these results. Cyclosporine is an immunosuppressive agent inhibiting CD8+ T cells. One study found a significant and beneficial effect of cyclosporine when compared to supportive care. Although it seems to be a promising treatment, it is contraindicated in patients with severe renal dysfunction, infection, malignancy, and sepsis. Patients with SJS/TEN often have secondary infection, organ dysfunction, and other comorbidities, which limits its use.

 Duong T, Valeyrie-Allanore L, Wolkenstein P, Chosidow O. Severe cutaneous adverse reactions to drugs. The Lancet. 2017;390(10106):1996–2011.
https://www.thelancet.com/journals/lancet/article/PIIS0140-6736(16)30378-6/fulltext

13.   Answer: F

14.   Answer: A

15.   Answer: E

16.   Answer: G

17.   Answer: H

Dermatological emergencies are usually accompanied by severe and often striking visual appearance and are often indicative of systemic illness with high morbidity and mortality, necessitating rapid diagnosis and treatment.

The SCARs (severe cutaneous adverse reactions) encompass a group of T-cell mediated, type IV hypersensitivity reactions which are often stimulated by medications or their metabolites. SCARs include Stevens-Johnson syndrome (SJS), toxic-epidermal necrolysis (TEN), drug rash with eosinophilia and systemic symptoms (DRESS), acute generalised exanthematous pustulosis (AGEP), and SJS/TENs overlap.

SJS and TEN are now recognised as two points on the spectrum of the same pathologic process. SJS and TEN are rare SCARs which are characterised by significant epidermal and mucosal loss. Typically, SJS/TEN will occur 7–10 days after initiation a culprit drug, and classically starts on the face and trunk and rapidly spreads over a few days – lesions can be macular or targetoid and desquamate over time. Nikolsky's sign, where rubbed skin leads to exfoliation of the outermost layer, is typically positive, and mucosal surfaces are often involved. Classification is by percentage of body area involved; less than 10% is SJS, between 10 and 30% is SJS/TEN overlap, and greater than 30% is TEN. Acute respiratory distress, bacteraemia, and other infections are common complications, and mortality is high. Treatment is by ceasing the offending drug, aggressive supportive care, and sometimes IVIG.

DRESS is characterised by a widespread rash – most typically a maculopapular morbilliform exanthem, i.e. the rash looks like measles – fever and visceral organ involvement. Hypereosinophilia is common as is facial oedema and lymphadenopathy – mucosa is spared. The rash usually develops greater than three weeks after starting a medication and persists after cessation. Cessation of the drug, supportive measures and prednisolone are the usual treatments. Fatality is lower than with SJS/TEN but approaches 10%.

AGEP has the lowest mortality of the SCARs, with some modern case series showing no fatalities. However, this drug rash is still striking, with widespread or skin fold erythema evolving to innumerable pinhead-sized sterile pustules, and typically resolving within two weeks of drug cessation. AGEP is thought to be mediated through T-cell activation of neutrophils. Spider bites have been thought to cause AGEP, and the rash shares similarities with pustular psoriasis, but with a more acute onset. Major morbidity and occasional mortality can usually be attributed to bacterial superinfection of the lesions.

Dermatological emergencies can also be caused by, or be indicative of, severe infection. Staphylococcal scalded skin syndrome (SSSS) is a highly feared complication of infection with *Staphylococcus aureus* secreting exfoliative toxin. Most commonly experienced by children, where fatality rates are lower, SSSS has high mortality rates in adults, of around 50%. Erythematous areas in SSSS typically develop around the face, neck, axilla, and perineum, and progress to flaccid bullae, mucous membranes are typically spared. Nikolsky's sign is positive. Treatment is with antibiotics and supportive care, usually involving intravenous fluids and nasogastric feeding.

Meningococcal septicaemia is characterised by rash, which is typically maculo-papular and blanching when seen very early in the disease course, and remains blanching in 10 to 15% of cases, and 5 to 10% of patients do not develop rash. However, around 70% of patients have the typical, non-blanching rash, which is either petechial or purpuric, on presentation to hospital. Given the severe nature of invasive meningococcal disease, other symptoms and signs need to be taken into account in presumptive diagnosis – the rash is not sensitive enough.

Necrotising fasciitis is a severe subcutaneous infection that requires surgical debridement in addition to antibiotics. Early diagnosis has positive impact on outcome, and typically, early infection resembles severe cellulitis except for severe tenderness, severe sepsis, and rapidly progressive rash, signs which should prompt a high index of suspicion for the disease. Type I necrotising fasciitis is typically polymicrobial with both aerobic and anaerobic bacteria, whereas type II is monomicrobial, and usually caused by Group A *Streptococcus*.

Disseminated candidiasis with skin lesions is a rare complication of profound immune suppression, most commonly neutropaenic patients with acute myeloid leukaemia during induction therapy. Diffuse maculopapular lesions predominate in cases caused by *Candida tropicalis,* and nodular or papular lesions in cases caused by *Candida krusei.*

Vashi N. The Dermatology Handbook. Cham: Springer International Publishing; 2019. https://link.springer.com/chapter/10.1007/978-3-030-15157-7_5

4 Endocrinology

Questions

Answers can be found in the Endocrinology Answers section at the end of this chapter.

1. A 48-year-old woman is referred by her GP with a 3-month history of headaches and night sweats for investigation. Her medical history includes difficult to control hypertension for 5 years which requires 3 agents; OSA on CPAP treatment, glucose intolerance, and total hysterectomy 7 years ago. On examination, BP is 156/95 mmHg, her hands are large, and she is no longer able to wear her ring. There is no hirsutism buts there is coarseness of her facial features. Her laboratory test results and MRI of head are shown below.

Tests	Results	Normal values
HbA1c	6.5%	<6.0%
Cortisol (9 am)	320 nmol/L	133–540
Free T4	15 pmol/L	10–20
Prolactin	278 mIU/L	90–630
Estradiol	48 pg/ml	15–350
Growth hormone (GH)	362 pmol/L	<226
Insulin like growth factor 1 (IGF-1)	748 ng/ml	<320

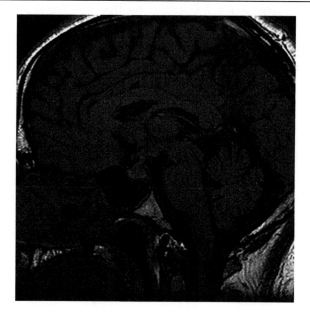

What is the most appropriate next step for this patient?
- **A.** Inferior petrosal sinus sampling for growth hormone.
- **B.** Measurement of growth hormone after insulin induced hypoglycaemia.
- **C.** Measurement of growth hormone releasing hormone (GHRH).
- **D.** Referral to neurosurgery.

How to Pass the FRACP Written Examination, First Edition. Jonathan Gleadle, Jordan Li, Danielle Wu, and Paul Kleinig.
© 2022 John Wiley & Sons Ltd. Published 2022 by John Wiley & Sons Ltd.

2. A 28-year-old woman presents to the emergency department with symptoms of nausea, vomiting, diarrhoea, severe lethargy, weakness, and drowsiness. Her BP is 85/45 mmHg, heart rate is 98 bpm, respiratory rate is 13/min, blood glucose level is 5.6 mmol/L [3.2–5.5 fasting], and temperature is 38°C. Her serum sodium level is 130 mmol/L [135–145] and potassium level is 5.8 mmol/L [3.5–5.2]. You find a MedicAlert necklace which says, 'Adrenal insufficiency'.

Which one of the following steps of management is **INCORRECT**?
   A. Administer IV hydrocortisone 100 mg stat followed by IV hydrocortisone 50 mg qid.
   B. Administer IV 0.9% normal saline 1 L within the first hour.
   C. Avoid giving corticosteroid due to the potential risks of worsening sepsis.
   D. Perform a septic screen and start empirical broad-spectrum antibiotics.

3. A 65-year-old woman was referred by her GP to the general medicine clinic with a 2.5 cm adrenal mass during investigation for abdominal discomfort. She reports no symptoms of headache, sweating, palpitations, significant weight changes, night sweats, fever, nausea, vomiting or proximal muscle weakness. She has a history of hypertension, type 2 diabetes, obesity, and osteoporosis.

Which one of the following investigations is **NOT** indicated at this stage?
   A. 24-hr urinary fractionated metanephrine and catecholamine collection.
   B. Overnight dexamethasone (1 mg) suppression test.
   C. Plasma aldosterone and plasma renin activity measurement.
   D. Positron-emission tomography (PET) scan.

4. A 65-year-old man is referred to the endocrine clinic with a 6-week history of unintentional weight loss (5 kg), diarrhoea, myopathy and lethargy. He has a history of atrial fibrillation, diagnosed one year previously. He was started on amiodarone and warfarin but he reverted to sinus rhythm spontaneously at which point the amiodarone was stopped 6 months prior to presentation. On examination, there is no obvious goitre. He has an irregularly irregular pulse at 90 bpm. His skin is warm and sweaty. His TSH level is 0.2 mIU/L [0.4–4.0], Free T4 level 30 pmol/L [9.0–25.0], and Free T3 10–pmol/L [3.5–7.8].

Which one of the following management strategies is correct?
   A. Commence carbimazole.
   B. Commence high-dose oral prednisolone.
   C. Commence carbimazole and high-dose oral prednisolone.
   D. Referral for thyroidectomy.

5. A 23-year-old woman presents to hospital because of a 3-day history of confusion, cough, white sputum and fever. She is diagnosed with a lower respiratory tract infection and commenced on intravenous penicillin and normal saline infusion. She was diagnosed with type 1 diabetes at age 6. She is currently receiving short acting insulin three times a day before meals and insulin glargine at night. She has had several hypoglycaemic episodes recently. She has been intermittently taking thyroxine 100 mcg daily for 5 years after being diagnosed with hypothyroidism. She has not been feeling well in the past 4 months, experiencing fatigue, nausea, poor appetite, and weight loss of approximately 7 kg. On examination, she is afebrile, BP is 85/50 mmHg and HR is 110 bpm, the rest of her physical examination is unremarkable. The initial investigation results are shown below.

Tests	Results	Normal values
Sodium	128 mmol/L	135–145
Potassium	5.5 mmol/L	3.5–5.2
Bicarbonate	24 mmol/L	22–32
Urea	28 mmol/L	2.7–8.0
Creatinine	123 μmol/L	45–90
Glucose	16.3 mmol/L	3.2–5.5
Calcium	2.95 mmol/L	2.1–2.6
Hb	140 g/L	115–155
WBC	7.1 x10⁹/L	4–11
CRP	7 mg/L	0–8
HbA1c	8.6%	<6%

What is the most appropriate immediate next treatment?
   A. Commence insulin infusion.
   B. Give double dose of thyroxine immediately.
   C. Give intravenous norepinephrine.
   D. Intravenous hydrocortisone.

6. Which one of the following is a characteristic of brown adipocytes?
   A. Adiponectin secretion.
   B. Leptin secretion.
   C. Storage of energy-yielding triglycerides.
   D. Uncoupling protein 1–containing mitochondria.

7. A 37-year-old woman is referred by her GP following a low energy fracture to her right distal radius. She is a current heavy smoker. She is diagnosed to have osteoporosis with bone mineral density Z score of –2.8 in the lumbar spine. She is obese with BMI 33 kg/m². BP is 150/95 mmHg. She has facial rubor and proximal muscle weakness. Her 24-hour urine free cortisol excretion is 55 µg [3.5–45]. Baseline serum 8 a.m. cortisol level is 320 µg/L [70–280] and is 310 µg/L the following morning after taking 1 mg dexamethasone. The baseline plasma level of adrenocorticotropic hormone (ACTH) is 8 pg/ml [10–90].
   Where is the most likely anatomical location of her clinical presentations?
   A. Adrenal cortex.
   B. Hypothalamus.
   C. Lung.
   D. Pituitary gland.

8. While treating a patient with stage 2 CKD due to diabetic nephropathy (DN) with significant proteinuria and hypertension, which one of the recommendations is appropriate?
   A. ACE inhibitor has better renoprotective effects in patients with DN than angiotensin II receptor blocker (ARB) and the renoprotective effect of ACE inhibitor is dose-related.
   B. Dual Renin-Angiotensin-Aldosterone System (RAAS) blockade with both ACE inhibitor and ARB should be prescribed as it has better antiproteinuric effect compared to monotherapy.
   C. Intensive glycaemic control in patients with type 2 diabetes reduces incidence and progression of DN and all-cause mortality.
   D. Intensive glycaemic control reduces progression of DN in type 1 diabetes; this benefit persists even after the patient returns to suboptimal glycaemic control.

9. A 32-year-old man presents to the emergency department with nausea, vomiting, and diffuse abdominal pain. He has had type I diabetes since age 7, which is treated with an intensive insulin regimen (insulin glargine 24 IU at bedtime and rapid-acting insulin analogue before each meal). On examination, he is febrile and tachypnoeic. HR is 106 bpm and BP is 90/60 mmHg; he also has dry mucous membranes and poor skin turgor. He is slightly confused. The result of the strip for ketone bodies in urine is strongly positive and the concentration of β –Hydroxybutyric acid (β–OHB) in serum is elevated at 3.5 mmol/L [<0.5]. His ABG at room air demonstrates pH 7.11, PO_2 95 mmHg, PCO_2 28 mmHg. His other initial investigation results are shown below.

Tests	Results	Normal values
Sodium	149 mmol/L	135–145
Potassium	4.5 mmol/L	3.5–5.2
Bicarbonate	11 mmol/L	22–32
Urea	28 mmol/L	2.7–8.0
Creatinine	143 µmol/L	60–110
Glucose	26.3 mmol/L	3.2–5.5
Calcium	2.85 mmol/L	2.10–2.60
Hb	138 g/L	135–175
WBC	17.1 x10⁹/L	4–11
CRP	57 mg/L	0–8
HbA1c	9.6%	–

Which one of the following resuscitation treatment plans suggested by the emergency department team is the **LEAST** appropriate?
   A. Intravenous 0.9% sodium chloride 1000 ml/hour.
   B. Intravenous 8.4% sodium bicarbonate 100 ml over 1 hour.
   C. Intravenous potassium replacement with second bag of 0.9% sodium chloride.
   D. Intravenous short acting insulin and hold long-acting insulin analogue.

10. A 58-year-old man is concerned regarding his inability to maintain an erection satisfactory for sexual intercourse over the past 6 months. He has had type 2 diabetes for 10 years, but his glycaemic control has been good with the most recent HbA1c at 7%. His other medical problems include hypertension, peripheral vascular disease, and hyperlipidaemia. His medication includes perindopril, gliclazide, metformin, amlodipine, and atorvastatin.

Which of the following is **INCORRECT** regarding the management of erectile dysfunction?
   A. Measure morning total testosterone levels.
   B. Perform an exercise stress echocardiogram.
   C. Sildenafil treatment increases overall cardiovascular risk.
   D. Sildenafil treatment has a 65% chance of enabling satisfactory intercourse.

11. Which of the following chemotherapeutic agents carries the highest risk for inducing premature ovarian failure?
   A. Cyclophosphamide.
   B. Doxorubicin.
   C. Gemcitabine.
   D. Paclitaxel.

12. A 70-year-old man presents for follow-up after recent initiation of citalopram for his depressed mood. He reports that his mood and sleep have improved, but his lethargy, low libido, and erectile dysfunction have not. He has a past history of type 2 diabetes. His BMI is 29 kg/m². His HbA1c is 8.2%. His other current medications are empagliflozin and metformin. His fasting serum total testosterone level is between 6.4 and 6.7 nmol/L [8–30] on repeated measures, serum prolactin is 120 mIU/L [<325].

Which of the following clinical benefits is he most likely to experience as a result of testosterone treatment?
   A. Better glycaemic control.
   B. Decreased fracture risk.
   C. Improved erectile function and libido.
   D. More energy.

13. A 35-year-old man with ESKD is on chronic haemodialysis. He has severe secondary hyperparathyroidism and has undergone a parathyroidectomy. Which one of the following biochemical abnormalities is the most likely to cause significant post-operative complications and will require intensive monitoring post-parathyroidectomy?
   A. Hypocalcaemia.
   B. Hypokalaemia.
   C. Hypomagnesaemia.
   D. Hypophosphataemia.

14. Which of the following metabolites is particularly important for macrophage and dendritic cell function?
   A. Citrate.
   B. Fumarate.
   C. Malate.
   D. Oxaloacetate.

15. A 29-year-old man has hypercalcaemia due to primary hyperparathyroidism which was treated with subtotal parathyroidectomy. During the perioperative period he complains of episodic headaches and palpitations. He is found to be hypertensive. Further investigations reveal that his 24-hour urinary noradrenaline and adrenaline are 615 nmol/L [0–450] and 750 nmol/L [0–100] respectively. His serum calcitonin is also elevated at 135.5 ng/L [0–5.5].

Which one of the following genes should be considered for mutational analyses?
   A. *CDNK1B* gene.
   B. *MEN1* tumour suppressor gene.
   C. *RET* proto-oncogene.
   D. *Von Hippel-Lindau (VHL)* gene.

16. Which one of the following tests is **LEAST** useful in distinguishing between type 1 diabetes and maturity-onset diabetes of the young (MODY)?
   A. C-Peptide levels.
   B. Insulin autoantibodies (IAA).
   C. Islet cell cytoplasmic autoantibodies (ICA).
   D. Ketonuria.

17. Which of the following options best describe the pathogenesis of Paget's disease of bone?
   A. Increased osteoclast and osteoblast activity.
   B. Increased osteoclast and reduced osteoblast activity.
   C. Reduced osteoclast and increased osteoblast activity.
   D. Reduced osteoclast and osteoblast activity.

18. Regarding painful diabetic neuropathy, which of the following is correct?
   A. Approximately 80% of patients with diabetic neuropathy will suffer from pain.
   B. The prevalence of painful neuropathy in type 2 diabetes is more than twice that seen in type 1 diabetes.
   C. The intensity of pain is proportional to the degree of neuropathy.
   D. Tight glycaemic control in type 2 diabetes reduces the occurrence of painful neuropathy.

19. Which of the statements describing the pathogenesis of diabetic gastroparesis is **INCORRECT**?
   A. Enteric neuropathy increases transient lower oesophageal sphincter relaxation.
   B. Hyperglycaemia induces pyloric contraction, antral hypomotility and delays gastric emptying.
   C. Loss of interstitial cells of Cajal is the commonest enteric neuropathological abnormality in diabetic gastroparesis.
   D. Vagal neuropathy leads to reduced pyloric relaxation and impaired antral contraction.

20. A 35-year-old woman is diagnosed with phenotype A polycystic ovarian syndrome. Which one of following is **NOT** an associated consequence?
   A. Associated with 80% of cases of anovulatory infertility.
   B. Associated with increased risk of breast cancer.
   C. Associated with increased risk of endometrial cancer.
   D. Associated with increased risk of non-alcoholic fatty liver disease.

21. A 63-year-old woman has resistant hypertension. She is currently taking four antihypertensive medications. She is referred to the general medicine outpatient clinic by her GP after the discovery of a mildly elevated plasma metanephrine level. The GP is concerned that she may have a phaeochromocytoma.
   What is the next most appropriate investigation?
   A. 24-hour urinary fractionated catecholamines and metanephrines.
   B. 24-hour urinary vanillylmandelic acid.
   C. Plasma catecholamines and metanephrines.
   D. MRI abdomen.

22. A 42-year-old woman with known type 1 diabetes presents to renal outpatient clinic for review of worsening renal function. Her type 1 diabetes is treated with glargine and short acting insulin Novorapid. She is waiting gynaecology appointment review for irregular vaginal bleeding, and also has chronic liver disease due to excessive alcohol consumption. You note her most recent HbA1c is 10.5% and her usual reading in the past is 8.5%. Her mean blood glucose measurement before meals in the past 3 months is 10.5mmol/L, which is consistent with an HbA1c of 8.3%.
   What is the most likely cause for the worsening of HbA1c in this patient?
   A. Chronic alcoholism.
   B. Chronic liver disease.
   C. Iron deficiency due to vaginal bleeding.
   D. Worsening of chronic kidney disease.

23. A 55-year-old woman presents with a 2-month history of frontal headache. She reports having two car accidents recently which she attributed to not being able to see the right side of her car as she changed lanes. She had menopause at age of 50 and has no significant medical history and is taking no medications. The neurological examination reveals a right superior temporal visual field deficit. Her MRI head is shown below. Further investigation reveals normal TSH and T4 levels. Her IGF-1, LH, FSH levels are also normal. Her early morning cortisol level is slightly low but the short Synacthen test demonstrates normal serum cortisol levels post-Synacthen. The prolactin level is 54 ng/mL [<20].

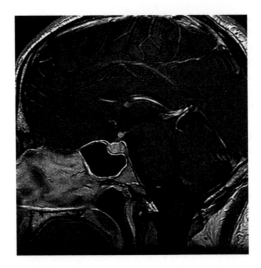

What is the most appropriate next step in her management plan?
- **A.** Consider transsphenoidal surgery.
- **B.** Start cabergoline.
- **C.** Start cortisol replacement.
- **D.** Watch and wait approach, repeat macroprolactin level.

24. A 27-year-old farmer suffers from brittle type 1 diabetes with impaired hypoglycaemic awareness. He is currently on a basal bolus regimen. His most recent HbA1c is 7.1%. You are considering real-time continuous glucose monitoring (RTCGM). Which one of the clinical statements regarding the usage of RTCGM in this patient is correct?
- **A.** RTCGM provides continuous accurate measurement at 1–5 min increments of blood glucose concentrations.
- **B.** RTCGM provides no benefit in this patient because he is not using an insulin pump.
- **C.** RTCGM reduces time spent in the hyperglycaemic ranges but not hypoglycaemic range due to less accurate measurement at lower glucose.
- **D.** RTCGM will benefit this patient despite having achieved good blood glucose control.

25. Which of the following complications is most clearly and often associated with treatment with dapagliflozin in comparison to other diabetic treatments?
- **A.** Acute kidney injury.
- **B.** Amputation.
- **C.** Diabetic ketoacidosis.
- **D.** Urinary tract infection.

26. A 32-year-old woman presents with fatigue and self-reported memory issues. She has no deficits on formal cognitive testing. She has no significant past medical or surgical history. Basic investigations reveal normal full blood examination, electrolytes, and liver function tests. Urine pregnancy test is negative. Thyroid function tests reveal FT4 of 12 pmol/L [10–20] and TSH of 6.7 mIU/L [0.5–4.5].
   Which of the following options represents the most appropriate next step?
- **A.** Initiate levothyroxine treatment.
- **B.** Measure thyroid stimulating antibodies.
- **C.** No further action required.
- **D.** Repeat TSH and T4 measurement in 1–3 months.

27. A 65-year-old woman has had a total thyroidectomy and radioactive iodine for treatment of papillary thyroid carcinoma. She had an excellent response to the initial treatment and is on an appropriate dose of thyroxine therapy. Six months later a neck ultrasound showed no residual thyroid disease.

What other investigation should be performed at this time?
   A. Anti-thyroperoxidase antibody.
   B. Anti-thyroid stimulating hormone receptor antibody.
   C. Thyroglobulin.
   D. Whole body bone scan.

28. In which of the following pathways are driver mutations most frequently found in thyroid cancer?
   A. Mitogen-activated protein kinase (MAPK).
   B. Myc.
   C. Phosphoinositide 3-kinase/protein kinase B/mechanistic target of rapamycin (PI3k/AKT/mTOR).
   D. Tumour protein p53.

29. A 38-year-old man presents to his GP with a 3 cm mobile thyroid nodule. His thyroid function tests are normal. A fine-needle aspirate is performed under ultrasound guidance. The cytologic findings are reported as non-diagnostic.
   What is the next most appropriate investigation?
   A. Analyse fine-needle aspirate for *BRAF* and *RAS* mutation.
   B. Measure serum calcitonin level.
   C. Repeat fine-needle aspiration within 3 months.
   D. Repeat thyroid ultrasound within 6 months.

30. A 37-year-old transgender (TGD) person is seeking feminising hormone therapy. Which one of the following should be avoided in the gender-affirming medical care?
   A. Anti-androgens should be avoided.
   B. Cyproterone acetate should be avoided.
   C. Gonadotrophin-releasing hormone analogues should be avoided.
   D. Progestins should be avoided.

QUESTIONS (31–34) REFER TO THE FOLLOWING INFORMATION

Match the clinical presentation, symptoms, and signs with metabolic and nutritional complications after bariatric surgery.
   A. Calcium deficiency.
   B. Copper deficiency.
   C. Iron deficiency.
   D. Vitamin A deficiency.
   E. Vitamin B1 deficiency.
   F. Vitamin B12 deficiency.
   G. Vitamin D deficiency.
   H. Zinc deficiency.

31. A 50-year-old man underwent a gastric banding because of OSA, type 2 diabetes. Post-surgery, he developed chronic inter-mittent nausea and vomiting. He is now admitted with high output heart failure.

32. A 48-year-old man underwent a gastric sleeve operation for his morbid obesity 12 months ago. On his annual outpatient review, he complains of tingling in fingers and toes. He states that his memory is very poor. He has a tendency to stumble. He is diagnosed to have depression by his GP recently despite the significant weight loss. His blood test arranged by his GP shows macrocytic anaemia and mild abnormal LFTs.

33. A 49-year-old woman reported flashes in the eyes with poor night vision and reduced visual acuity for 8 weeks. She had a Roux-en-Y gastric bypass surgery 3 years ago. Ophthalmology evaluations revealed bilateral visual acuity of 6/36. Humphrey visual fields showed peripheral constriction in both eyes without a central scotoma. Slit-lamp examination revealed conjunctival xerosis in both eyes. Bitot's spots and relative afferent papillary defects were absent. Fundoscopy examination revealed optic atrophy but normal appearing macula, vessels, and peripheral retina in both eyes.

34. A 48-year-old woman underwent a biliopancreatic diversion several years ago. She suffers skin or respiratory tract infections frequently. Her skin wound heals very slowly. She complains of blunting of taste sense, hair loss leading to alopecia. There is clinical evidence of glossitis.

QUESTIONS (35–5–36) REFER TO THE FOLLOWING INFORMATION
Match the clinical presentation with the appropriate endocrine investigations.
- **A.** 24-hour urinary catecholamines and metanephrines.
- **B.** 24-hour urinary cortisol.
- **C.** Blood renin/aldosterone ratio.
- **D.** Plasma vasopressin level.
- **E.** Saline infusion test.
- **F.** Thyroid function test.
- **G.** Urinary sodium and osmolality.
- **H.** Water deprivation test.

35. A 76-year-old woman presents with confusion. Her family reports her being constipated and gaining 5 kg weight in recent months. On examination, she is alert but disoriented in time and place. Her HR is 52 bpm and BP is 158/95 mmHg. There is non-pitting oedema in the bilateral low limbs. The CXR reveals cardiomegaly and bilateral small pleural effusions. Apart from mild hyponatraemia (serum sodium level 133 mmol/L), other biochemistry results are unremarkable. What is the next most appropriate investigation?

36. A 68-year-old woman presents after a two-day history of vomiting. She is found to have hypernatraemia but her elevated serum sodium concentration did not improve despite adequate fluid replacement. She has history of bipolar disorder and has been taking lithium for the past 8 years. What is the appropriate investigation after stabilizing this patient clinically?

Answers

1. Answer: D

This patient has typical clinical features of acromegaly. She has elevated insulin like growth factor 1 (IGF-1) and growth hormone (GH) levels. The MRI demonstrates a large pituitary tumour. There is NO need for further investigation. She needs referral for neurosurgery.

Acromegaly is a severe disease resulting from GH hypersecretion, usually caused by a pituitary adenoma. It is associated with cardiovascular, cerebrovascular, and respiratory disorders, malignancies, and a high mortality. The onset of acromegaly in adults is usually insidious. Typical physical examination findings include hand and foot enlargement, facial bone enlargement and acral/soft tissue changes.

Investigation in a suspected patient involves measurement of IGF-1 and GH. Elevated IGF-I levels in a patient with clinical features of acromegaly almost always indicate GH excess. In subjects with elevated or equivocal serum IGF-1 concentrations, guidelines recommended confirmation of the diagnosis with a lack of suppression of GH to less than 1 mcg/l following an oral glucose load. In a patient with signs and symptoms of acromegaly and a clearly elevated IGF-1 value, an oral glucose suppression test is not needed for diagnosis.

GH, produced by the somatotroph cells of the pituitary gland in a pulsatile fashion, circulates and stimulates hepatic secretion of IGF-1. A random GH measurement is not useful in diagnosis because of the lack of a well-defined normal range, although a markedly elevated random GH level is consistent with the disease.

After biochemical diagnosis of acromegaly, imaging studies are needed; a MRI scan of the head is the preferred modality and should be obtained to determine tumour size, location, and invasiveness. Visual field testing is performed if the tumour is touching or compressing the optic chiasm. A thorough ophthalmologic examination should be performed if the patient describes diplopia and the tumour is invading the cavernous sinus. Further endocrine testing is also necessary to determine general pituitary function and need for hormone replacement therapy.

Acromegaly is associated with diabetes, hypertension, OSA, and cardiovascular disease. There is also increased risk for colonic polyps and colonoscopy is indicated when acromegaly is diagnosed. Excess GH is also associated with an increase in thyroid nodules and thyroid cancer. A thyroid ultrasound may be performed if there is palpable thyroid nodularity.

The goals of therapy for acromegaly are to normalise GH and IGF-1 activity, reduce tumour size, prevent local mass effects, reduce signs and symptoms of disease, prevent or improve medical comorbidities, and prevent premature mortality. Surgery is the treatment of choice. Surgery is useful to debulk or resect the somatotroph adenoma, decompress local mass effects, and rapidly lower or normalise GH and IGF-1 values.

Surgery is recommended for all patients with microadenomas, and in experienced hands >85% are curable. Surgery is also recommended for all patients with macroadenomas and mass effects. Surgical cure rates for macroadenomas range from 40–50%, likely reflecting the high prevalence of extrasellar extension and parasellar invasion of the cavernous sinus. The transsphenoidal approach is the most common procedure, with craniotomy reserved for select cases involving large, extrasellar lesions. Transnasal endoscopic endonasal procedures offer improved visibility and are rapidly replacing microscopic transsphenoidal techniques.

Medical therapy is largely used in an adjuvant role for patients with residual disease following surgery. However, primary medical therapy may be considered in subjects with macroadenomas and extrasellar involvement (especially involving the cavernous sinus) but no evidence of local mass effects such as chiasmal compression. In this situation, surgery will unlikely be curative and primary medical therapy in lieu of surgery may be considered. Primary medical therapy may also be considered in patients, who are at high risk from surgery and according to patient preferences. In a patient who is undergoing primary medical therapy, surgery can always be reconsidered for tumour debulking to improve response to medical therapy. Somatostatin receptor ligands (SRLs) such as octreotide are the mainstay of medical treatment. Octreotide acts primarily on somatostatin receptor subtypes II and V, inhibiting GH secretion. Dopamine agonist such as cabergoline can also be used. Cabergoline monotherapy results in biochemical control rates of approximately 35%; similar benefits have also been seen with the addition of cabergoline to an SRL in patients with inadequate control on SRL therapy. GH receptor antagonist, pegvisomant monotherapy administered as second-line therapy yields biochemical control rates of 90% or more in clinical trials and closer to 60% in real-world surveillance studies. Radiation therapy is largely relegated to an adjuvant role.

Melmed, S., Bronstein, M., Chanson, P., Klibanski, A., Casanueva, F., Wass, J., Strasburger, C., Luger, A., Clemmons, D. and Giustina, A. (2018). A Consensus Statement on acromegaly therapeutic outcomes. Nature Reviews Endocrinology, 14(9), pp.552–561.
https://www.nature.com/articles/s41574-018-0058-5

2. Answer: C

The patient is likely to have a diagnosis of adrenal crisis with symptoms of nausea, vomiting, hypotension, severe lethargy, weakness, altered mental state, hyponatraemia, hyperkalaemia, and a known history of adrenal insufficiency. Her low BP suggests that she has adrenal crisis with haemodynamic instability, rather than adrenal insufficiency. Septic shock can clinically mimic adrenal insufficiency with symptoms of hypotension, fever, and gastrointestinal symptoms, thus it is important not to miss either the diagnosis of sepsis or adrenal crisis and initiate appropriate investigations and treatment. Administration of appropriate dosage of corticosteroids is imperative to avoid adverse sequalae.

In patients with vomiting and diarrhoea, administration of 100 mg IV hydrocortisone initially is recommended followed by IV hydrocortisone 100 mg qid then 50 mg qid the next day until it is safe to change to oral hydrocortisone after 24 hours. Oral hydrocortisone is usually prescribed at 2 to 3 times the normal oral hydrocortisone dose, with a gradual taper back to the patient's regular dose over the following 2 to 3 days. Administration of oral fludrocortisone is not required if the initial hydrocortisone doses exceed 50 mg over 24 hours for patients with primary adrenal insufficiency as high doses of hydrocortisone will exert mineralocorticoid activity. Oral fludrocortisone can be resumed once the patient is able to have oral hydrocortisone.

Biochemical abnormalities observed in patients with adrenal crisis include hyponatraemia, hyperkalaemia, hypercalcaemia, hypoglycaemia, neutropenia, lymphocytosis, eosinophilia, and mild normocytic anaemia. IV fluid resuscitation with 0.9% normal saline 1L within the first hour is recommended. If the patient is hypoglycaemic, intravenous dextrose 5% in normal saline is given.

It is important for patients with a medical history of adrenal insufficiency and adrenal crisis to have a sick day plan and ongoing education about the condition. Without appropriate recognition and treatment of adrenal crisis, patients may potentially take longer to diagnose, leading to poorer outcomes. MedicAlert bracelets, necklaces, easy access to intramuscular hydrocortisone, oral corticosteroid medications, ambulance services and hospitals are important measures to prevent subsequent adrenal crisis in patients with past history of adrenal crisis or insufficiency.

Rushworth R, Torpy D, Falhammar H. Adrenal Crisis. New England Journal of Medicine. 2019;381(9):852–861. https://www.nejm.org/doi/full/10.1056/NEJMra1807486?url_ver=Z39.88-2003&rfr_id=ori:rid:crossref.org&rfr_dat=cr_pub%3dpubmed

3. Answer: D

An 'adrenal incidentaloma' is an adrenal mass, greater than 1 cm in diameter, that is found serendipitously when a patient undergoes a radiological examination for reasons unrelated to adrenal disease. There has been an increased incidence of 'adrenal incidentalomas' due to the widespread use of CT and MRI. The prevalence of adrenal incidentalomas during autopsies ranges from 1 to 9% and increases with increasing age.

Most adrenal tumours are non-hypersecreting, benign adrenocortical adenomas. Adrenal masses, such as cortisol-secreting adrenocortical adenoma, unilateral or bilateral congenital adrenal hyperplasia, pheochromocytoma, adrenocortical carcinoma, and metastatic carcinoma, are also frequently described. Metastases to the adrenal glands are usually bilateral; primary malignancies that are commonly associated with adrenal metastasis include carcinoma of the lung, kidney, colon, breast, oesophagus, pancreas, liver, and stomach.

Focused history taking and clinical examination is important to rule out functioning and malignant adrenal tumours to diagnose the underlying medical conditions, e.g. Cushing's syndrome, pheochromocytoma, primary aldosteronism, adrenocortical carcinoma, and metastatic cancer.

In patients with a positive overnight dexamethasone (1 mg) suppression test, that is a morning serum cortisol >139 nmol/L, confirmatory tests including serum corticotropin, 24-hr urine cortisol collection, midnight salivary cortisol, and a formal 2-day high-dose dexamethasone suppression test, are required to establish the diagnosis of Cushing's syndrome.

The size of the adrenal tumour does not affect recommendations regarding biochemical testing. However, adrenal tumours that are greater than 4 cm in diameter raise concern for potential primary adrenocortical malignancy.

Due to its high cost and a greater (FDG-PET) uptake in a small percentage of benign adrenal lesions compared to the background uptake, PET scans are not routinely recommended to evaluate patients with adrenal incidentaloma without a history of malignancy.

Image-guided fine-needle aspiration (FNA) biopsy is generally not recommended to differentiate between adrenal vs non-adrenal tissues (metastases or infection), due to risks associated with possible biopsy of a phaeochromocytoma or seeding of metastasis. It is important to biochemically rule out pheochromocytoma before considering performing an FNA biopsy of the adrenal mass due to the potential hypertensive crisis and bleeding complications associated with pheochromocytoma.

Young W. The Incidentally Discovered Adrenal Mass. New England Journal of Medicine. 2007;356(6):601–610. https://www.nejm.org/doi/full/10.1056/NEJMcp065470

4. Answer: C

Amiodarone, is a potent class III antiarrhythmic drug and an iodine-rich compound with a molecular structure similar to thyroxine (T_4) and triiodothyronine (T_3). It has a long half-life (107 days), which allows effects to occur months after stopping treatment. Therapeutic doses of amiodarone contain much more iodine (up to 50–100 times), than the recommended daily iodine intake and significantly increases systemic and thyroidal iodine pools. Amiodarone can cause changes in thyroid function tests and serious thyroid dysfunction, such as amiodarone-induced hypothyroidism (AIH) and type I and type II amiodarone-induced thyrotoxicosis (AIT 1 and AIT 2, respectively) in patients with or without underlying thyroid disease.

AIH does not require cessation of amiodarone and is easily managed. In patients with overt hypothyroidism second to AIH, levothyroxine replacement is recommended. In patients with subclinical hypothyroidism, patients will require ongoing monitoring of the thyroid function; treatment is only required if there is overt hypothyroidism.

The diagnosis of AIT requires increased serum FT4 and FT3 and suppressed serum TSH levels. Anti-thyroid antibodies, such as anti-thyroid peroxidase antibodies, are often positive in AIT 1 and negative in AIT 2.

The clinical presentation of AIT is variable and there is poor correlation between the clinical findings and biochemical severity of the condition. Extreme weight loss and myopathy may indicate life-threatening thyrotoxicosis.

AIT 1 occurs in patients with pre-existing multinodular goitre or latent Graves' disease. The excess iodine from amiodarone provides increased substrate, resulting in enhanced thyroid hormone production. Treatment of AIT 1 includes antithyroid therapy with thionamides (carbimazole or propylthiouracil) that may be combined for a few weeks with sodium perchlorate to make the thyroid gland more sensitive to thionamides.

AIT 2 results from direct toxic effect on the thyroid cells by amiodarone causing thyroiditis in a normal thyroid gland without increased hormone synthesis and is treated with glucocorticoids. It occurs in patients without underlying thyroid disease.

Mixed forms of AIT 1 and AIT 2 exist secondary to underlying mechanisms. Mixed/indefinite forms of AIT are treated with thionamides. Empirical dual therapy with a high-dose glucocorticoid therapy and a high-dose antithyroid mediation can be started from the beginning if it is difficult to distinguish the subtypes of AIT. Urgent endocrinologist consultation and cardiologist opinion will be important to guide the diagnosis and treatment of AIT and discontinuation of amiodarone.

Serum thyroglobulin concentrations are higher in patients with AIT 1. Thyroid ultrasonography can assess thyroid volume, nodularity, parenchymal echogenicity, and vascularity. Overall, most evidence suggests that thyroid ultrasonography has low diagnostic value in AIT. The color flow Doppler sonography (CFDS) may distinguish AIT 1 (increased vascularity) from AIT 2 (absent vascularity). Nuclear medicine imaging using technetium-99m (99mTc)-sestamibi thyroid uptake and scintigraphy can help to distinguish AIT 1 (normal or increased) from AIT 2 (decreased). The presence of thyrotropin receptor antibodies suggests Graves' disease.

The diagnosis of AIT 2 is based on the absence of goitre, reduced radioiodine uptake in areas of iodine deficiency, absence of hypervascularity on CFDS, and, in most cases, anti-thyroid and anti-TSH receptor antibodies negativity. Patients who are refractory to antithyroid drug therapy after 4 to 6 weeks of medical treatment should be considered for thyroidectomy.

Bartalena L, Bogazzi F, Chiovato L, Hubalewska-Dydejczyk A, Links T, Vanderpump M. 2018 European Thyroid Association (ETA) Guidelines for the Management of Amiodarone-Associated Thyroid Dysfunction. European Thyroid Journal. 2018;7(2):55–66.
https://www.karger.com/Article/Pdf/486957

5. Answer: D

This patient has type 1 diabetes, and her general heath has been deteriorating with symptoms of fatigue, nausea, poor appetite and significant weight loss. She is now hypotensive after an infection. Investigations reveal hyponatraemia, hyperkalaemia, a disproportionally higher urea compared to serum creatinine, and hypercalcaemia which is likely secondary to dehydration. These features are highly suggestive of a diagnosis of primary adrenal insufficiency. She has type 1 diabetes, hypothyroidism, and Addison's disease which are features of type 2 autoimmune polyendocrine syndrome (APS). The coexistence of adrenal failure with either autoimmune thyroid disease and/or type 1 diabetes is known as Schmidt's syndrome. It is imperative to prescribe intravenous hydrocortisone when a patient is suspected of having Addison's disease/crisis. Her hypothyroidism may be undertreated as she has only been taking thyroxine intermittently but replacing thyroxine without adequate adrenal steroid replacement in a patient with hypothyroid and Addison's disease can predispose them to an adrenal crisis. Replacement of thyroxine increases the cortisol turnover rate in the liver, and this may further tax a failing adrenal gland.

APS comprises a diverse group of clinical conditions characterised by functional impairment of multiple endocrine glands due to loss of immune tolerance. There are three main syndromes.

Type 1 APS (APS-1) results from mutations in the AIRE gene on chromosome 21 and is inherited in an autosomal recessive manner. This mutation leads to the loss of central tolerance – a process by which developing T cells with potential reactivity for self-antigens are eliminated during early differentiation in the thymus. It is a very rare disease. It usually manifests in infancy or childhood with a persistent mucocutaneous candidiasis, the presence of acquired hypoparathyroidism, and Addison's disease. In most patients, mucocutaneous candidiasis precedes the other disorders, usually followed by hypoparathyroidism.

In type 2 APS (APS-2), alleles of HLAs determine the targeting of specific tissues by autoreactive T cells, which leads to organ-specific autoimmunity as a result of this loss of tolerance. Non-HLA genes also contribute to autoimmunity in APS-2 and, depending on the polymorphism, potentially predisposes to a loss of tolerance or influence which organ is specifically targeted.

The prevalence of APS-2 is 1:20,000. It is more frequently seen in women, and the peak incidence is between the age of 30 to 40 years. It is common for multiple generations to be affected by one or more components of disease. The inheritance of APS-2 is complex, with genes on chromosome 6 playing a predominant role. Within some families, autoimmune endocrine disease susceptibility appears to be inherited as an autosomal dominant form associated with a specific HLA haplotype. The presence of one autoimmune endocrine disease is associated with an increased risk of developing autoimmunity in other organs or tissues.

Each of these disorders is characterised by several stages beginning with active autoimmunity and followed by metabolic abnormalities and overt clinical disease. Type 1 diabetes is a very frequent component disorder of APS-2 and is often its first symptom. Other autoimmune diseases such as coeliac disease, autoimmune gastritis, pernicious anaemia, vitiligo, primary ovarian insufficiency, and alopecia areata may occur in APS-2.

Many of the endocrine disorders of APS can be adequately treated with hormonal replacement therapy. Subjects with pathological ACTH levels and increased levels of basal plasma ACTH require close clinical follow-up with repetition of the test every 6 months. Replacement therapy with hydrocortisone or cortisone acetate should be considered in the case of physiological stress.

IPEX (immune dysfunction, polyendocrinopathy, enteropathy, X-linked) syndrome results from mutations in the forkhead box protein P3 (FOXP3) gene, which is necessary for normal function of regulatory T cells, leading to severe autoimmunity and immune deficiency. IPEX is an extremely rare inherited syndrome characterised by early-onset type 1 diabetes, autoimmune enteropathy with intractable diarrhoea and malabsorption, dermatitis, eosinophilia, and elevated IgE levels. IPEX is frequently fatal in the first few years of life unless patients are promptly treated with immunosuppressants or, if possible, with allogeneic bone marrow transplantation, which can cure the disease.

Husebye E, Anderson M, Kämpe O. Autoimmune Polyendocrine Syndromes. New England Journal of Medicine. 2018;378(12):1132–1141.
https://www.nejm.org/doi/full/10.1056/NEJMra1713301

6. Answer: D

There are three types of adipocytes.

White adipocytes are the main cell type found in human adipose tissue. Energy-yielding triglycerides and cholesterol ester are stored within the large intracellular lipid droplets. They secrete leptin, adiponectin, and other adipokines. Large amounts of white adipocytes around the abdominal area are associated with a higher risk of metabolic syndrome.

Brown adipocytes contain many small lipid droplets, and a high number of uncoupling protein 1 (UCP1) and iron containing mitochondria. Deposits of brown adipocytes are observed within supraclavicular, paravertebral, and mediastinal regions. Compared to adults, newborns have a higher proportion of brown fat. Brown fat has more capillaries than white fat and requires higher oxygen consumption. Brown fat also has many unmyelinated nerves, providing sympathetic stimulation to the fat cells. Brown fat can be activated through sympathetic nervous system stimulation to generate heat by burning calories after cold exposure.

Thermogenic beige (brown-and-white) adipocytes are found scattered within white adipose tissue. They are characteriseds by multiple lipid droplets and uncoupling protein 1–containing mitochondria. 'Browning' of white adipose tissue can be induced with cold exposure, exercise, and some endocrine hormones.

Brown fat is emerging as a promising target for therapeutic intervention in obesity and metabolic syndrome. Activation of brown fat in humans is associated with marked improvement in metabolic parameters such as levels of free fatty acids and insulin sensitivity. Brown adipocytes possess a unique cellular mechanism to convert chemical energy into heat: UCP1, which can short-circuit the mitochondrial proton gradient.

Betz M, Enerbäck S. Targeting thermogenesis in brown fat and muscle to treat obesity and metabolic disease. Nature Reviews Endocrinology. 2017;14(2):77–87.
https://www.nature.com/articles/nrendo.2017.132

7. Answer: A

This patient's clinical features and investigation results are consistent with Cushing's syndrome. She has very low adrenocorticotropic hormone (ACTH) level which is indicative that the likely pathology is an adrenal adenoma.

Cushing's syndrome is characterised by endogenous hypercortisolism due to excessive ACTH production, or autonomous adrenal cortisol production. It is associated with significant comorbidities, including hypertension, diabetes, cardiovascular disease, infections, and osteoporosis. It can be difficult to recognises, especially when it is mild and the presenting features overlap with common conditions such as metabolic syndrome in the general population. However, there is a need to diagnose Cushing's syndrome at an early stage, as it tends to progress, accruing additional morbidity, and increasing mortality rates.

Two of three different screening tests are recommended: 24-hour urine free cortisol (UFC) excretion, late night/bedtime salivary cortisol levels and the 1 mg overnight dexamethasone suppression test (DST) or alternatively the 2 mg 2-day DST. The screening tests all reflect different physiologic abnormalities in Cushing's syndrome: high integrated daily cortisol production (UFC), loss of bedtime salivary or serum cortisol nadir, and impaired response to glucocorticoid negative feedback. Thus, they are complimentary, and the use of more than one test is extremely helpful, as the results generally should corroborate each other.

After establishing the diagnosis, its cause must be determined. The causes of Cushing's syndrome divide into disorders of ACTH excess (either from a pituitary or non-pituitary [ectopic] tumour) and disorders of ACTH-independent primary adrenal overproduction of cortisol (adenoma, carcinoma, or bilateral macronodular/micronodular hyperplasias), in which plasma ACTH values are low or undetectable. Those patients with low/undetectable values should next undergo adrenal gland imaging with CT and/or MRI to identify unilateral masses with adjacent and contralateral atrophy or bilateral disease. Those with normal or elevated ACTH levels should undergo additional testing, usually with pituitary MRI, inferior petrosal sinus sampling, corticotropin releasing hormone, and/or 8 mg dexamethasone suppression which can determine whether ACTH excess is coming from pituitary or ectopic tumour. The ideal treatment is surgical resection of the abnormal tissue or tumour which will induce remission of hypercortisolism and preserve the normal hypothalamic-pituitary-adrenal axis. If surgery is not possible or there is recurrent or metastatic disease, medical therapy is chosen to normalises cortisol levels.

Loriaux, D. (2017). Diagnosis and Differential Diagnosis of Cushing's Syndrome. New England Journal of Medicine, 376(15), pp.1451–1459.
https://www.nejm.org/doi/full/10.1056/NEJMra1505550

8. Answer: D

Diabetic nephropathy (DN) is the most common cause of end stage kidney disease in developed countries and is associated with increased cardiovascular morbidity and mortality.

Intensive glycaemic control can reduce the incidence and progression of DN in type 1 diabetes, and this benefit can persist even if the patient subsequently returns to suboptimal glycaemic control, termed the 'legacy' effect.

In patients with type 2 diabetes, several studies showed that intensive blood glucose control reduced the relative risk of developing microalbuminuria or worsening of albuminuria by 30–35% when compared to conventional control. However, mortality rates were not reduced or higher in one study in the intensive control group. This may be higher occurrence of significant hypoglycaemia, weight gain, increased use of medications of different classes, and higher use of insulin.

ACE inhibitors and ARBs have similar renoprotective effects in patients with DN but ACE inhibition has been shown to have superior cardiac benefits. Therefore, if a patient has DN and CCF, they should be treated with an ACE inhibitor in preference to an ARB.

The renoprotective effect of an ACE inhibitor or ARB is dose-related. If the medication is tolerated well the dose should be gradually increased to the maximum recommended dose. An initial 10% reduction in eGFR before plateauing is common after the commencement of ACE inhibitor or ARB and the drug should be continued unless there is further reduction of eGFR.

Dual renin–angiotensin–aldosterone system (RAAS) blockade with both ACE inhibitor and ARB has shown a superior antiproteinuric effect compared to monotherapy with either agent, but the effect on slowing DN progression is unknown. Significant rates of serious adverse events; including AKI, hyperkalaemia and need for dialysis were observed with dual therapy in the ONTARGET, ALTITUDE and VA-NEPHRON D trials with no significant benefit. Therefore, dual therapy is not currently recommended.

Umanath K. Update on diabetic nephropathy: Core Curriculum 2018. Am J Kidney Dis. 2018;71:884–95.
https://www.ajkd.org/article/S0272-6386(17)31102-2/fulltext

9. Answer: B

Diabetic ketoacidosis (DKA) is a life-threatening complication of type 1 diabetes. It can also occur in patients with type 2 diabetes and is known to occur in patients taking SGLT2 inhibitors; in this situation, blood glucose may not be elevated. In its classical form, DKA is a complex disordered metabolic state characterised by ketonaemia, hyperglycaemia, and metabolic acidosis. This results from absolute or relative insulin deficiency accompanied by an increase in counter-regulatory hormones (glucagon, epinephrine, cortisol, growth hormone). DKA is often triggered by other medical or surgical conditions such as sepsis and is associated with significant morbidity and mortality. Therefore, it must be diagnosed promptly and managed intensively.

The diagnostic criteria of DKA include:

1. Blood ketones ≥3 mmol/L or urine ketones ≥2+ on dipsticks.

2. Blood glucose >11 mmol/L or known diabetes.

3. Bicarbonate (HCO3⁻) <15 mmol/L and/or venous pH <7.3.

The goals of treatment for DKA include:

- Restoration of circulatory volume.
- Clearance of ketones.
- Correction of electrolyte losses (mainly hypokalaemia).
- Normalisation of blood glucose and prevention of hypoglycaemia.
- Prevention of other potential complications such as cerebral oedema, venous thromboembolism (VTE), and sepsis.

Intravenous 0.9% sodium chloride solution is the principal fluid to restore circulating volume and reverse dehydration. The first litre is administered over 1 hour. If the systolic BP remains <90 mmHg, 500 mL should then be administered over 15 min and reassessed. Caution should be exercised in the elderly or patients with CCF where too rapid rehydration may precipitate pulmonary oedema, but insufficient fluid resuscitation may fail to reverse AKI. Regular reassessment of cardiovascular status is mandatory.

Bag number	Time (hr)	Fluid	Infusion rate	Potassium replacement
1	0–1	0.9% sodium chloride	1000 ml/hour	May be required if >1000 ml of fluid has been given due to hypotension
2	1–3	0.9% sodium chloride	500 ml/hour	Monitor potassium level & replace with IV potassium chloride as per table below
3	3–5	0.9% sodium chloride	500 ml/hour	
4	5–9	0.9% sodium chloride	250 ml/jour	
5	9–13	0.9% sodium chloride	250 ml/hour	
6	13–19	0.9% sodium chloride	166 ml/hour	

Potassium level in first 24hrs (mmol/L)	Potassium replacement
>5.5	Nil
3.5–5.5	30 mmol
<3.5	ICU admission, replacement 10 mmol/L/hr

Intravenous insulin infusion with Actrapid should be started as soon as possible and boluses of insulin should be avoided unless there is significant delay (≥1 hour) in setting up an insulin infusion. Insulin infusion should not be stopped until the patient is eating and drinking normally and ketones <0.3 mmol/L, venous pH >7.35, and the patient has received a bolus of long-acting subcutaneous insulin as part of transition to subcutaneous basal bolus insulin regimen.

Sodium bicarbonate should not be administered in patients with DKA unless the arterial plasma pH falls below 7. However, this decision should be individualised. Most patients with DKA do not require the administration of sodium bicarbonate, since infused insulin will slow the rate of ketoacid production, and bicarbonate ions will be produced when ketoacid anions are oxidised.

Karslioglu French E, Donihi A, Korytkowski M. Diabetic ketoacidosis and hyperosmolar hyperglycemic syndrome: review of acute decompensated diabetes in adult patients. BMJ 2019;365:l1114
https://www.bmj.com/content/365/bmj.l1114

10. Answer: C

Erectile dysfunction (ED) is defined as persistent inability to achieve or maintain an erection adequate for satisfactory sexual activity. After premature ejaculation, it is the most common disorder of sexual function in men. ED is a natural part of ageing and prevalence increases with age. Due to its effects on blood vessels and nerves systemically and in the penis, diabetes is a common aetiology of ED. Men with diabetes are four times more likely to experience ED, and on average, ED develops 15 years earlier than in men without diabetes. ED and/or decreased libido are common side-effects of many medications; drugs which can cause this include β-blockers, hydrochlorothiazides, and SSRIs. The pathogenesis of organic ED is related to dysfunction of the endothelium.

Guidelines recommend screening for low testosterone with a morning total testosterone assay (08.00–11.00 a.m.) in men with ED and hypoactive sexual desire, incomplete response to phosphodiesterase type 5 (PDE5) inhibitors, delayed ejaculation, and in all men with known diabetes. The prevalence of low total testosterone levels in men with ED varies widely across studies and ranges from 12.5% to 35%. The threshold of testosterone to maintain an erection is low (< 5.5 nmol/L) and ED is usually a symptom of more severe cases of hypogonadism. If total testosterone level is ≥ 12 nmol/L, testosterone deficiency is unlikely. If total testosterone is < 12 nmol/L, a second morning venous blood sample drawn after an interval of at least one week, together with serum luteinising hormone and prolactin levels is required.

ED may be a precursor of cardiovascular disease. Men with proven or suspected vasculogenic ED or multiple vascular risk factors, especially diabetes, should be screened for silent myocardial ischaemia with exercise electrocardiography, a coronary artery calcium score, or coronary CT angiography.

Lifestyle modifications are the first-line therapy. Other treatment options include testosterone replacement therapy (TRT), PDE5 inhibitors, intracavernosal injection therapy, vacuum constriction devices (VCDs), intraurethral prostaglandin suppositories and surgical placement of a penile prosthesis. PDE5 inhibitors enhance blood flow in the corpora cavernosa. 60–65% of men who have ED, including those with hypertension, diabetes, spinal cord injury, and other comorbid medical conditions, can successfully complete intercourse in response to the PDE5 inhibitors. There is no evidence that currently approved ED treatments add to the overall cardiovascular risk in patients with or without previously diagnosed cardiovascular disease.

McMahon CG. Current diagnosis and management of erectile dysfunction. MJA 2019;210:469–76.
https://www.mja.com.au/journal/2019/210/10/current-diagnosis-and-management-erectile-dysfunction

11. Answer: A

Fertility preservation may be requested by women who experience disease processes or treatments that carry a risk of premature ovarian failure, thereby potentially extending their ability to have children. Treatments causing premature ovarian failure include alkylating chemotherapeutic agents, multi-agent chemotherapy, ovarian radiation therapy, and sometimes pelvic surgery. Alkylating agents include nitrogen-mustard agents such as cyclophosphamide, nitrosureas, and busulfan carry the highest risk of premature ovarian insufficiency, with increasing risk in a dose dependent manner. Other agents with alkylating like actions such as platinum containing agents also carry increased risk, as do other treatments for malignancy such as pelvic radiotherapy.

Counselling about risk of premature ovarian failure is recommended for women of childbearing age undergoing high risk treatments, and parents of children undergoing the same. The probability of premature ovarian failure following chemotherapy is dependent on individual ovarian reserve, which varies greatly between women. For prepubertal girls, ovarian tissue cryopreservation is most likely to result in successful outcome. In adults, this strategy is emerging in cases where there is an urgent indication to initiate treatment, leaving no time for oocyte or embryo cryopreservation. However, where treatment can be safely delayed, mature oocyte cryopreservation or embryo cryopreservation are currently the methods endorsed by the Clinical Oncology Society of Australia. Successful pregnancy rates are higher when larger numbers of oocytes are used, or where the donor is of younger age at the time of cryopreservation.

Donnez J, Dolmans M. Fertility Preservation in Women. New England Journal of Medicine. 2017;377(17):1657–1665.
https://www.nejm.org/doi/full/10.1056/NEJMra1614676

12. Answer: C

Hypogonadism is common in older age men and is most commonly due to functional suppression of sex hormones by chronic disease, medications, and obesity. Hypogonadism as a consequence of testicular or pituitary pathology (organic hypogonadism) is rarer in this age group and occurs in inverse frequency to the level of testosterone, BMI, and degree of comorbidity. First line treatment of functional hypogonadism is lifestyle advice as non-specific symptoms, including sexual dysfunction, responds well to exercise and weight loss.

Testosterone treatment, with the goal of keeping total serum testosterone within the normal range for a young male can be helpful for some symptoms. Libido and erectile function improved with testosterone in comparison to placebo, but its effect on erectile function is not as significant compared with phosphodiesterase-5 inhibitors. Poor glycaemic control is better treated with changes to diabetic medications over and above testosterone treatment. Effects on mood, vitality, and physical function are not consistently seen in randomised trials.

Testosterone treatment has some minor effects on muscle mass, fat mass, and bone mineral density, but it is unlikely that these changes are enough to be clinically relevant.

Snyder P, Bhasin S, Cunningham G, Matsumoto A, Stephens-Shields A, Cauley J et al. Effects of Testosterone Treatment in Older Men. New England Journal of Medicine. 2016;374(7):611–624.
https://www.nejm.org/doi/full/10.1056/NEJMoa1506119

13. Answer: A

Secondary hyperparathyroidism is a common complication in patients with CKD and ESKD. Despite optimised medical treatment, patients with severe secondary hyperparathyroidism may still require parathyroidectomy.

Severe, prolonged, and symptomatic hypocalcaemia is a common post-operative complication in patients following parathyroidectomy. 'Hungry Bone Syndrome' (HBS) is defined as prolonged and severe hypocalcaemia (corrected serum calcium level of 2.1 mmol/L or below) lasting 4 or more days, occurring anytime within 1 month of parathyroidectomy. The measurement of ionised calcium up to 2 to 4 times a day for the first few days postoperatively is preferred to total calcium since it is difficult to predict ionised calcium from total calcium in patients with CKD. Loading with calcitriol pre-operatively can reduce occurrence of severe hypocalcaemia.

Treatment strategies for hypocalcaemia include giving intravenous calcium, oral calcium, and Vitamin D supplementation such as calcitriol, and even providing haemodialysis treatment using a higher calcium dialysate (1.75 mmol/L) to avoid complications related to hypocalcaemia, such as paraesthesia, tetany, laryngeal spasm, seizures, cardiac arrhythmia, and heart failure.

Other biochemical abnormalities which can occur post-parathyroidectomy include hypomagnesaemia, hypophosphataemia, and hyperkalaemia. The correction of hypomagnesaemia may contribute to correction of the hypocalcaemia. The correction of hypophosphataemia in HBS is usually avoided since phosphate can bind to calcium and worsens hypocalcaemia unless the phosphate level is critically low (<0.16 to 0.32 mmol/L) or hypophosphataemia is associated with severe muscle weakness or heart failure. Hyperkalaemia is more common than hypokalaemia as a complication post-parathyroidectomy since this group of patients have ESKD and are often oliguric or anuric after chronic dialysis and can be managed post-operatively with dialysis.

Ho L, Wong P, Sin H, Wong Y, Lo K, Chan S et al. Risk factors and clinical course of hungry bone syndrome after total parathyroidectomy in dialysis patients with secondary hyperparathyroidism. BMC Nephrology. 2017;18(1).
https://www.ncbi.nlm.nih.gov/pmc/articles/PMC5223390/pdf/12882_2016_Article_421.pdf

14. Answer: A

The tricarboxylic acid (TCA) cycle, also known as the Krebs cycle or citric acid cycle, is important in cell metabolism. The Krebs cycle is a series of chemical reactions in mitochondria used by all aerobic organisms to release stored energy from carbohydrates, fats, and proteins through the oxidation of acetyl-CoA into adenosine triphosphate (ATP) and carbon dioxide. The cycle also generates precursors of some amino acids and reducing agent (NADH), that can be used in other reactions.

Citrate, a metabolite in the Krebs cycle, has been linked to fatty-acid synthesis and protein acetylation, which is important for macrophage and dendritic cells activation. Macrophages and dendritic cells play important roles in the innate immune system as the first line of defence against pathogens by producing inflammatory mediators, phagocytosis of pathogens, and releasing chemokines to recruit other inflammatory cells to the site of infection. Dendritic cells are also antigen presenting cells and play an important role in the adaptive immune response.

Itaconate is derived from citrate and has a direct antibacterial effect and is an important immunomodulator.

Williams N, O'Neill L. A Role for the Krebs Cycle Intermediate Citrate in Metabolic Reprogramming in Innate Immunity and Inflammation. Frontiers in Immunology. 2018;9.
https://www.frontiersin.org/articles/10.3389/fimmu.2018.00141/full

15. Answer: C

Multiple endocrine neoplasia (MEN) is characterised by the occurrence of tumours involving two or more endocrine glands. There are four major forms of MEN (Table 4.1), which are autosomal dominant disorders.

Table 4.1 Four major forms of MEN with their characteristics and associated genetic abnormalities.

Syndrome	Gene mutation	Encoded protein	Clinical criteria
MEN1	*MEN1* (tumour suppressor gene) mutation	Mentin	Parathyroid, pancreatic islet and anterior pituitary tumours
MEN2 (MEN2A)	Rearranged during transfection (*RET*) mutation	Tyrosine kinase receptor	Medullary thyroid carcinoma (MTC) in association with phaeochromocytoma and parathyroid tumours
MEN3 (MEN2B)	*RET* mutation	Tyrosine kinase receptor	MTC and phaeochromocytoma in association with a marfanoid habitus, mucosal neuromas, medullated corneal fibres and intestinal autonomic ganglion dysfunction, leading to megacolon
MEN4	*CDNK1B* mutation	Cyclin-dependent kinase inhibitor	Parathyroid and anterior pituitary tumours in possible association with tumours of the adrenals, kidneys, and reproductive organs

RET ('rearranged during transfection)' is located on chromosome 10 (10q11.2) and contains 21 exons. The *RET* proto-oncogene encodes a receptor tyrosine kinase for members of the glial cell line-derived neurotrophic factor family of extracellular signalling molecules. 'Loss of function' RET mutations are associated with the development of Hirschsprung's disease, while 'gain of function' germline mutations are associated with the development of various types of human cancers, including medullary thyroid carcinoma, MEN type 2A and 2B, phaeochromocytoma and parathyroid hyperplasia.

MEN2A is characteriseds by MTC, phaeochromocytoma and primary hyperparathyroidism. If MEN2A is suspected, the RET gene should be examined for an underlying mutation. Autosomal dominant inheritance of MEN2 means that the offspring of an affected person has a 50% chance of inheriting the mutated gene. Identification of the underlying genetic mutation also allows predictive testing in relatives, monitoring for early detection of disease in mutation carriers, and reassurance for non-carriers.

Von Hippel-Lindau (VHL) gene mutation is associated with renal cell cancer, phaeochromocytoma, retinal angioma and hae-mangioblastoma.

McDonnell J, Gild M, Clifton-Bligh R, Robinson B. Multiple endocrine neoplasia: an update. Internal Medicine Journal. 2019;49(8):954–961.
https://onlinelibrary.wiley.com/doi/full/10.1111/imj.14394

16. Answer: D

Maturity-onset diabetes of the young (MODY) is a group of inherited, non-autoimmune diabetes which usually present in adolescence or young adulthood. It is caused by single gene mutations related to beta cell development, regulation, and function. These defects lead to impaired glucose sensing and insulin release. MODY should be suspected in patients with early-onset diabetes in adolescence or young adulthood (typically age <35 years). They usually have atypical features for both type 1 and 2 diabetes.

Features atypical for type 1 diabetes:

- Absence of pancreatic islet autoantibodies
- Evidence of endogenous insulin production
- Measurable C-peptide in the presence of hyperglycemia
- Low insulin requirement for treatment (<0.5 U/kg/day)
- Lack of ketoacidosis when insulin is omitted from treatment.

Features atypical for type 2 diabetes:

- Onset of diabetes before age 45 years
- Lack of obesity (unless south-east Asian ethnicity, where type 2 diabetes occurs at lower BMIs)
- Normal triglyceride levels and/or HDL-C
- Mild, stable fasting hyperglycemia that does not progress or respond appreciably to pharmacologic therapy
- Extreme sensitivity to sulfonylureas.

Ketonuria is often seen in type 1 diabetes especially when the patient develops DKA. However, it can occur in MODY during other complications such as sepsis, acute myocardial infarction, excessive alcohol intake, and prolonged fasting and is therefore not a useful test to differentiate between type 1 diabetes and MODY.

There are at least 14 genes that are associated with MODY. The four most common causes of MODY are the following: GCK-MODY (MODY2) and HNF1A-MODY (MODY3), each accounting for 30%–60% of all MODY. While HNF4A-MODY (MODY1) and HNF1B-MODY (MODY5), together account for about 10% of all MODY. Approximately 20% of all MODY has been attributed to pathogenic variants in ten other genes.

Establishing a specific genetic cause of MODY can help in management of the proband, genetic counseling of family members, and medical surveillance of at-risk family members. Moreover, in certain cases, it can also assist in optimising diabetes therapy. A MODY multigene panel that includes the 14 known MODY-related genes and other genes of interest is most likely to identify the genetic cause of MODY at the most reasonable cost while limiting identification of variants of uncertain significance and pathogenic variants in genes that do not explain the underlying phenotype.

Bishay R, Greenfield J. A review of maturity onset diabetes of the young (MODY) and challenges in the management of glucokinase-MODY. The Medical Journal of Australia. 2016;205(10):480–485.
https://www.mja.com.au/journal/2016/205/10/review-maturity-onset-diabetes-young-mody-and-challenges-management-glucokinase

17. Answer: A

Paget's disease of bone (PDB) is a non-malignant bone disease, characterised by abnormal bone remodelling at one or multiple sites. Increased osteoblast activity leads to increased bone formation which is paired with increased osteoclast activity. Although bone formation is increased, it is disorganised, mechanically weak, and prone to deformity and fractures. Risk factors of PDB include increasing age, male sex (1.4:1), and certain ethnicities (most commonly in Caucasians). Genetic mutations in the *SQSTM1* gene, are identified in up to 50% patients with a family history of PDB and in 5–10% of patients without a family history of PDB.

This genetic mutation impairs the ability of p62 to bind ubiquitin, leading to activation of receptor activator of nuclear kappa B ligand (RANKL)-induced NF-kB which increases the osteoclast activity.

PDB most commonly affects the pelvis, spine, femur, tibia, and skull. Clinical symptoms, signs, and complications of PDB are the results of abnormal bone remodelling, enlarged bones, marrow fibrosis, and increased vascularity of bone. Depending on the affected sites, hearing loss, obstructive hydrocephalus, spinal canal stenosis, paraplegia, and high-output cardiac failure may occur. Although, bone pain is the most commonly presenting symptom, and classically presents with pain at rest and up to 25% of patients are asymptomatic.

Serum total ALP is recommended as a first-line screening biochemical test in combination with the liver function test to identify metabolically active PDB. Radionuclide bone scans, and targeted XX-ray of the abdomen, tibias, skull, and facial bones are recommended to determine the extent of active bone disease in patients with PDB. X-rays typically demonstrate a mixed pattern of osteolysis and sclerosis in keeping with disease pathophysiology.

The treatment aim in PDB is to relieve symptoms rather than achieving normalising ALP. Bisphosphonates, especially zolendronic acid, may help alleviate bone disease associated pain. Total hip or knee replacements are recommended in patients with PDB who develop osteoarthritis and in whom medical management is inadequate to manage symptoms.

Ralston S, Corral-Gudino L, Cooper C, Francis R, Fraser W, Gennari L et al. Diagnosis and Management of Paget's Disease of Bone in Adults: A Clinical Guideline. Journal of Bone and Mineral Research. 2019;34(4):e3657.
https://asbmr.onlinelibrary.wiley.com/doi/full/10.1002/jbmr.3657

18. Answer: B

Approximately 50% of patients who have had diabetes for >25 years will develop neuropathy. The most common form of diabetic neuropathy is distal symmetric, nerve-length-dependent polyneuropathy. Of these, approximately 50% will have pain as a symptom of neuropathy that is painful diabetic neuropathy (PDN). The prevalence of PDN in type 2 diabetes is more than twice that seen in type 1 diabetes.

Among patients with the same degree of neuropathy, some experience more pain than others. Pain is mediated by small fibresr, which may be damaged or destroyed in diabetic neuropathy, resulting in sensory loss. However, these small fibresr have the capacity to regenerate and to lead to ectopic generation of impulses and hyperexcitability, resulting in highly painful neuropathy in some patients. Moreover, pain nociception is complex and involves various other factors. Patients with normal findings on clinical examination and small-fibre testing may also experience painful neuropathy.

Tight glycaemic control in patients with type 1 diabetes reduced the occurrence of clinical neuropathy by 60% in 5 years according to the Diabetes Control and Complications Trial. But it appears not to be enough to ameliorate the onset and progression of the disease in patients with type 2 diabetes. One of the reasons could be that the neuropathic process starts early in type 2 diabetes. The underlying mechanisms for the development of neuropathy in type 1 diabetes and type 2 diabetes appear to be different.

Sundara Rajan R, de Gray L, George E. Painful diabetic neuropathy. Continuing Education in Anaesthesia Critical Care & Pain. 2014;14(5):230–235.
https://www.sciencedirect.com/science/article/pii/S1743181617300847?via%3Dihub

19. Answer: A

Gastroparesis is a syndrome characterised by delayed gastric emptying in the absence of mechanical obstruction of stomach. The main symptoms include post-prandial fullness, early satiety, bloating, nausea and vomiting. Gastroparesis is a serious complication of diabetes and is reported by 5 to 12% of patients with diabetes. It typically develops after at least 10 years of diabetes, and these patients generally have additional evidence of autonomic dysfunction. Other non-diabetic causes of gastroparesis are neurologic disorders, surgery, medication, and idiopathic causes.

Gastric emptying involves integration of fundic tone and antral phasic contractions with inhibition of pyloric and duodenal contractility. Gastric emptying requires interactions between smooth muscle, enteric nerves, vagus nerve, and specialised pacemaker cells, the interstitial cells of Cajal (ICC).

- Autonomic neuropathy: Vagal neuropathy results in reduced pyloric relaxation, impaired antral contraction, disturbed antropyloric coordination, and reduced gastric secretion.
- Enteric neuropathy: The enteric nervous system (ENS) is the myenteric plexus, a network of nerves that is layered between the longitudinal and circular muscle layer of the gut and coordinates gastric motor function. Pathological changes in these pathways due to hyperglycaemia affect motor control and may contribute to delay emptying, impaired accommodation, and gastric dysrhythmia.

- Loss of ICC: This is the most common enteric neuropathological abnormality in diabetic and idiopathic gastroparesis. ICC generate slow waves that control smooth muscle contractility, are involved in aspects of neurotransmission, set the smooth muscle membrane potential gradient. A range of diabetes related mechanisms induce ICCs damage including insulinopaenia, IGF-1 deficiency, and oxidative stress. Diabetes is a high oxidative stress state, which can cause loss of ICCs and delay gastric emptying.
- Glucagon like peptide-1 (GLP-1) treatment: Known causes of iatrogenic gastroparesis include vagal inhibition and pharmacological blockade such as GLP-1 receptor agonist in the treatment of type 2 diabetes.
- Fluctuations in blood glucose: Acute increases in blood glucose may further delay gastric emptying, which in turn exacerbates blood glucose fluctuations that can then further impair gastric emptying rate. Delayed emptying can be the result of the pyloric contractions and antral hypomotility induced by the hyperglycaemic state. Once established, diabetic gastroparesis tends to persist, despite amelioration of glycaemic control.

Grover M. Gastroparesis: A turning point in understanding and treatment. Gut Published Online First: 28 September 2019. https://gut.bmj.com/content/68/12/2238.abstract

20. Answer: B

Polycystic ovarian syndrome (PCOS) is the most common endocrinopathy in women and is associated with significant adverse sequelae that can affect overall health and well-being. Physicians need to have a good understanding of the complications and develop strategies to prevent long-term health morbidities for women who have been diagnosed with PCOS.

PCOS is diagnosed, after exclusion of other causes, and if the woman meets two of the following three features, including: (1) clinical and/or biochemical signs of hyperandrogenism, (2) oligo- or anovulation, and (3) polycystic ovaries (PCO) on abdominal USS. In adolescents or those within 8 years of menarche, ultrasound is not a reliable discriminator for PCOS. PCOS is classified into four phenotypes, which plays an important role in determining the metabolic and possibly long-term complications of PCOS. The phenotypes are differentiated based on presence and absence of the three criteria of hyperandrogenism, ovulatory dysfunction, and ultrasound features of PCO and outlined in the table below. Phenotypes A and B account for two-thirds of all cases.

	Hyperandrogenism	Oligomenorrhoea	Ultrasound features of PCO
Type A	Yes	Yes	Yes
Type B	Yes	Yes	No
Type C	Yes	No	Yes
Type D	No	Yes	Yes

Phenotypes A, B and C are associated with an increased risk of metabolic syndrome, whereas phenotype D is not associated with an increased metabolic risk as compared with the general population. Phenotypes A and B have higher rates of insulin resistance compared with the general population irrespective of BMI while the other phenotypes do not possess this characteristic, implying that hyperandrogenism contributes to insulin resistance. PCOS is responsible up to 80% of cases of anovulatory infertility. As women with PCOS have greater degrees of insulin resistance and secondary hyperinsulinemia than weight-matched controls, they are at greater risk of developing long-term complications including a higher lifetime risk of type 2 diabetes, non-alcoholic fatty liver disease, metabolic syndrome, hypertension, dyslipidaemia, and possibly vascular complications (coronary artery disease and CVA). Venous thromboembolism is also more common in women with PCOS.

Studies have demonstrated an increased risk of endometrial cancer in women with PCOS but no increased risk of breast cancer in association with PCOS. Evidence has been mixed regarding the association of PCOS and ovarian cancer risk. Multiple studies have also demonstrated a consistent link between PCOS and mental health issues, including an increased prevalence of depression, anxiety, and decreased sexual satisfaction and quality of life.

Escobar-Morreale H. Polycystic ovary syndrome: definition, aetiology, diagnosis and treatment. Nature Reviews Endocrinology. 2018;14(5):270-284.
https://www.nature.com/articles/nrendo.2018.24

21. Answer: A

Catecholamines produced by phaeochromocytomas are metabolised within chromaffin cells. Norepinephrine is metabolised to normetanephrine and epinephrine is metabolised to metanephrine. As conversion occurs within the tumour, independently of catecholamine release, phaeochromocytomas are best diagnosed by measurement of these metabolites rather than by measurement of the parent catecholamines.

Plasma fractionated metanephrines can be measured as a first-line test for phaeochromocytoma. The negative predictive value for this test is extremely high. However, despite a high sensitivity of 96%, specificity of plasma fractionated metanephrine is low at 85%, and falls to 75% in patients older than 60 years and taking multiple antihypertensive medications. One study suggested that 97% of patients with hypertension seen in a tertiary care clinic who have a positive plasma fractionated metanephrine measurement will not have a phaeochromocytoma.

As such, 24-hour urinary fractionated catecholamines and metanephrines should be performed first after a high level of plasma metanephrine. Specificity is highest for urinary epinephrine (99.9%), followed by urinary norepinephrine and dopamine (99.5% and 99.3%, respectively), and urinary total metanephrines (99.7%). If there is high clinical suspicion and elevated 24-hour urinary fractionated catecholamines and metanephrines, clonidine suppression test can be used as a confirmatory test.

Plasma catecholamines no longer have a role in investigation for phaeochromocytoma because of poor overall accuracy. The 24-hour urinary vanillylmandelic acid (VMA) excretion has poor diagnostic sensitivity and specificity compared with 24-hour urinary fractionated metanephrines.

Biochemical confirmation of the diagnosis should be followed by radiological evaluation to locate the tumour. About 10% of the tumours are extra-adrenal, but 95% are within the abdomen and pelvis. MRI can distinguish phaeochromocytomas from other adrenal masses: on T2-weighted images, phaeochromocytomas appear hyperintense whilst other adrenal tumours appear isointense, as compared with the liver. However, MRI lacks the superior spatial resolution of CT. If abdominal and pelvic CT or MRI is negative in the presence of clinical and biochemical evidence of phaeochromocytoma, a metaiodobenzylguanidine (MIBG) scan should be ordered. MIBG is a compound resembling norepinephrine that is taken up by adrenergic tissue. It can detect tumours not detected by CT or MRI, or multiple tumours when CT or MRI is positive.

Neumann H, Young W, Eng C. Pheochromocytoma and Paraganglioma. New England Journal of Medicine. 2019;381(6):552–565.
https://www.nejm.org/doi/full/10.1056/NEJMra1806651

22. Answer: C

Iron deficiency anaemia is a common cause of a falsely elevated HbA1c. HbA1c is a marker of the average blood glucose levels over a 90–120 day period (the average life span of a RBC). This is because haemoglobin, like other plasma proteins, glycate in response to glucose exposure, and the degree of glycation is proportional to the average plasma glucose concentration. HbA1c is subsequently used to both diagnose and monitor diabetes treatment efficacy.

HbA1c is advantageous as there is low biological variability, so HbA1c is relatively stable during states of fasting or fed, well or unwell, and whether a sample is processed quickly or delayed. However HbA1c is also reliant on stable haemoglobin concentration. When this is not the case it can be falsely elevated or depressed:

- Factors which falsely decrease HbA1c (expose haemoglobin to less glucose):
  o Decreased average RBC age, i.e. blood loss, haemolytic anaemia, CKD (chronic anaemia with decreased cell survival)
  o Increased RBC turnover, i.e. pregnancy, erythropoietin therapy, chronic liver disease (secondary to splenomegaly)
  o Decreased protein glycation, i.e. high dose vitamin C and E, alcohol, antivirals (e.g. ribavirin), antibiotics (e.g. trimethoprim)
- Factors which falsely increase HbA1c (expose haemoglobin to more glucose):
  o Increased average age of RBCs, e.g. asplenia
  o Decreased RBC turnover, e.g. anaemia secondary to iron deficiency, vitamin B12 and folate deficiency.
  o Increased protein glycation, e.g. iron deficiency anaemia.

In situations where HbA1c is not suitable for monitoring patients with diabetes, alternatives to consider include glucose profiling, total glycated haemoglobin, fructosamine, or glycated albumin.

Sodi, R., McKay, K., Dampetla, S. and Pappachan, J. (2018). Monitoring glycaemic control in patients with diabetes mellitus. BMJ, p.k4723.
https://www.bmj.com/content/363/bmj.k4723

23. Answer: A

This patient has a large symptomatic pituitary tumour and encroachment of surrounding structures resulting in visual field deficit. With pituitary tumours, prolactin levels correlate with the tumour size. In other words, the bigger the tumour size the higher the prolactin level. This patient has a large tumour but only slightly elevated prolactin level relative to the tumour size, so this tumour is unlikely to be a prolactinoma. Therefore, the appropriate management is surgical, not conservative management using cabergoline. In contrast, if the tumour is small but the prolactin level is very high, then it is likely a prolactinoma and a dopamine receptor agonist such as cabergoline treatment should be the first choice.

Based on its size, a pituitary adenoma can be classified as a microadenoma (<10 mm diameter) or a macroadenoma (>10 mm diameter). Approximately 50% are microadenomas. Prolactinomas are the most common hormone-secreting pituitary tumours accounting for 32 to 66% of adenomas. Symptoms and signs of prolactinomas are shown in Table 4.2. Female patients usually have small prolactinomas at diagnosis because the symptoms of galactorrhoea and amenorrhoea result in an early presentation. Patients may present with headaches which can have variable quality and location due to stretching of the dura.

Table 4.2   Clinical features for prolactinoma.

Female clinical features	Male clinical features	Both male and female features
Galactorrhoea	Hypogonadism	Headache
Amenorrhoea	Reduced libido	Visual field deficit
Infertility	Erectile dysfunction	Osteoporosis
	Gynaecomastia	
	Infertility	

Laboratory investigations for suspected prolactinoma include the following:
- Serum prolactin level and macroprolactin level if clinically needed
- Serum pregnancy test
- Serum TSH
- Serum testosterone or bioavailable testosterone: In males presenting with symptoms of hypogonadism
- Basal cortisol level and short Synacthen test in patients with a history suggestive of adrenal insufficiency or any patient before surgery
- Renal function tests, impaired renal function can lead to impaired prolactin clearance.

After performing biochemical and hormonal tests, MRI or CT head with contrast is used to determine if a mass lesion is present. If no mass lesion is present, it is also important to note that prolactin may be elevated due to a range of medications, including dopamine antagonists such as antipsychotics, drugs that affect gastric motility such as metoclopramide and domperidone and certain antihypertensives such as methyldopa.

Patients with pituitary adenomas should be identified at an early stage so that effective treatment can be planned. For all other pituitary adenomas, initial therapy is generally transsphenoidal surgery with medical therapy being reserved for those not cured by surgery. For prolactinomas, treatment is indicated if mass effects from prolactinoma and/or significant effects from hyperprolactinemia are present. The initial therapy is generally dopamine agonists, which not only decrease the synthesis and secretion of prolactin but also the rate of tumour cell division and the growth of individual cells. Cabergoline, an ergot derivative, is a long-acting dopamine agonist. It is usually better tolerated than bromocriptine and its efficacy profiles are superior to bromocriptine. It offers the convenience of twice-a-week administration, with a usual starting dose of 0.5 mg. Bromocriptine is an ergoline derivative and dopamine agonist. It had been used in the treatment of prolactinoma because of its long track record and safety. In macroprolactinomas, bromocriptine treatment results in some reduction of tumour size in up to 80–85% of the patients.

Transsphenoidal pituitary adenomectomy is the preferred surgical treatment in patients with macroprolactinoma and patients with microprolactinoma who fail to respond to medical treatment. A combination of surgery followed by postoperative medical treatment with bromocriptine or one of the other agents is used in patients with incomplete resolution of elevated prolactin levels and in patients with residual tumours seen on follow-up imaging studies.

Molitch ME. Diagnosis and treatment of pituitary adenomas A Review. JAMA. 2017;317:516–524.
https://jamanetwork.com/journals/jama/article-abstract/2600472

24. Answer: D

Two types of continuous glucose monitoring (CGM) systems are now available: real-time CGM (rtCGM) and intermittently scanned CGM (isCGM). Current rtCGM system automatically transmits a continuous stream of glucose data (trend and numerical) in real time to a receiver, smart watch, or smartphone and provides alerts and active alarms. The current isCGM system provides the same type of glucose data but requires the user to purposely scan the sensor to obtain information and does not have alerts and alarms. CGM systems provide continuous measurement at 1–5 min increments of glucose concentrations in the interstitial fluid, which correlate with blood glucose levels. The lag time between the interstitial fluid glucose measured by rtCGM and plasma glucose is a limitation to the real-time actionable data provided by devices. Moreover, all current systems for rtCGM are less accurate in the lower glucose ranges but are improving in this regard.

Numerous recent studies have demonstrated the clinical efficacy and other benefits of rtCGM use in individuals with type 1 diabetes (T1D) and type 2 diabetes (T2D) regardless of the insulin delivery method used. There is a modest reduction in HbA1c. rtCGM reduced the time spent in the hypoglycaemic (T1D only) and hyperglycaemic ranges and demonstrated reductions in moderate to severe hypoglycaemia in individuals with T1D and T2D compared with traditional self-monitoring of blood glucose (SMBG).

Recent studies have also demonstrated the benefits of rtCGM as an integrated component of sensor-augmented insulin pumps with predictive low glucose suspend functionality. Automatic insulin pump suspension can help individuals with T1D avoid hypoglycaemia without significantly increasing hyperglycaemia or the risk of diabetic ketoacidosis. Guidelines recommended the use of rtCGM in individuals with recurrent severe hypoglycaemia and/or impaired hypoglycaemia awareness. The beneficial effects of rtCGM use have not only been shown in poorly controlled T1D, but also in individuals who have achieved good control, by reducing glycaemic variability.

Individuals who could benefit from data sharing capability (e.g. paediatric patients, the elderly, patients with mental health illness and patients who travel alone) are also good candidates for rtCGM. Other candidates for rtCGM use include individuals who have a high HbA1c, are physically active, want to use insulin pump systems that offer predictive low glucose suspend functionality, experience hypoglycaemia fear, or desire tighter glucose control than obtained with their current monitoring system.

In summary, based upon the current evidence, use of rtCGM is now recognised as the standard of care for individuals with T1D and a subset of those with insulin-requiring T2D.

Edelman S, Argento N, Pettus J, Hirsch I. Clinical Implications of Real-time and Intermittently Scanned Continuous Glucose Monitoring. Diabetes Care. 2018;41(11):2265–2274.
https://care.diabetesjournals.org/content/41/11/2265.long

25. Answer: D

Multiple side effects have been identified for treatment with SGLT-2 inhibitors, including those listed as answer options as well as bone fracture. However, individual trials lack the power to detect significant differences in these rare adverse outcomes. As a result multiple meta-analyses have been performed with the intention of clarifying these post-marketing observations. The most recent of which showed no overall difference in fracture, or UTI – except that dapagliflozin alone independently increases the risk of UTI. Despite some reports, SGLT-2 inhibitors are strongly protective against AKI and recent evidence suggests it is protective against progression of chronic diabetic kidney disease. DKA can occur in the setting of acute physiological stress without hyperglycaemia when treated with SGLT-2 inhibitors, but the overall rate of DKA is not greater in treated patients. There is some suggestion that SGLT-2 inhibitors may increase the risk of limb amputation, although meta-analysis of available trial data is significantly underpowered to draw this conclusion, and absolute risk is very low.

Overall the fairly significant medium-term benefits of this class of drug are compelling reasons for significantly expanded use, and individual practitioners need to be aware of individual situations that pose excess risk for a patient on this class of medication. Two significant such situations are physiological stress and volume depletion, where relative insulin insufficiency and excess diuresis can lead to DKA and AKI, respectively.

Donnan J, Grandy C, Chibrikov E, Marra C, Aubrey-Bassler K, Johnston K et al. Comparative safety of the sodium glucose co-transporter 2 (SGLT2) inhibitors: a systematic review and meta-analysis. BMJ Open. 2019;9(1):e022577.
https://bmjopen.bmj.com/content/9/1/e022577

26. Answer: D

The tests are most indicative of subclinical hypothyroidism, which is most likely due to autoimmune (Hashimoto) thyroiditis. Randomised trial data suggests that treatment of subclinical hypothyroidism is not warranted in older adults, however observational data suggests that treatment may be considered in pregnant women, or if TSH is over 7.0 mIU/L. Treatment can also be considered in younger individuals, particularly females with a possibility of becoming pregnant and patients with multiple symptoms attributable to hypothyroidism. Certainly, there is a general recommendation for treatment in individuals with TSH equal to or greater than 10.0 mIU/L. Other possible indications for treatment are thyroid peroxidase antibody positivity or presence of a goitre.

Observational data also suggest that individuals with subclinical hypothyroidism have a greater prevalence of heart failure, coronary heart disease mortality and fatal stroke.

Diagnosis of subclinical hypothyroidism requires measurement of normal FT4 despite elevated TSH. As levels fluctuate for an individual, repeat measurements are required to confirm subclinical hypothyroidism or progression to hypothyroidism. For measurements of TSH between 4.5 and 14.9 mIU/L, reassessment should be conducted in 1–3 months to maximise clinical relevance. However, if the TSH is over 14.9 mIU/L, assessment should be repeated more expediently as a transition to overt hypothyroidism is more likely.

If treatment is initiated for subclinical hypothyroidism, TSH should be measured after six weeks of levothyroxine therapy in order to adjust the dosage accordingly. Annual measurements of TSH are generally sufficient thereafter.

Biondi B, Cappola A, Cooper D. Subclinical Hypothyroidism. JAMA. 2019;322(2):153.
https://jamanetwork.com/journals/jama/article-abstract/2737687

27. Answer: C

Papillary thyroid carcinoma (PTC) is the most common form of thyroid cancer, and the most common form of thyroid cancer caused by exposure to radiation. Total thyroidectomy is the mainstay of treatment in patients with PTC. Radioactive iodine ablation and long-term TSH suppression using thyroxine are also important adjuvant therapies.

An excellent response to the initial treatment is defined by an undetectable serum thyroglobulin, the absence of both thyroglobulin antibodies and abnormal findings on neck ultrasound.

The purpose of follow-up is for early detection and treatment of persistent or recurrent locoregional or distant PTC. Most local recurrences develop within the first 5 years after treatment. However, in a few cases, local or distant recurrence may develop within 10–20 years after the initial treatment.

Three months after initial treatment, TFTs should be done to check the adequacy of thyroxine suppressive therapy. Follow-up at six to twelve months should ascertain whether or not the patient is free of disease. This follow-up should include a physical examination, neck ultrasound, and a check of basal and recombinant human TSH (rhTSH)-stimulated serum thyroglobulin measurement. At this time, about 80% of the patients will have a normal neck ultrasound, an undetectable (<1.0 ng/ml) stimulated serum thyroglobulin in the absence of serum thyroglobulin antibodies, and will be classified in the low-risk category or in complete remission. The rate of subsequent recurrence is very low (<1.0% at 10 years). Diagnostic whole-body bone scan does not add any clinical information in this setting and is not required.

Recently, new methods for obtaining serum thyroglobulin measurement with functional sensitivity below 0.1 ng/ml have become available. An undetectable basal serum thyroglobulin (<0.1 ng/ml) may give the same information as a stimulated thyroglobulin test, thus negating the need for thyroglobulin stimulation. However, the higher negative predictive value of these tests comes at the expense of a very low specificity, and risks exposing large numbers of patients, who are probably free of disease, to extensive testing and/or unnecessary treatment.

In clinical practice, when basal serum thyroglobulin is ≤0.1 ng/ml and neck ultrasound is unremarkable, patients may be considered free of disease (negative predictive value, NPV = 100%) and a rhTSH stimulation can be avoided. However, if basal serum thyroglobulin is between 0.1 ng/ml and 1.0 ng/ml, it is not possible to distinguish between the absence or presence of disease; rhTSH stimulation testing is then necessary.

The subsequent follow-up of patients considered free of disease at 6–12 months should consist of physical examination, basal serum thyroglobulin measurement on thyroxine and neck ultrasound once per year.

Patients with a high risk of disease recurrence who do not respond excellently to treatment should be followed up with serum TSH, thyroglobulin and anti-thyroglobulin antibody determination and neck ultrasound every 6–12 months.

Measurement of the serum thyroglobulin level with anti-thyroglobulin antibodies to validate accuracy of the thyroglobulin assay is important. In the absence of residual normal thyroid tissue (after surgical and radioiodine ablation), thyroglobulin is a marker of residual or recurrent papillary or follicular thyroid carcinoma.

Lamartina L, Grani G, Durante C, Borget I, Filetti S, Schlumberger M. Follow-up of differentiated thyroid cancer – what should (and what should not) be done. Nature Reviews Endocrinology. 2018;14(9):538–551.
https://www.nature.com/articles/s41574-018-0068-3

28. Answer: A

The vast majority of driver mutations in thyroid carcinoma come from the MAPK pathway, which dominates the oncogenesis of both papillary and follicular thyroid cancers, and together account for around 85% of thyroid cancer diagnoses. Of these mutations, alterations in BRAF V600E accounts for the majority, and less commonly RAS, NTRK, ALK, or RET. Anaplastic thyroid cancers have high mutational variation involving multiple pathways, but are rare, and associated with poor mean survival. Medullary thyroid cancers are typically associated with gain-of-function mutations in RET, a proto-oncogene in the MAPK pathway.

 Fagin J, Wells S. Biologic and Clinical Perspectives on Thyroid Cancer. New England Journal of Medicine. 2016;375(11):1054–1067.
https://www.nejm.org/doi/10.1056/NEJMra1501993

29. Answer: C

Thyroid nodules are common in the general population. They are palpable in 4–7% of the population and have been detected using ultrasound in up to 60% of adults. The majority of nodules are benign but approximately 7–15% of thyroid nodules are thyroid cancer.

TFTs should be performed in all patients with a thyroid nodule on examination. While most patients will be euthyroid, a suppressed TSH level indicates a hyperfunctioning nodule and the risk of malignancy is extremely low. Serum calcitonin levels should only be requested when a medullary thyroid carcinoma is suspected.

The ultrasound assessment provides key information regarding the size and sonographic features of the nodules, which form the basis for risk stratification. A decision to proceed to fine-needle aspiration (FNA) is typically made based on ultrasound appearance. Features taken into consideration include size and shape of the nodule and other features including homogeneity, presence of micro-calcifications and vascularity. Ultrasound-guided FNA is the most sensitive and cost-effective method to assess the nature of thyroid nodules and the need for surgery. The Thyroid Imaging Reporting and Data System (TIRADS) score and size of the nodule are used to guide whether FNA should be performed. Guidelines recommend FNA for nodules ≥1 cm that have a high pattern of suspicion on ultrasound, ≥1.5 cm that have a moderate suspicion pattern on ultrasound, and nodules ≥2.5 cm that have a mildly-suspicion pattern on ultrasound. If the cytologic findings are interpreted as non-diagnostic, FNA should be repeated within 3 months to obtain sufficient cells for a more definitive diagnosis.

Molecular analysis should be performed in patients with atypia of undetermined significance, follicular lesions of undetermined significance (AUS/FLUS), follicular neoplasm or suspicious for a follicular neoplasm in FNA. One molecular approach is to analyse the specimen by means of a gene-expression classifier to rule out cancer. The other molecular approach is to directly assess the FNA for *BRAF* and *RAS* mutations. If the FNA is positive for a *BRAF* mutation, the chance of cancer is close to 100%, and if the FNA is positive for a *RAS* mutation, the chance of cancer is 80 to 90%.

 Durante C, Grani G, Lamartina L, Filetti S, Mandel S, Cooper D. The Diagnosis and Management of Thyroid Nodules. JAMA. 2018;319(9):914–924.
https://jamanetwork.com/journals/jama/article-abstract/2673975

30. Answer: C

Transgender (TGD) people are individuals whose gender identity is markedly and persistently incongruent with their sex assigned at birth. About 0.6% of the population identifies as TGD in Western countries. Gender-affirmation treatment should be multidisciplinary and include diagnostic assessment, psychotherapy, counselling, real-life experience, hormone therapy, and surgical therapy.

Hormonal therapy is effective at aligning physical characteristics with gender identity and improving mental health symptoms.
- Masculinising hormone therapy options include transdermal or intramuscular testosterone at standard doses.
- Feminising hormone therapy options include transdermal or oral estradiol. Additional anti-androgen therapy with cyproterone acetate or spironolactone is typically required.

No data exists on gradual versus rapid titration or comparison of formulations in feminising TGD individuals. The value of biochemical monitoring is uncertain; when performed, trough estradiol levels should be used. Target estradiol levels should be between 250–600 pmol/L and total testosterone levels is < 2 nmol/L. Despite anecdotal reports that progestins increase breast growth, no data supports their use. Furthermore, progestins can increase risk of coronary artery disease, thrombosis, and weight gain. Cyproterone acetate, a commonly used anti-androgen agent, has progestogenic effects. Anti-androgens are often required in addition to estradiol therapy to lower endogenous testosterone levels or inhibit testosterone effects. Spironolactone (100–200 mg daily) or cyproterone acetate (12.5–25 mg daily) are both effective. Gonadotrophin-releasing hormone analogues are used as puberty blockers in adolescents only.

Hormonal therapy can impair fertility and patients should receive counselling for this prior to commencing gender affirming treatment. Sperm cryopreservation should be discussed before estradiol therapy due to expected changes in spermatogenesis. Oocyte storage can be considered; however, ovulation typically resumes on cessation of testosterone therapy.

Cheung A, Wynne K, Erasmus J, Murray S, Zajac J. Position statement on the hormonal management of adult transgender and gender diverse individuals. Medical Journal of Australia. 2019;211(3):127–133.
https://www.mja.com.au/journal/2019/211/3/position-statement-hormonal-management-adult-transgender-and-gender-diverse

31. Answer: E

32. Answer: F

33. Answer: D

34. Answer: H

Obesity is a complex, multifactorial disorder that has genetic, biological, and environmental origins. Traditional treatments consist of counseling, restrict calories intake, and lifestyle changes such as eating a nutrient-dense diet, participating in regular physical activity, and other behaviour modifications. Medications commonly used in the treatment of obesity include orlistat, phentermine, topiramate, naltrexone, and liraglutide. Many patients with severe obesity (BMI≥40) are unable to lose and maintain significant weight loss. Bariatric surgery is an effective treatment morbid obesity because it leads to sustained weight loss, reduction of obesity-related comorbidities and mortality, and improvement of quality of life.

There are three types of bariatric surgery:

1. Restrictive: Laparoscopic sleeve gastrectomy (LSG), laparoscopic adjustable gastric banding (LAGB, a restrictive procedure to induce early satiety through reduction of gastric capacity).

2. Malabsorptive: Biliopancreatic diversion (BPD) with or without duodenal switch comprises this category of bariatric surgery. Each has only a minimal restrictive component that involves the creation of a sleeve like stomach.

3. Restrictive Malabsorptive: Proximal Roux-en-Y gastric bypass (RYGB) is a restrictive-malabsorptive technique. Gastric capacity is reduced by 90%. The section of the gastrointestinal tract bypassed is called the biliopancreatic limb, which includes the majority of the stomach, the duodenum, and part of the jejunum. This limb drains bile, digestive enzymes, and gastric secretions to assist digestion and absorption further down the gastrointestinal tract. The proximal to mid-end of the jejunum is anastomosed to the gastric pouch for malabsorption. This creates the common limb. The food and enzymes ingested are mixed only in the small area of the common limb, compromising absorption of certain nutrients.

Macro- and micronutrient deficiencies are common in patients after obesity surgery. It is estimated that BPD with or without duodenal switch can cause a 25% decrease in protein absorption and a 75% reduction in fat absorption. Ten vitamins and minerals that depend on fat absorption for optimal bioavailability, such as vitamins A, D, E, and K and zinc, will have impaired absorption. Moreover, the delay in gastrointestinal transit time may increase the risk of many other micronutrient deficiencies, including iron, calcium, vitamin B12, and folate. Low serum levels of fat-soluble vitamins (vitamin A, K and E) have been found after BPD and RYGB. Water-soluble vitamins such as thiamine deficiency can occur in up to 49% of patients after surgery as a result of bypass of the jejunum, where it is primarily absorbed, or in the presence of impaired nutritional intake from persistent, severe vomiting. Patients may have preexisting thiamin deficits. Thiamin deficiency can cause high-output heart failure, wet beriberi. Gastric banding patients also may be at risk, particularly if they experience intractable vomiting because thiamin has a short half-life, meaning that thiamin stores last only a few days in the body.

A vitamin B12 deficiency is uncommon among gastric banding patients. A study found a 10 to 26% prevalence of vitamin B12 deficiency among gastric sleeve patients. Clinical manifestation of vitamin B12 deficiency includes paraesthesias, difficulty maintaining balance, poor memory, depression, loss of proprioception and vibratory sensation, peripheral neuropathy, gait abnormalities, cognitive impairment, glossitises, and macrocytic anemia.

Zinc is a mineral that helps maintain the immune system and is associated with cell division, cell growth, wound healing, and carbohydrate metabolism. A zinc deficiency also exacerbate hair loss, which is common within the first six months after bariatric surgery. Furthermore, patients who are zinc deficient may experience a metallic taste in their mouths. Studies had shown that BPD and RYGB patients are more likely to be at risk of zinc deficiency. However, one study found that 34% of gastric sleeve patients experienced zinc deficiency post-surgery.

During routine clinic follow-up after bariatric surgery, it is important to monitor weight loss progress and complications each visit, monitor adherence to appropriate diet and physical activity levels, review medications (avoid NSAIDs, adjust antihypertensives, cholesterol-lowering medications, and diabetes medications as appropriate). Changes in drug absorption and bioavailability in post-bariatric surgery patients make dosage adjustment important for some of the prescribed medications. The requirement for diabetes medications often reduced after bariatric surgery.

In terms of nutritional supplements, patients should be taking adult multivitamin and multimineral which contain iron, folic acid, thiamine, vitamin B12 (doses: two tablets daily for LSG or RYGB; one daily for adjustable LAGB), calcium 1200–1500 mg/day, titrate 25-OH vitamin D levels >30 ng/mL, typical dose of Vitamin D required is 3000 IU/day. Additional iron and vitamin B12 supplementation is usually required and dosage is based on lab results. Laboratory assessments should include FBE, urea, creatinine and electrolytes, LFTs, uric acid, glucose, lipids (every 6–12 months), 25-OH vitamin D, PTH, calcium, albumin, phosphate, B12, folate, iron studies annually, more frequently if deficiencies identified.

Lee P, Dixon J. Bariatric–metabolic surgery: A guide for the primary care physician. Austral Family Physician. 2017;46(7):465–471.
https://www.racgp.org.au/download/Documents/AFP/2017/July/AFP-Focus-Bariatric-metabolic-surgery-2017.pdf

35. Answer: F

36. Answer: H

Hypothyroidism is one of the most common endocrine disturbances alongside diabetes. It may present in the elderly with very non-specific symptoms and signs. It should be considered in the differential diagnosis of anyone presenting with confusion (so-called part of the 'dementia' screen) and general deterioration with no readily identifiable cause. It should not be missed as a cause of a range of symptoms from neurological signs, typically bradykinesia, reduced deep tendon reflexes, and paraesthesias from nerve entrapment (especially carpal tunnel syndrome) to abdominal pain from chronic constipation to mental disturbance manifest as confusion and apparent memory impairment. Other subtle signs of hypothyroidism include loss of the outer one-third of the eyebrows with male-pattern frontal balding, hypothermia, bradycardia, non-pitting oedema (myxoedema), and dry, coarse skin.

TFTs are usually diagnostic and demonstrate a low free thyroxine (T4) with a high TSH in primary hypothyroidism. Very occasionally a low TSH and a low free T4 may be seen in the context of panhypopituitarism and assay of levels of sex hormones, ACTH, and other pituitary hormones will confirm the diagnosis.

Lithium is used in the treatment of bipolar disorder. It can cause major disturbance in water balance, manifest by polyuria and secondary polydipsia. This is because of decreasing urinary concentrating ability resulting from impaired responsiveness of the distal nephron to anti-diuretic hormone (ADH) which is known as nephrogenic diabetes insipidus. In most cases there is a correlation between impaired urinary concentrating ability and duration of lithium therapy or total lithium dose.

Nephrogenic diabetes insipidus in adults is usually partial with mild symptoms. Usually the serum sodium is normal or mildly elevated, the plasma osmolality is within normal range, the urine osmolality is low (<300 mOsmol/kg) and the urine volume is between 2.5 and 6 L/day. However when patients are fluid depleted, there is a marked rise in serum sodium, a rise in plasma osmolality urine osmolality that may exceed that of plasma. The water deprivation test is useful in diagnosis: the urine osmolality is usually <300 mOsmol/kg after dehydration with no further or a minimal (<95) rise after desmopressin. In partial nephrogenic diabetes insipidus, the urine osmolality is between 300 and 750 mOsmol/kg after dehydration and is <750 mOsmol/kg after desmopressin. Lithium-induced nephrogenic diabetes insipidus is usually reversible on stopping therapy but a few patients remain symptomatic long after the lithium has been discontinued. If the urine volume exceeds 4 L/day, treatment with thiazides and amiloride has been advocated. Preventive measures include education of patients and their carers about maintaining adequate hydration. The serum lithium level should be kept between 0.5 and 0.8 mmol/L. Annual measurement of 24-hour urine volume is a simple and effective screening test.

Gitlin M. Lithium side effects and toxicity: prevalence and management strategies. International Journal of Bipolar Disorders. 2016;4(1).
https://journalbipolardisorders.springeropen.com/articles/10.1186/s40345-016-0068-y

5 Epidemiology, Statistics, and Research

Questions

Answers can be found in the Epidemiology, Statistics, and Research Answers section at the end of this chapter.

1. You have developed a new method to measure a biomarkers in blood for oxidative stress. Most of the measurements range from 30–50 ng/L. However, there are several samples which measure 200–300 ng/L.

Which measure of central tendency would be the most distorted by the outlier results?
- **A.** Arithmetic mean.
- **B.** Geometric mean.
- **C.** Median.
- **D.** Mode.

2. While using non-parametric testing for your research data, which one of the following statements is true?
- **A.** It can be applied to ordinal data.
- **B.** It can only be used for data that is normally distributed.
- **C.** It has greater statistical power than a parametric test.
- **D.** It is only suitable for large sample sizes.

3. During a double-blind randomised placebo-controlled clinical trial for a new medication which treats severe sepsis involving 1200 participants in each arm, 156 participants receiving standard care died in the hospital and 108 participants died receiving the new medication on top of the standard care. The number needed to treat (NNT) for this new medication in this trial is:
- **A.** 25
- **B.** 48
- **C.** 50
- **D.** 100

4. You are conducting a case-control study to see whether there is an association between taking 'Livelonga' herbal medicine and the development of CKD. In the study group, there are 500 participants who have been taking Livelonga herbal medicine for more than 2 years. 50 participants develop CKD and 450 do not develop CKD. In the control group, there are 10 participants who do not take the herbal medicine and develop CKD; the remaining 490 do not develop CKD.

What is the odds ratio (OR) of having CKD in patients taking Livelonga for more than 2 years?
- **A.** 4.5
- **B.** 5.5
- **C.** 12.5
- **D.** Not enough information to calculate OR

5. You are an associate investigator in a randomised controlled drug trial which is being conducted in your unit. Which one of the following types of biases will be reduced by randomisation in your trial?
- **A.** Ascertainment bias.
- **B.** Bias in handling dropouts.
- **C.** Recall bias.
- **D.** Selection bias.

How to Pass the FRACP Written Examination, First Edition. Jonathan Gleadle, Jordan Li, Danielle Wu, and Paul Kleinig.
© 2022 John Wiley & Sons Ltd. Published 2022 by John Wiley & Sons Ltd.

6. In a pilot study to evaluate a new urine test for bladder cancer, a cohort of 35 participants is investigated. This new test is positive in 15 of the 35 participants. Bladder cancer is confirmed by conventional 'gold standard' test cystoscopy plus biopsy in 6 of the 35 participants. Of the 15 participants with a positive result from the new test, 6 are shown to have bladder cancer by the conventional 'gold standard' test. The new test is negative in 20 of the 35 participants and none of them are subsequently shown to have bladder cancer by the conventional test.

What is the main issue for the new urine test for bladder cancer?
- **A.** The performance of the new test cannot be interpreted as the prevalence of bladder cancer is too high.
- **B.** The negative predictive value of the new test is 40%.
- **C.** The sensitivity of the new test is too low.
- **D.** The specificity of the new test is too low.

7. The frequency of attendance of 120 final year medical students at a weekly 'Transition to Internship Program' teaching session is recorded over a six-month period. The students are assessed at the end of this period with 100 multiple choice questions (MCQs).

Which of the following statistical tests is the most appropriate to evaluate the effectiveness of students' attendance on improving MCQ scores?
- **A.** Chi-square test.
- **B.** Fisher's exact test.
- **C.** Spearman's rank correlation test.
- **D.** Student's t test.

8. Range, standard deviation (SD), and variance are common measures of dispersion. Which one of the following is correct concerning measures of dispersion?
- **A.** In a normal distribution, 70% of the values will fall between one SD above and below the mean value.
- **B.** Range is the difference between 75th and 25th percentiles, and the most commonly used measure of dispersion.
- **C.** The range gives the width of the entire distribution and the pattern of the distribution.
- **D.** Variance is the standard deviation squared.

9. You are organising a study to investigate the association between low birth weight and maternal alcohol intake during pregnancy sin a Maori population. The alcohol intake history is obtained during the routine prenatal visits. The birth weight is recorded at delivery and assigned according to the alcohol use history.

What type of study is this?
- **A.** Case-control study.
- **B.** Clinical trial.
- **C.** Cross-sectional study.
- **D.** Prospective cohort study.

10. A study is testing the effects of a new drug on hypertension. Two groups of hypertensive patients are recruited. One group is treated with the drug for 6 months while the other is given a placebo. The study evaluated the reduction of blood pressure after treatment between the two groups.

What is the most appropriate statistical test to use for this study?
- **A.** Paired t-test.
- **B.** Unpaired t-test.
- **C.** Mann Whitney U-test.
- **D.** Chi-square test.

11. A 52-year-old woman has peritoneal metastasis from ovarian cancer. Pressurized IntraPeritoneal Aerosol Chemotherapy (PIPAC) treatment is planned as part of a clinical trial. To obtain her informed consent, which one of the following is **NOT** essential?
- **A.** Inform patient of the alternatives to the PIPAC treatment.
- **B.** Inform patient of the consequences if the PIPAC treatment is not given.
- **C.** Inform patient of the nature, goal, benefits and risks of the PIPAC treatment.
- **D.** Obtain patient's next of kin written consent.

12. Which method can be used to evaluate the possibility of publication bias in a meta-analysis?
   A. Chi squared test.
   B. Confidence interval.
   C. Funnel plot.
   D. I^2 test.

QUESTIONS (13–15) REFER TO THE FOLLOWING INFORMATION
   A. Attack rate.
   B. Case fatality.
   C. Crude rate.
   D. Incidence rate.
   E. Population attributable risk.
   F. Prevalence.
   G. Risk.
   H. Survival.

13. What is the most appropriate measure to estimate the proportion of the South Australians who suffered from obesity in 2018?

14. Which is the best measure to describe the risk of death among patients with a confirmed diagnosis of Ebola haemorrhagic fever?

15. Which is the best measure to define the proportion of patient following head or neck radiation treatment who will develop thyroid cancer?

QUESTIONS (16–18) REFER TO THE FOLLOWING INFORMATION
For each of the following medical research projects in your hospital, select the type of error that is most likely to occur.
   A. Cohort effect.
   B. Confounding.
   C. Differential misclassification.
   D. Ecologic fallacy
   E. Non-differential misclassification.
   F. Random errors.
   G. Recall bias.
   H. Selection bias.

16. In a case-control study of the relationship of urine albumin-creatinine ratio (ACR) to risk of developing CKD, 90-day-old stored frozen urine samples are used to measure ACR among cases and controls. While in transport and storage, the samples have deteriorated resulting in artificially low ACR.

17. In a cohort study of daily calcium supplement and the risk of developing coronary artery disease, high socioeconomic status is associated with both use of calcium supplement and the risk of developing coronary artery disease.

18. In a case-control study of the relationship between a new lipid-lowering drug, and the risk of developing cancer, control subjects are sampled from voluntary participants in a health screening program of a large state government department.

Answers

1. Answer: A

The measure of central tendency is a statistic that summarises the entire quantitative set of data in a single value (a representative value for the data set) having a tendency to concentrate somewhere in the centre of the data. The summary value of central tendency is also known as the measure of location or position, or average.

The measure of central tendency should be somewhere within the range of the data set. It should remain unchanged by a rearrangement of the observations in a different order. The mean, median, and mode are all valid measures of central tendency, but under different situations, some measures of central tendency become more appropriate to use than others.

The arithmetic mean: The sum of all measurements divided by the number of observations in the data set. It uses all the data values, but it is distorted by outliers and skewed data as seen in this question.

The geometric mean: The arithmetic mean is an inappropriate measurement of central tendency or location if the data is skewed. If the data is skewed to the right, a distribution that is more symmetrical can be calculated if one takes the logarithm of each value of the variable in the data set. The arithmetic mean of the log values is a measure of location for the transformed data. This will generate the geometric mean which is appropriate for right skewed data.

Median is the middle value in the data set when all of the values (observations) in a data set are arranged in ascending or descending order of magnitude. Median is also considered as a measure of central tendency which divides the data set in two halves, where the first half contains 50% observations below the median value and 50% above the median value. If in a data set there are an odd number of observations (data points), the median value is the single most middle value after sorting the data set. When the number of observations in a data set is even then the median value is the average of two middlemost values in the sorted data. The median is less affected by extreme values in the data set, so median is the preferred measure of central tendency when the data set is skewed or not symmetrical.

Mode represents the most frequently occurring value in the data set and it is therefore not sensitive to outliers, just like the median. Since mode is the most frequently occurring score, it can be determined directly from a frequency distribution or a histogram. It is possible that there may be more than one mode or it may also be possible that there is no mode in a data set. Usually mode is used for categorical data. If any of the data points don't have the same values then the mode of that data set will not exist or not be meaningful. A data set having more than one mode is called multimode or multimodal.

Tenny S, Hoffman M. Median [Internet]. Statpearls.com. 2019 [cited 18 February 2020]. Available from: https://www.statpearls.com/kb/viewarticle/34516/

2. Answer: A

Non-parametric tests, also known as distribution-free tests are used when the data is not normally distributed, or the distribution of the data is unknown. If the data has approximately normal distribution, then one should use parametric statistical tests. Therefore, the key is to figure out the distribution of data.

If at all possible, one should use parametric tests, as they are more accurate. Parametric tests have greater statistical power, which means they are likely to find a true significant effect. Use non-parametric tests only if necessary (i.e. you know that assumptions like normality are being violated).

Other reasons to use non-parametric tests:
- The study result is better represented by the median rather than mean.
- The sample size is too small to run a parametric test.
- The data is ordinal data, ranked data.
- The data has outliers that cannot be removed.

The common parametric tests include ANOVA and Student's T test. Both these tests assume that the population data has a normal distribution. Non-parametric tests do not assume that the data is normally distributed. One common non-parametric test is the Chi-square test. Other examples include: the Kruskal Willis test, which is a non-parametric alternative to the One-way ANOVA, and the Mann Whitney, which is the non-parametric alternative to the two-sample t-test.

In summary, non-parametric tests have several advantages when compared to parametric tests:
- Greater statistical power when assumptions for the parametric tests have been violated.
- Fewer assumptions (i.e. the assumption of normality does not apply).

- Small sample sizes are acceptable.
- They can be used for all data types, including nominal variables, interval variables, or data that has outliers or that has been measured imprecisely.

Whitley E, Ball J. Statistics review 6: Nonparametric methods. Critical Care. 2002;6(6):509.
http://ccforum.com/content/6/6/509

3 Answer: A

The benefit of an intervention or treatment can be expressed by the number needed to treat (NNT), meaning the number of patients who need to be treated for one patient to benefit. The NNT is the inverse of the absolute risk reduction (ARR). The ARR is the absolute difference in the rates of events between a given intervention or treatment relative to a control activity or treatment, i.e. control event rate (CER) minus the experimental event rate (EER), or ARR = CER − EER. In this case, the control mortality is 156/1200 = 13% and the treatment group mortality is 108/1200 = 9%. Therefore, NNT = 1/13% − 9% = 25. Or expressed another way 156 − 108 = 48 out of 1200 participants benefitted from the new medication, so the NNT is 1200/48 = 25.

The NNT provides a more clinically useful measure of the relative benefit of an active treatment over a control than the use of the relative risk, the relative risk reduction (RRR) or the odds ratio. The ideal NNT would be 1, which means all patients treated will benefit. NNTs can be used either for summarising the results of a therapeutic trial or for medical decision-making about an individual. NNT allows a simple explanation of the likelihood of benefit, which may be used in helping patients reach a decision about whether to start a medication. An analogous calculation can be made to look at harm, e.g. side effects in the number needed to harm.

NNT cannot be used for performing a meta-analysis. Pooled NNTs derived from meta-analyses can be seriously misleading because the baseline risk often varies appreciably between the trials. NNT cannot be used to calculate the risk/benefit ratio for an individual person, it gives the information for the population as a whole. The concept expresses the number of individuals who must be treated for one to benefit but not the degree of benefit, which will vary across conditions and circumstances.

Mendes D, Alves C, Batel-Marques F. Number needed to treat (NNT) in clinical literature: an appraisal. BMC Medicine. 2017;15(1).
https://bmcmedicine.biomedcentral.com/articles/10.1186/s12916-017-0875-8

4. Answer: B

The odds ratio (OR) is a measure of how strongly an event is associated with exposure. OR is a ratio of two sets of odds: the odds of the event occurring in an exposed group versus the odds of the event occurring in an unexposed group. OR = (odds of the event in the exposed group) / (odds of the event in the non-exposed group).

$$\text{Odds in exposed group} = (\text{taking Livelonga with CKD}) / (\text{taking Livelonga without CKD}) = 50 / 450 = 0.11$$

$$\text{Odds in non-exposed group} = (\text{no herbal medicine with CKD}) / (\text{no medicine without CKD}) = 10 / 490 = 0.02$$

$$\text{Odds ratio} = (\text{odds in exposed group}) / (\text{odds in unexposed group}) = 0.11 / 0.02 = 5.5$$

ORs are commonly used to report case-control studies but can also be used in cross-sectional and cohort study designs. The OR helps identify how likely an exposure is to lead to a specific event. The larger the OR, the higher odds that the event will occur with exposure, and thus the exposure may be considered a risk factor. OR less than one implies the event has fewer odds of happening with the exposure and may suggest the exposure is a protective factor.

The 95% confidence interval (CI) is used to estimate the precision of the OR. A large CI indicates a low level of precision of the OR, whereas a small CI indicates a higher precision of the OR. It is important to note however, that unlike the p value, the 95% CI does not report a measure's statistical significance. In practice, the 95% CI is often used as a proxy for the presence of statistical significance if it does not overlap the null value (e.g. OR = 1). Nevertheless, it would be inappropriate to interpret an OR with 95% CI that spans the null value as indicating evidence for lack of association between the exposure and outcome.

5. Answer: D

A central doctrine of many clinical trials is randomisation. Subjects are randomised in a trial to ensure that the groups are as similar as possible. It reduces systematic differences between intervention groups in factors, known and unknown, that may affect outcome of the trial other than the intervention. Randomisation means that each subject has a predetermined chance of being allocated to each group, but the group to be allocated cannot be predicted. This will minimise any selection bias.

Ascertainment bias occurs when the results of a trial are systematically distorted by the knowledge of which intervention each participant is receiving. This type of bias is minimised by blinding of researchers, clinicians, and participants.

Loss of some participants to follow-up and dropout occurs in any clinical trial. Bias caused by dropouts occurs because characteristics of subjects who left the trial before completion may be different from those who do not. This type of bias is minimised by appropriate analysis such as intention to treat analysis.

Recall bias occurs when the subjects' recall of past events is distorted and inaccurate. This type of bias occurs mainly in retrospective studies such as case control studies rather than randomised controlled trials.

 Munnangi S, Boktor S. Epidemiology Of Study Design [Internet]. Statpearls.com. 2020 [cited 18 February 2020]. Available from: https://www.statpearls.com/kb/viewarticle/21207/

6. Answer: D

		Gold standard test		
		TCC	No TCC	Total
New test	Positive	6 TP	9 FP	15
	Negative	0 FN	20 TN	20
	Total	6	29	35

TCC: Transitional cell cancer, TP: True positive, TN: True negative,
FP: False positive, FN: False negative, PPV: Positive predictive value,
NPV: Negative predictive value

$$\text{Sensitivity} = TP / (TP + FN) = 6 / (6 + 0) = 100\%$$

$$\text{Specificity} = TN / (TN + FP) = 20 / (20 + 9) = 69\%$$

$$PPV = TP / (TP + FP) = 6 / (6 + 9) = 40\%$$

$$NPV = TN / (FN + TN) = 20 / (20 + 0) = 100\%$$

The prevalence of a disease is the number of people with the disease in the test population at the time of testing. In this instance, the prevalence of TCC in this cohort is 6/35 = 17%. The performance of the new test should not be influenced by the prevalence.

Sensitivity and specificity are two statistical test characteristics to describe a population under test. They are often inversely related. Sensitivity is the proportion of subjects with the disease showing a positive test result while specificity is the proportion of subjects without the disease showing a negative test result. In this instance, the sensitivity is 100% which is excellent.

The false negative rate can be calculated as the number of false negatives divided by all those who have disease (i.e. the number of true positives plus the false negatives). False negative rate is also equal to 1 − sensitivity.

The specificity is 69% in this study. Positive predictive value is the proportion of those subjects testing positive who actually have the disease while negative predictive value is the proportion of those subjects testing negative who do not truly have the disease. In this instance, the negative predictive value is 100% which is excellent, but the positive predictive value of the new test is only 40%. There is thus a high false positive result with the new test: 9/15 = 60%. This is the biggest challenge for this new test which means many patients with a positive result using the new urine test will have to undergo invasive cystoscopy but up to 60% of these patients will not have bladder cancer.

7. Answer: C

Spearman's rank correlation is a non-parametric measure of statistical dependence between two variables. It assesses how well the relationship between two variables can be described using a monotonic function. If there are no repeated data values, a perfect Spearman correlation of +1 or −1 occurs when each of the variables is a perfect monotone function of the other.

The Chi-squared test is most often used in situations where raw data is being examined for effect and is similar to the paired student's t-test in generating p values, however, the latter is used for comparison of the means of two populations.

Fisher's exact test is a statistical significance test used in the analysis of contingency tables. It is employed when sample sizes are small, it is valid for all sample sizes. It is one of a class of exact tests, so called because the significance of the deviation from a null hypothesis (e.g. P-value) can be calculated exactly, rather than relying on an approximation that becomes exact in the limit as the sample size grows to infinity, as with many statistical tests.

8. Answer: D

Range, standard deviation (SD), and variance are common measures of dispersion. The SD is the most widely used measure of the spread of data about their mean. The larger the SD, the more spread out the distribution of the data about the mean. The range is the measurement of the width of the entire distribution and is found simply by calculating the difference between the highest and lowest value. The range gives no information about the distribution of the value. Interquartile range (IQR), also called the midspread, middle 50%, is another measure of statistical dispersion. It equal to the difference between 75th and 25th percentiles, or between upper and lower quartiles, IQR = Q3 − Q1. In other words, the IQR is the first quartile subtracted from the third quartile. In skewed distributions, the extreme values will affect the mean to a larger degree than they will affect the median. In normal distributions, 68% of the values should fall between one SD in either direction and over 95% of the values should be fall between two SDs in either direction. The variance is the measurement of the variation among all the subjects in the sample. The variance is simply the square of the SD.

 Kroussel-Wood M, Chambers R, Muntner P. Clinicians' guide to statistics for medical practice and research: part I. The Ochsner Journals. 2006;6(2):68–83.
https://www.ncbi.nlm.nih.gov/pmc/articles/PMC3121570/

9. Answer: D

This study is a prospective cohort study. The research participants are categorised on the basis of alcohol exposure or non-alcohol exposure then are followed forward in time to determine the occurrence of a particular outcome (low birth weight).

Clinical trial is research investigation in which participants volunteer to test new treatments, interventions or tests as a means to prevent, detect, treat, or manage various diseases or medical conditions but in this case there in no new intervention or treatment.

Cross-sectional study is a type of observational study that analyses data from a cohort, or a representative subset, at a specific point in time. The exposure and outcome are measured at the same time point.

Case–control study is a type of observational study in which two existing groups differing in outcome are identified and compared on the basis of some supposed causal attribute.

 Kroussel-Wood M, Chambers R, Muntner P. Clinicians' guide to statistics for medical practice and research: part I. The Ochsner Journals. 2006;6(2):68–83.
https://www.ncbi.nlm.nih.gov/pmc/articles/PMC3121570/

10. Answer: B

In the unpaired (Student's) t-test, two groups can be independent of each other, i.e. individuals randomly assigned into two groups, measured after an intervention and compared with the other group.

In the paired t-test, each member of one sample has a unique relationship with a particular member of the other sample, e.g. the same people measured before and after a new treatment.

The Mann Whitney U-test is used for non-parametric (not normal distribution) analysis. In this study, it is assumed that both groups have normal distributed BP values.

A chi-square test is commonly used for testing relationships between expected frequencies and the observed frequencies in categorical variables. The null hypothesis of the Chi-Square test is that no relationship exists between the categorical variables in the population.

Whitley E, Ball J. Statistics review 6: Nonparametric methods. Critical Care. 2002;6(6):509.
http://ccforum.com/content/6/6/509

11. Answer: D

The main purpose of the informed consent process is to protect the patient. Informed consent is based on the moral and legal premise of patient autonomy: You as the patient have the right to make decisions about your own health and medical conditions. For many types of interactions (for example, a physical exam with treating doctor, attend a blood test), implied consent is assumed. For more invasive tests or for those tests or treatments with significant risks or alternatives, the patient will be asked to give explicit (written) consent.

There are four components of informed consent:

1. Patient must have the capacity (or ability) to make the decision.
2. The treating doctors must disclose information on the treatment, test, or procedure in question, including the expected benefits and risks, and the likelihood (or probability) that the benefits and risks will occur. Appropriate alternatives should also be disclosed. Consent for enrolment in clinical trials should always be obtained.
3. Patient must comprehend the relevant information.
4. Patient must voluntarily grant consent, without coercion or duress.

Consent may be obtained verbally but it must be documented in the case notes. Written consent is not always required but it is done for most major interventions such in this case. It provides proof that some degree of discussion or consultation occurred between the treating doctor and a patient. Written consent is not an absolute protection against liability or proof that information was comprehensive and understood. Written consent should be obtained from the patient with capacity.

12. Answer: C

Publication bias refers to the over representation of studies with positive, significant effects in the systemic reviews. Funnel plots can detect publication bias. The funnel plot is a graphical representation of the size of trials plotted against the effect size they report. As the size of the trial increases, trials are likely to converge around the true underlying effect size. One would expect to see an even scattering of trials either side of this true underlying effect. A symmetric inverted funnel shape that arises from a systemic review data set indicates that publication bias is unlikely. When publication bias has occurred, one expects an asymmetry in the scatter of small studies with more studies showing a positive result that those showing a negative result.

Heterogeneity in meta-analysis refers to the variation in study outcomes between studies. There are two statistical methods to measure heterogeneity.

Chi-squared (χ^2) test

This test assumes the null hypothesis that all the studies are homogeneous, or that each study is measuring an identical effect, and gives us a p-value to test this hypothesis. If the p-value of the test is low we can reject the hypothesis and heterogeneity is present. Because the test is often not sensitive enough and the wrong exclusion of heterogeneity happens quickly, many scientists use a p-value of <0.1 instead of <0.05 as the cut-off.

I^2 statistic test

This test describes the percentage of variation across studies that is due to heterogeneity rather than chance. It represents the percentage of the total variation across studies due to heterogeneity. Thresholds for the interpretation of I^2 can be misleading since the importance of inconsistency depends on several factors. A rough guide to interpretation is as follows:

0%: No heterogeneity
25%: Low heterogeneity
50%: Moderate heterogeneity
75%: High heterogeneity

Sterne Jonathan A C, Sutton Alex J, Ioannidis John P A, Terrin Norma, Jones David R, Lau Joseph et al. Recommendations for examining and interpreting funnel plot asymmetry in meta-analyses of randomised controlled trials BMJ 2011; 343:d4002.
https://www.bmj.com/content/343/bmj.d4002

13. Answer: F

14. Answer: B

15. Answer: G

There are several commonly used epidemiological measurements to describe the occurrence of disease.

Prevalence measures the proportion of individuals in a defined population that have a disease or other health outcomes of interest at a specified point in time (point prevalence) or during a specified period of time (period prevalence).

$$\text{Point Prevalence} = \frac{\text{Number of cases in a defined population at one point in time}}{\text{Number of persons in a defined population at the same point in time}}$$

In contrast to prevalence, incidence is a measure of the number of new cases of a disease (or other health outcome of interest) that develops in a population at risk during a specified time period. There are two main measures of incidence:

Risk is the proportion of individuals in a population (initially free of disease) who develop the disease within a specified time interval. Incidence risk is expressed as a percentage (or if small as per 1000 persons).

$$\text{Incidence Risk} = \frac{\text{Number of new cases of disease in a specified period of time}}{\text{Number of disease-free persons at the beginning of that time period}}$$

Incidence Rate also measures the frequency of new cases of disease in a population. However, incidence rates take into account the sum of the time that each person remained under observation and the time at which they were at risk of developing the outcome under investigation.

$$\text{Incidence Rate} = \frac{\text{Number of new cases of disease in a given time period}}{\text{Total person-time at risk during the follow-up period}}$$

Case Fatality is the proportion of persons within a population affected by a particular disease that die from the disease within a specified period of times.

Attack Rate is the measure of frequency of morbidity, or speed of spread, in an at-risk population. It is the proportion of people who become ill with (or who die from) a disease in a population initially free of the disease. The term attack rate is sometimes used interchangeably with the term incidence rate. Attack rates typically are used in the investigation of acute outbreaks of disease, where they can help identify exposures that contributed to the illness (e.g. consumption of a specific food). The attack rate is calculated as the number of people who became ill divided by the number of people at risk for the illness. In order to calculate an attack rate, a case definition, or set of criteria to define the disease of interest, must first be developed. The number of people who meet the case definition is represented in the numerator of the attack rate. The denominator of the attack rate is the number of people who are at risk of becoming ill. At-risk individuals are those persons who had the opportunity to be exposed to the disease – for example, all individuals who ate a certain food item.

Population Attributable Risk (PAR) is the proportion of the incidence of a disease in the population (exposed and unexposed) that is due to exposure. It is the incidence of a disease in the population that would be eliminated if exposure were eliminated. PAR measures the potential impact of control measures in a population and is relevant to decisions in public health. PAR is calculated by subtracting the incidence in the unexposed from the incidence in the total population (exposed and unexposed). PAR is usually expressed as a percentage. The PAR% is calculated by dividing the PAR by the incidence in the total population. In order to calculate PAR, the prevalence of exposure in the study population must be known or estimated (PAR = AR × prevalence of exposure to risk factor in the population).

Crude rates are calculated by dividing the total number of cases in a given time period by the total number of persons in the population. The problem with this comparison is that the crude rate is an overall average rate of disease, but it does not take into account possible confounding factors. A confounding factor is another risk factor for the outcome of interest that is also unequally distributed among the populations being compared and age is one of the most common confounding factors.

Chapter 2. Quantifying disease in populations | The BMJ [Internet]. Bmj.com. 2019 [cited 24 March 2019]. Available from: https://www.bmj.com/about-bmj/resources-readers/publications/epidemiology-uninitiated/2-quantifying-disease-populations

16. Answer: E

17. Answer: B

18. Answer: H

Bias is a systematic error in a study that leads to a distortion of the results. Bias can occur in any research but is of particular concern in observational studies because the lack of randomisation increases the chance that study groups will differ with respect to important characteristics. Bias often is subdivided into different categories, based on how bias enters the study. The most common classification divides bias into three categories:

1. Selection Bias

A variety of procedures can be used to select subjects for a study. The selection process itself, however, may increase or decrease the chance that a relationship between exposure and disease of interest will be detected. Selection bias is of particular importance in case-control studies in which the investigator must select two study groups, cases, and controls.

2. Information Bias

Information (or misclassification) bias can occur when there is random or systematic inaccuracy in measurement. If the errors in classification of exposure or disease status are independent of the level of the other variables, then the misclassification is termed non-differential. Differential misclassification, on the other hand, occurs when errors in the information about one variable are affected by the status of another variable.

3. Confounding

Confounding is concerned with the mixing of the primary effect of interest with the effects of one or more extraneous factors. In clinical studies such as scenario 2, the problem of confounding is reduced by randomisation, which tends to balance the study groups with respect to both known and unknown determinants of outcome.

Delgado-Rodriguez M. Bias. Journal of Epidemiology & Community Health. 2004;58(8):635–641.
https://jech.bmj.com/content/58/8/635

6 Gastroenterology

Questions

Answers can be found in the Gastroenterology Answers section at the end of this chapter.

1. An 84-year-old woman presents with acute abdominal pain of one hour's duration, with a background history of atrial fibrillation and peripheral vascular disease. Her pain is sharp, intense and she describes it as the 'worst pain ever'. Her medications are aspirin, perindopril, and atorvastatin. She is mildly tender over her epigastrium and right iliac fossa, but she does not have rebound or percussion tenderness. Her HR is 125 bpm and BP is 90/55 mmHg. Blood tests show no major abnormality. CT angiography shows occlusion of her superior mesenteric artery.

Which of the following measures is **LEAST LIKELY** to be part of appropriate initial management?
- **A.** Fasting.
- **B.** Intravenous antibiotics.
- **C.** Systemic anticoagulation.
- **D.** Vasopressors.

2. A 45-year-old man presents with epigastric pain to the emergency department. His lipase is elevated and an abdominal CT scan with contrast is consistent with acute pancreatitis, but no gallstones are present. He does not drink alcohol and has no history of diabetes, hyperlipidaemia, or ischaemic heart disease.

Which one of the following is **LEAST LIKELY** to be associated with the aetiology of his pancreatitis?
- **A.** A history of ANCA associated vasculitis on maintenance treatment with azathioprine and low dose prednisolone.
- **B.** A history of CKD due to biopsy proven IgG4 disease but not on prednisolone.
- **C.** A history of primary hyperparathyroidism awaiting parathyroidectomy.
- **D.** A history of Whipple's disease and just completed 7 days ceftriaxone treatment.

3. A 65-year-old man is brought to the emergency department by police after he is found lying on the floor in a shopping centre with a few empty beer bottles. He consumes high quantities of alcohol regularly. He reports abdominal pain in the epigastric area associated with nausea and vomiting for the last 2 days but he continues to consume alcohol. He also complains of dizziness when standing. Examination reveals tenderness in the epigastrium and right hypochondrium. A reddish discolouration is noted in the flanks and he cannot recall any previous falls or injuries. He is afebrile with BP 90/60 mmHg and HR 110 bpm. His initial laboratory results are shown below.

Tests	Results	Normal values
Sodium	132 mmol/L	135–145
Potassium	3.5 mmol/L	3.5–5.2
Urea	18 mmol/L	2.7–8.0
Creatinine	178 μmol/L	60–100
Albumin	21 g/L	38–48
Bilirubin	2.95 mmol/L	2–24
ALP	238 IU/L	30–110
GGT	159 IU/L	0–60
ALT	179 IU/L	0–55
AST	213 IU/L	0–45
Hb	101 g/L	135–175
WBC	16.3 x 10⁹/L	4.0–11.0
Platelet	765 x 10⁹/L	150–450
Lipase	830 IU/L	0–60

How to Pass the FRACP Written Examination, First Edition. Jonathan Gleadle, Jordan Li, Danielle Wu, and Paul Kleinig.
© 2022 John Wiley & Sons Ltd. Published 2022 by John Wiley & Sons Ltd.

Which of the following investigation results is most likely?
- **A.** His abdominal ultrasound is likely to demonstrate a pancreatic pseudocyst.
- **B.** His contrast abdominal CT is likely to demonstrate severe necrotising pancreatitis.
- **C.** His MRCP is likely to demonstrate choledocholithiasis.
- **D.** His plain AXR is likely to demonstrate pancreatic calcification.

4. A 56-year-old man is admitted for paracentesis due to recurrent ascites refractory to low salt diet and a combination of frusemide and spironolactone. This is his fifth paracentesis in the past 6 months. He is known to have cirrhosis secondary to hepatitis B infection which has been complicated by one episode of GI bleeding and one episode of encephalopathy. He is also taking propranolol and pantoprazole. On examination, he is mildly confused but afebrile. His BP is 90/60 mmHg, HR is 72 bpm, and BMI is 22 kg/m². He is jaundiced. There are signs of large ascites, chronic liver disease stigmata and peripheral oedema. His investigation results are presented below.

Tests	Results	Normal values
Sodium	128 mmol/L	135–145
Potassium	3.5 mmol/L	3.5–5.2
Bicarbonate	31 mmol/L	22–32
Urea	10.3 mmol/L	2.7–8.0
Creatinine	143 umol/L	60–110
Albumin	24 g/L	34–48
Bilirubin	5.5 umol/L	2–24
ALP	230 U/L	30–110
GGT	125 U/L	5–50
ALT	59 U/L	0–55
AST	73 U/L	0–45
Hb	70 g/L	135–175
WBC	7.1 x 10⁹/L	4–11
Platelet	95 x 10⁹/L	150–450
INR	3.1	0.9–1.3
AFP	4 ng/mL	<10

What is the next best treatment for this patient?
- **A.** Automated low-flow ascites (ALFA) pump.
- **B.** Liver transplant.
- **C.** Peritoneal dialysis.
- **D.** Transjugular intrahepatic portosystemic shunt (TIPS).

5. A 62-year-old woman presents with lethargy, nausea, abdominal pain, vomiting, and jaundice. On examination, there is no evidence of ascites or hepatic encephalopathy. All of the following serological markers are suggestive of a diagnosis of autoimmune hepatitis (AIH), **EXCEPT** which?
- **A.** Anti-smooth muscle antibodies (ASMA).
- **B.** Anti-soluble liver antigen/liver pancreas antibodies (Anti-SLA/LP).
- **C.** Cytoplasmic antineutrophil cytoplasmic antibodies (cANCA).
- **D.** Liver kidney microsome type 1 antibodies (Anti-LKM1).

6. A 50-year-old Caucasian man has a 10-year history of GORD for which he is intermittently taking ranitidine. He is a current heavy smoker and consumes 3 standard drinks of alcohol every day. He underwent an endoscopy due to epigastric pain. His endoscopy is shown below.

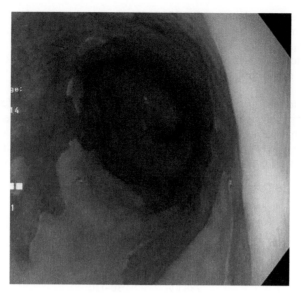

Which one of the following is correct in regarding this lesion?
- **A.** A biopsy will show columnar to squamous metaplasia.
- **B.** The most likely location of this lesion is the upper third of the oesophagus.
- **C.** This is a precursor to adenocarcinoma of the oesophagus.
- **D.** This is a precursor to adenocarcinoma of the stomach.

7. The brush border microvilli of intestinal epithelial cells **DO NOT** contain which one of the followings:
- **A.** Alkaline phosphatase.
- **B.** Amylase.
- **C.** Disaccharidases.
- **D.** Peptidases.

8. A 46-year-old man is referred by his urologist for investigation of recurrent renal calculi. He is known to have Crohn's disease but has been in remission for the past three years while on sulfasalazine. He has had several abdominal operations in the past. The proximal colon and 90 cm of the distal ileum were removed. His serum electrolytes, PTH, and urate level are normal.

Which one of the following appearances is most likely on urine microscopy examination?

(A)
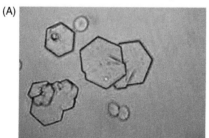

(B)
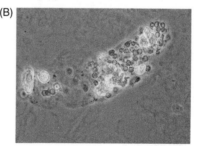

(C)
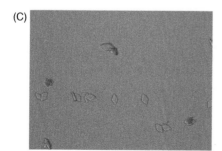

(D)
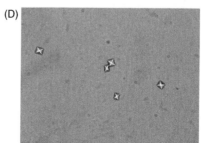

9. Which one of the statements regarding cirrhosis is **INCORRECT**?

    A. Direct oral anticoagulants may safely be used to prevent portal vein thrombosis in select patients.

    B. Once chronic liver disease progresses from a compensated to a decompensated state, it is no longer reversible.

    C. Statins have been shown to improve survival in patients who survive an episode of variceal bleeding.

    D. Transient elastography is a non-invasive way to diagnose cirrhosis.

10. A 65-year-old man presents to the emergency department (ED) with abdominal discomfort and breathlessness. He has a medical history of idiopathic cirrhosis complicated by recurrent large ascites which requires repeat paracentesis. On examination, he is haemodynamically stable with an oxygen saturation of 95% on room air. There is clinical evidence of large volume ascites. He wants to have a paracentesis to relieve his dyspnoea. The ED physician is concerned that he may have a PE and is arranging a CTPA. His initial investigation results are displayed below:

Tests	Results	Normal values
Sodium	128 mmol/L	135–145
Potassium	3.5 mmol/L	3.5–5.2
Urea	7.6 mmol/L	2.7–8.0
Creatinine	89 µmol/L	60–100
Albumin	21 g/L	38–48
Bilirubin	29 mmol/L	2–24
ALP	238 IU/L	30–110
GGT	159 IU/L	0–60
ALT	179 IU/L	0–55
AST	213 IU/L	0–45
Hb	101 g/L	135–175
WBC	7.1×10^9/L	4.0–11.0
Platelet	59×10^9/L	150–450
INR	1.8	0.9–1.2

What is the appropriate advice for the ED team?

    A. Arrange platelet transfusion until platelet $>100 \times 10^9$/L then proceed with paracentesis.

    B. Cancel CTPA as he is coagulopathic and PE is therefore unlikely.

    C. Give intravenous eltrombopag, a thrombopoietin receptor agonist, then proceed with paracentesis.

    D. Proceed with paracentesis without FFP and platelet infusion.

11. A 55-year-old woman is confirmed to have coeliac disease by small bowel biopsy after she presents with a 2-year history of intermittent poor appetite, abdominal distention, and weight loss. She is started on a gluten free diet. Her mother died of breast cancer at age of 67. Your appropriate follow up management plan is:

    A. Arrange for pneumococcal vaccination.

    B. Arrange screening for endometrial and ovarian cancer.

    C. Repeat endoscopy in 6 months to ensure mucosal healing.

    D. Repeat serology in 3 months to monitor mucosal healing.

12. A 55-year-old man underwent a colonoscopy because he had a positive FOBT which was performed via the Australian government bowel cancer screening program. There is no family history of bowel cancer. Several polyps were removed.

Which of the following types of polyps from his histopathology report is associated with the greatest risk of malignant transformation?

    A. Hyperplastic polyp.

    B. Mixed tubulovillous adenoma.

    C. Tubular adenoma.

    D. Villous adenoma.

13. A 56-year-old man had a normal colonoscopy following a positive screening for a FOBT sent by the Australian government. His father was diagnosed with bowel cancer at aged 82. He asks if there is anything he can do to reduce his risk of bowel cancer in the future.

Which one of the following is associated with a reduced risk of bowel cancer?

    A. Avoidance of processed meats.

    B. Drinking red wine.

    C. Low fibre diet.

    D. Smoking.

14. A 54-year-old woman has a 5-year history of chronic idiopathic constipation. She is taking prucalopride. This medication is a:
   A. 5-HT$_4$ receptor agonist.
   B. Osmotic laxative.
   C. Prosecretory agent.
   D. Stimulant laxative.

15. A 46-year-old man presents with a four month history of intermittent heartburn, solid food dysphagia and food impaction. His other medical history includes asthma and rhinitis. He is a current smoker. He undergoes an endoscopy where biopsies are taken. The results are shown below:

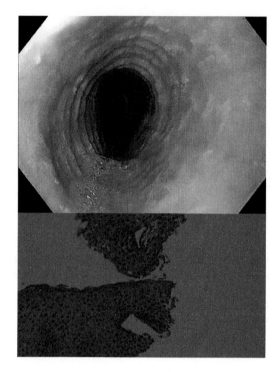

What is the mainstay of treatment for this condition?
   A. Gluten-free diet.
   B. Oral liquid budesonide.
   C. Oral prednisolone.
   D. Oral proton-pump inhibitor.

16. Which one of the following accurately describes the extraintestinal manifestations of inflammatory bowel disease (IBD)?
   A. Anti-TNF biological agents have no benefit for extraintestinal manifestations of IBD.
   B. Episcleritis, scleritis and uveitis are the most common extraintestinal manifestations of IBD.
   C. Extraintestinal manifestations of IBD only develop after the diagnosis of IBD.
   D. The likelihood of developing extraintestinal manifestations increases with IBD duration.

17. In regarding the use of faecal calprotectin in the diagnosis and management of inflammatory bowel disease, which one of the recommendations is **INAPPROPRIATE**?
   A. Calprotectin is specific for inflammatory bowel disease.
   B. Calprotectin is used as a diagnostic screening test.
   C. Calprotectin predicts imminent clinical relapse of inflammatory bowel disease.
   D. Calprotectin predicts mucosal healing of inflammatory bowel disease.

18. A 36-year-old woman undergoes gastrectomy for gastric cancer. Histopathology report describes the resected stomach as diffusely thickened without a lesion. Microscopic examination shows an infiltration of signet-ring tumour cells. She was also diagnosed 2 years ago to have left lobular breast cancer, oestrogen- and progesterone-receptor positive, for which she was treated with a nipple-sparing mastectomy. Her mother died of breast cancer at age of 45.

What gene is most likely mutated in this patient?
   A. APC.
   B. BRCA2.
   C. CDH1.
   D. PMS2.

19. Which of one of the following can cause unconjugated hyperbilirubinaemia?
   A. Dubin-Johnson syndrome.
   B. Gilbert's syndrome.
   C. Oral contraceptive pill.
   D. Primary biliary cirrhosis.

20. A 32-year-old man presents with a one-month history of epigastric discomfort. His endoscopy demonstrates a small duodenal ulcer and the biopsy shows the presence of *Helicobacter pylori*. He is treated with pantoprazole, clarithromycin and amoxicillin for 7 days. However, he still has mild epigastric discomfort and the urea breath test for *H. pylori* remains positive one month after treatment.

What second line treatment would you consider most appropriate in Australia or New Zealand at this stage?
   A. Amoxicillin, levofloxacin, and pantoprazole.
   B. Bismuth, metronidazole, pantoprazole, and tetracycline.
   C. Clarithromycin, trimethoprim-sulfamethoxazole, and pantoprazole.
   D. Sequential treatment with amoxicillin and pantoprazole then clarithromycin and pantoprazole.

21. A 55-year-old man with a past medical history of alcoholic liver disease, cirrhosis, and portal hypertension has repeated episodes of hepatic encephalopathy requiring admission. He is not responding to lactulose therapy. He last consumed alcohol 5 months ago.

What is the next best treatment strategy for this patient?
   A. Insertion of transjugular intrahepatic portosystemic shunt (TIPS).
   B. Liver transplantation.
   C. Protein restriction.
   D. Rifaximin.

22. A 32-year-old man has recently been diagnosed with HIV infection and is about to start treatment with highly active antiretroviral therapy (HAART). CD4 count is 450/μL. His social history includes prior intravenous drug use and unprotected sex with both male and female partners. He and his family were born in New Zealand and have not travelled extensively. As part of his treatment planning, he is screened for evidence of chronic hepatitis infection. His results for Hepatitis B infection screening are shown below:

Hepatitis B surface antigen (HBsAg)	-ve
Hepatitis B surface antibody (anti-HBs)	-ve
Hepatitis B core antibody (anti-HBc)	+ve
Hepatitis B e antibody (anti-HBe)	-ve
Hepatitis B core IgM	-ve
Hepatitis B DNA	absent

What is the most appropriate next step in management?
   A. Hepatitis B immunisation.
   B. Hepatitis B treatment prior to HAART treatment.
   C. Initiate HAART treatment and retest anti-HBc in one month.
   D. Treat hepatitis B and HIV concurrently.

23. A 55-year-old man is diagnosed with hepatitis C. His LFTs are mildly abnormal. His liver ultrasound demonstrates early cirrhotic changes.

Which one of the following statements regarding the direct-acting antiviral (DAA) treatment and follow up plan is **INCORRECT**?

- **A.** After successful hepatitis C virus (HCV) eradication treatment, there is no need for hepatocellular carcinoma surveillance.
- **B.** DAA treatment reduces the risk of cryoglobulinaemic vasculitis.
- **C.** Sustained virologic response should be confirmed at 24 weeks after successful eradication.
- **D.** There are DAA treatments against all 6 major HCV genotypes.

24. Which one of the following statements regarding hepatitis E infection is correct?

- **A.** Acute and chronic hepatitis E can be reliably diagnosed by detection of IgM and IgG antibodies to hepatitis E virus (HEV).
- **B.** Chronic HEV hepatitis can develop in immunocompromised patients.
- **C.** HEV causes a self-limiting acute hepatitis only; it does not cause fulminant hepatitis.
- **D.** HEV is transmitted by the faecal-oral route; it cannot be transmitted by blood transfusion.

25. Which of the following modes of transmission is most common in cases of hepatitis E acquired in developed countries?

- **A.** Blood transfusion.
- **B.** Contaminated food products.
- **C.** Intravenous drug use.
- **D.** Sexually transmitted.

26. In regard to screening for hepatocellular carcinoma, which one of the following is **INAPPROPRIATE**?

- **A.** Abdominal ultrasound every 6 months with serum alpha-fetoprotein level.
- **B.** Patients on the active liver transplant waiting list should be screened, regardless of the waiting time.
- **C.** Patient with cirrhosis and eligible for curative treatment should be screened, regardless of cause.
- **D.** Patient with non-alcoholic steatohepatitis without cirrhosis should be screened.

27. Hereditary haemochromatosis is associated with which of the following?

- **A.** Hepcidin deficiency.
- **B.** Increased insulin production.
- **C.** Reduced serum ferritin level.
- **D.** Reduced transferrin saturation.

28. A 30 year-old-man is referred to a Gastroenterology clinic. He has a six-year history of bloating and intermittent loose stools accompanied by crampy abdominal pain, with a maximum of three loose bowel actions a day. These symptoms have been stable over the last three years and are having a significant impact on his quality of life. He has no weight loss, fever, melaena, or tenesmus. There is no significant past medical history or family history. He has tried eliminating gluten and lactose entirely from his diet without any significant effect. His abdominal examination and digital rectal examination are normal. Basic blood tests show normal serum biochemistry and full blood examination.

Which of the following is the most appropriate investigation?

- **A.** An upper gastrointestinal endoscopy with small bowel biopsy.
- **B.** Colonoscopy.
- **C.** Faecal calprotectin.
- **D.** Sigmoidoscopy.

29. A 22-year-old woman presents to the Internal Medicine outpatient clinic with a 2-month history of nausea, bloating, diarrhoea, and abdominal cramps after consuming dairy products. Physical examination is non-contributory.

Which one of the following tests is **NOT** helpful in confirming your provisional diagnosis of lactose intolerance?

- **A.** Genetic test for lactase mutation.
- **B.** Hydrogen breath test.
- **C.** Milk specific IgE RAST test.
- **D.** Small bowel biopsy.

30. Which one of the following is the commonest indication for liver transplantation in patients with chronic liver disease in Australia and New Zealand?
  A. Alcoholic liver disease (ALD).
  B. Hepatitis B-related cirrhosis.
  C. Hepatitis C-related cirrhosis.
  D. Non-alcoholic steatohepatitis (NASH).

31. A 75-year-old man underwent a coronary artery angiogram and a drug eluting stent was inserted into his left anterior descending artery after he presented with chest pain and was found to have a STEMI. He was started on ticagrelor plus aspirin. His medical history includes type 2 diabetes, hypertension, stage 3A CKD with baseline serum creatinine 130 µmol/L [60–110], and gout. On day 5 of hospitalisation, he was found to have approximately 300 ml of rectal bleeding. He was haemodynamically stable with BP 120/70 mmHg. Haemoglobin was 106 g/L [135–175].
  The recommended management is to:
  A. Perform an abdominal CT angiogram urgently.
  B. Perform an upper endoscopy to exclude upper GI bleeding urgently.
  C. Stop aspirin and ticagrelor indefinitely.
  D. Transfuse two units of RBC immediately.

32. A 77-year-old man presents with a 6-month history of epigastric and umbilical abdominal pain, especially following meals. This is associated with nausea but no vomiting. There is no change of bowel movements and no melaena. He has lost 5 kg in 6 months as he tries to avoid eating. His other medical history includes IHD, PVD, diet-controlled type 2 diabetes, smoking related COPD and he is a current smoker. On examination, BP is 140/90 mmHg, oxygen saturation on room air is 93% and BMI is 18 kg/m². There is mild epigastric tenderness on palpation. Bowel sounds are normal. Abdominal ultrasound demonstrates no gallstones or evidence of cholecystitis. His recent FOBT is negative.
  The next appropriate investigation is:
  A. Capsule endoscopy.
  B. CT angiography of the abdomen.
  C. Colonoscopy.
  D. Gastric emptying study.

33. A 61-year-old man presents with a one-month history of non-specific epigastic discomfort. His medical history includes hypertension, hypercholesterolemia, obstructive sleep apnoea, gout, and obesity (BMI 42 kg/m²). He is currently taking ramipril, allopurinol, and atorvastatin. He does not drink alcohol. His physical examination is unremarkable except for central obesity. His liver ultrasound revealed features of hepatic steatosis. His laboratory investigation results are displayed below:

Tests	Results	Normal values
Urea	10.1 mmol/L	2.7–8.0
Creatinine	109 µmol/L	60–110
Albumin	36 g/L	34–48
Bilirubin	2.95 mmol/L	2–24
ALP	220 U/L	30–110
GGT	78 U/L	0–60
ALT	58 U/L	0–55
AST	53 U/L	0–45
Hb	146 g/L	135–175
WBC	7.1 x 10⁹/L	4.00–11.00
Platelet	59 x 10⁹/L	150–450
INR	1.1	0.9–1.2

He was referred for investigation and management of his hepatic steatosis. Apart from lifestyle interventions, you should advise:
  A. He can continue taking atorvastatin.
  B. He needs a liver biopsy before considering any treatment.
  C. He should be started on metformin.
  D. He should be started on ursodeoxycholic acid.

34. Which one of the following is an indication for oesophageal high-resolution manometry?
  A. Patients presenting with dysphagia for investigation.
  B. Patients with confirmed achalasia.
  C. Patients with suspected rumination syndrome.
  D. Patients with suspected gastro-oesophageal reflux disease.

35. Which one of the following additional findings is suggestive of oesophageal dysphagia instead of oropharyngeal dysphagia?
  A. Aspiration pneumonia.
  B. Coughing.
  C. Regurgitation.
  D. Speech disturbance.

36. Which one of the following is **NOT** a risk factor for paracetamol hepatotoxicity while using oral paracetamol at the recommended normal dose for headaches?
  A. Concomitant administration of oral and intravenous paracetamol.
  B. Concomitant use of drugs that induce cytochrome P450 2D6.
  C. Fasting.
  D. Induction of cytochrome P450 2E1 by alcohol.

37. Which one of the following is **NOT** associated with the long-term use of proton-pump inhibitors (PPIs)?
  A. Increased risk of chronic kidney disease.
  B. Increased risk of fracture.
  C. Increased risk of gastric cancer.
  D. Increased risk of hypomagnesaemia.

38. A 56-year-old woman presents to outpatient clinic with a 6-month history of fatigue, pruritus, dry eyes, dry mouth, and right upper abdominal discomfort. Physical examination is noncontributory. Initial blood test results are shown below:

Tests	Results	Normal values
Urea	13 mmol/L	2.7–8.0
Creatinine	109 µmol/L	60–110
Albumin	32 g/L	34–48
Bilirubin	43 mmol/L	2–24
ALP	720 U/L	30–110
GGT	780 U/L	0–60
ALT	58 U/L	0–55
AST	53 U/L	0–45
Hb	145 g/L	135–175
WBC	7.7 x 10⁹/L	4.00–11.00
Platelet	159 x 10⁹/L	150–450
INR	1.3	0.9–1.2

Which of the following serological markers is likely to be positive in this patient?
  A. Antibodies to liver kidney microsome type 1 (Anti-LKM1).
  B. Anti-smooth muscle antibodies (ASMAs).
  C. Anti-mitochondrial antibodies (AMAs).
  D. Atypical perinuclear antineutrophil cytoplasmic antibodies (atypical pANCAs).

39. A 75-year-old woman undergoes an internal fixation for right neck of femur fracture after a fall. As the orthogeriatric registrar, you note progressive painless abdominal distension in the last 3 days post operatively. She has minimal oral intake. Her pain is under control with oral oxycodone. Her vital signs are stable. Bowel sounds are decreased. There are no electrolytes disturbances. Her AXR is shown below:

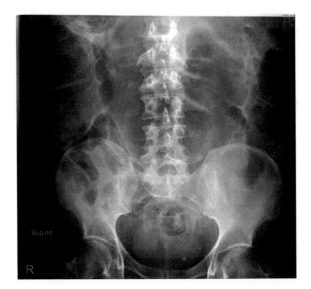

Which of the following statements is true concerning her diagnosis and management?
- **A.** A rectal tube as the primary treatment is generally not successful.
- **B.** After successful colonoscopic decompression, recurrence is unlikely.
- **C.** Intravenous patient-controlled analgesia should be used to hasten her recovery.
- **D.** Regular intravenous metoclopramide will hasten her recovery.

40. Which of the following laboratory results is most likely to be observed in a patient with severe small bowel bacterial overgrowth?

	Mean corpuscular volume	Folate level	Vitamin B$_{12}$ level
A	High	Low	Low
B	Normal	High	Normal
C	Normal	Normal	High
D	High	High	Low

41. Tacrolimus administration after liver transplantation does **NOT** cause which one of the following adverse effects?
- **A.** Bone marrow suppression.
- **B.** Diabetes mellitus.
- **C.** Hyperkalaemia.
- **D.** Seizures.

42. What is the mechanism of action of terlipressin in treatment of patients with hepatorenal syndrome?
- **A.** Acting through V1a receptors, causing insertion of aquaporin 2 to increase renal blood flow.
- **B.** Acting through V1a receptors, causing splanchnic vasoconstriction and increased renal blood flow.
- **C.** Acting through V2 renal receptors, causing insertion of aquaporin 2 to increase renal blood flow.
- **D.** Acting through V2 renal receptors, causing splanchnic vasoconstriction and increased renal blood flow.

43. A 62-year-old man presents to the emergency department with melaena, dizziness, and abdominal discomfort. His medical history including hypertension and diet-controlled type 2 diabetes. He is taking perindopril and aspirin. On examination, his BP is 86/40 mmHg and HR is 110 bpm. Haemoglobin is 96 g/L [135–175]. He undergoes an urgent endoscopy which reveals a gastric ulcer as shown below. He is treated with an adrenaline injection and thermal therapy. Biopsy is negative for *H. pylori* infection.

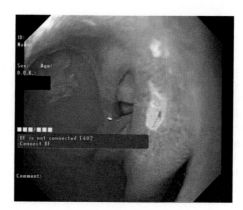

Which of the following is the most appropriate management after endoscopy?
- **A.** Give pantoprazole intravenously with a bolus followed by continuous infusion for 72 h.
- **B.** Keep patient fasted for 48 h after endoscopy.
- **C.** Repeat endoscopy 24 h after initial endoscopic haemostatic therapy.
- **D.** Resume enteric coated aspirin after 7 days given his cardiovascular risk factors.

44. A 45-year-old man is diagnosed with hypergastrinaemia due to Zollinger-Ellison syndrome associated with multiple endocrine neoplasia syndrome type 1 (MEN1).

Which one the following findings would likely be present in this patient?
- **A.** Decrease in lower esophageal sphincter (LES) pressure.
- **B.** Decrease in pepsinogen secretion.
- **C.** Increase in gastric motility.
- **D.** Inhibition of gastric mucosal growth.

QUESTIONS (45–50) REFER TO THE FOLLOWING INFORMATION

Match the gastrointestinal (GI) hormone with its main function.
- **A.** Gastrin.
- **B.** Cholecystokinin (CCK).
- **C.** Secretin.
- **D.** Glucose-dependent insulinotropic peptide (GIP).
- **E.** Glucagon-like peptide-1 (GLP-1).
- **F.** Motilin.
- **G.** Vasoactive intestinal peptide (VIP).
- **H.** Somatostatin.
- **I.** Ghrelin.

45. This peptide stimulates insulin secretion and induces satiety. In large doses, it decreases gastric acid secretion and decreases the motor activity of the stomach to slow gastric emptying when the upper small intestine is full. It also stimulates the activity of lipoprotein lipase in adipocytes. It protects beta-cells of the pancreas from destruction by apoptosis.

46. This hormone inhibits gastrin, acid secretion and growth of stomach mucosa. The hormone also stimulates biliary secretion of bicarbonate and fluid, and increases secretion of bicarbonate from the pancreas. It has a trophic effect on the exocrine pancreas.

47. This peptide decreases gastric emptying and induces satiety. It also increases sensitivity of pancreatic beta-cells to glucose.

48. This hormone is responsible for the inhibition of secretion and the function of many GI hormones.

49. This hormone stimulates the release of growth hormone from the pituitary and plays an important role in the regulation of food intake, energy homeostasis, gastric emptying and acid secretion.

50. This neuropeptide regulates gut mucosal growth. It is a potent vasodilator, and it regulates smooth muscle activity, epithelial cell secretion, and blood flow in the gastrointestinal tract.

Answers

1. Answer: D

Mesenteric ischaemia is an uncommon cause of acute abdominal pain but carries a high mortality. Females are more commonly affected than males. Early diagnosis is critically important for better outcomes. High serum lactate, acidosis, and hyperkalaemia are late signs and should not be relied upon for diagnosis. The typical presentation of pain out of proportion to examination findings is thought to be due to lack of peritoneal inflammation in early disease, and to the older age of the typical patient (around 70 years), in whom marked tenderness, percussion, and rebound tenderness are less likely in acute abdominal pathology. Causes of acute ischaemia are embolic events (which is most likely in this case), acute thrombosis of stenosed vessels, venous ischaemia due to thrombus, and non-occlusive disease, in which the dominant pathology is global hypoperfusion on stenosed or small calibre vessels.

Oral intake can exacerbate acute mesenteric ischaemia, so fasting is important in early management. Early supportive care involves fluid resuscitation, which may require fairly high volumes, even more so after revascularisation. Close monitoring of electrolytes is also important. Intravenous antibiotics and anticoagulation improve outcomes. Vasopressors should be avoided if possible as they can worsen ischaemia. Definitive management will often involve endovascular repair, or open embolectomy plus or minus arterial bypass. Non-viable organs are typically resected, and 'second look' operations are common to recheck areas of questionable viability. Chronic arterial ischaemia is most commonly treated with stenting, and nutritional support is highly relevant, as many patients will be malnourished. The mainstay of treatment of venous mesenteric ischaemia is anticoagulation, and long-term anticoagulation is often warranted. Failure of anticoagulation alone is only seen in around 5% of cases, and mechanical thrombectomy, thrombolysis, and directed arterially administered thrombolysis are often used for these cases. Addressing haemodynamic instability while minimising systemic vasoconstrictors is key in non-occlusive mesenteric ischaemia, and catheter directed vasodilatory medications have been used.

Smoking cessation, blood pressure control, and statins are recommended long term after an episode of mesenteric ischaemia. Lifelong aspirin is recommended, as well as clopidogrel for 1 to 3 months after endovascular repair. Atrial fibrillation and mesenteric venous thrombosis are indications for long term anticoagulation, either indefinitely or until the underlying cause has resolved.

Clair D, Beach J. Mesenteric Ischemia. New England Journal of Medicine. 2016;374(10):959–968.
https://www.nejm.org/doi/full/10.1056/NEJMra1503884

2. Answer: D

Acute pancreatitis is usually caused by either alcohol abuse or gallstones. Other causes of acute pancreatitis include:
- ERCP which can be complicated by acute pancreatitis in 5–20% of cases
- Diabetic ketoacidosis
- Severe hypercalcaemia
- Severe hypertriglyceridaemia
- Trauma
- Pancreatic cancer causing obstruction
- Biliary microlithiasis
- Medications
  - ✓ 5-aminosalicylic acid (5-ASA) derivatives
  - ✓ Antibiotics: Tetracycline, sulphonamides
  - ✓ Azathioprine
  - ✓ Diuretics: thiazides and frusemide
  - ✓ Oestrogens
  - ✓ Sodium valproate.

Whipple's disease is a systemic disease caused by a gram-positive bacterium, *Tropheryma whippelii*. It usually manifests as a malabsorption syndrome with small intestine involvement, but the disease also affects the joints, the central nervous system, and the cardiovascular system. It is not associated with acute pancreatitis. The standard initial treatment is intravenous ceftriaxone 2 g once daily for 14 days. After the initial treatment is completed, 1 year of maintenance therapy follows in the form of oral double-strength trimethoprim-sulfamethoxazole twice daily. This patient has not completed ceftriaxone treatment and has not started on sulphonamides.

Azathioprine can cause pancreatitis. Patients with hyperparathyroidism waiting for surgery may have severe hypercalcaemia which can cause pancreatitis.

IgG4-related disease (IgG4-RD) is a systemic fibroinflammatory disease characterised by dense infiltration of IgG4-positive plasma cells in the affected tissue(s) with or without elevated plasma levels of IgG4. The inflammatory infiltration along with a characteristic storiform fibrosis can lead to the development of chronic damage and dysfunction that may affect any organ. Common features include IgG4-related autoimmune pancreatitis, sclerosing cholangitis, retroperitoneal fibrosis, tubulointerstitial nephritis, and lung pseudotumour. Treatment is mainly with glucocorticoids, while multiple immunosuppressive medications can be used as adjuvant agents. Rituximab has shown promising results.

 Olson E, Perelman A, Birk J. Acute management of pancreatitis: the key to best outcomes. Postgraduate Medical Journal. 2019;95(1124):328–333.
https://pmj.bmj.com/content/95/1124/328

3. Answer: B

This patient's history and clinical features including abdominal pain, epigastric tenderness, hypotension, and Grey Turner's sign are suggestive of acute pancreatitis with pancreatic necrosis due to alcohol abuse. Hence a contrast CT scan of the abdomen is likely to reveal severe necrotising pancreatitis. Areas of necrosis are seen as non-enhancing low attenuating regions within the pancreas. Acute necrotising pancreatitis (ANP) often affects both the pancreas and peripancreatic tissues. Rarely it will affect only the peripancreatic tissues in isolation. Foci of gas may also be present in more extreme cases; extraluminal gas is highly suggestive of superimposed infection.

ANP is a subtype of acute pancreatitis (AP). Necrosis usually tends to occur early in AP, within the first 24–48 hours. ANP is defined by single or multiple organ failure lasting >48 hours and is diagnosed when >30% of the gland is affected by necrosis. ANP accounts for 10% of AP cases and is associated with a higher mortality (up to 25%) and morbidity. ANP may become infected in up to 40% cases, more commonly after the first week.

The revised Atlanta classification of AP should be used to predict severity and guide future management in all patients with severe AP. This classification is based upon both:
- Local factors (pancreatic necrosis)
- Systemic factors (organ failure)

In addition, based on CT imaging, the revised Atlanta classification divides AP and associated fluid collections into:
- Interstitial oedematous pancreatitis
  o within four weeks – acute peripancreatic fluid collections
  o after four weeks – pseudocyst
- Necrotising pancreatitis
  o within four weeks – acute necrotic collections (ANCs)
  o after four weeks – walled off necrosis (WON)

 Goodchild G, Chouhan M, Johnson G. Practical guide to the management of acute pancreatitis. Frontline Gastroenterology. 2019;10(3):292–299.
https://fg.bmj.com/content/10/3/292.full

4. Answer: B

Ascites is one of the most common complications of cirrhosis. Development of ascites is associated with poor prognosis. Approximately 60% of patients will develop ascites within 10 years after diagnosis of cirrhosis. Refractory ascites, which develops in 5–10% of all patients with cirrhotic ascites, has a 1–year mortality of 50%. Ascites can be treated by large-volume paracentesis (LVP), transjugular intrahepatic portosystemic shunt (TIPS), vasoconstrictive drugs, and an automated low-flow ascites (ALFA) pump, but liver transplantation is the most effective treatment modality.

The following are criteria for diagnosing refractory ascites:
1. Treatment duration, intensive diuretic therapy: spironolactone (400 mg/day) and frusemide (160 mg/day) for at least 1 week with a salt-restricted diet;
2. Lack of response, mean weight loss of <0.8 kg over 4 days and a urinary sodium output less than sodium intake;
3. Early recurrence of ascites, reappearance of grade 2 or 3 ascites within 4 weeks of initial mobilisation;
4. Diuretic-induced complications:
   a. Diuretic-induced hepatic encephalopathy
   b. Diuretic-induced renal impairment is defined as an increase in the serum creatinine level of >100% to a value of >2 mg/dL in patients with treatment-responsive ascites
   c. Diuretic-induced hyponatraemia is defined as a decrease in the serum sodium level of >10 mmol/L or a serum sodium level of <125 mmol/L
   d. Diuretic-induced hypokalaemia or hyperkalaemia is defined as a change in serum potassium of <3 mmol/L or >6 mmol/L, despite appropriate measures

LVP, defined as direct aspiration of >5 L of ascites, is the first-line treatment for refractory ascites but it has no effect on the mortality rate. Removal of a large volume of ascites can be associated with paracentesis-induced circulatory dysfunction, which can be prevented by an infusion of 7–8 g of albumin per litre of fluid tapped. Patients with refractory ascites should continue to receive diuretics if tolerated, unless there are major complications.

TIPS is indicated if ≥4 paracentesis procedures are performed within 6 months, or paracentesis is not tolerated or contraindicated. TIPS can relieve refractory ascites by directly reducing portal venous pressure. The most common non-surgical complication of TIPS is development of hepatic encephalopathy, which occurs in 15–48% of cases. History of previous hepatic encephalopathy is a relative contraindication for TIPS such as in this case. Appropriate use of TIPS in patients with refractory ascites increases their survival rate.

The ALFA pump is subcutaneously implanted and battery-powered. It moves ascites from the peritoneal cavity to the urinary bladder to facilitate removal of fluid by urination. Compared with repeated LVP, the ALFA pump is more acceptable for patients with refractory ascites and improves the quality of life. The ALFA pump is indicated in patients who are contraindicated for TIPS, those who previously failed TIPS, or patients with portal thrombosis. However, the ALFA pump system is a potential source of infection which may lead to severe sepsis, acute on chronic liver failure, and hampering of liver transplantation.

Liver transplantation can radically reverse portal hypertension. All patients with ascites should be considered as potential candidates for liver transplantation. Patients with refractory ascites, spontaneous bacterial peritonitis, or hepatorenal syndrome should be prioritised based on their Model for End-Stage Liver Disease (MELD) score. There is a remarkable improvement in the survival rate after liver transplantation.

 European Association for the Study of the Liver. EASL Clinical Practice Guidelines for the management of patients with decompensated cirrhosis. Journal of Hepatology 2018;69 j:406–460.
https://www.journal-of-hepatology.eu/article/S0168-8278(18)31966-4/fulltext

5. Answer: C

Autoantibodies, such as anti-smooth muscle antibodies (ASMA), ANA (most useful when found with ASMA, with a diagnostic accuracy of 74%), anti-soluble liver antigen/liver pancreas antibody (Anti-SLA/LP), liver kidney microsome type 1 antibody (Anti-LKM1), and atypical perinuclear antineutrophil cytoplasmic antibodies (pANCA) are seen in patients with autoimmune hepatitis (AIH).

AIH is a rare autoimmune disease and has variable clinical features, ranging from no symptoms, lethargy, nausea, vomiting, abdominal pain, anorexia, jaundice, to decompensated liver disease with variceal bleeding, hepatic encephalopathy, and ascites. AIH can affect children and adults of all ages.

There is a strong association of DRB1*0301 haplotype with AIH. Liver inflammation, fibrosis, and cirrhosis is via T cell-mediated activation of B cells that produce autoantibodies directed against liver antigens.

Diagnosis of AIH requires a high index of suspicion. It is important to exclude AIH in patients who present with acute or chronic hepatitis, since without treatment, patients with subclinical disease may develop decompensated liver disease in the long run and most of the patients respond to current standard treatment and expect near normal life expectancy and a reasonable quality of life.

Biochemistry shows a predominantly elevated aminotransferases and sometimes mild elevation of serum ALP and serum gamma globulins, especially elevated IgG level. If gamma globulins are negative, the diagnosis of AIH should be questioned since it is usually positive in 90% of the patients with AIH.

Liver biopsy is required to diagnose AIH and guide therapeutic decisions. Characteristic histology findings of AIH include interface hepatitis characterised by inflammation at the parenchymal portal junction, hepatocyte rosette formation, dense plasma cell rich infiltrate and emperipolesis (active penetration of lymphocytes into hepatocytes). In patients with severe disease, multi acinar and bridging necrosis areare found on histology.

Treatment should be considered in all patients with AIH since regression of scarring has been reported in patients with advanced fibrosis or even cirrhosis unless the risks outweigh benefits in patients with decompensated liver disease or in whom there are little or no disease activities on histology.

Current first-line treatment for AIH is combined tapering dose of oral prednisolone plus azathioprine after excluding patients with contraindications to the treatment. More studies are required in this rare and heterogenous disease to individualise immunosuppressive regimen.

 Lowe D, John S. Autoimmune hepatitis: Appraisal of current treatment guidelines. World Journal of Hepatology. 2018;10(12):911–923.
https://www.wjgnet.com/1948-5182/full/v10/i12/911.htm

6. Answer: C

Barrett's oesophagus (BO) is a complication of long-standing GORD and is a precursor of oesophageal adenocarcinoma (OAC). The most common location is in the lower third of the oesophagus. This patient's endoscopy shows a salmon-pink coloured columnar epithelium extending above the gastro-oesophageal junction which is typical for BO. BO is columnar metaplasia of the oesophageal squamous epithelium (squamous-to-columnar) and biopsies from the oesophageal columnar epithelium show evidence of intestinal metaplasia, with the presence of mucin-containing goblet cells. Under Australian guidelines, patients with a columnar-lined oesophagus on endoscopy but no evidence of intestinal metaplasia on biopsy do not meet the definition for BO.

Screening for BO with endoscopy in unselected patients with GORD is NOT recommended and NOT cost-effective. Currently, most guidelines suggest endoscopic screening for BO in patients with chronic GORD symptoms and multiple risk factors (i.e., 50 years of age or older, white race, male gender, obesity, history of smoking, family history for BO or OAC) or in men older than 60 years with reflux symptoms for 10 years.

Only observational studies have shown that patients with BO receiving an OAC diagnosis during endoscopic surveillance have earlier-stage tumours and higher survival rates than those whose tumours are discovered because of symptoms. However, the annual risk of progression from BO to OAC is only approximately 0.3% per year. Most guidelines recommend surveillance endoscopy every 2–5 years for non-dysplastic BO. For patients with indefinite for dysplasia (IND), low grade dysplasia (LGD) or high- grade dysplasia (HGD), the surveillance interval is shown in the algorithm in the reference.

The control of reflux is important in the management of BO because of a significantly lower rate of progression to LGD, HGD, or OAC in patients with a history of antireflux surgery or PPI use. There is no evidence to support the use of high dose PPI and oesophageal pH monitoring to titrate the PPI dosage in patients with BO. In terms of endoscopic resection/ablation management in patients with IND, LGD, and HGD please see the reference. In HGD, there is a high rate of progression to OAC (6%–19% per year), and endoscopic therapy is a well-established therapy for these cases. Surgery is the treatment of choice in early OAC.

Whiteman D, Kendall B. Barrett's oesophagus: epidemiology, diagnosis and clinical management. Medical Journal of Australia. 2016;205(7):317–324.
https://www.mja.com.au/system/files/issues/205_07/10.5694mja16.00796.pdf

7. Answer: B

The columnar epithelial cells of the intestine are responsible for absorption. These cells exhibit a striated luminal border or brush border appearance due to microvilli. The microvilli greatly increase the absorption surface of the epithelial cell. In addition to increasing surface area the microvilli perform an important digestive function including terminal digestion and absorption of nutrients. The microvillus membrane possesses a large complement of integral membrane proteins, many of which are glycoproteins and have been identified with specific brush border enzymes. The brush border contains disaccharidases in high concentration. The other brush border enzymes include peptidase and alkaline phosphatase. In coeliac disease the microvilli are abnormally short, irregular, and sparse and the terminal web is incompletely developed. Brush border enzymes are reduced to about 10% of normal but recover on a gluten free diet, except for 3-glucosidase and lactase which show a slower and less complete response.

Hooton D, Lentle R, Monro J, Wickham M, Simpson R. The Secretion and Action of Brush Border Enzymes in the Mammalian Small Intestine. Reviews of Physiology, Biochemistry and Pharmacology. 2015; 59–118.
https://www.ncbi.nlm.nih.gov/pubmed/26345415

8. Answer: D

Image A shows cystine crystals which are flat colourless plates and have a characteristic hexagonal shape with equal or unequal sides. They often aggregate in layers.

Image B shows a RBC cast which is indicative of glomerular disease and should not been seen in a patient with recurrent renal calculi with haematuria.

Image C shows uric acid crystals. They are variably sized, small to medium, with some large forms. They are yellow, red-brown, or brown, rarely colourless. They are variable in shape: rhomboid to diamond crystals, often with pointed ends, hexagonal flat crystals, rosettes, barrel shapes, or needles (uncommon).

Image D shows calcium oxalate dihydrate crystals. They are typically colourless squares whose corners are connected by intersecting lines (resembling an envelope). Calcium oxalate monohydrate crystals vary in size and may have a spindle, oval, or dumbbell shape. They indicate supersaturation of the urine with calcium and oxalate.

Crohn's disease (CD) is a chronic, granulomatous bowel disease. Urolithiasis is a common extraintestinal manifestation. Nephrolithiasis is more common after small bowel surgery: 4–5.5% (before) versus 15.0–30.5% (after), predominantly with calcium oxalate stones. This is because bile salt malabsorption in the diseased or resected distal ileum leads to fat malabsorption. Fat binds to calcium leading to a decrease in the amount of calcium bound to oxalate and an increase in oxalate absorption and deposition in the kidney, where it can form into stones. In the long term, recurrent urolithiasis and calcium-oxalate deposition can cause severe chronic interstitial nephritis and, as a consequence, CKD, ESKD, renal disease, and systemic oxalosis often develop early, especially in those patients with multiple bowel resections.

The risks for oxalate stone formation include hyperoxaluria (urine oxalate excretion > 45 mg/day), low urine volume due to chronic diarrhoea, acidic urine, lower urinary concentrations of magnesium, and citrate (stone inhibitors).

Urate stone or pure uric acid crystals can also occur. This type of stone develops in acidic urine and is caused by increased uric acid absorption in the injured colon.

Treatment of enteric hyperoxaluria is directed toward reducing intestinal oxalate absorption, a high fluid intake, potassium citrate or bicarbonate supplement to correct metabolic acidosis if present, and oral calcium with meals to bind oxalate in the intestinal lumen.

Corica D, Romano C. Renal Involvement in Inflammatory Bowel Diseases. Journal of Crohn's and Colitis. 2015;10(2): 226–235.
https://academic.oup.com/ecco-jcc/article/10/2/226/2392033

9. Answer: B
Cirrhosis is the fourth cause of death worldwide based on large studies. Cirrhosis is the pathologic end-stage of any chronic liver disease and the main causes of cirrhosis are alcohol abuse, viral hepatitis, and non-alcoholic fatty liver disease with the increased prevalence of metabolic syndrome. Contrary to previous thought, cirrhosis is now considered a dynamic disease able to progress or regress between decompensated and compensated states. Risk stratification, early diagnosis, and management of the underlying aetiology of chronic liver disease are important to prevent chronic liver disease progression. Once a patient with cirrhosis develops signs of decompensation, survival is significantly reduced.

The diagnosis of liver cirrhosis can be made on imaging studies such as ultrasound abdomen, CT abdomen, MRI abdomen, and more recently transient elastography. If the cause(s) of chronic liver failure are unclear, a liver biopsy may be indicated to identify the underlying cause(s) of liver disease and the extent and severity of the liver damage. The diagnosis of clinically significant portal hypertension is made possible by transient elastography, where the hepatic venous pressure gradient (HVPG) is equal or greater than 10 mmHg.

The management of cirrhosis is aimed at treating underlying liver disease, avoiding superimposed injury, and managing complications. Non-pharmacological measures include alcohol abstinence, lifestyle modifications such as weight loss if overweight and exercise. Early diagnosis and pharmacological primary and secondary prophylaxis of cirrhosis complications are key to optimizing cirrhosis management. Oesophageal varices should be screened for early at signs of decompensation, and treated with non-selective beta-blockers to prevent bleeds. Ascites detected clinically should undergo diagnostic paracentesis to establish cause and exclude spontaneous bacterial peritonitis (SBP). Ascites should subsequently be treated with mineralocorticoid receptor antagonist, diuretics, large volume paracentesis, and transjugular intrahepatic portosystemic shunt (TIPS) if refractory. TIPS can also reduce variceal bleeds. If SBP is detected, empiric antibiotic treatment should be commenced with consideration of long term secondary antibiotic prophylaxis, for example with norfloxacin. Rifaximin is often prescribed in cirrhotic patients for refractory hepatic encephalopathy, however there is new evidence it may also reduce SBP. Anticoagulants such as low molecular-weight heparin or direct oral anticoagulants can be used to prevent portal vein thrombosis and prevent venous thromboembolic disease in a procoagulant stage associated with cirrhosis.

Six-monthly abdominal ultrasound and serum alpha-fetoprotein tests may be considered in patients with a high risk of developing hepatocellular carcinoma as ongoing surveillance. Timely referral for liver transplantation may be the only curative treatment option for patients with decompensated cirrhosis.

Statins have been shown to prevent hepatic decompensation in large epidemiological surveys in patients with hepatitis B and C virus cirrhosis. The use of statins has also been associated with a decreased risk of hepatocellular carcinoma and an improved survival in patients who survived an episode of bleeding from esophageal varices.

Berzigotti A. Advances and challenges in cirrhosis and portal hypertension. BMC Medicine. 2017;15(1).
https://bmcmedicine.biomedcentral.com/articles/10.1186/s12916-017-0966-6

10. Answer: D

Coagulopathy is common in advanced cirrhosis and liver failure, constituting a key part of MELD scores. Bleeding tendency in patients with cirrhosis is multifactorial, including:

1. Thrombocytopenia due to splenic sequestration, shortened survival, decreased thrombopoietin (TPO) and/or inadequate bone marrow response.
2. Platelet dysfunction.
3. Hyperfibrinolysis.
4. Diminished liver-derived procoagulant factors levels such as Factors V, VII, and X, causing prolongation of the prothrombin time (PT).

However, inappropriate clotting attributed to changes in the haemostatic balance is now recognised in patients with advanced cirrhosis. It is seen especially in portal and mesenteric vein thrombosis (PVT) but also in DVT and PE. These often warrant challenging considerations of anticoagulant therapy or prophylaxis.

Diminished liver derived procoagulant factors are significantly offset by increased endothelial derived von Willebrand factor (vWF); reduced liver derived anticoagulant factors such as protein C; and elevated endothelial derived Factor VIII. These changes lead to a relatively hypercoagulable state and, together with relative venous stasis and endothelial injury (Virchow's triad), contribute to the risk of VTE in cirrhosis patients. The incidence of VTE in patients with cirrhosis is not decreased compared to those without cirrhosis. In fact, population-based data reports increased relative risk (1.7-fold) for VTE in cirrhosis. Despite this risk, use of VTE prophylaxis in hospitalized cirrhotic patients is significantly lower than non-cirrhotic. While there is no data to guide specific strategies, there is no evidence that prophylactic anticoagulation is associated with increased risk for bleeding complications in cirrhotic patients. PVT is the most common VTE event in cirrhosis.

Although prospective, randomised, controlled, and blinded trials are generally lacking, consideration of both DVT prophylaxis in hospitaliseds liver disease patients and full dose anticoagulation in cirrhotic patients with acute PVT and VTE is indicated. Heparin or low molecular weight heparin (LMWH) is recommended for acute VTE but there are unresolved issues regarding monitoring of both the anti-Xa assay and the APTT due to cirrhosis related antithrombin deficiency (heparin cofactor).

Paracentesis, thoracentesis, and routine upper endoscopy for variceal ligation have low risk of bleeding even in patients with a combined elevation in INR due to hepatic synthetic dysfunction and thrombocytopenia. Therefore, clinicians should not routinely correct thrombocytopenia and coagulopathy prior to paracentesis as the risks of transfusion greatly outweigh the potential benefit. This however, does not apply to pharmacologically anticoagulated and renal failure patients, who may be at increased risk for bleeding from the above procedures.

The following transfusion thresholds to improve haemostasis are for management of active bleeding or high-risk procedures in advanced liver disease: haematocrit ≥25%, platelet count >50,000/uL, and fibrinogen >120 mg/dL. The commonly utilised threshold value for INR correction (<1.5) is not supported by evidence.

The life span of a normal platelet is 7–10 days and one third are sequestered in the spleen. The half-life of transfused platelets is about 3 days. When procedures are planned in advance, a thrombopoietin (TPO) receptor agonist is a good alternative to platelet transfusion as it has the advantage of elevating platelets for longer than transfusions can but also requires more time (about 10 days) to elevate platelet levels.

Tranexamic acid is rarely used prophylactically before procedures, but is more commonly used as a rescue measure should bleeding occur after procedures. Desmopressin (DDAVP) releases vWF as its primary haemostatic mechanism. As this factor is usually elevated in cirrhosis, DDAVP lacks a sound evidence base for use in cirrhosis but may be useful in patients with concomitant severe renal failure. Evidence is also lacking for the identification of hospitalised patients with cirrhosis who may benefit from vitamin K therapy as well as optimal dosing and route of administration.

The large volume of FFP required to reach an arbitrary INR target, its minimal effect on thrombin generation, and adverse effects on portal pressure significantly limit the utility of this agent. The 4-factor Prothrombin Complex Concentrate (PCC) contains both pro- and anticoagulant factors which offer an attractive low volume therapeutic to re-balance a disturbed haemostatic system.

 O'Leary J, Greenberg C, Patton H, Caldwell S. AGA Clinical Practice Update: Coagulation in Cirrhosis. Gastroenterology. 2019;157(1):34–43.e1.
https://www.gastrojournal.org/article/S0016-5085(19)35694-X/fulltext

11. Answer: A

Coeliac disease is an immune-mediated chronic, small-intestinal enteropathy initiated by exposure to gluten in genetically predisposed individuals and is characteriseds by specific autoantibodies against tissue transglutaminase 2 (anti-tTG2), endomysium, and/or deamidated gliadin peptide. In Australia, it is estimated that the prevalence is 1.2% in adult men (1:86) and 1.9% in adult women (1:52).

A strict gluten-free diet is the only available treatment for coeliac disease. Nutritional markers should be evaluated at diagnosis, and abnormal findings should be reassessed after 1 year of adherence to a gluten-free diet. Recommendations also support a baseline bone density scan at diagnosis for patients at high risk of osteoporosis, especially in those with malabsorption or with a long delay in diagnosis, such as in this case. It should be repeated at 5-year intervals or shorter (2–3 years) with low bone density on index measurement or poor dietary adherence.

Newly diagnosed patients should receive the pneumococcal vaccine due to their increased risk of hyposplenism.

In patients with coeliac disease, the proportion of deaths from malignancy (30.4%) was higher than in the general population (23.6%), and was the second most common cause of death in patients with coeliac disease after cardiovascular disease. The overall risk of incident malignancy is similar in patients with coeliac disease and the general population, with the exception of lymphoproliferative malignancy and gastrointestinal cancer. This excess risk is particularly high in individuals with persistent villous atrophy and poor dietary adherence. Women with coeliac disease seem to be at lower risk of ovarian, endometrial, and breast cancer than the general population.

Mucosal healing in coeliac disease takes a considerable time: studies show that this can take up to 2 years in children and up to 8 years in adults. A recent Australian study showed that adherence to a gluten free diet improves both mucosal healing (85% of patients showed improvement and 53% showed remission) and consequences of nutritional deficiency at 5 years, while serology is poorly predictive of duodenal mucosal damage.

Non-responsive coeliac disease can be defined as primary if there is no response to a gluten free diet at 12 months, and secondary if, after an initial response, the symptoms relapse.

First-degree family members of patients with coeliac disease have a 15- to 25-fold higher frequency of developing coeliac disease, compared with individuals without a first-degree family member with coeliac disease. For that reason, guidelines suggest screening first-degree family members with or without signs or symptoms concerning for coeliac disease. However, the US Preventive Services Task Force recently released recommendations that screening asymptomatic patients with or without a known increased risk of coeliac disease, inclusive of family members, is not recommended, based on inadequate evidence regarding benefits and risks of this screening.

 Walker M, Ludvigsson J, Sanders D. Coeliac disease: review of diagnosis and management. Medical Journal of Australia. 2017;207(4):173–178.
https://www.mja.com.au/journal/2017/207/4/coeliac-disease-review-diagnosis-and-management

12. Answer: D

Colon cancer is one of the leading causes of cancer-related morbidity and mortality worldwide especially in developed countries. The number of colorectal polyps removed is increasing due to colorectal cancer screening programmes. Hyperplastic polyps have no risk of malignant transformation. It is well known that colorectal cancers arise from precursor adenomatous polyps, which have three histologic types: tubular, tubulovillous, and villous adenomas. Tubular adenomas represent 75–85% of adenomatous polyps and have <5% chance of harbouring a malignancy. Mixed tubulovillous adenomas have a risk of 22%. Villous adenomas have the highest risk of malignant transformation at 40%.

 Salmo E, Haboub N. Adenoma and malignant colorectal polyp: pathological considerations and clinical applications. EMJ Gastroenterol. 2018;7[1]:92–102.
https://www.emjreviews.com/gastroenterology/article/adenoma-and-malignant-colorectal-polyp-pathological-considerations-and-clinical-applications/

13. Answer: A

The WHO recently reclassified processed meat as a Group 1 carcinogen, and red meat as a Group 2A (probably carcinogenic). The Cancer Council of Australia recommends eating no more than 1 serve of lean red meat per day or 2 serves 3–4 times per week, and to cut out processed meat altogether.

A recently published study found that consumption of red and processed meats was associated with an increased risk of colorectal cancer. Participants who reported consuming an average of 76 g/day of red and processed meat compared with 21 g/day had a 20% higher risk of colorectal cancer. Alcohol was also associated with an increased risk of colorectal cancer, whereas fibre from bread and breakfast cereals was associated with a reduced risk. Alcohol was associated with an 8% higher risk per 10 g/day higher intake. Participants in the highest fifth of intake of fibre had a 14% lower risk.

The strongest risk factor for the development of colorectal cancer remains age, with the increased risk rising significantly over the age of 50 years. There is a higher risk for people of African descent than Caucasians, and lower risk for Hispanics compared to non-Hispanics. Smoking, alcohol, obesity, and presence of previous polyps are associated with increased risk, whereas consumption of fruit and vegetables, exercise, and hormone-replacement therapy may be protective.

 Bradbury K, Murphy N, Key T. Diet and colorectal cancer in UK Biobank: a prospective study. International Journal of Epidemiology. 2019.
https://academic.oup.com/ije/article/49/1/246/5470096

Strum W. Colorectal Adenomas. New England Journal of Medicine. 2016;374(11):1065–1075.
https://www.nejm.org/doi/full/10.1056/NEJMra1513581

14. Answer: A

Constipation may occur either in isolation, chronic idiopathic constipation, or secondary to another underlying disorder (e.g, Parkinson's disease). The median prevalence of constipation is 16% in adults overall and 33.5% in adults aged 60–100 years.

Lifestyle modifications, such as increasing dietary fibre, probiotics, adequate hydration and exercise are the first step in managing constipation. Pharmacological treatments include:

- *Osmotic laxatives*, such as polyethylene glycol and lactulose are the first-line drug treatment. In individual RCTs, polyethylene glycol is superior to both lactulose and prucalopride, a 5-HT$_4$ receptor agonist, when compared directly. Lactulose may be poorly tolerated, as it frequently causes bloating and occasionally GI bleeding.

- *Stimulant laxatives*, such as bisacodyl, glycerin suppositories, and sodium picosulfate, induce propagated colonic contractions and appear safe even with long-term use; bisacodyl and sodium picosulfate also have antiabsorptive plus secretory effects. It is used if there is no response to osmotic laxatives.

- *Prosecretory agents* stimulate net efflux of ions and water into the intestinal lumen, secretagogues accelerate transit and also facilitate ease of defecation. Both secretagogues for chronic constipation (i.e. lubiprostone and linaclotide) increase intestinal chloride secretion by activating channels on the apical (luminal) enterocyte surface.

- *5-HT$_4$ receptor agonists* induce fast excitatory postsynaptic potentials in intrinsic neurons, release neurotransmitters such as the excitatory acetylcholine, and induce mucosal secretion by activating submucosal neurons. Serotonin 5-HT$_4$ receptors are widely distributed on enteric neurons. Prucalopride is a selective 5-HT$_4$ receptor agonist which stimulates gastrointestinal and colonic motility. It is well tolerated; common side effects include diarrhoea and headache. The dose should be reduced to 1 mg once daily in older patients or those with renal or hepatic impairment. It should be considered in patients with constipation who have not responded to two different laxatives for 6 months. It has had promising effects in some patients who did not respond to conventional laxatives but up to 2/3 of patients will not. It should be ceased if ineffective after 4 weeks of treatment.

- *Bile acid transporter inhibitors,* elobixibat, induces a state of bile acid malabsorption in the terminal ileum, which leads to retrograde flow into the colon, where they are deconjugated and dehydroxylated by colonic microbiota to produce secondary bile acids such as deoxycholic acid, which induce colonic secretion.

Black C, Ford A. Chronic idiopathic constipation In adults: epidemiology, pathophysiology, diagnosis and clinical management. Medical Journal of Australia. 2018;209(2):86–91.
https://onlinelibrary.wiley.com/doi/abs/10.5694/mja18.00241

15. Answer: B

Eosinophilic esophagitis (EoE) is one of the most common conditions diagnosed during the evaluation of dysphagia and food impaction in adults. EoE is a chronic, immune-mediated or antigen mediated esophageal disease. Symptoms of EoE include intermittent solid food dysphagia, food particle impaction, vomiting, and epigastric discomfort. Risk factors for EoE include food allergy, coeliac disease, a family history and lower socioeconomic status.

The history of asthma, rhinitis, intermittent dysphagia, and food impaction in this patient is suggestive of EoE together with the esophageal rings on endoscopy and eosinophils on biopsy. Diagnosis of EoE is by endoscopy and biopsies of 2–4 samples from the proximal, mid, and distal oesophagus due to the patchy nature of the disease. The most common endoscopic findings are white specks (representative of eosinophilic exudates), mucosal edema, linear furrows, esophageal rings, and strictures as seen in this case. An increased number of eosinophils in the esophageal epithelium is the histologic hallmark of EoE. A cutoff value of at least 15 eosinophils per high-power field is thought to approach a sensitivity of 100% and specificity of 96% for establishing the histologic diagnosis of EoE.

The treatment goals include the alleviation of symptoms, control of inflammation and restoration of function. Three approaches are diet, drugs, and dilation. Elimination of causative allergens/antigens from the diet can be highly effective. A lack of response to PPIs is usual. Glucocorticoids target key mechanisms in EoE. Liquid budesonide is the mainstay of pharmacologic therapy. The efficacy of these topical medications in improving symptoms and histologic abnormalities after 2–12 weeks of use ranges from 53 to 95%. Systemic steroids are limited to very severe cases. Dilatation of the esophagus may be required in patients with rings or high-grade strictures.

Furuta GT, Katzka DAN Eosinophilic Esophagitis. N Engl J Med 2015;373:1640–8.
https://www.ncbi.nlm.nih.gov/pmc/articles/PMC4905697/

16. Answer: D

Extraintestinal manifestations (EIMs) of IBD encompass a wide range of potential symptoms and can involve nearly any organ. EIMs can occur as manifestations of the same pathogenesis of IBD or as separate disease processes. Development of one EIM increases the risk of a second EIM. The likelihood that a patient will develop EIMs increases with IBD duration. EIMs can present at any time during the course of the disease, including prior to onset of GI symptoms. Peripheral and axial musculoskeletal syndromes are the most common EIMs of IBD, occurring in approximately 30% of patients. Eye disease is the third most common EIM of IBD, occurring in up to 5% of patients with IBD. Anti-TNF agents are effective and the treatment of choice for EIMs.

Vavricka S, Schoepfer A, Scharl M, Lakatos P, Navarini A, Rogler G. Extraintestinal Manifestations of Inflammatory Bowel Disease. Inflammatory Bowel Diseases. 2015;21(8):1982–1992.
https://academic.oup.com/ibdjournal/article/21/8/1982/4602969

17. Answer: A

Faecal calprotectin (FC) is one of the useful tools for clinical diagnosis and management of IBD.

Calprotectin is a calcium and zinc binding protein, which represent about 60% of soluble proteins of the cytoplasm of granulocytes. Functions of calprotectin include: competitive inhibition of zinc-dependent enzymes, potential biostatic activity against microbes through chelation of zinc ions, apoptosis induction in malignant cells, and regulation of the inflammatory process. Calprotectin remains stable in stools for up to 7 days at room temperature. Many different methods of measurement have been developed, most of them based on ELISA, with different cut-offs suggested for different clinical settings. A cut-off value of 50 µg/g of FC has been the most commonly adopted both in literature and by commercially available ELISA kits to differentiate IBD from other forms of inflammation and IBS. In patients with intestinal symptoms, due to a high negative predictive value, a normal FC level reliably rules out active IBD. FC can be used as a diagnostic screening test for IBD.

A high FC concentration could identify those IBD patients in remission who were at risk of early relapse. FC is a stronger predictor of clinical relapse in ulcerative colitis than in Crohn's disease.

Many studies have shown that FC is a good non-invasive marker for assessing mucosal inflammation. There is a strong correlation between FC levels and mucosal healing and histological findings in patients with IBD. FC assessment can be helpful in monitoring disease activity and response to therapy as well as in predicting relapse, post-operative recurrence or pouchitis. FC is a more sensitive marker than CRP for detection of mild mucosal inflammation.

In clinical practice, 'Treat-To-Target' is currently considered the most important strategy for therapy adjustment which leads to a better outcome than clinically-based therapy adjustment in patients with IBD. In the biologic era, many studies have confirmed the role of FC in monitoring the effectiveness of therapy.

FC is inflammation-specific, but not disease-specific. Almost every colonic disease and many small bowel diseases are associated with inflammation, and hence, test positive for FC. However, most of these diseases such as NSAID enteropathy, are associated with low-grade inflammation and the FC level is low. A further limitation of FC is a low specificity in discriminating ulcerative colitis from Crohn's disease, and active IBD from non-IBD intestinal inflammation as seen in infections, drug-related damage, bowel cancer, and diverticulitis.

Bjarnason I. The use of faecal calprotectin in inflammatory bowel disease. Gastroenterology & Hepatology 2017;13: 53–6.
https://www.ncbi.nlm.nih.gov/pmc/articles/PMC5390326/

18. Answer: C

Gastric cancer (GC) is divided into intestinal, diffuse, and mixed subtypes. Intestinal GC is associated with chronic inflammation and is frequently associated with *H. pylori* infection. In developed countries, the incidence of intestinal GC has decreased as a result of improvements in hygiene, food conservation, and treatment of *H. pylori* infection in the last 50 years. About 3% of GCs arise as a result of inherited cancer predisposition syndromes such as Lynch syndrome, MUTYH-associated adenomatous polyposis (MAP), and E-cadherin 1 (*CDH1*) germline mutations associated hereditary diffuse gastric cancer (HDGC)

HDGC syndrome is defined on the basis of family history of diffuse gastric cancer (DGC), particularly early onset of the disease or presence of DGC associated with lobular breast cancer (LBC). The genetic alteration is a germline mutation of the E-cadherin 1 (*CDH1*) gene. Its product, endothelial cadherin, is an adhesion molecule crucial for maintaining epithelial cell polarity and architectural structure. The syndrome is characterised by an autosomal dominant inheritance and in common with many inherited cancer predispositions requires a second 'hit' (mutation, loss of heterozygosity, methylation) to inactivate the wild-type allele.

Hereditary cancer syndromes are rare compared with sporadic cancer, but their investigation is crucial, due to different clinical management that mutation carriers warrant and the implications for disease-free relatives. Families in whom a deleterious genetic mutation occurs require genetic counselling, clinical surveillance and the possible recommendation of prophylactic surgery. HDGC is characterised by a lifetime DGC risk of over 80%. The following table summarises the common oncogenes and associated cancers.

Protein Function	Oncogene	Associated Cancer
Transforming growth factor α	TGFα	Melanoma
EGF-receptor	ERB-B2	Breast and ovarian cancers
Non-receptor tyrosine kinase	ABL	CML
RAS signal transduction	BRAF	Melanoma
Negative regulator of the signalling pathway	APC	Adenomatous polyposis coli (APC), most colon cancers
Components of DNA repair systems	BRCA1 BRCA2	Familial breast and ovarian cancer
E-cadherin, a cell adhesion molecule	CDH1	Hereditary diffuse gastric cancer & lobular breast cancer
Transcription factor and protein kinase	MEN1	Multiple endocrine neoplasia & many metastatic cancers
Transcription factor; guardian of the genome	P53	Most frequently mutated in human cancers
Ubiquitin ligase	VHL	Renal cell carcinoma
DNA mismatch repair protein Msh2	MSH2	Hereditary nonpolyposis colorectal cancer (HNPCC)
Mismatch repair endonuclease	PMS2	Colon cancer

van der Post R, Vogelaar I, Carneiro F, Guilford P, Huntsman D, Hoogerbrugge N et al. Hereditary diffuse gastric cancer: updated clinical guidelines with an emphasis on germline CDH1 mutation carriers. Journal of Medical Genetics. 2015;52(6):361–374.
https://www.ncbi.nlm.nih.gov/pmc/articles/PMC4453626/

19. Answer: B

Unconjugated hyperbilirubinemia can result from increased production, impaired conjugation, or impaired hepatic uptake of bilirubin. The common causes include:

- Gilbert syndrome
- Crigler-Najjar syndrome type 1 and 2
- Ineffective erythropoiesis
- Physiologic and non-physiologic neonatal jaundice.

Gilbert's syndrome (GS) consists of chronic, mild, unconjugated hyperbilirubinemia in the absence of overt haemolysis or evidence of structural or functional liver disease. GS is an inherited disorder in which decreased levels of the enzyme uridine-diphosphoglucuronate glucuronosyltransferase (UDPGT or UGT1A1) of at least 50% results in impaired conjugation of bilirubin. It may affect as many as 5% of population and is commonly inherited in an autosomal-recessive manner.

Patients with GS have elevated unconjugated bilirubin, while conjugated bilirubin is usually within the normal range and is <20% of the total. The serum bilirubin level fluctuates but can rise to 3–4 times above normal range especially during prolonged fasting, physical exercise, stress, intercurrent illness, or menstruation. GS is often recognised around puberty, which is related to the inhibition of bilirubin glucuronidation by endogenous steroid hormones.

The diagnosis is generally clinical and can be confirmed by documenting a two-fold to three-fold rise in unconjugated bilirubin during a 24-hour fast with normal LFTs. Tests can also detect DNA mutations of UGT1A1 by PCR.

Affected individuals are generally asymptomatic. GS is a benign and clinically inconsequential entity, requiring neither treatment nor long-term follow-up. Its clinical importance lies in the fact that the mild hyperbilirubinemia may be mistaken for a sign of occult, chronic, or progressive liver disease and the patient is subjected to extensive and invasive investigation.

Dubin-Johnson syndrome is a rare autosomal recessive condition. It is characterised by conjugated hyperbilirubinemia with normal liver transaminases, a unique pattern of urinary excretion of heme metabolites (coproporphyrins), and the deposition of a pigment that gives the liver a characteristic black colour. It is due to defective bilirubin excretion into bile.

Oestrogen and oral contraceptive pills (OCPs) can cause mild inhibition of bilirubin excretion, leading to jaundice. It can also induce a clinically apparent cholestatic liver injury that typically arises during the first few cycles of therapy. The characteristic pattern is bland intrahepatic cholestasis with liver biopsy showing little inflammation or hepatocyte necrosis. Resolution may be delayed after cessation of OCPs.

Primary biliary cirrhosis (PBC) is a chronic progressive cholestatic granulomatous and destructive inflammatory lesion of small intralobular and septal bile ducts, caused by an autoimmune mechanism. Jaundice is an important clinical symptom of PBC especially in end-stage disease. It occurs as the disease progresses leading to increased blood levels of conjugated bilirubin. When jaundice is an initial manifestation of PBC, the patient exhibits a more rapid development of end-stage disease, with lower survival rates than those with its anicteric type.

King D, Armstrong M. Overview of Gilbert's syndrome. Drug and Therapeutics Bulletin. 2019;57(2):27–31.
https://dtb.bmj.com/content/57/2/27

20. Answer: A

H. pylori infection is common and it is estimated to affect more than 50% of the worldwide population. It is also associated with significant morbidity: gastritis, gastroduodenal ulcer disease, gastric cancer, and gastric mucosa-associated lymphoid tissue lymphoma (MALT).

The gold standard for diagnosis is via endoscopic biopsy, where histology and rapid urease test taken from two different locations in the stomach represents the most accurate means of diagnosis. Urea breath test is also highly sensitive and specific, and is the preferred diagnostic test in patients without an indication for endoscopy. Faecal antigen tests and serology are less sensitive and specific.

Treatment of *H pylori* infection involves antibiotics and protein pump inhibitors (PPIs). In Australia, first line therapy is PPI, amoxicillin, and clarithromycin for 1 week. Treatment failure is associated with medication non-compliance, smoking, and clarithromycin resistance. In Australia, clarithromycin resistance is low: 6–8%. Metronidazole, which is a first line treatment in other countries, is not recommended initially in Australia due to very high resistance up to 50%. Amoxicillin resistance is effectively non-existent, and is not a cause of treatment failure.

Failure of clarithromycin-based triple therapy occurs in up to 20% of cases, so it is recommended to test for *H pylori* clearance at least 4 weeks after therapy. Urea breath test is the diagnostic test of choice, unless an endoscopy is otherwise indicated when biopsy testing is preferred. False negatives can occur, especially with recent antibiotic use within 4 weeks, and recent PPI use within 1–2 weeks.

Second line 'salvage eradication therapy' in Australia is typically levofloxacin-based triple therapy with PPI, amoxicillin, and levofloxacin. Expected failure rate is <4%. A more effective regimen is quadruple therapy with bismuth subcitrate, PPI, tetracycline and metronidazole, with an ideal expected failure rate <1%. However, this option is less preferred: medication compliance is an issue with 4 × daily dosing required, and bismuth is not available on PBS, only from TGA through Special Access Scheme.

Mitchell H, Katelaris P. Epidemiology, clinical impacts and current clinical management of Helicobacter pylori infection. Medical Journal of Australia. 2016;204(10):376–380.
https://www.mja.com.au/journal/2016/204/10/epidemiology-clinical-impacts-and-current-clinical-management-helicobacter

21. Answer: D

Hepatic encephalopathy is a complication of chronic liver disease. Colonic bacterial digestion of protein releases ammonia into the gut which then enters the portal circulation of the liver and is converted to urea through the urea cycle. Ammonia and other toxic metabolites accumulate and are shunted into the systemic circulation. High ammonia levels in the blood result in neuronal dysfunction, causing hepatic encephalopathy. Brain oedema may occur due to this rapid rise in ammonia levels, particularly in patients with acute liver failure.

For patients with severe acute encephalopathy, ammonia level can be reduced by administering 30 mL of lactulose 1 to 2 hourly to induce a rapid laxative effect. When the laxative effect is achieved, reduce lactulose dosing frequency to 3 to 4 times daily. To prevent recurrent hepatic encephalopathy, or to treat patients with chronic hepatic encephalopathy, prescribe 30 mL of lactulose orally, 3 to 4 times daily, aiming for 2 or 3 semisoft stools per day. For patients with repeated episodes of hepatic encephalopathy despite lactulose therapy, add rifaximin 550 mg orally, twice daily.

Even though protein breakdown via the urea cycle can cause hyperammonaemia, protein restriction is not recommended for recurrent or chronic encephalopathy because patients with chronic liver disease are often significantly malnourished. In general, encourage patients to have a good protein intake.

Patients with chronic hepatic encephalopathy should be assessed for large portosystemic shunts. Patients with recurrent or chronic hepatic encephalopathy should also be referred for consideration of liver transplantation.

Wijdicks E. Hepatic Encephalopathy. New England Journal of Medicine. 2016;375(17):1660–1670.
https://www.nejm.org/doi/10.1056/NEJMra1600561

22. Answer: A

HBsAg positivity is the hallmark of active hepatitis B infection. However, several hepatitis B infection states are possible in the absence of HBsAg positivity. Hepatitis B surface antibody can be detectable following successful immunisation or following clearance of past infection. Presence of core antibody without surface antigen positivity can represent cleared 'past infection' whether the clearance was spontaneously or through treatment, the window phase of acute infection, false-positive core antibody results, or false negative surface antigen results, or surface antigen level below the limit of detection of the test. In patients undergoing HIV treatment, chemotherapy or immunosuppressive therapy, presence of core antibody should be screened for as patients are at risk of reactivation of chronic infection with therapy. Presence of detectable HBV DNA in peripheral blood in the setting of an isolated core antibody indicates HBV infection, and presence of core IgM would be suggestive of acute infection.

It is recommended that patients undergoing HIV treatment who have isolated core antibody and do not have HBV infection should receive the hepatitis B vaccine, as 60–80% of patients become surface antibody positive with 3 or 4 vaccinations. This is possible regardless of whether the cause of core antibody positivity is false positivity or past infection. Vaccination can be effective if CD4 counts exceed 200/μL. Vaccination can also be considered for patients with isolated core antibody who do not have HBV infection undergoing stem-cell transplant for haematological malignancy, or prior to chemotherapy. Patients with isolated positive anti-HBc who are from high-risk countries but who are not at risk of reactivation do not require immunisation, as the anti-HBc likely represents cleared past infection. Screening recommendations for chronic hepatitis B infection include patients from high-risk countries, infants born to HBsAg positive mothers, and those at risk of sexually transmitted or blood borne disease.

Terrault N, Lok A, McMahon B, Chang K, Hwang J, Jonas M et al. Update on prevention, diagnosis, and treatment of chronic hepatitis B: AASLD 2018 hepatitis B guidance. Hepatology. 2018;67(4):1560–1599.
https://aasldpubs.onlinelibrary.wiley.com/doi/full/10.1002/hep.29800

23. Answer: A

Direct-acting antiviral (DAA) therapy eradicates HCV and prevents progression to cirrhosis, liver failure, hepatocellular carcinoma (HCC), the need for liver transplant, and death. DAA treatment also reduces the risk of extrahepatic diseases, including cryoglobulinemic vasculitis. DAAs target multiple mechanisms of the HCV replication cycle. They are safe and well tolerated, including in patients with HIV infection, severe renal and hepatic impairment, and history of organ transplantation.

All patients infected with HCV should receive DAA treatment to reduce liver-related and all-cause morbidity and mortality and to prevent HCV transmission, unless their life expectancy is less than 1 year due to non–HCV-related comorbidities. Patients co-infected with HIV and HCV can be treated in the same way as patients with HCV alone.

Prior to therapy, patients with detectable HCV RNA should undergo a clinical evaluation Including:
• HCV genotype/subtype testing
• HIV testing
• Vaccination for hepatitis A and B virus for individuals who are not immune
• Glomerular filtration rate measurement
• Pregnancy testing
• Assessment of liver fibrosis using transient elastography
• Radiologic screening for HCC for patients with cirrhosis.

Current HCV treatment is 12 weeks in duration. HCV infection is considered cured if HCV RNA is undetectable 12 weeks after completion of DAA therapy which is termed sustained virologic response (SVR). If detectable HCV RNA returns within 12 weeks of treatment discontinuation, it is considered a relapse which is likely due to resistance to some or all of the drugs. Relapse after SVR beyond 12 weeks is rare (<2 in 1000), guidelines recommend confirming SVR 24 to 48 weeks after therapy. More often, viraemia after SVR at 12 weeks represents a reinfection (new exposure and HCV acquisition).

The mechanism of DAAs includes inhibition of the non-structural 5B RNA polymerase, non-structural 5A protein, and serine non-structural 3/4A protease. Current regimens include drugs that target 2 to 3 mechanisms to overcome the highly replicative capacity and lack of proof reading of the error-prone polymerase. Two regimens are active against all 6 major genotypes.

Studies reveal the increased risk of HCC recurrence remains for up to 3.6 years after achieving virological cure and remains particularly high in patients with cirrhosis. Therefore, HCC surveillance needs to be continued in patients with cirrhosis even after successful HCV eradication.

Marks K, Naggie S. Management of Hepatitis C in 2019. JAMA. 2019;322(4):355.
https://jamanetwork.com/journals/jama/article-abstract/2734262

24. Answer: B

Hepatitis E virus (HEV) infects humans and belongs to the Hepeviridiae family, Orthohepevirus genus, A species, Genotypes 1–4. Genotypes 1 and 2 only infect humans and are spread by the faecal–oral route in countries with poor sanitary infrastructure, i.e., Asia, Africa, Mexico. Genotypes 3 and 4 are zoonotic infections endemic in higher income countries with the primary host of pigs, spread to humans via the consumption of infected food and iatrogenically via infected blood products. HEV is an icosahedral, positive-strand RNA virus.

Young adults are most commonly affected, especially the 15–35 age group, and men are more likely to be infected than women. The typical presentation is acute hepatitis, with deranged liver enzymes, jaundice, and nonspecific symptoms including fatigue, itch and nausea. Acute hepatitis occurs in 20% of patients exposed to HEV genotypes 1 and 2, and pregnant women have mortality rates up to 25%. By contrast, acute hepatitis presents in less than 5% of patients infected with HEV genotypes 3 and 4, who are typically older males. Chronic hepatitis has only been reported with HEV genotypes 3 and 4 in immunosuppressed patients. Extrahepatic manifestations can be neurological including neuralgic amyotrophy, Guillain-Barré syndrome, and meningoencephalitis, and renal including membranoproliferative and membranous glomerulonephritis and IgA nephropathy. Detection is important, as complications may represent an indication to treat.

HEV infection can be diagnosed by serological detection of anti-HEV antibodies (IgM, IgG, or both) and HEV RNA by nucleic acid amplification (NAT). However, serological and NAT testing both have wide variations in specificity of different assays, and anti-HEV antibodies are often undetectable in chronic hepatitis E, so testing both together is preferable.

Acute HEV infection does not usually require antiviral therapy, however ribavirin can be considered in cases of severe acute hepatitis E or acute on chronic liver failure.

Dalton H, Kamar N, Baylis S, Moradpour D, Wedemeyer H, Negro F. EASL Clinical Practice Guidelines on hepatitis E virus infection. Journal of Hepatology. 2018;68(6):1256–1271.
https://www.journal-of-hepatology.eu/article/S0168-8278(18)30155-7/fulltext

25. Answer: B

Hepatitis E virus (HEV) typically causes a self-limited illness of less than one-month with nausea, anorexia, malaise, fatigue and jaundice. Mortality is low, around 1–2% in immunocompetent patients, unfortunately reaching 25% if contracted in the third trimester of pregnancy, and is also higher in children under 2 years of age. However, HEV probably affects tens of millions of people worldwide, making the virus an important global health issue. Immune compromised patients often develop a chronic hepatitis, with rapid progression to cirrhosis. HEV has been linked to extra-hepatic syndromes such as pancreatitis, Guillain-Barré syndrome, glomerulonephritis and mixed cryoglobulinaemia.

In developing countries, the predominant route of transmission is faecal–oral, and HEV testing is recommended in the case of a returned traveller with jaundice. This mode of transmission commonly results in infection with genotypes 1 and 2. Genotypes 3 and 4 predominate in sporadic or clustered cases of infection in developed countries, and are mostly transmitted through undercooked meat, most commonly pork. HEV can be transmitted through blood transfusion, however, screening of blood products is not currently undertaken in Australia.

Ribavirin is a commonly used treatment for chronic hepatitis in immunocompromised patients. However, as the pathogenesis and intracellular molecular mechanisms behind the replication and life cycle of HEV are poorly understood, direct antiviral agents have not been developed to date. There is some evidence that vaccination can prevent infection in high-risk groups.

Nimgaonkar I, Ding Q, Schwartz R, Ploss A. Hepatitis E virus: advances and challenges. Nature Reviews Gastroenterology & Hepatology. 2017;15(2):96–110.
https://www.nature.com/articles/nrgastro.2017.150

26. Answer: D

Hepatocellular carcinoma (HCC) is an important cause of cancer-related death worldwide. If HCC is detected at early stages, the treatment is more likely to be curative and improves survival. However, no high-quality randomized, controlled trials have evaluated the effect of HCC surveillance in patients with cirrhosis. Nonetheless, mathematical models, a low-quality clinical trial, meta-analysis of cohort studies all show survival benefits of surveillance. This evidence informs the recommendation of surveillance by major hepatology professional societies. Furthermore, HCC surveillance should be put into practice because all of the criteria for effective surveillance testing are met: (i) HCC has a major impact on public health, (ii) the detection of HCC at an early stage improves outcomes, (iii) there are known groups at high risk for HCC, (iv) tests are available for surveillance, (v) these tests can detect HCC at an early stage, (vi) the tests are cost-effective and acceptable to physicians and patients, (vii) an algorithmic approach to recall and diagnosis after the detection of findings is available, and (viii) there are effective treatments for confirmed cases of HCC.

The target population for surveillance is patients with cirrhosis, regardless of cause. The annual incidence of HCC among these patients surpasses the threshold of 1.5% that renders surveillance cost-effective. Patients with cirrhosis and advanced liver dysfunction, who would not be eligible for a curative treatment, are not candidates for surveillance. Surveillance for patients on the transplant waiting list is to ensure that HCC does not develop that may preclude transplantation in some cases. Some patients who have liver disease without cirrhosis such as chronic HBV infection with high level of viral replication should also be enrolled in surveillance programs. Surveillance is not recommended for patients who have non-alcoholic fatty liver disease (NAFLD) without cirrhosis.

Abdominal ultrasonography every 6 months is the recommended method for surveillance, with or without measurement of serum levels of alpha-fetoprotein. The results are operator-dependent, with a sensitivity of 47–84% and a specificity higher than 90%.

Villanueva A. Hepatocellular Carcinoma. New England Journal of Medicine. 2019;380(15):1450–1462.
https://www.nejm.org/doi/full/10.1056/NEJMra1713263

27. Answer: A

Hereditary haemochromatosis (HH) is a common autosomal recessive condition in Caucasians with an estimated 1/200 people homozygous for the C282Y mutation in the *HFE* gene. C282Y homozygotes have the highest risk of developing total body iron overload, and the consequences of iron overload involving multiple organs, such as liver fibrosis, liver cirrhosis, hepatocellular carcinoma, cardiomyopathy, cardiac arrhythmias, diabetes, arthropathy, hypogonadism, and skin hyperpigmentation. C282Y/H63 compound heterozygotes have a much lower risk of total body iron overload.

HH is a metabolic condition of iron homeostasis associated with hepcidin deficiency. Hepcidin is a peptide hormone synthesized by the liver. It inhibits absorption of iron and release of iron by macrophages. It achieves this by regulating levels of ferroportin, a cellular iron export protein expressed on duodenal enterocytes and macrophages which is responsible for scavenging iron from red blood cells. Hepcidin binding to ferroportin initiates the internalization and degradation of ferroportin.

Only 10% of patients with elevated serum ferritin levels have the diagnosis of HH. The other 90% of patients have elevated serum ferritin levels associated with metabolic syndrome, obesity, diabetes, liver cirrhosis, inflammatory conditions, malignancy, chronic alcohol consumption, etc. Elevations of serum ferritin in the range 300–1000 µg/L is often associated with the presence of the above-mentioned complications. If serum ferritin level is >1000 µg/L, referral to a gastroenterologist or a haematologist with an interest in iron overload is important. Careful interpretation of the iron studies is important to avoid unnecessary referral for therapeutic venesection. Transferrin saturation >45% is sensitive and fairly specific for diagnosis of HH. There is increasing specificity when the transferrin saturation is >55%. Eligibility criteria for therapeutic venesection includes evidence of hereditary haemochromatosis with C282Y homozygosity or C282Y/H63D compound heterozygosity, evidence of clinical iron overload on FerriScan MRI or liver biopsy, polycythaemia ruba vera, and porphyria cutanea tarda.

Therapeutic venesection tries to achieve a target serum ferritin level of ~50 µg/L at the iron unloading phase, which may take many months or even years to unload excess iron. It is important to ensure pre-venesection haemoglobin level is >120 g/L to avoid anaemia. Monitor serum ferritin level every 4 to 6 venesections. Oral vitamin B12 and folate supplements are given to support erythropoiesis during frequent venesections. Lifelong maintenance phase has a target serum ferritin of ~50–100 µg/L. The frequency of venesections varies between individuals, often between 2 to 5 venesections per year. Serum ferritin level needs to be monitored every year.

Goot K, Hazeldine S, Bentley P, Olynyk J, Crawford D. Elevated serum ferritin – what should GPs know? Australian Family Physician. 2012;41(12):945–949.
https://www.ncbi.nlm.nih.gov/pubmed/23210117

28. Answer: C

The patient has classical symptoms of irritable bowel syndrome (IBS) which is a functional bowel disorder with complex pathophysiological origins, and is probably due to multiple pathological states. However, the distinction of IBS is useful in terms of its relatively benign course without severe physical debility and mortality. BS presents with pain, change in frequency of stool and change in appearance of stool – the symptoms must be present for at least one day a week over at least three months (Rome IV criteria). IBS can be diagnosed with these symptoms plus the absence of warning signs such as older age, overt gastrointestinal bleeding, or unintentional weight loss. A positive diagnosis rather than relying on exclusion of other diagnoses with unnecessary invasive procedures is good medical practice supported by the natural history of large cohorts of patients with suspected IBS by these criteria. Faecal calprotectin is a sensitive and specific test to rule out inflammatory bowel disease in patients with diarrhoea predominant symptoms.

Treatment of IBS revolves around an empathic and professional doctor–patient relationship, which improves follow-up and decreases unnecessary testing. Multiple medical treatments have a positive effect in IBS, but given the heterogeneity of illness, personalised medicine is essential. Effective treatments include dietary fibre, prosecretory agents in constipating disease, dietary interventions, tricyclic antidepressants, 5HT-3 receptor antagonists, antihistamines, rifaximin, and probiotics in diarrhoeal or mixed disease. A sobering fact is that in one study of patients with IBS, patients would trade-off over a decade of life-expectancy for a cure to the disease, highlighting its profound effect on quality of life.

 Ford A, Lacy B, Talley N. Irritable Bowel Syndrome. New England Journal of Medicine. 2017;376(26):2566–2578. https://www.nejm.org/doi/full/10.1056/NEJMra1607547

29. Answer: C

Lactose is found only in mammalian milk and is hydrolysed into glucose and galactose by lactase in the small intestine. Lactose intolerance is defined as the onset of abdominal symptoms such as abdominal pain, bloating, and diarrhoea after lactose ingestion by an individual with lactose malabsorption (LM). LM is inefficient absorption of lactose caused by lactose maldigestion due to lactase deficiency as lactose cannot be absorbed in the undigested form. Lactase deficiency is classified as:

1. Congenital lactase deficiency (alactasia).
2. Primary lactase deficiency (adult-type hypolactasia) is caused by the non-persistence of lactase, with enzyme levels progressively reducing starting from the age of 2–5 years, depending on ethnicity.
3. Secondary hypolactasia involves the loss of the lactase enzyme due to other clinical conditions affecting the intestinal tract such as bacterial or viral enteritis, coeliac disease, inflammatory bowel diseases, and severe malnutrition.

Approximately 65% of the world's population have LM, but most are asymptomatic. Approximately 30% of lactose malabsorbers develop symptoms of lactose intolerance. The threshold of lactose tolerance varies significantly among patients and is dependent on several factors including the dose of lactose consumed, residual lactase expression, food matrix (ingestion with other dietary components), gut-transit time, and enteric microbiome composition. In other word, LM is the precondition of lactose intolerance. In clinical practice, some people with lactose intolerance can consume milk and dairy foods without developing symptoms, whereas others will need lactose restriction.

The following tests can confirm lactose maldigestion/malabsorption:

1. Lactose tolerance test (LTT):
   It consists of administering oral lactose (1 to 1.5 g/kg body weight) and obtaining serial blood glucose levels. The test is positive if intestinal symptoms occur and the blood glucose level increases <1.1 mmol/L above the fasting level. However, false-positive and false-negative test results occur in 20% of normal subjects because of the influence of variable gastric emptying and glucose metabolism.
2. Hydrogen breath test:
   This test is based on the principle that carbohydrates in the colon are detectable in pulmonary excretion of hydrogen and other gases. A rise in breath hydrogen concentration >20 ppm over baseline after 50 g of lactose ingestion suggests hypolactasia. It is more sensitive and specific than LTT. It is positive in 90% of patients with LM.
3. Small bowel biopsy:
   Tests for lactase enzymatic activities on intestinal biopsies will detect primary and secondary LM. It is regarded as the gold standard for determining lactase activity but it is invasive.
4. Genetic test:
   Genetic tests apply real-time PCR or sequencing on DNA extracted from a venous blood or buccal swab sample. In Caucasians, lactase persistence is nearly uniformly mediated by the LCT-13910:C/T polymorphism, and genetic testing can detect genetic lactase non-persistence (LNP).

It is important to remember that whereas lactase deficiency and malabsorption can be objectively measured, demonstration of lactose intolerance relies on subjective self-reporting of symptoms, which are very common even in the absence of lactose ingestion and are also highly susceptible to the placebo effect.

Lactose intolerance is not cow's milk allergy. Lactose intolerance results from a reduced ability to digest lactose. It is a 'non-immune-mediated adverse food reaction', while cow's milk allergy is one of the most common forms of immune-mediated food allergy. Cow's milk allergy may be due to IgE, non-IgE mediated, or mixed reactions. After food intake, IgE-mediated reactions typically occur within 2 hours, whereas non-IgE-mediated reactions develop after 2–48 hours or days after the food ingestion.

Treatment of lactose intolerance should not be primarily aimed at reducing malabsorption but rather at improving gastrointestinal symptoms. Restriction of lactose intake is recommended. Lactase enzyme replacement is another important approach in patients with 'isolated' lactose intolerance that wish to enjoy dairy products.

Misselwitz B, Butter M, Verbeke K, Fox M. Update on lactose malabsorption and intolerance: pathogenesis, diagnosis and clinical management. Gut. 2019;:gutjnl-2019–318404.
https://gut.bmj.com/content/early/2019/08/19/gutjnl-2019-318404.long

30. Answer: C

In Australia and New Zealand, the most common indication for liver transplant (LT) is hepatitis C–related cirrhosis with or without concomitant hepatocellular carcinoma (HCC) (28%). Other indications for LT for patients with chronic liver disease include HCC (14%), alcoholic liver disease (ALD) (13%), non-alcoholic steatohepatitis (NASH) (6%), hepatitis B (3%), hepatitis B/C/D (2%), and other diseases (34%).

In recent years, the endemic hepatitis B in Maori and Pacific Island population in New Zealand has increased the incidence of LT for hepatitis B. There is also an increasing trend of patients with NASH receiving LT, corresponding to the increasing burden of obesity, type 2 diabetes, and metabolic syndrome observed in Australia and New Zealand. Addressing these risk factors to prevent multiorgan complications is important. Given the limited availability of donor organs, eligibility of LT is restricted to patients for whom quality and quantity of life is expected to be improved by LT or if their liver disease poses an imminent threat to patients' survival.

In Australia and New Zealand, adult patients with chronic liver disease with life-threatening complications and a Model for End-Stage Liver Disease (MELD) score of greater or equal to 15 are the main indications for LT. The MELD Score is used to estimate relative disease severity and likely survival of patients awaiting LT.

$$MELD\,Score = 10 * ((0.957 * \ln(Creatinine)) + (0.378 * \ln(Bilirubin)) + (1.12 * \ln(INR))) + 6.43$$

The maximum serum creatinine is 4.0 mg/dL (354 umol/L). This includes those patients on dialysis. All cirrhosis patients should be screened for HCC with serum AFP and by appropriate imaging to see if they meet 'standardised MELD exceptions'.

When prioritising HCC patients, the unit in New Zealand makes use of the North American 'HCC MELD score', whereas Australian units prioritise on the basis of tumour progression despite locoregional therapy, provided such patients remain within UCSF criteria.

Adults with MELD score of <15 may be eligible for LT if they fit any of the following criteria:

- HCC that fulfils the University of California, San Francisco (UCSF) criteria
- Liver disease that would result in a two-year mortality risk of >50% without LT
- Diuretic-resistant ascites
- Recurrent hepatic encephalopathy
- Recurrent spontaneous bacterial peritonitis
- Recurrent or persistent gastrointestinal haemorrhage
- Intractable cholangitis (in primary or secondary sclerosing cholangitis patients)
- Hepatopulmonary syndrome
- Portopulmonary hypertension
- Metabolic syndromes (with severe or life-threatening symptoms) that are curable with LT (e.g. familial amyloidosis, urea cycle disorders, oxalosis etc.)
- Polycystic liver disease with severe or life-threatening symptoms
- Intractable itch secondary to cholestatic liver disease
- Hepatoblastoma in children.

McCaughan G, Munn S. Liver transplantation in Australia and New Zealand. Liver Transplantation. 2016;22(6):830–838.
https://aasldpubs.onlinelibrary.wiley.com/doi/full/10.1002/lt.24446

31. Answer: A

In patients with major lower GI bleeding (LGIB) localisation of the site of bleeding is the first priority which can be most quickly, and least invasively, achieved via CT angiography. In patients who are haemodynamically unstable, resuscitation should be commenced, and CT angiogram should proceed as soon as patient is stable. If CT angiography is positive, the patient should, when indicated and as soon as possible, undergo catheter angiography with a view to embolisation, to achieve maximum chance of success. If there is haemodynamic instability associated LGIB, and initial CT angiography reveals no bleeding source, an upper endoscopy should be performed immediately, since there may be an upper GI bleeding source. Patients should not, except under exceptional circumstances, proceed to emergency laparotomy unless an exhaustive effort has been made, via radiologic and/or endoscopic modalities, to localise bleeding.

The concern of contrast induced nephropathy (CIN) is not a contraindication for angiogram especially in a medical emergency. The frequency of CIN is not as high as previously thought. Furthermore, the majority of CIN is reversible.

Restrictive RBC thresholds (a Hb trigger of 70 g/L and an Hb concentration target of 70–90 g/L after transfusion) are appropriate for clinically stable patients who need RBC transfusion. In patients with a history of cardiovascular disease, however, the trigger and target should be 80 g/L and 100 g/L, respectively.

Routine cessation of dual antiplatelet therapy with a P2Y12 receptor antagonist and aspirin is not recommended in patients with coronary stents in situ, and a cardiologist should be involved in management. If administration of the P2Y12 receptor antagonist is interrupted in the context of unstable haemorrhage, aspirin therapy should be continued. Treatment with the P2Y12 receptor antagonist should recommence within 5 days.

Oakland K, Chadwick G, East J, Guy R, Humphries A, Jairath V et al. Diagnosis and management of acute lower gastrointestinal bleeding: guidelines from the British Society of Gastroenterology. Gut. 2019;68(5):776–789. https://gut.bmj.com/content/68/5/776.long

32. Answer: B

This patient's presentation is typical of chronic mesenteric ischaemia, especially postprandial abdominal pain, fear of eating, and weight loss. He is a current smoker and has clinical features of vasculopathy. CT angiography of the abdomen is the investigation of choice for diagnosing mesenteric ischaemia. The symptoms of gastroparesis can be similar to mesenteric ischaemia. The importance of timely diagnosis to avoid an acute ischaemic event means that a gastric emptying study is inappropriate at this stage.

Mesenteric ischemia can be classified as acute or chronic. Acute mesenteric ischemia is a surgical emergency. It is associated with embolic occlusion in 40–50% of cases with thrombotic occlusion of a previously stenotic mesenteric vessel in 20–35% of cases, and with dissection or inflammation of the artery in <5% of cases. More than 90% of cases of chronic mesenteric ischemia (CMI) are related to progressive atherosclerotic disease that affects the origins of the visceral vessels.

CMI is often underdiagnosed and the diagnosis is often delayed due to the low index of suspicion. Arteriogram is the gold standard for the diagnosis of CMI. Typically, the arteriogram shows occlusion of two visceral branches of the aorta, with severe stenosis of the remaining visceral branch, usually the coeliac trunk or the superior mesenteric artery (SMA). CT angiogram (CTA) has a sensitivity of 96% and a specificity of 94% for detecting CMI and is the first-line investigation if the renal function is normal. Mesenteric duplex ultrasound may be a useful initial screening tool for CMI but this is limited by operator training, bowel gas patterns, and obesity. Magnetic resonance angiography (MRA) is the second-line imaging modality.

After the diagnosis of CMI is confirmed with angiography, patients should undergo open or endovascular revascularisation because of the risk of continued weight loss, acute infarction, perforation, sepsis, and death. Because of the high rate of thrombosis, medical management as the sole therapy is warranted only when the risks of revascularisation outweigh the benefits. Nitrate therapy may provide short-term relief but is not curative.

Clair D, Beach J. Mesenteric Ischemia. New England Journal of Medicine. 2016;374(10):959–968. https://www.nejm.org/doi/full/10.1056/NEJMra1503884

33. Answer: A

In the absence of alcohol intake, hepatic steatosis is most likely related to non-alcoholic fatty liver disease (NAFLD) in the setting of morbid obesity. NAFLD is the most common chronic liver disease in developed countries. NAFLD represents a spectrum of liver disease severity. It starts with the accumulation of triacylglycerol in the liver (steatosis), and is defined by hepatic fatty infiltration of >5% by liver weight, or the presence of >5% of hepatocytes loaded with large fat vacuoles. Approximately 25% of patients with NAFLD will progress with the development of liver inflammation to non-alcoholic steatohepatitis (NASH). NASH can cause ongoing liver injury and cell death resulting in fibrosis, cirrhosis, and, but rarely, hepatocellular carcinoma.

Clinicians should consider a potential diagnosis of NAFLD in patients with features of metabolic syndrome, diabetes or abnormal LFTs. A liver ultrasound is the first-line investigation (sensitivity 85%, specificity 95%) to diagnose hepatic steatosis in NAFLD and to exclude other liver pathology.

Currently there is no reliable and non-invasive method to identify the progression of steatosis to NASH. Identifying NASH is important due to its progressive nature and efficacy of new drugs to induce resolution of NASH is a key end-point in clinical trials. However, the presence of NASH per se does not predict liver outcomes but rather the presence of liver fibrosis on biopsy.

FibroScan uses pulsed-echo ultrasound to evaluate the liver's reduced elasticity, due to deposition of fibrotic tissue in hepatic parenchyma, and produces a liver stiffness measurement (kPA) as a surrogate marker of fibrosis. This technique has been validated for several aetiologies of chronic liver disease including NAFLD. It has a sensitivity of 87% and specificity of 91% in detecting cirrhosis. It also has very high negative predictive value and can therefore be used to reliably exclude advanced fibrosis.

Liver biopsy however, is the gold standard for diagnosing hepatic steatosis, NASH and liver fibrosis. Liver biopsy should be considered in all patients in whom the diagnosis remains uncertain after initial investigations. Additionally, in those with a high probability of liver fibrosis, a biopsy can be used to confirm the diagnosis.

As the patient has no liver-related signs or symptoms, has very mildly abnormal LFTs, and the diagnosis is suggestive on liver ultrasound, a liver biopsy is not recommended.

Current management of NAFLD is largely focused on lifestyle interventions to achieve weight loss and to modify both metabolic and cardiovascular risk factors. Even relatively small amounts of weight loss (3–5%) can result in significant reductions in liver fat percentage, improved insulin sensitivity, improvements in cardiometabolic risk factors and better long-term outcomes.

Many drugs to limit the development and progression of NAFLD have been trialled, but none are, to date, specifically licensed for the treatment of NAFLD. One such drug, pioglitazone, targets both adipose tissue metabolism and inflammation, acting through the transcription factor peroxisome proliferator-activated receptor gamma (PPARγ). Pioglitazone reduces hepatic steatosis through increased uptake of fatty acids by adipocytes, and therefore reduces the flux of fatty acids to the liver.

Metformin has no significant effect on liver histology and is not recommended as a specific treatment for NAFLD or NASH. Ursodeoxycolic acid is also not recommended for the treatment of NAFLD. Given the lack of evidence to show that patients with NAFLD and NASH are at increased risk for serious drug-induced liver injury from statins, statins can be used to treat dyslipidaemia in patients with NAFLD and NASH.

Diehl A, Day C. Cause, Pathogenesis, and Treatment of Nonalcoholic Steatohepatitis. New England Journal of Medicine. 2017;377(21):2063–2072.
https://www.nejm.org/doi/full/10.1056/NEJMra1503519?url_ver=Z39.88-2003&rfr_id=ori%3Arid%3Acrossref.org&rfr_dat=cr_pub%3Dpubmed

34. Answer: B

High resolution manometry (HRM) is superior to standard manometry in terms of reproducibility, speed of performance and ease of interpretation. The addition of impedance to HRM is helpful to 'visualise' bolus movement and peristalsis effectiveness; however, its utility in clinical practice and impact on therapeutic decision making is not yet clear.

In patients with confirmed achalasia, HRM provides information on achalasia subtype which is predictive of clinical outcome. Patients presenting with dysphagia should undergo endoscopy with oesophageal biopsies to rule out and treat mucosal and structural disorders prior to manometry. Among patients with major motility disorders other than achalasia (diffuse oesophageal spasm, hypercontractile oesophagus, absent peristalsis), HRM, compared with standard manometry, may provide increased diagnostic and functional information changing intervention.

Patients with symptoms suspected to be due to GORD should undergo a therapeutic trial of a PPI as the initial diagnostic approach. Only if the symptoms are not responding to twice daily PPIs, should HRM be performed. Furthermore, HRM should be performed in advance for all patients being considered for anti-reflux surgery to rule out lower oesophageal sphincter (LOS) dysfunction (ie, achalasia), as well as major motor disorders of the oesophageal body such as diffuse oesophageal spasm.

Rumination syndrome is characterised by rapid onset of regurgitation after most meals and can be confidently diagnosed clinically on the basis of a typical history, but if the diagnosis is unclear, the patient needs convincing of the diagnosis or objective evidence is required prior to therapy, HRM with impedance after a test meal can be utilised to identify diagnostic features.

Trudgill N, Sifrim D, Sweis R, Fullard M, Basu K, McCord M et al. British Society of Gastroenterology guidelines for oesophageal manometry and oesophageal reflux monitoring. Gut 2019;68:1731–1750.
https://gut.bmj.com/content/68/10/1731.full

35. Answer: C

Symptoms associated with oesophageal dysphagia are chest pain, regurgitation, and water brash. It is often caused by oesophageal motor disorders or cancer. Symptoms associated with oropharyngeal dysphagia include aspiration pneumonia, weakness, speech disturbance, coughing, or choking during swallowing.

In elderly patients, 80% of oropharyngeal dysphagia is caused by neuromuscular disorders such as CVA, Parkinson's disease, myasthenia gravis; while 20% is caused by structural abnormalities such as cancer. Brain stem CVA is more likely to cause oropharyngeal dysphagia than a hemispheric CVA. Approximately 25–50% of CVA will result in oropharyngeal dysphagia and most of these cases will improve spontaneously within the first 2 weeks. Unnecessary diagnostic tests or intervention such as percutaneous endoscopic gastrostomy (PEG) insertion should be avoided immediately after CVA. Oropharyngeal dysphagia is best investigated by videofluoroscopic swallowing study known as a modified barium swallow. Simultaneous occurrence of oesophageal dysphagia and oropharyngeal dysphagia is extremely rare for any underlying disease process except infection.

Jansson-Knodell CL, Codipilly DC, Leggett CL. Making Dysphagia Easier to Swallow: A Review for the Practicing Clinician. Mayo Clin Proc. June 2017;92(6):965–972
https://www.mayoclinicproceedings.org/article/S0025-6196(17)30272-0/fulltext

36. Answer: B

At normal doses of paracetamol, concomitant use of drugs which induce cytochrome P450 2D6 have not been demonstrated to increase the risk of paracetamol hepatotoxicity.

Paracetamol elimination occurs via three major pathways:

1. 90% of paracetamol is metabolised by hepatic UDP-glucuronosyltransferases (UGT1A1 and 1A6) and sulfotransferases (SULT1A1, 1A3/4, 1E1) into glucorinide and sulfate conjugates respectively, which are excreted in urine.
2. 5% of paracetamol is excreted into the urine unchanged.
3. 5% of paracetamol is metabolised by hepatic cytochrome P450 enzymes (predominantly CYP2E1, to a lesser extent CYP1A2, CYP3A4) into N-acetyl-p-benzoquinonemine (NAPQI).
   a. If sufficient hepatic glutathione stores: NAPQ1 binds to hepatic glutathione spontaneously and via glutathione-S-transferases, forming non-toxic cysteine and mercaptate compounds, which are excreted in urine
   b. If depleted hepatic glutathione stores: NAPQ1 accumulates causing hepatotoxicity.

It has been reported that up to 40% of accidental paracetamol poisonings occur in patients taking 4 g paracetamol/day or less. In fasting and chronic alcohol use, paracetamol conjugates and hepatic glutathione stores are already depleted prior to paracetamol intake. In paracetamol overdose, and use of alcohol and other drugs which induce CYP450 2E1, a greater fraction of paracetamol is metabolized to NAPQI, depleting hepatic glutathione stores quicker during paracetamol administration. Depleted paracetamol conjugates and hepatic glutathione prevents NAPQI metabolism, predisposing to NAPQ1 accumulation and hepatotoxicity. A reduced daily dose of paracetamol is recommended in people who are fasting, heavy users of alcohol, and taking medications that induce cytochrome P450 2E1.

Caparrotta T, Antoine D, Dear J. Are some people at increased risk of paracetamol-induced liver injury? A critical review of the literature. European Journal of Clinical Pharmacology. 2018;74(2):147–160.
https://link.springer.com/article/10.1007/s00228-017-2356-6

37. Answer: C

PPIs are among the most commonly prescribed classes of drugs, and their use is increasing, in particular for long-term treatment for GORD and peptic ulcers. PPIs are generally well tolerated, with only rare and mild side effects in short-term use. However, the potential adverse effects related to PPI longer-term therapy are also coming to light. The possible associations between long-term PPI treatment include:

- Hypomagnesaemia has been associated with long-term PPI use according to systematic reviews and a meta-analysis of nine observational studies. PPI should therefore be discontinued in severe, persistent hypomagnesaemia. Resolution of hypomagnesaemia occurs after 1 to 2 weeks following PPI withdrawal with GI malabsorption and renal wasting being the likely mechanisms.
- Increased cardiovascular risk in patients on antiplatelet therapy following acute coronary syndrome and percutaneous coronary intervention who are prescribed PPIs to prevent GI bleeding. A potential interaction between PPIs and clopidogrel leading to an attenuated antiplatelet effect is associated with increased risk of cardiovascular events, including higher overall mortality.
- Hypocalcaemia: absorption of calcium compounds can be significantly reduced in the presence of achlorhydria, implicating PPIs as a potential cause for calcium malabsorption. A weak association exists between long-term PPI use and a higher incidence of bone fractures.
- Acute interstitial nephritis is observed in PPI users, and weak association exists between long-term PPI treatment and induced CKD.
- Fundic gland polyps: PPI use is significantly associated with a two-fold increased risk of fundic gland polyps.
- *C. Difficile* infection risk: statistically significant association between PPI use and the risk of *clostridium difficile* infection was found in two meta-analyses, but high heterogeneity among studies and publication bias weakened the results.

Currently, there is no clear evidence that long-term PPI use is associated with following conditions:

- Increased risk of gastric cancer
- Increased risk of community acquired pneumonia
- Increased risk of iron malabsorption and anaemia
- Increased risk of developing dementia.

Eusebi L, Rabitti S, Artesiani M, Gelli D, Montagnani M, Zagari R et al. Proton pump inhibitors: Risks of long-term use. Journal of Gastroenterology and Hepatology. 2017;32(7):1295–1302.
https://onlinelibrary.wiley.com/doi/full/10.1111/jgh.13737

38. Answer: C

This patient has symptoms and biochemical tests consistent with primary biliary cholangitis (PBC), previously known as primary biliary cirrhosis. However, patients with PBC can also present without symptoms or with complications of decompensated liver disease.

Anti-LKM1 is a serologic marker for type 2 autoimmune hepatitis (AIH), anti-smooth muscle antibodies (ASMAs) are serological markers of type 1 AIH along with ANAs, and atypical pANCAs are found in patients with type 1 AIH and are associated with primary sclerosing cholangitis and ulcerative colitis.

PBC is a chronic autoimmune cholestatic liver disease that has a female preponderance of 10:1, with presentation mainly in the 5th and 6th decades. The circulating antimitochondrial antibodies (AMAs) selectively damage intrahepatic cholangiocytes, leading to progressive cholestasis and chronic liver disease. The diagnostic criteria for PBC include positive AMAs, an abnormal ALP level for over 24 weeks, nonsuppurative cholangitis, and interlobular bile duct injury findings on liver biopsy. Without treatment, patients are likely to develop chronic liver disease. Associated autoimmune conditions include Sjogren's syndrome, thyroid disease, coeliac disease, and systemic sclerosis.

First-line therapy to slow disease progression of PBC is ursodeoxycholic acid (UDCA). Side effects of UDCA include weight gain in the first 12 months, hair loss, and gastrointestinal discomfort. If patients do not achieve an adequate biochemical response on UDCA a farnesoid X receptor agonist, obeticholic acid, can be trialed as a second-line medication. Off-label use of peroxisome proliferator-activated receptor agonists, including the fibrate class of drugs, such as fenofibrate, are also recognised as options for patients. Therapeutic options for pruritus include cholestyramine and rifampicin.

Liver transplant referral may be considered in patients with a Model for End-Stage Liver Disease (MELD) score of at least 15, whose bilirubin levels are above 50 μmol/L, and with refractory pruritus.

Lowe D, John S. Autoimmune hepatitis: Appraisal of current treatment guidelines. World Journal of Hepatology. 2018;10(12):911–923.
https://www.ncbi.nlm.nih.gov/pmc/articles/PMC6323516/

39. Answer: A

This patient's clinical features and AXR are consistent with acute pseudo-obstruction or ileus of the colon, known as Ogilvie's syndrome. It is a paralytic ileus of the large bowel characterised by rapidly progressive abdominal distension often without associated pain. AXR may reveal air in the small bowel and distension of discrete segments of the colon (cecum or transverse colon) or the entire colon. Distension can become marked, often in chronic cases colonic distension in excess of 15 cm can be observed without evidence of colon perforation or wall ischemia.

Major risk factors for the development of Ogilvie's syndrome include systemic infection, cardiovascular disease, severe blunt trauma, orthopaedic trauma or procedures, coronary bypass surgery, stroke or neurosurgical procedures, electrolyte disturbances, and medications with an anticholinergic effect.

Initial management includes:

- Intravenous fluids to maintain normovolaemia and correct electrolyte abnormalities.
- Patients should be given nothing by mouth.
- Medications that can decrease colonic motility such as opiates, calcium channel blockers and medications with anticholinergic side effects should be stopped.
- Discontinuation of and avoidance of laxatives.
- A nasogastric tube is indicated if the patient is vomiting and will prevent swallowed air from passing distally.
- If distension is painless and the patient shows no signs of toxicity or bowel ischemia, expectant management can be successful in half of cases.
- Neostigmine should be considered in patients at risk of perforation and those who have failed conservative therapy.
- If distension worsens so that the cecal diameter increases beyond 12 cm or persists for > 48 hours, colonoscopy is recommended.
- Endoscopic decompression is successful in 60–90% of cases, but colonic distension may recur in up to 40%.
- To prevent the recurrence of colon dilation, more than one endoscopic decompression procedure and/or endoscopic placement of a decompression tube is often required.
- Rectal tubes are ineffective in managing distension of the proximal colon such in this case; however, such tubes may be useful after colonoscopy.

The use of intravenous patient controlled analgesia has no benefit for the recovery of Ogilvie's syndrome ileus when compared to other route of narcotic administration. There has been little success in the use of prokinetic agents to shorten recovery times of Ogilvie's syndrome.

Haj M, Haj M, Rockey D. Ogilvie's syndrome. Medicine.2018;97(27):e11187.
https://journals.lww.com/md-journal/fulltext/2018/07060/Ogilvie_s_syndrome__management_and_outcomes.8.aspx

40. Answer: D

Small bowel bacterial overgrowth is defined as the presence of $>10^5$ CFU/mL of bacteria in the proximal small bowel or $>10^3$ CFU/mL of isolates routinely found in colonic flora. Conditions that causes reduced gastric acid, structural abnormalities (e.g. small bowel diverticula) and dysmotility syndromes are associated with small bowel bacterial overgrowth. The following diseases are associated with small bowel bacterial overgrowth:

- Achlorhydria due to chronic atrophic gastritis and long-term proton pump inhibitors use
- Autonomic neuropathy in diabetes mellitus
- Cirrhosis
- Coeliac disease
- Crohn's disease
- Exocrine pancreatic insufficiency
- Scleroderma
- Short bowel syndrome.

Clinical manifestations may vary but can include diarrhoea, anorexia, nausea, weight loss, and anaemia. Malabsorption can result in hypocalcaemia, night blindness due to vitamin A deficiency, vitamin K deficiency, and osteomalacia. Vitamin B12 deficiency is common with severe overgrowth. Anaemia may be megaloblastic and macrocytic as a result of vitamin B12 deficiency. Luminal bacteria tend to consume cobalamin but produce folate resulting in low vitamin B12 and high folate levels.

Krajicek E, Hansel S. Small Intestinal Bacterial Overgrowth. Mayo Clinic Proceedings. 2016;91(12):1828–1833.
https://www.mayoclinicproceedings.org/article/S0025-6196(16)30589-4/pdf

41. Answer: A

Liver transplant is a lifesaving treatment for patients with acute liver failure, end stage liver disease and its complications, and some hereditary metabolic disorders. Recipients of orthotopic liver transplants have excellent survival rates (85–90% for 1 year and 75% for 5 years).

Tacrolimus is superior to cyclosporin in improving patient and graft survival and preventing acute rejection. Common side effects include:

- Increased risk of post-transplant diabetes: the diabetogenic effect of tacrolimus is greater than cyclosporin.
- Nephrotoxic effect at high levels: tacrolimus causes afferent renal arteriolar vasoconstriction leading to renal dysfunction and tubular injury. This vasoconstrictor effect is dose-dependent and reversible. However, these agents may also play a role in inducing CKD.
- Electrolyte disturbances including hyperkalaemia, hypophosphataemia, hypomagnesaemia, and metabolic acidosis.
- Hypertension.
- Hyperlipidaemia.
- Increased risk of infection.
- Neurotoxicity: mild manifestations include tremors, insomnia, sleep disturbances, headaches, and paraesthesia; serious adverse neurological effects include seizures, speech disorders, cortical blindness, encephalopathy, and central pontine myelinolysis. Tacrolimus has a significantly higher incidence of neurotoxicity than cyclosporin.
- Alopecia.

Tacrolimus does not cause bone marrow suppression, gingival hyperplasia or hirsutism.

Muduma G, Saunders R, Odeyemi I, Pollock R. Systematic Review and Meta-Analysis of Tacrolimus versus Ciclosporin as Primary Immunosuppression After Liver Transplant. PLOS ONE. 2016;11(11):e0160421.
https://journals.plos.org/plosone/article?id=10.1371/journal.pone.0160421

42. Answer: B

Terlipressin is a vasopressin analogue acting through V1a receptors, found on vascular smooth muscle within the splanchnic circulation, causing splanchnic vasoconstriction. The splanchnic vasoconstriction then increases renal blow flow and has beneficial effects on hepatorenal syndrome and reduces portal pressure and the risk of oesophageal varices bleed.

Terlipressin also stimulates the V2 renal receptors leading to insertion of aquaporin 2, a vasopressin-regulated water-channel protein, at the apical plasma membrane of the renal collecting duct and thus leading to increased free water absorption. The solute free water absorption can potentially result in profound and life-threatening hyponatraemia and patients treated with terlipressin need to be closely monitored.

A retrospective Australian study found using terlipressin and albumin infusion together can be an effective therapy for profound hyponatraemia in patients with liver cirrhosis. Terlipressin can potentially worsens asthma and COPD and is contraindicated in unstable angina, recent myocardial infarction (terlipressin causes vasoconstriction and fluid retention) and in pregnancy (may stimulate uterine contraction). Terlipressin should be used with caution in patients with cardiac disease, arrhythmias, uncontrolled hypertension, cerebral or peripheral vascular disease, or atherosclerosis.

Papaluca T, Gow P. Terlipressin: Current and emerging indications in chronic liver disease. Journal of Gastroenterology and Hepatology. 2018;33(3):591–598.
https://onlinelibrary.wiley.com/doi/full/10.1111/jgh.14009

43. Answer: A

Haemodynamic status should be assessed and resuscitation should begin immediately upon presentation of overt upper gastrointestinal bleeding (UGIB). Blood transfusions should target haemoglobin ≥70 g/L, with higher haemoglobin levels targeted in patients with comorbidities such as coronary artery disease.

Risk assessment should be performed. The Blatchford score predicts the need for therapy and admission. Patients are unlikely to need treatment and therefore may not require admission if they satisfy the following criteria:

- Urea <6.5 mmol/L
- Haemoglobin >130 g/L (men) or 120 g/L (women)
- Systolic BP >110 mmHg
- HR<100 beats/min (excluding those with syncope).

The Rockall score is used for risk categorisation before and after endoscopy. This predicts rates of re-bleeding and mortality and can be used in management algorithms. Pre-endoscopic intravenous PPI may decrease the proportion of patients who have higher risk stigmata of haemorrhage at endoscopy. Haemodynamically stable patients with UGIB should undergo endoscopy within 24 h of admission and within 12 hours for patients with haemodynamic instability that persists despite resuscitation. In patients who are low risk, haemodynamically stable, and without serious comorbidities, endoscopy should still be performed as soon as possible in a non-emergent setting to identify the substantial proportion of patients with low-risk endoscopic findings who can be safely discharged.

During endoscopy, stigmata of recent haemorrhage should be recorded as they predict risk of further bleeding and guide management decisions. The stigmata, in descending risk of further bleeding, are:

- Active spurting
- Non-bleeding visible vessel
- Active oozing
- Adherent clot
- Flat pigmented spot
- Clean base.

Endoscopic haemostatic therapy should be undertaken in patients with higher risk stigmata of haemorrhage including active spurting or oozing bleeding or a non-bleeding visible vessel. Thermal therapy with bipolar electrocoagulation or heater probe and injection of sclerosant (eg absolute alcohol) are recommended. Adrenaline therapy should not be used alone.

After successful endoscopic haemostasis, intravenous PPI therapy with pantoprazole 80 mg bolus followed by 8 mg/h continuous infusion for 72 h should be given to patients who have an ulcer with active bleeding, a non-bleeding visible vessel, or an adherent clot. The patient in this question has a non-bleeding visible vessel in the gastric ulcer. Routine second-look endoscopy, in which repeat endoscopy is performed 24 h after initial endoscopic haemostatic therapy, is not recommended. Repeat endoscopy should only be performed in patients with clinical evidence of recurrent bleeding.

Patients with high-risk stigmata should generally be hospitalised for 3 days assuming no re-bleeding and no other reason for hospitalisation. They can be fed clear liquids soon after endoscopy. Patients with *H. pylori*-associated bleeding ulcers should receive *H. pylori* therapy. After documentation of eradication, maintenance PPI therapy is not needed unless the patient also requires NSAIDs or antithrombotics.

There is NO evidence to support using aspirin as primary prevention of cardiovascular events in diabetic patients. Therefore, there is no indication to resume aspirin in this case especially given the UGIB and negative *H. pylori*.

Sverdén E, Markar S, Agreus L, Lagergren J. Acute upper gastrointestinal bleeding. BMJ. 2018;:k4023.
https://www.bmj.com/content/363/bmj.k4023.long

44. Answer: C

Gastrin is released by gastric G cells, classically when stimulated by food intake to facilitate digestion. Gastrin works on cholecystokinin receptors to stimulate parietal and pepsin cells to produce stomach acid and pepsinogen respectively, to increase gastric mucosal blood flow, and to stimulate gastric, duodenal, and colonic mucosa growth. Meanwhile gastrin release is inhibited by increased stomach acidity, fasting, and somatostatin secreted from gastric D cells.

Hypergastrinaemia can be physiological or pathological. Physiological hypergastrinaemia occurs with neutral gastric pH in conditions with decreased acid production, for example with PPI therapy, *Helicobacter pylori* infection, atrophic gastritis, and renal failure. Pathological hypergastrinaemia occurs with an already acidic pH, for example with Zollinger Ellison syndrome (ZES), retained antrum syndrome, or antral G cell hyperplasia.

ZES is characterized by hypersecretion of gastrin from gastrinomas, a type of neuroendocrine tumour. ZES typically presents with diarrhoea and abdominal pain secondary to multiple recurrent ulcers refractory to PPIs and often in atypical locations throughout the gastrointestinal tract. ZES diagnosis is confirmed with a secretin stimulation test, where elevated gastrin >200 pg/ml after administration of 1–2 micrograms/kg of body weight of secretin is diagnostic. Surgical resection is curative, and generally recommended as first line treatment.

ZES is most often sporadic, but 20–38% of gastrinomas are also associated with multiple endocrine neoplasia type 1 (MEN1.) Gastrinomas are invariably multiple, and found predominantly in the duodenum (85–100%), pancreas (0–15%), and often with lymph node metastases (40–65%). MEN1 gastrinoma management is primarily conservative with PPIs and H2 histamine antagonists to control gastric acid hypersecretion with regular radiological monitoring. Whipple resection is the only recognised cure and is generally not recommended due to high complication rate.

The main functions of the gastrin are:
1. Increases hydrochloric acid secretion (via parietal cells).
2. Simulates growth of gastric mucosa.
3. Increases gastric motility.
4. Increases lower oesophageal sphincter pressure (preventing reflux).
5. Lowers ileocecal sphincter pressure (allows defaecation).
6. Increases pepsinogen secretion.

Dacha S, Razvi M, Massaad J, Cai Q, Wehbi M. Hypergastrinemia. Gastroenterology Report. 2015;3(3):201–208. https://academic.oup.com/gastro/article/3/3/201/613199

45. Answer: D

46. Answer: C

47. Answer: E

48. Answer: H

49. Answer: I

50. Answer: G

The GI system is the largest endocrine organ in the body. The most important function of the GI system is to provide nutrients to our bodies via the process of ingestion, motility, secretion, digestion, and absorption. Currently there are more than 50 GI hormones and bioactive peptides identified. They function as endocrine, paracrine, and neurocrine. Some of the common GI hormones and their main functions are described as above.

Rao J, Wang J. Regulation of Gastrointestinal Mucosal Growth. San Rafael: Morgan & Claypool Life Sciences; 2010. Role of GI Hormones on Gut Mucosal Growth. Available from: https://www.ncbi.nlm.nih.gov/books/NBK54093/#!po=48.8095

7 General and Geriatric Medicine

Questions

Answers can be found in the General and Geriatric Medicine Answers section at the end of this chapter.

1. A 37-year-old male is being investigated for a febrile illness over the past two weeks. On his second clinic visit, he reports a painful, red right eye over the past 3 days. There has been no discharge and the lids are not stuck on awakening. On examination, there is anisocoria with the left pupil measuring 4 mm and the right 2 mm. There is diffuse engorgement of deeper and superficial vessels, without other obvious abnormality to the naked eye. Pen torch shone into the ipsilateral and contralateral eye causes right eye pain, as does accommodation. Visual acuity is not affected. Test results from the first clinic visit one week ago show normal CXR; blood culture and urine culture are negative.

Which of the following steps is most appropriate?
- **A.** Referral to an ophthalmologist.
- **B.** Right eye swab adenovirus PCR.
- **C.** Right eye swab culture.
- **D.** Start topical antibiotics.

2. Which one of the following describes a normal physiological change of ageing?
- **A.** Decreased renal mass with medullary loss greater than cortical loss.
- **B.** Increased basal renin level.
- **C.** Reduced renal cellular oxidative stress and increased nitric oxide.
- **D.** Reduction in aldosterone level and increased risk of hyperkalaemia.

3. A 78-year-old woman is admitted to the Acute Assessment Unit after a fall at home as she cannot see very clearly and tripped over a small box. She has a fracture of her pelvic rami. She tells you that her vision has been poor over the past 3 months. You ask for an ophthalmology consult. A diagnosis of exudative form of macular degeneration is made.

Which of the following statements is true regarding this condition and its impact on discharge planning?
- **A.** The exudative form is usually more severe with more rapid visual loss than the non-exudative form.
- **B.** The exudative form typically causes peripheral visual loss and central vision is preserved.
- **C.** The non-exudative is typically associated with drusen and neovascularisation.
- **D.** There is no treatment available for the exudative form of macular degeneration.

4. Which of the following are the main metabolites of alcohol oxidative metabolism?
- **A.** Acetaldehyde, acetate.
- **B.** Fatty acid ethyl esters.
- **C.** Phosphatidylethanol.
- **D.** Pyruvate, beta-hydroxybutyrate.

5. A 48-year-old man has a left distal radius fracture, and a plaster cast has been applied. He is in pain and has been give intravenous morphine and oral oxycodone in the emergency department. He had significant alcohol intake yesterday and had a fight with his mate, before falling in a pub. He has presented to emergency department several times this year due to alcohol withdrawal syndrome and had one seizure in the past. He is a heavy smoker and denies taking any medications or other substances. His vital signs are stable with an oxygen saturation of 95% on room air. His blood alcohol level is 0.19g/100ml. His initial blood test results are presented below.

How to Pass the FRACP Written Examination, First Edition. Jonathan Gleadle, Jordan Li, Danielle Wu, and Paul Kleinig.
© 2022 John Wiley & Sons Ltd. Published 2022 by John Wiley & Sons Ltd.

Tests	Results	Normal values
Magnesium	0.35 mmol/L	0.7–1.1
Potassium	3.5 mmol/L	3.5–5.2
Glucose	3.8 mmol/L	3.2–5.5
Urea	2.6 mmol/L	2.7–8.0
Creatinine	55 µmol/L	60–110
Albumin	31 g/L	34–48
Bilirubin	2.95 umol/L	2–24
ALP	458 U/L	30–110
GGT	621 U/L	0–60
ALT	130 U/L	0–55
AST	360 U/L	0–45
Hb	101 g/L	135–175
WBC	7.1 x 10^9/L	4.0–11.0
Platelet	89 x 10^9/L	150–450

Whilst reviewing the clerking by a junior doctor, which one of the following management orders would you change?
A. Give intravenous thiamine first before giving intravenous 5% glucose.
B. Give oral diazepam 10mg, 8 hourly on a regular basis.
C. Give intravenous magnesium replacement.
D. Oxygen administration.

6. A 59-year-old man presents to the emergency department with a 6-hour history of central chest pain. An initial ECG is shown below in Figure 7.1A and his previous ECG taken two months ago is shown in Figure 7.1B. His BP is 120/70 mmHg with a HR of 72 bpm. You are performing a cardiovascular examination while the patient is waiting for urgent blood test results and a CXR.
   Which one of the following signs is unlikely to be present?

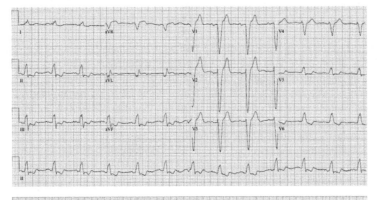

Figure 7.1A

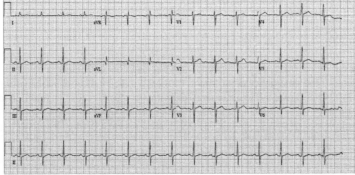

Figure 7.1B

A. Fourth heart sound.
B. Pansystolic murmur in the apex area.
C. Pericardial rub.
D. Third heart sound.

7. Which one of the following is **NOT** an indication for radioisotope bone scan?
  A. Evaluation of bone viability in avascular necrosis.
  B. Evaluation of osteolytic lesions in multiple myeloma.
  C. Evaluation of prosthetic joint infections.
  D. Evaluation of vertebral insufficiency fracture.

8. Which of the following valvular lesions is most common in patients with carcinoid heart disease?
  A. Aortic stenosis.
  B. Mitral regurgitation.
  C. Pulmonic stenosis.
  D. Tricuspid regurgitation.

9. Which of the following is characterised by down-regulation of the hypothalamic-pituitary-adrenal (HPA) axis?
  A. Chronic fatigue syndrome.
  B. Cushing's disease.
  C. Major depression.
  D. Schizophrenia.

10. A 73-year-old woman is admitted to a teaching hospital in South Australia with urosepsis complicated by hypoactive delirium. She is known to have dementia with a previous Mini-mental state examination (MMSE) score of 23/30 three months ago. Just before discharging her back to her retirement village, you discover she is a regular driver and often takes her friends bowling. She tells you she will pick up her car from a crash repairer early next week due to a 'minor accident' three weeks ago.
  The most appropriate advice for your patient is:
  A. A driving co-pilot is recommended for patients with dementia, especially with a crash record.
  B. Patients with a diagnosis of dementia should stop driving regardless.
  C. Patients with dementia should have a neuropsychological assessment before a decision is made about driving.
  D. Patients with dementia, are legally obliged to inform the driver licensing authority in Australia.

11. Which one of the following is **NOT** a feature of dementia with Lewy bodies?
  A. Fluctuating cognition with variations in attention and alertness.
  B. Focal neurological signs.
  C. Severe antipsychotic sensitivity.
  D. Spontaneous features of parkinsonism.

12. Which one of the following statements is true regarding elder abuse?
  A. Elder abuse is defined as any pattern of behaviour that causes physical harm to an elder.
  B. It is mandatory to report elder abuse in all states and territories.
  C. The majority of abusers of the elderly are non-family members.
  D. There is no difference in the rates of abuse for men and women.

13. A 55-year-old man with known smoking-related COPD is considering switching from cigarette smoking to electronic cigarettes. Which of the following advice is correct?
  A. Electronic cigarettes can be used in public smoke-free areas.
  B. Electronic cigarettes can lead to lower motivation to quit smoking.
  C. Electronic cigarettes provide long-term health benefits for lung function compared with cigarette smoking.
  D. Electronic cigarettes are nicotine free.

14. A 52-year-old man complains of diminished libido. Examination shows bilateral gynaecomastia. He has a history of type 2 diabetes, hypertension, hypercholesterolaemia, and gastroparesis. His regular medications include metformin, empagliflozin, Optisulin insulin, hydrochlorothiazide, atorvastatin, and metoclopramide. Laboratory testing shows a mildly elevated serum prolactin level.
  Which one of this patient's regular medications is the most likely cause of his bilateral gynaecomastia?
  A. Atorvastatin.
  B. Empagliflozin.
  C. Hydrochlorothiazide.
  D. Metoclopramide.

15. An 80-year-old woman who lives alone at home is concerned that she may get heat exhaustion because the temperature has been 35 to 37 °C over the last 3 days and her air conditioner has broken down. She has a headache, but her skin is cool and dry. Her vital signs are within the normal range. She has hypertension treated with a low salt diet and enalapril; she is obese with a BMI of 32 kg/m².

Which one of the following is most accurate regarding her concern?

A. Aggressive fluid resuscitation is recommended.

B. Anhidrosis is essential for diagnosis of heat stroke.

C. She is at risk of heat-related illness only if the temperature >38 °C.

D. She is at high risk of heat-related illness because she is on a low salt diet.

16. A 26-year-old woman is referred for investigation of hypoglycaemia. She has no history of diabetes and takes no medications or supplements. She reports episodes of sweats and light-headedness. She checked her finger prick blood glucose level (BGL) at work and found that it was 3.0 mmol/L. She had some fizzy cordial and felt better, and her BGL had improved to 5.1 mmol/L 20 minutes later.

She reports several of these episodes over the past few months which tend to occur two hours after meals. She brings in a spreadsheet detailing the carbohydrate content of her diet, and the timing of symptoms. She is trying to snack regularly to keep her sugars up and requests a letter for her employer to ensure she has regular breaks during the day. On examination, her BMI is 24 kg/m²; BP is 128/70 mmHg with no postural drop. Electrolytes are normal.

She undergoes a 72 hour fast and develops dizziness and sweating at 9am on day 2, with a plasma BGL of 3.9 mmol/L. Her insulin and C peptide level are low. Fasting cortisol level at 9am is at the upper limit of normal. She is discharged but represents with ongoing symptoms and the test is repeated, with symptoms at 12pm on day one of fasting. Her BGL is 4.1 mmol/L with low normal insulin and C peptide.

What is the most likely diagnosis?

A. Insulinoma.

B. Postprandial hypoglycaemia.

C. Pseudohypoglycaemia.

D. Sulfonylurea ingestion.

17. A 64-year-old woman has had difficulty falling asleep for 45 years. Her medical and psychiatric histories include obesity, type 2 diabetes, ischaemic heart disease, and generalised anxiety disorder. She awakens three to four times per night and lies in bed for around half an hour each time. She spends 10 hours in bed, from 10 p.m. to 8 a.m. but has a poor quality of sleep.

Which of the following is the first-line therapy for insomnia in this lady?

A. Cognitive behaviour therapy.

B. Diphenhydramine.

C. Mirtazapine.

D. Temazepam.

18. A 75-year-old woman has recurrent bilateral venous leg ulcers which have been complicated by cellulitis on several occasions, necessitating intravenous antibiotics and hospitalisation. She has history of heart failure with reduced ejection fraction, hypertension, and obesity but no diabetes. Her mobility is poor. Her recent ankle-brachial index is 0.92.

Best management for this patient is:

A. Daily wound dressing by district nurse.

B. Prophylactic oral antibiotics to prevent recurrent cellulitis.

C. Use of graded compression from toe to knee.

D. Long-term wound dressing containing silver nanoparticles.

19. A 25-year-old man experiences sudden onset of severe back pain radiating down his left leg while gardening. He is in severe pain and having trouble walking. He is reviewed by you one week later and is still having trouble walking, only managing short distances. He is having trouble dressing himself. Neurological examination is normal, and gait is antalgic. Straight leg raise test is positive at 20 degrees on the left, and he is tender over the lower lumbar area. On discussion he feels as though the pain will improve, he is happy to keep moving as much as possible and is not worried about it. He does however rate his pain as 'extremely troubling.'

Which of the following strategies is most appropriate in managing his pain?
A. MRI of the lumbosacral spine and referral to a spinal surgeon.
B. Non-steroidal anti-inflammatory drugs plus as required opioids.
C. Reassurance and advice on activities, acupuncture, no follow-up required.
D. Reassurance and advice on activities, plus regular follow-up.

20. A 63-year-old lady is admitted to hospital following a fall which resulted in a fractured neck of femur. You are asked to review her by the surgical team to optimise her medically prior to a planned surgical procedure tomorrow. You note a history of oestrogen, treated with bisphosphonates and hypertension for which is treated with an ACE-inhibitor. She is taking combined oestrogen and progesterone hormone replacement therapy (HRT) which was prescribed 8 years ago for severe vasomotor symptoms. She has previously trialled a break from HRT 2 years ago but had recurrence of severe hot flushes. She has no personal or family history of breast cancer and has no history of thrombosis.
Which of the following statements is apply?
A. Her current risk of breast cancer is twice the risk of other women her age who are not taking HRT.
B. Her risk of breast cancer will immediately reduce if she stops her HRT now.
C. Oestrogen therapy should be continued for her bone health.
D. She should change to oestrogen-only therapy which has a lower risk of breast cancer.

21. A 43-year-old woman presents with a 3-day history of dyspnoea and ankle oedema. Two weeks ago, she was diagnosed with a lower respiratory tract infection due to influenza A, which was confirmed by a nasopharyngeal swab PCR test. She has now been diagnosed with fulminant myocarditis.
Which of the following medications should be avoided when treating this patient?
A. Eplerenone.
B. Nitroglycerin.
C. Naproxen.
D. Ramipril.

22. A 48-year-old man presents with dizziness and occipital headache. You suspect a cervicogenic headache. Which one of the following is accurate regarding this condition?
A. C5–6 facet joint injury is the most common cause of referred cervicogenic headache.
B. Degenerative discs contain a low level of inflammatory cytokines.
C. Dizziness may result from injury to facet joints that are supplied with proprioceptive fibres.
D. The presence of gait spasticity suggests cervical radiculopathy.

23. You are seeing a 70-year-old man who is going to have an elective right knee replacement for moderate osteoarthritis in the pre-admission clinic. His right knee pain is 2 to 3 out of 10 and needs regular paracetamol. He is able to mobilise without walking aids. His past medical history includes STEMI, requiring drug-eluting stent (DES) placement 3 months ago, ischaemic stroke, poorly controlled type 2 diabetes (HbA1c 9%), hypertension, hyperlipidaemia, ex-smoker (20 pack-year history) and obesity with a BMI of 35 kg/m². Medications include aspirin, clopidogrel, metformin, Optisulin insulin, perindopril, and simvastatin.
Regarding his perioperative management, which one of the following is correct?
A. Consult his orthopedic surgeon and cardiologist about delaying the operation.
B. Continue both aspirin and clopidogrel.
C. Stop both aspirin and clopidogrel pre-operatively.
D. Stop clopidogrel but continue with aspirin.

24. An 85-year-old man who lives in a nursing home presents to the emergency department with confusion, hallucination, agitation, dry mouth, and urinary retention. His medical history includes dementia, benign prostate hypertrophy, urge incontinence, insomnia, IHD, osteoarthritis, hypertension, type 2 diabetes, GORD, AF, CCF, stage 3 CKD, falls, depression and hyperlipidaemia. His medications include oxybutynin 5mg nocte, temazepam 10mg nocte prn, aspirin 100mg daily, warfarin variable dose daily, metoprolol 50mg bd, digoxin 125mcg daily, isosorbide mononitrate 60mg daily, irbesartan 300mg daily, metformin 1gm bd, pantoprazole 40mg daily, frusemide 40mg daily, mirtazapine 60mg nocte, ibuprofen 200mg tds prn, Panadeine forte 30mg/500mg x2 qid prn, and atorvastatin 80mg nocte.

Which medication is the most likely to account for his symptoms?
A. Digoxin.
B. Oxybutynin.
C. Oxycodone.
D. Temazepam.

25. A 75-year-old man presents with frequent postural dizziness and lightheadedness. He has a medical history of recurrent falls, fractured right neck of femur, and hypertension. His lying BP is 120/75 mmHg and standing BP is 90/60 mmHg despite taking adequate dose of fludrocortisone. You start him on midodrine for treatment of postural hypotension and explain to the intern that midodrine acts as a:
A. α1-adrenergic agonist.
B. Inotrope.
C. Mineralocorticoid.
D. Vasoconstrictor.

26. An 82-year-old nursing home resident with mild dementia and type 2 diabetes was admitted to the medical ward for left lower lobe pneumonia. She is being treated with intravenous ceftriaxone and oral doxycycline and is improving slowly. She is assessed to be malnourished by the malnutrition universal screening tool (MUST). Her BMI is 16 kg/m² and subsequently she has been commenced on oral nutritional supplementation. Two days later, she has a seizure. Her urgent blood test results during the MET call are displayed below.

Tests	Results	Normal values
Magnesium	0.55 mmol/L	0.70–1.10
Potassium	3.5 mmol/L	3.5–5.2
Phosphate	0.3 mmol/L	0.75–1.5
Glucose	6.8 mmol/L	3.2–5.5
Urea	2.6 mmol/L	2.7–8.0
Creatinine	55 µmol/L	60–100 µmol/L
Albumin	28 g/L	34–48
Hb	101 g/L	115–155
WBC	13.5 x 10⁹/L	4.0–11.0
Platelet	489 x 10⁹/L	150–450

What is the most appropriate immediate treatment?
A. Intravenous levetiracetam.
B. Intravenous magnesium.
C. Intravenous phenytoin.
D. Intravenous phosphate.

27. Regarding the evidence-based treatment of sarcopenia, which of the following is correct?
A. Growth hormones can be used as an anabolic agent to increase muscle mass and strength.
B. Ghrelin agonist can be used to increase muscle strength.
C. Leucine essential amino acid supplement can be used to increase muscle mass.
D. Testosterone can be used by older men with hypogonadism to increase muscle strength.

28. Which one of the following patients should be screened or treated for asymptomatic bacteriuria?
A. A 60-year-old man who will undergo a retrograde cystoscopy and biopsy for suspected bladder cancer.
B. A 70-year-old man with a 10-day old indwelling urethral catheter for urinary retention planned for trial of void.
C. A 60-year-old woman who received a renal transplant presenting for a 3-month review.
D. A 60-year-old woman with spinal cord injury who lives in a long-term care facility.

29. A 46-year-old woman presents with poor concentration, drowsiness, and confusion. She has a medical history of intellectual disability, epilepsy, and urinary incontinence. She takes the following medications: sodium valproate, topiramate, and carbamazepine. On examination, GCS is 13 (E4, V4, M5) and other vital signs are normal. She has asterixis and is disoriented to time, place, and person. She is unable to follow commands but is able to localise pain. There are no stigmata of chronic liver disease. Her investigation results are showed below. Urine and blood cultures are pending. CXR and CT head are normal.

Tests	Results	Normal values
WBC count	5 x 10⁹/L	4–11
CRP	4 mg/L	0–8
ALP	40 U/L	30–110
GGT	23 U/L	0–60
ALT	30 U/L	0–55
AST	34 U/L	0–45
Albumin	40 g/L	34–48
Total protein	70 g/L	60–80
Bilirubin	14 umol/L	2–24
INR	1.0	0.9–1.3
Ammonia	65 umol/L	0–49 umol/L

What is the best choice from the following interventions?
- **A.** Administer lactulose.
- **B.** Stop carbamazepine.
- **C.** Stop sodium valproate.
- **D.** Stop topiramate.

30. A malnourished 86-year-old man presents with confusion following a fall. He lives alone. He has a history of a severe oesophageal stricture which requires regular dilatation. He also has hypertension, smoking-related COPD, and osteoarthritis. His medications include amlodipine, pantoprazole, and inhaled salbutamol. On examination, he is haemodynamically stable. Gum hypertrophy and bleeding are evident (Figure 7.1). His skin is dry and flaky with non-healing venous ulcers on both legs. There are multiple bruises over his forearms (Figure 7.2). There is no family history of bleeding disorders. There is no lymphadenopathy or organomegaly. CT head reveals no acute pathology. His initial investigation results are displayed below.

Tests	Results	Normal values
Urea	2.5 mmol/L	2.7–8.0
Creatinine	41 μmol/L	60–110
Albumin	29 g/L	34–48
ALP	208 IU/L	30–110
GGT	44 IU/L	0–60
ALT	39 IU/L	0–55
AST	22 IU/L	0–45
Hb	110 g/L	135–175
WBC	7.1 x 10⁹/L	4.0–11.0
Platelet	139 x 10⁹/L	150–450
MCV	78 fL	80–98
INR	1.2	0.9–1.2

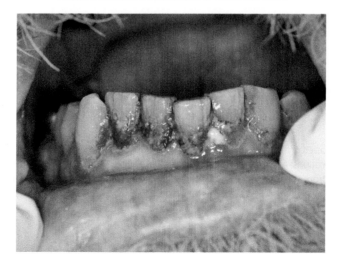

Figure 7.1

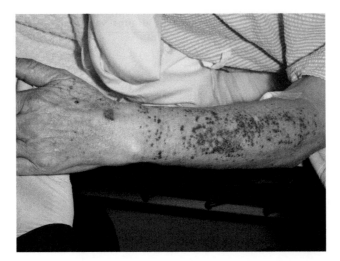

Figure 7.2

Which is the next most appropriate test?
  A. Bone marrow biopsy.
  B. Light transmission platelet aggregometry.
  C. Vitamin C level.
  D. von Willebrand disease (vWD) screen.

31. A 32-year-old Aboriginal and Torres Strait Islander woman presents to local community health service with a 2-month history of intermittent diarrhoea, vague abdominal pain, and weight loss of 6kg. She also tells you she has had an irritating cough and wheeze which is not responding to salbutamol puffer. She is known to have lupus nephritis and is taking 25mg prednisolone daily. Her stool culture is reported to be positive for a parasite. Which of the following parasitic infections is the most likely?
  A. Amoebiasis.
  B. Enterobiasis.
  C. Giardiasis.
  D. Strongyloidiasis.

QUESTIONS (32–36) **REFER TO THE FOLLOWING INFORMATION**
Match the clinical features of hypertension in the following cases and the initial screening tests for the possible cause of secondary hypertension:
  A. 24-hour urinary fractionated metanephrines or plasma metanephrines.
  B. CT renal artery angiogram.
  C. Echocardiogram.
  D. Kidney biopsy.
  E. Overnight 1-mg dexamethasone suppression test.
  F. Plasma aldosterone/renin ratio.
  G. Polysomnography.
  H. Urinary drug screen.

32. A 45-year-old woman has suffered from hypertension for 3 years. Her GP has found her BP is difficult to control. She is now taking five antihypertensive medications: atenolol, amlodipine, telmisartan, prazosin, and methyldopa. She has a permanent pacemaker inserted for sick sinus syndrome but no other medical history. She presents to emergency department with acute dyspnoea with BP 195/105 mmHg. Her BMI is 32 kg/m². Her serum creatinine is 135µmol/L [45-90]. Urinalysis shows + protein. Her CXR is shown below.

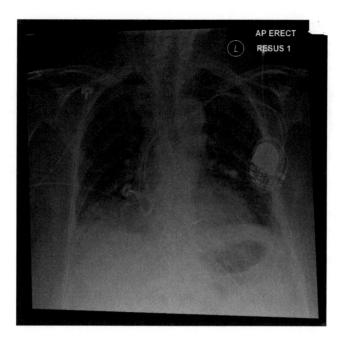

33. A 45-year-old man is referred because of resistant hypertension. He has been prescribed amlodipine, hydralazine, nebivolol, and candesartan. He reports these medications and other previous antihypertensive medications make him feel very weak and cause muscle cramps. On examination, his BP is 160/100mmHg and BMI is 33 kg/m². His initial investigation results and ECG showed below.

Tests	Results	Normal values
Sodium	135 mmol/L	135–145
Potassium	3.0 mmol/L	3.5–5.2
Bicarbonate	28 mmol/L	22–32
Urea	12 mmol/L	2.7–8.0
Creatinine	124 µmol/L	60–110
Glucose	16.3 mmol/L	3.2–5.5
Calcium	2.2 mmol/L	2.1–2.6
Hb	140 g/L	135–175
WBC	6.1 x 10⁹/L	4–11
CRP	7 mg/L	0–8
Urine analysis	+ protein	

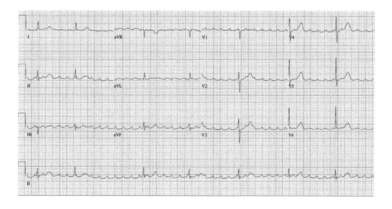

34. A 55-year-old man who works as a truck driver is referred by his GP because of difficult to control hypertension, stage 3B CKD with serum creatinine 150 µmol/L [60-110], type 2 diabetes for 7 years. He complains of fatigue and intermittent headaches. He is a current smoker. He is taking three antihypertensive medications: atenolol, irbesartan, and indapamide. On examination, his BP is 160/95 mmHg. BMI is 35 kg/m². Urine analysis shows ++ protein.

35. A 34-year-old man presents with a severe headache and BP 190/100 mmHg to his GP. He has been taking cephalexin for a sore throat since yesterday. On examination, there is a purpuric rash of both lower limbs. Urine analysis is positive for blood and +++ protein. He is anaemic and serum creatinine is 245 µmol/L [60-110]. His BMI is 30 kg/m².

36. A 35-year-old woman presents to the emergency department with a severe headache, nausea, vomiting, and abdominal pain. She is agitated, apprehensive, restless, and cannot stay on the hospital trolley to be examined. On examination, her BP is 170/95 mmHg, HR 110 bpm, and she has a tremor. Urinalysis is normal. Her BMI is 18 kg/m².

QUESTIONS (37–39) REFER TO THE FOLLOWING INFORMATION
Match the clinical features of the following case with the clinical diagnosis:
- **A.** Alzheimer's dementia.
- **B.** Creutzfeldt–Jakob disease.
- **C.** Frontotemporal dementia.
- **D.** Lewy body dementia.
- **E.** Multiple system atrophy.
- **F.** Normal pressure hydrocephalus.
- **G.** Progressive supranuclear palsy.
- **H.** Vascular dementia.

37. A 75-year-old woman presents to the emergency department with acute right visual disturbance. She describes it as 'a grey curtain that progresses from the periphery and moves toward the centre' lasting for 5 minutes. The left eye is normal. She says that she has had several similar episodes this year. Her daughter reports her memory has worsened and she often forgets to take her medications for her ischaemic heart disease, hypertension, hyperlipidaemia, poorly controlled type 2 diabetes and an unhealed ulcer on her right shin. Her mobility is poor because she complains of leg pain if she walks too much.

38. A 60-year-old man is seen in the clinic for review of his type 2 diabetes which is well controlled with metformin. His daughter notes gradual progression of memory loss over the past year. He also has inappropriate behaviour, disinhibition, as well as showing apathy and a lack of empathy. He has impaired fluency in speech and speech pathologist reported findings of semantic paraphasia.

39. A 65-year-old woman is seen in the clinic because of urinary incontinence. She has type 2 diabetes, hypertension, and peripheral vascular disease. Her son notes that she has progressive memory loss, difficulty in planning, organisation, attention, concentration, keeping track of appointments, paying bills, and daytime sleepiness over the past 12 months. On examination, you find bradykinesia and a broad-based and shuffling gait. The rest of the neurological examination seems normal.

Answers

1. Answer: A

Basic clinical findings can be useful in determining the likelihood of serious eye conditions in the acute red eye. Vision threatening problems such as anterior uveitis, scleritis, acute angle closure glaucoma, and corneal ulcer are suggested by findings of anisocoria and photophobia. Although loss of visual acuity can herald more permanent vision loss, normal vision does not preclude severe vision threatening diagnoses. The presence or absence of pain is not a helpful indicator, although patients presenting with severe eye pain should be investigated more thoroughly. Where a vision threatening diagnosis is suspected, specialist examination of the eye is required to refine the diagnosis.

Purulent exudate and bilaterally matted eyes are most suggestive of a bacterial cause, as is redness obscuring the tarsal vessels. The tarsal vessels are the usual vessels seen on the retracted inner membrane of the eyelids. Conjunctival papillae or follicles may be less useful in determining aetiology, but the traditional triad of follicles, adenopathy, and scant watery discharge suggesting a viral cause may be useful if present. Past medical history of conjunctivitis and itchy eyes are both highly suggestive of allergic conjunctivitis.

Treatment of the acute red eye depends on the cause, which, in the majority of severe cases, will probably only be diagnosed after specialist consultation. Bacterial conjunctivitis benefits from topical antibiotics, and it is reasonable to treat suspected foreign body or a corneal erosion/ulcer with topical antibiotics as well, pending specialist review. Treatment of allergic conjunctivitis can be achieved with oral antihistamines, and occasionally topical steroids are required.

 Narayana S, McGee S. Bedside Diagnosis of the 'Red Eye': A Systematic Review. The American Journal of Medicine. 2015;128(11):1220–1224.e1.
https://www.amjmed.com/article/S0002-9343(15)00577-X/fulltext

2. Answer: D

Changes in kidney function during normal ageing are among the most dramatic of any organ system. Progressive structural and functional deterioration of the kidney can occur with normal ageing.

Renal mass declines to less than 300 g by the ninth decade, correlating with reduction in body surface area. Loss of renal mass is primarily cortical with relative sparing of medulla. Age related changes in several hormonal systems controlling sodium excretion play a role in the impaired ability to conserve sodium, levels of plasma renin and of blood and urinary aldosterone fall significantly.

A continuous increase in cellular oxidative stress results in production of vasoactive mediators and the loss of anti-inflammatory and growth-inhibitory mediators such as nitric oxide and prostacyclin with ageing. Aldosterone response to hyperkalaemia is impaired in the ageing kidney and together with reduced activity of the renin–angiotensin system in the elderly; this may serve to enhance the risk of hyperkalaemia especially in the setting of increased use of NASIDs and ACE inhibitors in elderly. Some ageing-related changes in physiology are summarised below:

Cardiovascular system
- Cardiac output and cardiac index at rest is largely unchanged.
- Increased myocardial hypertrophy.
- Decreased arterial elasticity.
- Reduced heart rate responsiveness to stress and respiration.

Respiratory system
- Reduced lung volume due to loss of elastic recoil.
- Reduction in FEV1 and FVC.
- Increased residual volume.
- Increased V/Q mismatch.
- Decreased ventilatory response to hypoxia and hypercapnia.
- Reduced mucociliary clearance.

Gastrointestinal system and liver
- Decreased oesophageal peristalsis.
- Delayed gastric emptying.

- Decreased pancreatic enzyme secretion.
- Reduced liver volume, weight and blood flow.
- No change to LFTs.

Renal and urinary tract system
- Decreased renal mass, cortical loss > medulla.
- Decreased renal blood flow and GFR.
- Increased nocturnal polyuria.

Endocrine system
- Increased insulin resistance.
- Increased incidence of autoimmune thyroiditis.
- Increased vasopressin with increased risk of hyponatraemia.
- Decreased basal renin level.
- Decreased aldosterone and increased risk of hyperkalaemia.
- Increased in FSH /LH.

Immune system
- Immunoglobulin level tend to remain stable.
- Diminished antibody response.
- Impaired T cell response, especially to viral infections.

3. Answer: A

This question shows the importance of diagnosing the underlying medical conditions which may contribute to falls. Impaired vision is a common cause of fall or recurrent falls. It also has impact on safe discharge planning and prevention of readmission.

Age related macular degeneration (AMD) is the most common cause of blindness in the developed world. AMD is divided into early and late stages. The early stage, also referred to as age-related maculopathy (ARM), is characterised by yellow/white deposits (drusen) beneath the retinal pigment epithelium, and areas of hyperpigmentation or hypopigmentation. Later stages may take one of two forms:
- Neovascular (wet or exudative) AMD, characterised by growth of new blood vessels beneath the retina with a tendency to leak, causing sudden visual loss.
- Nonexudative (dry) age-related macular degeneration which comprises more than 90% of patients diagnosed with AMD.

Drusen can be detected early in this disease without visual loss. As dry AMD progresses, retinal atrophy, and central retinal degeneration occurs leading to loss of central vision. Generally, non-exudative AMD has a much slower progressive visual loss relative to exudative AMD. Patients with AMD have central visual loss. Less commonly, patients may report distortion of central vision. They may describe straight lines as appearing 'bent' or 'wavy'. Visual distortion in an elderly person is highly suggestive of the wet form of AMD.

For most patients with non-exudative AMD, little specific treatment beyond risk factor control is available. Antioxidant vitamin and mineral supplements may be helpful. Management of exudative AMD may include the following:
- Intravitreal injection with ranibizumab, bevacizumab, aflibercept, or pegaptanib. Vascular endothelial growth factor (VEGF) is a key mediator in ocular angiogenesis. The above VEGF inhibitors, delivered via intravitreal injection, block or neutralise VEGF expression. Multiple clinical trials have demonstrated their efficacy in slowing vision loss.
- Photodynamic therapy (PDT) with verteporfin. PDT is the current laser treatment of choice for subfoveal disease and shows a significant reduction in severe visual loss. A photosensitising dye (Verteporfin) is infused intravenously and passes to the choroid where it is preferentially absorbed by the rapidly dividing vessels of the neovascular membrane. A diode laser activates the dye and free radicals are released causing endothelial damage and thrombosis of affected vessels. The membrane is thus selectively destroyed, sparing the surrounding retina, although there will be resultant scotoma.
- Thermal laser photocoagulation surgery

Mitchell P, Liew G, Gopinath B, Wong T. Age-related macular degeneration. The Lancet. 2018;392(10153):1147–1159.
https://www.thelancet.com/pdfs/journals/lancet/PIIS0140-6736(18)31550-2.pdf

4. Answer: A

Oxidative metabolism of alcohol in the liver involves two enzymes, alcohol dehydrogenase (ADH) and aldehyde dehydrogenase (ALDH), and produces acetaldehyde and acetate. ADH metabolises alcohol to acetaldehyde which is highly toxic substance and a known carcinogen. However, in the healthy individual, most of the acetaldehyde is further metabolised to a less active by-product called acetate, which then is broken down into water and carbon dioxide for elimination. The residual amount circulates to peripheral tissues and is transformed into Acetyl CoA.

Chronic alcohol consumption results in high levels of acetaldehyde which leads to glutathione depletion, oxidative stress, lipid peroxidation and formation of adducts with proteins, making this metabolite highly toxic to the body. Non-oxidative derived metabolites included fatty acid ethyl esters (FAEE) and phosphatidylethanol.

 Zakhari S. Overview: How Is Alcohol Metabolized by the Body? [Internet]. National Institute of Alcohol Abuse and Alcoholism. 2019 [cited 9 November 2019]. Available from: https://pubs.niaaa.nih.gov/publications/arh294/245–255.htm

5. Answer: B

Alcohol withdrawal syndrome can occur when a person who is tolerant to alcohol stops drinking alcohol or drinks substantially less alcohol. It is a syndrome of CNS hyperactivity characterised by some or all of the following signs and symptoms:
- Hypersensitivity to stimulation
- Anxiety and/or agitation
- Perspiration, tremor
- Increased pulse, blood pressure
- Seizures
- Confusion and/or hallucinations

Patients at risk of withdrawal from alcohol are those whose last drink was less than 10 days ago and also meet at least one of the following criteria:
- Average daily alcohol consumption >80g/day for males and >60g/day for females
- Previous history of alcohol withdrawal syndrome
- CAGE questionnaire score >2
- Admitted with breath or blood alcohol (BAC) >0.15 g/100ml

Chronic alcoholics are at a high risk for thiamine deficiency, which increases risk for Wernicke–Korsakoff Syndrome, cerebellar degeneration, and cardiovascular dysfunction. The current protocol for alcohol withdrawal treatment includes: thiamine 100 mg IV 3 times a day for 3 days then oral 3 times a day until discharge. Thiamine should be given prior to IV glucose as pyruvate is unable to enter the TCA cycle in thiamine deficiency, causing the cell to convert the pyruvate to lactate instead in order to maintain glycolysis at a minimum rate. Therefore, giving glucose before giving the needed thiamine to complete ATP generation will increase lactate production leading to acidosis.

Lorazepam should be used instead of diazepam when LFT are severely abnormal and especially when synthetic liver function is impaired, this is because lorazepam has no active metabolites. Lorazepasm 0.5 mg is approximately equivalent to diazepam 5 mg. It should be given orally not by IM or IV injection.

Patient with a history of alcohol withdrawal seizures and abnormal LFTs should be given lorazepam 0.5 mg every 8 hours for 48 hours.

The combination of a benzodiazepine with opioids, antipsychotics (e.g. quetiapine, olanzapine) or sedating antihistamines (e.g. promethazine) will significantly increase the risk of respiratory failure. The benzodiazepine dose should be reduced by 50% to decrease the risk of excessive sedation or respiratory failure. Sedation scores should be monitored on a regular basis and the patient's Richmond Agitation and Sedation Scale (RASS) kept below −1 (−1 = easy to rouse but cannot stay awake). Oxygen administration is mandatory if patient also receiving an opioid or if sedation score ≥ −1.

 Gortney J, Raub J, Patel P, Kokoska L, Hannawa M, Argyris A. Alcohol withdrawal syndrome in medical patients. Cleveland Clinic Journal of Medicine. 2016;83(1):67–79. https://www.ccjm.org/content/83/1/67

6. Answer: C

This patient has an acute myocardial infarction (AMI). He has acute central chest pain. ECG shows new left bundle bunch block. There are no specific cardiovascular examination findings in patients with AMI. However, a S3 gallop represents severe systolic dysfunction in patients with large AMI. A S4 reflects myocardial non-compliance due to ischaemia. A new apical pansystolic murmur is usually due to mitral regurgitation caused by ischaemic papillary muscle dysfunction. Pericardial rub is not a finding in patient with acute AMI unless the chest pain is caused by pericarditis.

7. Answer: B

Bone scans are a sensitive and non-invasive modality for diagnosing a number of skeletal conditions. Technetium-99m labelled bisphosphonates, the most common radioactive tracer used, bind to hydroxyapatite at sites of active bone formation (osteogenesis), in proportion to local blood flow and degree of osteoblast/osteoclast activity. Increased radioactive tracer uptake is a very sensitive marker of metabolic bone changes, detecting significant lesions up to months prior to conventional radiology, with relatively modest radiation exposure.

Bone scans are indicated for three main reasons, to assess a suspected specific bone disease, predominantly oncologic, rheumatic, infective, or orthopaedic, to investigate unexplained symptoms including arthritis, arthralgia, abnormal biochemistry or radiology, and for the metabolic assessment prior to commencement of therapy such as radiation synovectomy, corticosteroid injection, and bisphosphonates in Paget 's disease.

However, osteogenesis is a nonspecific response of bone to a range of stimuli, such as physiological growth/turnover, mechanical stress or injury, fractures, infection and involvement by tumour. For example, increased focal uptake in striated muscle can occur in tumours and infections, as well as sites of repeated IM iron injections, haematomas, necrosis, sickle cell anaemia, rhabdomyolysis, myositis, and hypercalcemia. Importantly, bone scans have low diagnostic sensitivity for tumours confined to the marrow, and purely osteolytic lesions including multiple myeloma.

Bone scans are not subsequently indicated for bone lesions with known inconsistent bone scan findings such as plasmacytoma, multiple myeloma, chordoma, or Ewing's sarcoma, or for benign bone lesions or degenerative joint disease already characterised on other radiological imaging.

Van den Wyngaert T, Strobel K, Kampen W, Kuwert T, van der Bruggen W, Mohan H et al. The EANM practice guidelines for bone scintigraphy. European Journal of Nuclear Medicine and Molecular Imaging. 2016;43(9):1723–1738. https://www.eanm.org/publications/guidelines/EANM_Bone_Scintigraphy_GL_2016.pdf

8. Answer: D

Carcinoid heart disease occurs as a result of deposition of plaque like fibrous tissue on cardiac valves. The primary pathology is metastatic serotonin-secreting neuroendocrine tumour most commonly with hepatic metastases. High levels of circulating serotonin, but also changes to the metabolism of serotonin and its receptors are proposed to have an influence on the development of carcinoid heart disease. Carcinoid heart disease is the presenting problem in up to 20% of patients diagnosed with carcinoid syndrome, and affects up to 50% of patients during the course of their disease. Regurgitation is more common than stenosis in valvular lesions, and right-sided lesions are more common than left-sided lesions, thought to be due to the inactivation of humoral substances in the pulmonary vascular bed. Tricuspid regurgitation is the most common lesion (possibly present to a degree in all patients), followed by pulmonic regurgitation. Left sided lesions occur in 5–10% of patients, and can be due to intracardiac shunting, widespread hepatic metastases, or with bronchial carcinoid tumours. In around 4% of patients with metastatic carcinoid disease, cardiac metastases can occur.

Treatment of carcinoid heart disease involves treatment of the underlying condition predominantly with somatostatin analogues, and control of the tumour generally. Medical management of carcinoid heart disease involves palliation of symptoms and control of fluid balance. This is in practice mostly limited to the provision of loop diuretics and opioids for fluid balance and breathlessness, respectively. Surgical treatment of carcinoid heart disease can be successfully achieved with valve replacement in cases where the tumour is well controlled, and mechanical valves are usually necessary as bioprosthetic valves undergo accelerated degradation. Anaesthesia can precipitate carcinoid storm, which must be taken into account when assessing surgical plan and risks.

Hassan S, Banchs J, Iliescu C, Dasari A, Lopez-Mattei J, Yusuf S. Carcinoid heart disease. Heart. 2017;103(19):1488–1495. https://heart.bmj.com/content/103/19/1488.info

9. Answer: A

Chronic fatigue syndrome (CFS) is a debilitating and common illness of unclear aetiology. However, since its first observation as a clinical entity in the 1980s, significant progress has been made in elucidating a biological mechanism for the illness. Currently, it is hypothesised that chronic neuroglial inflammation triggers an evolutionarily preserved response to down-regulate metabolic activity. In synergy to hibernation for mammals such as the bear, it is felt that by doing so; the animals preserve survival at the expense of function. This causes decreased energy utilisation, expressed clinically as poor cognition and neuronal functioning, adverse response to physical and cognitive stimuli, and experienced by the individual as fatiguability and post-exertional malaise – typically after a delay of 12–48 hours.

Observed biological parameters that are consistent with this hypothesis include a vast array of measures that are abnormal in people with CFS compared with healthy controls. Down-regulation of HPA axis is commonly seen in CFS, whereas most severe psychiatric conditions have normal or increased HPA activity – with the exception of post-traumatic stress disorder, in which normal or decreased HPA activity can be observed. Punctate high-T2 signal areas on MRI are commonly observed in CFS, and functional MRI shows altered responses to sensory challenges, and tests of working memory. Positron emission tomography and MRI spectroscopy show widespread neuroinflammation, choline-creatinine ratios and lactate that correlate with fatigue severity. Cerebral blood flow is impaired, and cellular metabolism is downregulated from multiple sources. These metabolic abnormalities are more prominent on a re-challenge of exercise 24 hours after the first. It is currently felt that there are probably multiple causes of the underlying neural inflammation leading to the abnormal physiological response, but chronic viral infection, altered gut microbiota, neurotoxins and autoantibodies in combination with altered immune response are potential candidates in initiating this process.

Komaroff A. Advances in Understanding the Pathophysiology of Chronic Fatigue Syndrome. JAMA. 2019;322(6):499. https://jamanetwork.com/journals/jama/article-abstract/2737854

10. Answer: D

Dementia frequently leads to progressively impaired visuospatial skills, attention, memory and judgement and driving is a very complex task which requires such functions. Many patients with dementia continue to drive after the diagnosis has been made and only stop driving after they have had one or more crashes. There is no doubt that driving skills deteriorate with increasing dementia severity. Older drivers in general tend to have relatively few crashes however, when the number of accidents per distance travelled is calculated, the crash risk of drivers over the age of 75 years is similar to that of drivers aged 16–24 years.

It is not reasonable to suspend a patient's licence based solely on a diagnosis of mild dementia as such patients may drive safely. Studies have shown 69% of drivers with mild dementia and 88% of drivers with very mild dementia can pass on-road driving assessments. A driving co-pilot is not a recognised safe practice for reducing safety risk in dementia. Stopping driving may be voluntary or involuntary. If the patient is not accepting your advice of stopping driving, an occupational therapy on-road, formal driving test is a good alternative and is accepted as a 'gold standard' assessment. The results of a neuropsychological assessment generally do not sufficiently or consistently correlate with on-road driving performance. Regular review (at least 6 monthly) of safe driving capacity is required in patients who retain a driving licence in early dementia.

According to Austroads guidelines, a patient with dementia cannot hold an unconditional drivers' licence. Furthermore, all drivers in Australia with a condition which may impact on their ability to drive, such as dementia, are legally obliged to inform the driver licensing authority. Both South Australia and the Northern Territory have legislation that requires doctors to mandatorily report a patient with dementia who is at risk to themselves or others. Mandatory reporting is not required in other states or the Australian Capital Territory.

Patients with dementia and cognitive impairment should not drive according to the 'Medical aspects of fitness to drive – A guide for health practitioners' published by the New Zealand Transport Agency.

Position statement no. 11. Driving and dementia. Revised 2009. [Internet]. Australian and New Zealand Society for Geriatric Medicine. 2020 [cited 6 April 2020]. Available from: https://anzsgm.org/wp-content/uploads/2019/02/PS11DrivingandDementiaapproved6Sep09.pdf

Medical aspects of fitness to drive: a guide for health practitioners [Internet]. NZ transport agency. 2020 [cited 6 April 2020]. Available from: https://nzta2.cwp.govt.nz/driver-licences/getting-a-licence/medical-requirements/dementia-and-driving/

11. Answer: B

Dementia with Lewy bodies (DLB) is the second most common form of degenerative dementia after Alzheimer's disease. Diagnosis of DLB requires cognitive impairment usually without prominent memory impairment, and at least one core clinical feature with at least one indicative biomarker, or at least two core clinical features irrespective of biomarkers:

- Core clinical features
  - ✓ Fluctuating cognition
  - ✓ Recurrent visual hallucinations
  - ✓ REM sleep behaviour disorder
  - ✓ Spontaneous parkinsonism (at least one of): bradykinesia, rest tremor, rigidity
- Indicative biomarkers
  - ✓ Reduced dopamine transporter uptake in basal ganglia on SPECT or PET
  - ✓ Abnormal (low uptake) iodine MIBG myocardial scintigraphy
  - ✓ REM sleep without atonia on polysomnography
- Supportive clinical features
  - ✓ Severe sensitivity to antipsychotic agents
  - ✓ Postural instability
  - ✓ Repeated falls
  - ✓ Syncope or other transient episodes of unresponsiveness
  - ✓ Severe autonomic dysfunction ie. constipation, orthostatic hypotension, urinary incontinence
  - ✓ Hypersomnia
  - ✓ Hyposmia
  - ✓ Hallucinations in other modalities
  - ✓ Systematised delusions
  - ✓ Apathy
  - ✓ Anxiety
  - ✓ Depression
- Supportive biomarkers
  - ✓ Relative preservation of medial temporal lobe structures on CT/MRI
  - ✓ Generalised low uptake on SPECT/PET perfusion/ metabolism scan with reduced occipital activity +/− cingulate island sign on FDG-PET imaging
  - ✓ Prominent posterior slow wave activity on EEG with periodic fluctuations in pre alpha- theta range

Characteristic variations in attention and alertness in DLB are often associated with marked fluctuation in functional ability. In DLB, visual hallucinations are recurrent, vivid and realistic perceptions, seldom frightening and often of humans and creatures. Parkinsonian features are often present in DLB. Most patients with DLB have Lewy body pathology in key dopaminergic brain structures and some may have spontaneous Parkinsonism. Even if they do not have Parkinsonism they may be especially vulnerable to the adverse dopamine blocking effects of these anti-psychotic drugs. Patients with DLB may develop very significant and potentially dangerous parkinsonian or other extrapyramidal adverse effects even on low doses of antipsychotic drugs. Patients with DLB usually do not have focal neurological signs.

 McKeith I, Boeve B, Dickson D, Halliday G, Taylor J, Weintraub D et al. Diagnosis and management of dementia with Lewy bodies. Neurology. 2017;89(1):88–100.
https://n.neurology.org/content/89/1/88

12. Answer: D

Elder abuse is any pattern of behaviour which causes physical, psychological, financial harm or neglect to an older person. Elder abuse occurs in the context of a relationship of trust between the older person and the abuser, and this therefore excludes self-abuse and self-neglect, crime or assault in the street or at home by strangers, and discrimination in the provision of goods and services from the definition.

Forms of elder abuse	Definition	Example
Physical Abuse	Infliction of physical pain or injury	Hitting, slapping, pushing, burning, physical restraint, overmedication and sexual assault
Psychological Abuse	Infliction of mental anguish, involving actions that cause fear of violence, isolation or deprivation, and/or feelings of shame, indignity and powerlessness	Humiliation, emotional blackmail, blaming, swearing, intimidation, name calling, and isolation from friends and relatives

Forms of elder abuse	Definition	Example
Financial/ Economic Abuse	Illegal or improper use of the older person's property or finances	Misappropriation of money, valuables or property, forced changes to a will or other legal documents, and denial of the right of access to, or control over, personal funds
Neglect	Failure to provide adequate food, shelter, clothing, medical or dental care	Abandonment, failure to provide food, clothing or shelter, inappropriate use of medication and poor hygiene or personal care.

The prevalence of elder abuse is increasing. Aged Care Assessment Teams (ACAT) have reported that up to 5% of community dwelling patients referred to the Teams were victims of abuse. The abuser can be a family member, friend, neighbour, paid carer, health care worker or other person in close contact with the elder. The majority of abusers are family members, including spouses, adult children or a close relative, and they usually live with the victim. They may be financially dependent on the older person they are abusing. Personality characteristics of the abuser such as alcoholism, drug abuse, psychiatric illness and cognitive impairment are a major factor in the mistreatment of the older person.

Elders who are helpless or dependent on others for assistance due to physical impairments such as dementia, Parkinson's disease or stroke are vulnerable to abuse. Marital conflict resulting in spousal abuse often continues into old age, and in many cases of elder abuse there has been a long past history of domestic violence. Carer stress is another important risk factor for elder abuse.

Carer abuse or reverse abuse occurs when the carer is abused by the person they are caring for. Usually it is the wife being abused by her husband, and there has either been a long history of domestic violence, or a recent onset of dementia in the older person. There is no difference in the rates of abuse for men and women.

The medical profession plays an important role in the detection and intervention in cases of elder abuse. Mandatory reporting has not been introduced in Australia. A multidisciplinary team, led by geriatric health service or Aged Care Assessment Team, should be involved in both the assessment of cases where abuse is suspected or confirmed, and intervention. The doctor needs to balance the right of the older person to refuse any assistance with the physician's duty of care: unless the older person possesses a mental impairment sufficient to affect judgement, that person is able to make decisions and that right must be respected. Options for intervention includes crisis care, community support services, respite, counselling, alternative permanent accommodation such as nursing home, and legal interventions.

Lachs M, Pillemer K. Elder Abuse. New England Journal of Medicine. 2015,373(20).1947–1956.
https://www.nejm.org/doi/full/10.1056/NEJMra1404688

13. Answer: B

E-cigarettes, or electronic nicotine delivery systems (ENDS), are battery-operated products that deliver a nicotine-containing aerosol (commonly called vapor) to users by heating a solution typically made up of propylene glycol or glycerol (glycerin), nicotine, and flavouring agents. Using an e-cigarette is referred to as 'vaping'. E-cigarettes have been suggested as a potential aid for smoking cessation, but many questions about their efficacy and safety remain unanswered. Hazardous substances, such as acetaldehyde, formaldehyde, and acrolein, have been found in the aerosol produced by e-cigarettes, which are known to cause lung cancer and cardiovascular disease. Acrolein can cause acute lung injury, asthma, COPD, and lung cancer. Propylene glycol and vegetable glycerin are toxic to cells. Clinicians must support a smoker's quit attempt and try to ensure any that advice given does not undermine their motivation to quit. Counselling plus approved pharmacotherapies is the first-line smoking cessation therapy.

Multiple systematic reviews, including by the WHO and Cochrane collaboration, have failed to find clear evidence to support E-cigarettes as an aid to smoking cessation. It is well established that even low-level cigarette use is harmful, and there is no evidence that smoking reduction (compared to cessation) provides long-term health benefits for lung function, lung cancer or cardiovascular risk. Patients should quit smoking cigarettes entirely. Framing E-cigarettes as a legitimate harm reduction tool may lead to a false sense of security for smokers, leading to lower motivation to quit, delaying, or abandoning serious attempts to quit and increasing more harmful inhalation behaviour.

E-cigarettes are banned in public smoke-free areas in Australia. Currently, it is illegal to sell e-cigarettes that contain nicotine in Australia.

Dinakar C, O'Connor G. The Health Effects of Electronic Cigarettes. New England Journal of Medicine. 2016;375(14):1372–1381.
https://www.nejm.org/doi/10.1056/NEJMra1502466

14. Answer: D

Gynaecomastia is the benign proliferation of glandular breast tissue in men, resulting in breast enlargement, and rarely secretion of milk. It can occur physiologically in adolescents and elderly man. The most common cause of physiologic gynaecomastia is attributed to an imbalance of sex hormones or the tissue responsiveness to them. Non-physiologic gynaecomastia can be caused by chronic disease such as cirrhosis, hypogonadism, CKD, HIV, tumours including hCG producing tumours and use of medications (Table 7.1). Many cases of gynaecomastia are idiopathic. Gynaecomastia usually can be diagnosed by examination, occasionally ultrasound is needed to confirm the diagnosis.

Medications cause 10–20% of cases of gynaecomastia. Some act directly on the breast tissue, while others lead to increased secretion of prolactin from the pituitary by blocking the actions of dopamine on the lactotrope cell groups in the anterior pituitary. Medications used in the treatment of prostate cancer, such as antiandrogens and GnRH analogues can also cause gynaecomastia. Stopping these medications can lead to regression of the gynaecomastia.

Increased oestrogen levels can cause gynaecomastia which can be seen in certain testicular tumours, and hyperthyroidism. Certain adrenal tumours cause elevated levels of androstenedione which is converted by the enzyme aromatase into oestrogen. Other tumours that secrete hCG such as RCC and large cell lung cancer can also increase oestrogen. A decrease in oestrogen clearance can occur in chronic liver disease leading to gynaecomastia in cirrhosis. Obesity also tends to increase oestrogen levels. Decreased testosterone production in congenital or acquired testicular failure, such as Klinefelter Syndrome, diseases of the hypothalamus or pituitary can also cause gynaecomastia.

Treating the underlying cause of the gynaecomastia may lead to improvement in the condition. An alternative medication which has no or less gynaecomastia side-effects, may be used to treat the primary condition such as using eplerenone instead of spironolactone.

Table 7.1   Medications commonly associated with gynaecomastia

Medications with antiandrogenic properties
   Spironolactone
   Alkylating agents
   Bicalutamide
   Flutamide
   Ketoconazole
   Marijuana
   Metronidazole
Medications with oestrogenic properties
   Gonadotropin-releasing hormone agonists
   Oestrogens or oestrogen agonists
   Anabolic steroids
   Diazepam
Medications which induce hyperprolactinaemia
   Haloperidol
   Metoclopramide
Medications with unknown mechanism
   Amiodarone
   Calcium channel blockers
   Angiotensin-converting enzyme inhibitors
   Finasteride
   Antidepressants: Venlafaxine, tricyclic antidepressants, paroxetine, mirtazapine
   Minoxidil

Gretchen D. Gynecomastia. Am Fam Physician. 2012;85:716–722.
https://www.aafp.org/afp/2012/0401/p716.pdf

15. Answer: D

It is predicted that the incidence of heat related illness will increase because of global warming. Heat related illness is a continuum of illnesses due to the body's inability to cope with heat. It ranges from minor illnesses, such as heat rash, heat cramps to heat exhaustion and heat stroke. Heat stroke is the most severe heat related illness and is defined as a body temperature ≥41 °C associated with neurologic dysfunction. There are two forms of heat stroke (1). Exertional heat stroke (EHS) occurs in young individuals who engage in strenuous physical activity for a prolonged period in a hot environment. (2). Classic heat stroke more commonly affects sedentary elderly individuals and patients with chronic disease. Heat stroke is associated with high morbidity and mortality especially if the treatment is delayed. AKI is a common complication of heat stroke and may be due to hypovolemia, low cardiac output, and myoglobinuria from rhabdomyolysis.

Symptoms of heat exhaustion include heavy sweating, pallor, muscle cramps, fatigue, dizziness, headache, nausea, vomiting and syncope. If untreated, it will develop into heat stroke when the body can't control its temperature by normal cooling mechanisms such as sweating. Symptoms and signs of heat stroke include high body temperature ($\geq 41^{\circ}$C), anhidrosis, tachycardia, altered mental status, seizures, and unconsciousness. Anhidrosis has been cited as a key feature of heat stroke, but some patients with heat stroke can present with profuse sweating. Because of variable presentations, a high index of suspicion is needed to avoid delays in diagnosis. In another word, anhidrosis is not essential for diagnosis of heat stroke.

Older adults can be at risk for heat-related illness at lower temperatures, particularly if the air is humid. High humidity makes it harder for sweat to evaporate from the body. Patients are at higher risk of developing heat-related illness if they are following a salt-restricted diet as treatment for hypertension, due to the volume depleted state. Patients receiving multiple medications, particularly diuretics, are also at higher risk for heat-related illness. Obese patients are at higher risk of developing a heat-related illness due to an impairment of body temperature regulation as well as the retention of body heat.

Treatment for heat related illness is to rapidly lower the core temperature to about 38° while avoiding overshooting and rebound hyperthermia. Patients with heat stroke are invariably volume-depleted; cooling alone may improve hypotension and cardiac function by allowing blood to redistribute centrally. Aggressive fluid resuscitation is generally not recommended because it may lead to pulmonary oedema.

Epstein Y, Yanovich R. Heatstroke. New England Journal of Medicine. 2019;380(25):2449–2459.
https://www.nejm.org/doi/full/10.1056/NEJMra1810762

16. Answer: C

Hypoglycaemia in non-diabetic patients, who are otherwise healthy and well, can be challenging to investigate and manage. True hypoglycaemia requires the presence of Whipple's Triad: low BGL (<3 mmol/L), symptoms suggestive of hypoglycaemia, and improvement of symptoms with normalisation of BGL.

The Endocrine Society recommend only investigating patients in whom all three of Whipple's criteria are met. The history is vital and should include questions about the timing of symptoms in relation to food, symptoms that may suggest adrenal insufficiency, and a thorough history of medications and alcohol intake. Surreptitious insulin or sulphonylurea administration should also be considered.

To confirm the presence of hypoglycaemia, and to investigate further, either a prolonged fast or mixed meal test is required. For patients with suspected insulinoma, sulfonylurea ingestion or insulin administration, a prolonged fast is the preferred test, as patients typically experience fasting hypoglycaemia. When symptoms of hypoglycaemia develop, blood can be sent for glucose level, insulin, proinsulin, C peptide, beta hydroxybutyrate, insulin antibodies and sulfonylurea screening. Patients with insulinoma will have high insulin, C peptide, and a low BGL. Those with insulin administration will have a low BGL, high insulin and low C-peptide as endogenous insulin secretion is suppressed

For patients with suspected post prandial hypoglycaemia, a mixed meal test is the recommended investigation. This involves consumption of a typical precipitating meal to provoke symptoms, and regular measurements of BGL, insulin and C-peptide to prove (or exclude) true hypoglycaemia.

This patient has autonomic symptoms that she attributes to hypoglycaemia, and whilst initially it seems that she meets criteria for Whipple's triad, it is likely that the finger prick BGL measurement is inaccurate. She develops symptoms with a normal serum BGL on repeated prolonged fasts, therefore true hypoglycaemia is unlikely, and no further testing is recommended. It is likely this patient has pseudohypoglycaemia, which describes the development of autonomic symptoms with normal BGL, and often occurs 2–5 hours after a meal. The symptoms occur due to enhanced catecholamine release following food, or increased sensitivity to normal postprandial catecholamine release.

Answers A, B and C all require proven hypoglycaemia for diagnosis. Sulfonylurea ingestion should also be considered if hypoglycaemia is proven and is more common in young females working in healthcare environments with potential access to medications. Insulinoma is not suspected given the normal BGL and low insulin and C peptide, and it is a very rare condition.

Cryer P, Axelrod L, Grossman A, Heller S, Montori V, Seaquist E et al. Evaluation and Management of Adult Hypoglycemic Disorders: An Endocrine Society Clinical Practice Guideline. The Journal of Clinical Endocrinology & Metabolism. 2009;94(3):709-728.
https://academic.oup.com/jcem/article/94/3/709/2596247

17. Answer: A

Seven hours is considered an adequate amount of sleep and insomnia is defined as the inability to initiate or maintain sleep, or lack of refreshing sleep. Acute insomnia may occur in anyone with a short-term stressor (e.g. emotional, physical, financial stress, etc.), whereas insomnia is regarded as chronic if the duration is greater than 30 days.

Insomnia is the most common sleep disorder, with a prevalence of 10% in general population and is more common in women than in men. The condition is reported more by patients who work irregular shifts, with disabilities, with medical conditions that cause dyspnoea, pain, nocturia, gastrointestinal symptoms, poor mobility, and psychiatric conditions such as major depressive disorder, generalised anxiety disorder, and post-traumatic stress disorder. Insomnia may affect the quality of life, work performance, complex cognitive processes, concentration, attention, memory, workplace performance, and cause depression and increased suicide rates. Chronic insomnia is associated with increased risks of acute myocardial infarction, heart failure, coronary artery disease, hypertension, and diabetes, especially when the combined sleep times of less than 6 hours per day.

Patients with insomnia may experience hyperarousal during the day and night time, manifested as an increased whole-body metabolic rate, elevated cortisol levels, increased whole-brain glucose consumption during both the waking and the sleeping states, increased BP and high-frequency electroencephalographic activity during sleep.

This lady suffers from chronic insomnia since the duration of poor sleep quality has lasted for more than 30 days. Cognitive behaviour therapy (CBT) is the first-line management strategy for patients with insomnia. CBT addresses dysfunctional beliefs and behaviours about sleep that contributes to insomnia. If CBT is unavailable due to the lack of qualified provider with the expertise, shorter therapies and internet-based CBT can be considered with similar efficacy compared to that of longer and face-to-face delivery of CBT. The treatment goals are to improve sleep quality and quantity, and to relieve insomnia-related daytime symptoms. A sleep diary can assist patients with chronic insomnia to monitor their sleep time, duration, and habits, which are helpful for clinicians to identify causes of insomnia.

If CBT is unsuccessful, pharmacological treatment can be trialed with temazepam or zolpidem or melatonin, but side effects of these hypnotic medications include reduced daytime alertness and impairment of driving, increased risks of dangerous complex sleep-related behaviours, hallucinations, acute rage, and agitation. Melatonin is an endogenous hormone associated with the control of circadian rhythms and sleep regulation, which is available in Australia as a prolonged-release formulation for treatment of primary insomnia in patients aged 55 years or older.

Sedating antihistamines are also frequently used to improve sleep but there is no evidence for their efficacy. They can also cause significant side effects such as reduced daytime alertness, impaired cognitive function, delirium and paradoxical agitation. Benzodiazepine use in the older population is associated with increased falls and cognitive impairment, medication dependence, confusion, and incontinence. Sedating antidepressants, such as tricyclic antidepressants, mirtazapine, are sometimes used to improve sleep in patients with a concurrent depressive disorder.

Polysomnography is not indicated in the evaluation of insomnia unless other sleep disorders such as sleep apnoea, restless leg syndrome, periodic limb movement disorder, or an injurious rapid-eye-movement (REM) sleep behavior disorder is suspected, or usual treatment approaches fail.

Winkelman J. Insomnia Disorder. New England Journal of Medicine. 2015;373(15):1437–1444.
https://www.nejm.org/doi/10.1056/NEJMcp1412740

18. Answer: C

Venous disease is the most common cause of leg ulcers with prevalence of 1–1.5% of the adult population and 3.5% in people older than 65 years. Other signs associated with venous ulcers include lower extremity varicosities, oedema, venous dermatitis with hyperpigmentation, and lipodermatosclerosis.

Venous disease, arterial disease, and neuropathy cause over 90% of lower limb ulcers. Venous ulcers most commonly occur above the medial or lateral malleoli. Arterial ulcers often affect the toes or shin or occur over pressure points. Neuropathic ulcers tend to occur on the sole of the foot or over pressure points. The possibility of malignancy such as basal cell carcinoma, squamous cell carcinoma, and melanoma, particularly in ulcers that fail to heal after appropriate treatment, should always be kept in mind.

Multiple RCTs have not supported the routine use of prophylactic systemic oral antibiotics for lower limb venous ulcers. Many advanced dressings may be left in place for up to a week unless they are malodorous or saturated with exudate. Daily dressing may impair the wound healing. Dressings in combination with antiseptic agents such as silver nanoparticles can be helpful in the short-term to reduce the concentration of bacteria when infection is present, but they are not recommended for long-term use. No specific wound dressing has been shown to be superior.

Compression is the mainstay of treatment. Graded multi-component compression systems are more effective than single component ones. It promotes the healing of venous ulcer and reduces the risk of recurrence. Compression therapy should be modified if patients have mild to moderate peripheral vascular disease (PVD) with ABI 0.6–0.9. In patients with severe PVD with ABI <0.6, compression therapy is contraindicated. Surgery can help to promote healing and subfascial endoscopic perforator vein surgery has been shown to reduce recurrence.

Singer A, Tassiopoulos A, Kirsner R. Evaluation and Management of Lower-Extremity Ulcers. New England Journal of Medicine. 2017;377(16):1559–1567.
https://www.nejm.org/doi/full/10.1056/NEJMra1615243

19. Answer: D

Low back pain and sciatica can cause high levels of disability and dysfunction. Patients with a low level of physical symptoms and a low level of psychological distress surrounding their injury generally only require reassurance and advice around physical activity. Patients with severe symptoms and low level of psychological distress are at medium risk of a complicated clinical course, and frequent follow-up after initial advice is warranted. Patients at highest risk are those with high symptom burden and high levels of distress, and such patients benefit from prescribed exercise plans or classes, plus or minus psychotherapeutic intervention. The Keele STarT Back Screening Tool is an example of a validated risk stratification tool in this area.

Massage or spinal manipulation can be considered as part of treatment, but only in conjunction with exercise. Additionally, NSAIDs are a reasonable analgesia for low back pain in conjunction with standard therapies. Electrotherapies, such as transcutaneous electrical nerve stimulation (TENs) or ultrasound, show no benefit over standard therapies. Opioids should not be prescribed routinely. Imaging and invasive therapies have little role in the management of acute low back pain or sciatic pain, as most episodes improve with conservative measures. Symptoms and signs suggestive of malignancy, infection, spinal injury or spondyloarthritis require a different investigative and therapeutic approach.

Low back pain and sciatica in over 16s: assessment and management [Internet]. Nice guidance. 2020 [cited 6 April 2020]. Available from: https://www.nice.org.uk/guidance/ng59/chapter/Recommendations

20. Answer: A

The average age of onset of menopause in women is 51 years, with the vast majority occurring between 45 and 55 years of age. Hormone replacement therapy (HRT) is used to ameliorate symptoms of menopause such as hot flushes, vulvovaginal atrophy and dyspareunia. The potential adverse effects of HRT and optimal duration of HRT have long been debated.

The Endocrine Society guidelines recommend assessing the patient's individual risk factors prior to prescribing HRT. This takes into account the risk of hormone dependent cancers such as breast cancer, VTE, and cardiovascular disease. HRT is recommended in symptomatic women under 60 years of age (or within ten years of onset of menopause) who are at low risk of breast cancer, with annual review to consider if cessation is appropriate.

A large meta-analysis of all eligible prospective studies in 2019 examined over 100,000 women with postmenopausal breast cancer and evaluated the association between different types of HRT. The relative risk of breast cancer was found to increase with increasing duration of HRT and was highest in the combined oestrogen and progesterone cohort. They also found that some excess risk of breast cancer persisted for up to ten years following cessation of treatment. Oestrogen-only therapy is associated with a lower risk of breast cancer than combined therapies, however in the presence of an intact uterus would place the patient at risk of endometrial cancer.

The risk of VTE in women taking oral HRT is estimated to be twice that of women who are not on HRT, however, transdermal HRT is associated with reduced VTE risk. Cardiovascular disease and stroke risk are higher in women who start HRT after 60 years old or 10 years after the onset of menopause, leading the current recommendations for timing of initiation.

Oestrogen is not recommended for prevention of osteoporosis, particularly in the absence of other menopausal symptoms. The risks and benefits of continued HRT need to be clearly explained to the patient before a decision can be made.

Stuenkel C, Davis S, Gompel A, Lumsden M, Murad M, Pinkerton J et al. Treatment of Symptoms of the Menopause: An Endocrine Society Clinical Practice Guideline. The Journal of Clinical Endocrinology & Metabolism. 2015;100(11): 3975–4011.
https://academic.oup.com/jcem/article/100/11/3975/2836060

Type and timing of menopausal hormone therapy and breast cancer risk: individual participant meta-analysis of the worldwide epidemiological evidence. The Lancet. 2019;394(10204):1159–1168.
https://www.thelancet.com/journals/lancet/article/PIIS0140-6736(19)31709-X/fulltext

Pinkerton J. Hormone Therapy for Postmenopausal Women. New England Journal of Medicine. 2020;382(5):446–455.
https://www.nejm.org/doi/full/10.1056/NEJMcp1714787

21. Answer: C

The clinical presentation of acute myocarditis is highly variable, ranging from asymptomatic, dyspnoea, orthopnoea, peripheral oedema, palpitations to cardiogenic shock and even sudden cardiac death. There are no pathognomonic clinical features. In fulminant myocarditis, it can follow a viral prodrome or infection with distinct onset of decompensated CCF/acute pulmonary oedema or cardiogenic shock.

In approximately 50% of cases, no cause can be identified; hence, myocarditis is classified as idiopathic. In patients with an identified cause, it can be classified into infectious and non-infectious. The most common aetiology in infectious cause is viral and enteroviruses, notably Coxsackie B, are the most common. Other viral pathogens include HIV, adenovirus, and hepatitis C. Other infectious causes include bacterial (diphtheria or tuberculosis), helminths, or fungal. Non-infectious causes of myocarditis include granulomatous inflammatory diseases (sarcoidosis or giant cell myocarditis), SLE, eosinophilic myocarditis, polymyositis and dermatomyositis.

Management is primarily supportive but also includes treating any identifiable cause. Patients with heart failure should receive standard anti-heart failure treatment including angiotensin-converting enzyme inhibitors or angiotensin II receptor blockers, β-blockers, aldosterone receptor antagonists, nitroglycerin and diuretics. However, β-blockers should be avoided in the acutely decompensating phase of illness. Inotropic drugs (e.g. dobutamine, milrinone) may be necessary for severe decompensation. In severe cases, mechanical support devices such as an intra-aortic pump or left ventricular assist devices also can be used, with consideration of heart transplant as well.

Although myocarditis may be immune mediated, immunosuppressive therapy has not shown clinical benefit and therefore should not be used routinely except in patients who have underlying systemic autoimmune or granulomatous inflammatory diseases. Furthermore, viral aetiology is the most commonly identified cause, the efficacy of antiviral therapy is unknown and routine antiviral therapy is not recommended. NSAIDs should be avoided in the acute setting as they may impair healing of the myocardium.

Fung G, Luo H, Qiu Y, Yang D, McManus B. Myocarditis. Circulation Research. 2016;118(3):496–514.
https://www.ahajournals.org/doi/full/10.1161/circresaha.115.306573

22. Answer: C

Neck pain is one of the most common musculoskeletal presentations. Approximately 85% of neck pain results from acute or repetitive neck injuries or from chronic stresses and strain. Headache especially occipital headache is a frequent symptom of cervical strain termed cervicogenic headaches and facet joints and intervertebral disc damage have been implicated in the pathology of headaches caused by neck injury.

The C2–3 facet joint injury is the most common source of referred pain in patients with occipital headache (60%). The C5–6 region is the most common source of cervical, axial, and referred arm pain. Dizziness may be caused by the injury to facet joints that are supplied with proprioceptive fibres. Degenerative discs contain high level of inflammatory cytokines. Treatment with NSAIDs can be effective. The presence of spasticity and spasticity gait pattern implies an upper motor neuron dysfunction hence cervical myelopathy.

Cohen S, Hooten W. Advances in the diagnosis and management of neck pain. BMJ. 2017;:j3221.
https://www.bmj.com/content/358/bmj.j3221

23. Answer: A

Observational studies have shown patients who have had previous coronary artery disease requiring coronary artery stent placement are at increased risks of peri-operative major adverse cardiac events (MACE), moderated by stent type (DES vs. bare metal stent [BMS]), operative urgency, early discontinuation of antiplatelet therapy, and time from coronary intervention. There is an increased risk of thrombosis for 5 weeks after BMS placement and up to 12 months after DES placement. Current American College of Cardiology (ACC) and American Heart Association (AHA) guidelines recommend delaying non-cardiac surgery until 1 month after BMS placement and ideally 6 months after DES placement unless the benefits of the operation exceed the risks for earlier operation.

There are also concerns about increased risks of bleeding complications in patients who are on dual antiplatelet therapy (DAPT). The ACC/AHA recommend that patients receiving DAPT to stop the P2Y$_{12}$ inhibitor pre-operatively and continue with aspirin through the peri-operative period and to restart P2Y$_{12}$ inhibitor as soon as possible after surgery to avoid perioperative MACE.

 Childers C, Maggard-Gibbons M, Shekelle P. Antiplatelet Therapy in Patients With Coronary Stents Undergoing Elective Noncardiac Surgery. JAMA. 2017;318(2):120.
https://jamanetwork.com/journals/jama/article-abstract/2633647

24. Answer: B

Oxybutynin is used in this patient to treat urge incontinence. Oxybutynin inhibits the muscarinicactions of acetylcholine and has antispasmodic effects on smooth muscle and is indicated for detrusor over activity. It has strong anticholinergic effect and can cause confusion, hallucination, delirium, dry mouth, pupil dilatation, blurred vision, urinary retention, constipation, tachycardia and arrhythmias.

Aspirin in combination of ibuprofen, a NSAID, and warfarin in an elder patient with stage 3 CKD increase the risks of severe bleeding complications, e.g., intracranial bleeding in a patient with a history of falls. The patient is also on a combination of an NSAID (ibuprofen), an angiotensin receptor blocker (irbesartan), and a diuretic (frusemide), with a background of stage 3 CKD, this combination of medications is likely to worsen his renal function. Reviewing of the medical conditions and current symptoms to stop unnecessary medications is imperative to avoid complications.

Digoxin toxicity may happen at a lower digoxin level in elderly patients with an impaired renal clearance and in patients with electrolyte disturbance. If heart rate is controlled for atrial fibrillation, dose reduction, close monitoring of digoxin concentration, or cessation of digoxin may be appropriate. Common side effects of digoxin include anorexia, nausea, vomiting, diarrhoea, blurred vision, drowsiness, dizziness, headache, rash, bradycardia, and arrhythmia.

Because active/toxic metabolites accumulate in renal impairment, avoid use of codeine and pethidine. Panadeine forte can cause similar side effects as described in the clinical vignette above.

Benzodiazepine use increases sensitivity to central nervous system effects in CKD, use a lower dose in patients with severe renal impairment. Benzodiazepine also increase risks of over-sedation, ataxia, confusion, memory impairment, falls, fractures, motor vehicle accidents, and respiratory depression in the elderly. If a benzodiazepine is required, use short term and in low doses, and avoid long-acting benzodiazepines.

Older patients are in general on more medications than younger patients due to multiple medical conditions. A higher total number of medications is associated with increasing risks of drug-drug-interactions, medication non-adherence, adverse drug reactions, financial burden and worse outcomes. Doctors caring for elderly need to weigh the benefits vs. risks of drug therapy. Guidelines for treatment of medical conditions may not have included the appropriate study subjects in the right age group in some cases and treatment should be tailored to patients' age, symptoms, comorbidities, liver function, renal function, functioning level, life expectancy, values, preference, and goals of treatment.

It is important to have a periodic comprehensive review of the patient's medications, especially when there is transition of care. Due to the age-related changes in pharmacokinetics and pharmacodynamics, worsening renal function, decline in functional or mobility status, medical comorbidities, a more cautious approach is required to avoid medication-related complications.

The Beers criteria and the Screening Tool of Older Persons' Potentially inappropriate prescriptions (STOPP): selected warnings and recommendations or Screening Tool to Alert Doctors to Right Treatment (START) criteria can be useful tools to avoid prescribing inappropriate medications in older patients.

A geriatrician has developed the Beers criteria: Selected drugs to avoid in older adults and recommended to avoid the following medications in older nursing home patients: first-generation antihistamines, antispasmodics, antidepressants (highly anticholinergic), antiparkinsonian agents such as benztropine (not recommended for prevention of extrapyramidal symptoms with antipsychotics), conventional or atypical antipsychotics (increased risk of stroke and death in patients with dementia), skeletal muscle relaxants (most muscle relaxants are poorly tolerated by older adults), benzodiazepine, nonbenzodiazepine and benzodiazepine hypnotics (adverse events similar to those of benzodiazepines in older adults), and proton pump inhibitors (risk of Clostridium difficile infection, bone loss, and fractures).

In addition to the medications that need to be avoided recommended by the Beers criteria, the STOPP criteria also suggest to avoid tricyclic antidepressants in patients with dementia, narrow-angle glaucoma, cardiac conduction abnormality, prostatism, or history of urinary retention and to avoid antimuscarinic drugs in patients with overactive bladder with concurrent dementia or chronic cognitive impairment.

 Kim L, Koncilja K, Nielsen C. Medication management in older adults. Cleveland Clinic Journal of Medicine. 2018;85(2):129–135.
https://www.ccjm.org/content/85/2/129

25. Answer: A

Postural hypotension is defined as a sustained reduction in systolic BP ≥ 20 mmHg or a reduction in diastolic BP ≥ 10 mmHg from supine to standing position after 3 minutes or head up tilt to an angle of 60 degrees, a drop in systolic BP ≥ 30 mmHg in hypertensive patients, or upright systolic BP < 90mmHg and symptomatic in those with low baseline BP.

Postural hypotension is a common problem that is frequently observed in older patients, patients with neurodegenerative disorder, Parkinson's disease, diabetes mellitus, adrenal insufficiency, or treated hypertension.

Some patients have postural hypotension in the morning and supine hypertension at night which makes the management of BP difficult.

Patients should be advised to stand up in stages to prevent postural hypotension and to bend forward when standing to increase abdominal compression to increase venous return.

Some guidelines suggested using fludrocortisone, a synthetic mineralocorticoid, as the first-line treatment for postural hypertension. However, due to its effect of increasing blood volume and improve blood vessel sensitivity to pressor agents, it is not recommended for patients with nocturnal hypertension and CCF.

Midodrine is an α1-adrenergic agonist, increasing blood pressure by stimulating arterial and venous adrenoceptors to increase peripheral resistance. Midodrine can be used in the morning and seldom causes problems with hypertension at night due to its short half-life of 2–4 hours. It should not be taken 4 hours before bedtime to avoid supine hypertension. It may be used where standard treatment is not adequate. It has recently been approved by the TGA for severe symptomatic orthostatic hypotension due to autonomic dysfunction.

 Chisholm P, Anpalahan M. Orthostatic hypotension: pathophysiology, assessment, treatment and the paradox of supine hypertension. Internal Medicine Journal. 2017;47(4):370–379.
https://onlinelibrary.wiley.com/doi/abs/10.1111/imj.13171

26. Answer: D

Refeeding syndrome (RFS) is defined as potentially life-threating derangements in serum electrolytes, vitamin deficiency, and fluid occurring in malnourished patients after initiation of artificial refeeding whether enterally or parenterally. It arises from the switch from a catabolic to an anabolic state after prolonged starving. After the commencement of the nutritional therapy, carbohydrates become the main energy source, and blood glucose levels suddenly increase. The insulin secretion subsequently increases and stimulates the anabolic processes. Intracellular shifts of glucose and electrolytes including phosphate, potassium and magnesium occur. These shifts result in hypophosphataemia, hypokalaemia and hypomagnesaemia which can cause arrhythmias, rhabdomyolysis, paresis, confusion and respiratory failure. Along with the increased insulin secretion, the kidneys tend to retain sodium and water leading to extracellular volume expansion, peripheral oedema and acute pulmonary oedema.

Phosphate is important for the intracellular metabolism of macronutrients for both energy productions, as glucose must be phosphorylated to enter glycolysis, and energy transfer. Hypophosphataemia is the most common definitional criterion of RFS. Although mild hypophosphataemia is usually asymptomatic, severe hypophosphataemia can cause muscle weakness, disorientation, seizures, haemolytic anaemia, heart failure and respiratory failure.

Electrolyte disturbance occurs primarily within the first 72 hours after the start of nutritional therapy and causes a rapid progression. Patients at risk of RFS should have electrolytes checked daily and aggressive replacement should be administered. These patients include those with:
- Poor oral intake for more than 5 days
- Existing electrolyte disturbance
- Low BMI (<16)
- Recent unintentional significant weight loss
- History of alcohol abuse

This patient's seizure is likely caused by hypophosphataemia in the context of RFS, therefore it is inappropriate to use anticonvulsants. Severe hypophosphataemia (<0.3 mmol/L) in critically ill, intubated patients or in those with clinical sequelae of hypophosphataemia such as seizures, should be managed with intravenous replacement therapy (0.08–0.16 mmol/kg) over 2–6 hours. Rapid administration can result in hypocalcaemia, tetany, hypotension, metastatic calcification, hyperkalaemia associated with potassium-containing supplements, and volume excess.

McCray S, and Parrish C. Refeeding the malnourished patient: lessons learned. Practical gastroenterology. 2016;XL(9);56–66.
https://practicalgastro.com/2019/09/02/refeeding-the-malnourished-patient-lessons-learned/

27. Answer: D

Sarcopenia is a progressive and generalised skeletal muscle disorder involving the accelerated loss of muscle mass and function which may predispose to adverse outcomes including falls, functional decline, frailty, and mortality. It is an age-related process, influenced not only by contemporaneous risk factors, but also by genetic and lifestyle factors present throughout life. Sarcopenia can also occur during mid-life in association with a range of disorders.

A diagnosis of sarcopenia requires a combined measurement of muscle mass, muscle strength, and physical performance. The three main differential diagnoses are malnutrition, cachexia, and frailty. Most cases of sarcopenia go undiagnosed however, universal screening for sarcopenia is not recommended because screening tools are not accurate and the effect of such screening on relevant outcomes is not proven. Therefore, a case-finding approach is recommended practice. This approach involves looking for sarcopenia when relevant symptoms are reported. These symptoms may include falling, weakness, slowness, self-reported muscle wasting, or difficulties carrying out daily life activities. Case finding is particularly relevant in care settings where a higher prevalence of sarcopenia might be expected, such as prolonged hospital stays, rehabilitation settings, or nursing homes. The SARC-F is a commonly recommended case finding instrument with evidence to support its use.

At present, the evidence-based treatment of sarcopenia is resistance exercise as no specific drugs have been approved for the treatment of sarcopenia. Drugs that have potential, but not evidence to treat sarcopenia include myostatin antibodies, activin receptor antibodies and the ghrelin agonist, anamorelin. The use of leucine essential amino acids and/or β-hydroxybutyrate has not been clearly established. Interest has also been concentrated in the role of β-blockade, some ACE inhibitors and sarconeos, which activates the MAS (angiotensin-1) receptor.

Though evidence for pharmacological intervention is lacking, supplements have shown some promise to counteract sarcopenia Vitamin D was shown to have a beneficial effect on strength and physical performance in women with low baseline levels (<25 nmol/l) and testosterone demonstrated a positive effect on muscle mass (more than strength or function) in men with low serum testosterone levels (<200–300 ng/dl). However, findings from the high-profile Testosterone Trials suggest limited benefit of testosterone for physical function, particularly in those with a slow walking speed, and caution should be taken regarding the cardiovascular and prostate side-effect profile.

Cruz-Jentoft A, Sayer A. Sarcopenia. The Lancet. 2019;393(10191):2636–2646.
https://www.thelancet.com/journals/lancet/article/PIIS0140–6736(19)31138-9/fulltext

28. Answer: A

Asymptomatic bacteriuria (ASB) is a common finding in many populations, including healthy women and patients with many underlying medical conditions. ASB is defined as the presence of 1 or more species of bacteria growing in the urine at specified quantitative counts (≥10^5 colony-forming units [CFU]/mL or ≥10^8 CFU/L), irrespective of the presence of pyuria, in the absence of signs or symptoms attributable to UTI.

Non-screening and/or non-treatment of ASB is an important opportunity for decreasing inappropriate antimicrobial use. Clinical Practice Guideline for the Management of Asymptomatic Bacteriuria: 2019 Update by the Infectious Diseases Society of America provides detailed recommendations for the management of ASB in adults and children in different medical conditions and presentations. It includes recommendations that patients undergoing endourological procedures should be screened or treated for ASB but not patients with an indwelling urethral catheter, not individuals with impaired voiding following spinal cord injury and not in patients who have received a kidney transplant more than a month previously.

Nicolle L, Gupta K, Bradley S, Colgan R, DeMuri G, Drekonja D et al. Clinical Practice Guideline for the Management of Asymptomatic Bacteriuria: 2019 Update by the Infectious Diseases Society of America. Clinical Infectious Diseases. 2019.
https://academic.oup.com/cid/article/68/10/e83/5407612

29. Answer: C

This patient has a diagnosis of valproic acid (VPA)-induced hyperammonaemia and the most effect treatment strategy is to stop sodium valproate. VPA treatment can lead to increasing blood ammonia levels and encephalopathy by direct inhibition of N-acetyl glutamate in the urea cycle pathway, the principal pathway for nitrogen metabolism.

If discontinuation of VPA is not clinically feasible, levocarnitine and lactulose may be similarly effective in treating VPA-induced hyperammonaemia.

A high index of suspicion and familiarity of the VPA side effect is crucial to make the accurate diagnosis. There is no evidence of chronic liver disease in this case from the physical examination and investigation results. Symptoms of hyperammonaemia include lethargy, altered mental status, confusion, delirium, disorientation, vomiting, seizure and eventually stupor. Ammonia levels should be checked in patients on VPA when there are symptoms suggesting the diagnosis of VPA-induced hyperammonaemia. Patients only require treatment of VPA if they are symptomatic.

Risk factors for VPA-induced hyperammonaemia include intellectual disability, concurrent topiramate use, urea cycle disorder, and carnitine deficiency.

Baddour E, Tewksbury A, Stauner N. Valproic acid–induced hyperammonemia: Incidence, clinical significance, and treatment management. Mental Health Clinician. 2018;8(2):73–77.
https://mhc.cpnp.org/doi/full/10.9740/mhc.2018.03.073

30. Answer: C

This patient's clinical features are suggestive of vitamin C deficiency, which commonly manifests with ecchymoses, bleeding gums, cockscrew hairs, perifollicular bleeding, poor wound healing and malaise. Take a careful dietary history and measure blood vitamin C level to exclude scurvy in patients with unexplained mucocutaneous bleeding.

In modern days, scurvy is more common than appreciated. Contrary to the misconception that scurvy is non-existent in developed countries; the diagnosis of scurvy in certain at-risk groups may be overlooked unless there is a high index of suspicion. These include elderly patients, patients with poor or limited diet, patients with malabsorption and patients in social isolation. Good sources of vitamin C include citrus fruits, peaches, capsicum, papaya, strawberry, broccoli, and Brussel sprouts.

Vitamin C (ascorbic acid) is an essential nutrient involved in several biologic and biochemical functions. Vitamin C plays an important role in collagen synthesis. It enhances iron absorption and functions as an antioxidant. Recent population-based studies have shown that vitamin C deficiency ranges from 3% in control populations to 26% in low socioeconomic populations. The Australian NHMRC recommends that adult males consume 40 milligrams, and females consume 30 milligrams of Vitamin C daily.

Vitamin C deficiency is common in elderly and malnourished people. A large number of elderly patients are on antiplatelet medications and a significant number are on anticoagulants. Concomitant vitamin C deficiency can potentially increase the risk of bleeding. Low mood and depression are both recognised associated features common among elderly patients with vitamin C deficiency. Replacement of vitamin C, which is cheap, safe, and well tolerated, will reduce the risk of bleeding and may improve depressive symptoms without the side effects associated with antidepressants.

This patient has no clinical feature to suggest other haematological disorders. Therefore, there is no indication for bone morrow biopsy. vWD is a common, inherited, genetically and clinically heterogeneous haemorrhagic disorder due to deficiency or dysfunction of von Willebrand factor. The most common presentations of vWD are epistaxis, prolonged bleeding from trivial wounds, easy bruising and haematomas. This patient has no past history or family history of easy or excessive bleeding, which makes vWD less likely. Light transmission aggregometry (LTA) is the gold standard for evaluating platelet function and is based on the principle that light transmission increases with platelet aggregation. It is used for diagnosing platelet defects and monitoring antiplatelet treatment effect. It is not appropriate for this patient.

Goebel L, July M. Scurvy treatment & management [Internet]. Medscape. 2020 [cited 31 March 2020]. Available from: https://emedicine.medscape.com/article/125350-treatment

31. Answer: D

Strongyloidiasis is one of the most neglected tropical diseases. It is estimated 370 million people worldwide are infected with *S. stercoralis*. Strongyloidiasis is endemic, defined as prevalence >5%, in tropical and subtropical regions where warmth, moisture and poor sanitation favour its spread. It exists in Australia, particularly in some remote Aboriginal and Torres Strait Islander (ATSI) communities, which have had a prevalence of up to 60%. In Australia, clinicians should consider strongyloidiasis in residents of endemic areas, immigrants (including older patients from southern Europe), refugees, workers and travellers returning from endemic areas and all patients who are to receive immunosuppressive therapy (especially corticosteroids and chemotherapy).

Patients who are immunocompromised, such as those with diabetes, SLE, human T-cell lymphotropic virus type 1 (HTLV-1), or organ transplant recipients, as well as patients who are malnourished are at risk of infection and dissemination. ATSI patients from rural and remote areas in Australia should not be given immunosuppressive treatment without being tested or treated prophylactically for strongyloidiasis.

The autoinfective larvae of *S. stercoralis* can invade any organ of the body, including the central nervous system, through random migration. Signs and symptoms vary with the location and number of worms, and whether the autoinfective larvae have carried bacteria to extraintestinal locations (Table 7.2). This makes the diagnosis challenging. Clinicians should have high index of suspicion in particular for patients who have lived in an endemic area or have unexplained eosinophilia and must be checked for the presence of the parasite before initiation of corticosteroid or immunosuppressive therapy. These patients, if infected, may develop hyperinfective syndrome, which has a high mortality rate.

Table 7.2   Common manifestation of strongyloidiasis.

Gastrointestinal
Diarrhoea, protein-losing enteropathy, malnutrition, weight loss, abdominal pain, peritonitis, melaena, and haematochezia
Hepatic
Hepatomegaly, hepatic abscess, abnormal LFTs
Respiratory
Dyspnoea, bronchospasm, haemoptysis, bronchopneumonia, pleural effusion, lung abscess and interlobular septal fibrosis
Haematological
Eosinophilia is present in 10–70% of chronic strongyloidiasis
Central nervous system (CNS)
Bacterial meningitis and abnormal CNS signs
Skin
Erythematous serpiginous lesions appear and move rapidly, pruritus, recurrent urticaria or a 'rash that comes and goes'
Sepsis
Gram-negative septicaemia or sepsis in any organ may occur due to enteric bacteria
Multiple organ failure
An outcome of disseminated strongyloidiasis

Amoebiasis can present with chronic diarrhoea or hepatomegaly months to years after the initial infection. The diarrhoea is usually acute, bloody, mucoid (amoebic dysentery) with fever, and mild abdominal discomfort. Pinworm infection, also called enterobiasis, is caused by *Enterobius vermicularis* and is primarily a paediatric condition. The manifestation includes itching or prickling pain in the anal area, restless sleep or difficulty sleeping, and, rarely, abdominal discomfort or loss of appetite. Most patients, however, are asymptomatic. Giardiasis is a potential differential diagnosis however it does not account for the presence of pulmonary symptoms.

Corti M. Strongyloides stercoralis in Immunosuppressed Patients. Archives of Clinical Infectious Diseases. 2016;11(1). http://archcid.com/en/articles/20968.html

32. Answer: B
This patient's clinical features including resistant hypertension despite taking five antihypertensive medications and flash pulmonary oedema are suggestive of renal artery stenosis as a cause of secondary hypertension. Fibromuscular hyperplasia is especially common in young women. In patients with advanced age, other cardiovascular risk factors, atherosclerotic disease of the renal artery is most common. It is important to confirm the diagnosis given the presentation of APO. The best investigation is renal artery CT angiogram despite the renal impairment. Renal artery duplex ultrasound is not helpful given her obesity and is operator dependent.

33. Answer: F
This patient is likely to have primary aldosteronism ('Conn's syndrome') as a cause of secondary hypertension. The increased aldosterone hormone causes hypertension, cardiovascular and renal impairment, sodium retention, suppressed plasma renin level, and increased potassium excretion and eventually hypokalaemia if the effect of aldosterone is prolonged and severe. However, hypokalaemia is absent in many cases. Around 50% of patients with primary aldosteronism has unilateral aldosterone-producing adenoma and the remaining 50% of patients have bilateral adrenal hyperplasia. It is an underdiagnosed condition and is the cause of hypertension in about 10% of the patients with resistant hypertension. Initial screening test is plasma aldosterone/renin ratio (correction of hypokalaemia and withdrawal of aldosterone antagonists for 4 to 6 weeks). Intravenous normal saline infusion test

with plasma aldosterone measurement at 4 hour of infusion, adrenal CT scan, and adrenal vein sampling are used to confirm the diagnosis and identify the hyperfunctioning adrenal gland for further surgical consideration. Severe hypokalaemia can cause muscle weakness, cramps and predisposed patient to have atrial fibrillation or atrial flutter such as in this ECG.

34. Answer: G

Obstructive sleep apnoea (OSA) has been identified as a cause of resistant hypertension. This patient's history excessive daytime sleepiness, fatigue, obesity are suggestive of OSA. Sleep study with polysomnography should be considered in patients who have difficult-to-control hypertension and risk factors of OSA.

35. Answer: D

The patient presents with synpharyngitic glomerulonephritis following an upper respiratory tract infection, There are clinical features of nephritic syndrome including haematuria, significant proteinuria and renal impairment which may be chronic given he has anaemia. This is likely to be due to IgA nephropathy/Henoch Schonlein purpura and the patient would benefit from a kidney biopsy to confirm the diagnosis and provide prognosis.

36. Answer: H

This patient presents with acute onset of hypertension and symptoms suggestive of substance use, likely cocaine in this case. A urine drug screen could help to exclude/confirm recreational drug use.

Whelton P, Carey R, Aronow W, Casey D, Collins K, Dennison Himmelfarb C et al. 2017 ACC/AHA/AAPA/ABC/ACPM/AGS/APhA/ASH/ASPC/NMA/PCNA Guideline for the Prevention, Detection, Evaluation, and Management of High Blood Pressure in Adults: A Report of the American College of Cardiology/American Heart Association Task Force on Clinical Practice Guidelines. Hypertension. 2018;71(6).
https://www.acpjournals.org/doi/10.7326/M17-3203

37. Answer: H

38. Answer: C

39. Answer: F

Dementia is an acquired loss of cognition in multiple cognitive domains, including memory, language, attention, visuospatial cognition, executive function, and mood. The diagnosis of different types of dementia is easier at the earlier stages as the severity of the dementia at later stages makes it difficult to differentiate between aetiologies. The diagnosis of dementia is usually supported by history of cognitive decline and impact on daily function (from patients or their caregivers) as well as physical examination, especially cognitive assessment, neurologic and cardiovascular examination.

In patients with atypical presentation of earlier onset dementia (< 65 years of age), rapid symptom onset, or impairment in multiple cognitive domains, it is important to further investigate common causes of reversible pseudodementia such as hypothyroidism, vitamin B12 deficiency and depression. Consider performing screening thyroid function tests, vitamin B12 level, metabolic, infection, autoimmune screen, and cerebrospinal fluid (CSF) examination if indicated.

CT or MRI of the brain is essential for initial assessment to identify underlying neuropathology and potentially treatable pathologies such as normal pressure hydrocephalus or space occupying lesions. Brain imaging may show characteristic changes to help identifying the cause(s) of dementia, such as generalised or focal cortical atrophy (usually asymmetric, hippocampal atrophy) in Alzheimer's dementia; brain infarcts or white matter lesions in vascular dementia; or frontal lobe or anterior temporal lobe atrophy in frontotemporal dementia. Additional neurologic or medical testing may be required if specific aetiologies are suspected: EEG, head and neck MR angiogram or CT angiogram.

In patients with normal pressure hydrocephalus, there is ventriculomegaly and normal CSF pressure (with higher nocturnal pressures reported). Improvement of gait and cognitive function may be observed after ventriculoperitoneal shunt placement in suitable surgical candidates.

Multiple system atrophy (MSA) is a sporadic, rapidly progressive, multisystem, neurodegenerative fatal disease of undetermined aetiology, characterised clinically by varying severity of parkinsonian features; cerebellar, autonomic, and urogenital dysfunction; and corticospinal disorders. Neuropathological hallmarks of MSA are cell loss in the striatonigral and olivopontocerebellar structures of the brain and spinal cord accompanied by profuse, distinctive glia cytoplasmic inclusions (GCIs) formed by fibrillised alpha-synuclein proteins.

Creutzfeldt–Jakob disease (CJD) is a rare, uniformly fatal neurodegenerative disease manifested by rapidly progressive dementia, myoclonus, ataxia, visual disturbances, extrapyramidal and pyramidal involvement, and akinetic mutism. The pathogenesis is that prions convert into insoluble aggregates in nervous tissue and result in neuronal loss, astrocytic proliferation, spongiform change and abnormal disease-related, protease-resistant prion protein (PrP) in tissues. CJD is difficult to diagnose because of non-specific clinical manifestations. Definitive diagnosis requires identification of PrP in a brain biopsy. Suggestive investigation with CSF protein 14-3-3 has a sensitivity and specificity of 92% and 80% respectively. MRI, either diffusion-weighted MRI or fluid attenuation inversion recovery (FLAIR), features have 91–92.3% and 93.8–95% sensitivity and specificity respectively.

Progressive supranuclear palsy is a neurodegenerative disease whose characteristics include supranuclear, initially vertical, gaze dysfunction accompanied by extrapyramidal symptoms and cognitive dysfunction.

Arvanitakis Z, Shah R, Bennett D. Diagnosis and Management of Dementia: Review. JAMA. 2019;322(16):1589.
https://jamanetwork.com/journals/jama/article-abstract/2753376

8 Genetic Medicine

Questions

Answers can be found in the Genetic Medicine Answers section at the end of this chapter.

1. A 30-year-old Greek woman is investigated for coeliac disease because of anaemia but is found to have beta-thalassaemia trait. Her husband was informed by the Red Cross recently that he is not suitable for blood donation because of mild anaemia due to beta-thalassaemia trait.
   What is the probability of their 3-year-old son being unaffected?
   A. 0.1.
   B. 0.25.
   C. 0.5.
   D. 0.75.

2. Which of the following statements is correct in regard to a patient with cystic fibrosis?
   A. Pancreatic insufficiency usually spares islet cell function and diabetes is rare.
   B. Panopacification of the sinuses is rare in patients with cystic fibrosis.
   C. Beneficial treatments are available which increases CFTR channel opening or amount of the CFTR protein.
   D. Nosocomial transmission of *Burkholderia cepacia* is very rare.

3. Which variation of Down's syndrome does not increase in incidence with maternal age?
   A. Displacement.
   B. Duplication of a portion of chromosome 21.
   C. Mosaicism.
   D. Translocation.

4. Which one of the following descriptions regarding Duchenne muscular dystrophy (DMD) is true?
   A. DMD is caused by point mutations, deletions, or duplications, of one or more exons of the DMD gene.
   B. DMD is caused by defective production of myotrophin.
   C. DMD gene mutation has no impact on cardiac muscle.
   D. The gene affected in DMD is located on chromosome 8.

5. The maturation of monocytes requires the expression of new segments of DNA. The expression of these genes is mediated by demethylation of the needed DNA sequences. What is the name of this process?
   A. Alternative splicing.
   B. DNA splicing.
   C. Epigenetic modification.
   D. Translational modification.

6. A 54-year-old man has ESKD due to diabetic nephropathy with diabetes diagnosed at age 16. He is assessed for simultaneous pancreas and kidney transplant, but the serum C-peptide level is very high. He is diagnosed with maturity onset diabetes of the young (MODY) instead of type I diabetes. He subsequently undergoes a genetic test of a panel of genes which can be mutated

---

How to Pass the FRACP Written Examination, First Edition. Jonathan Gleadle, Jordan Li, Danielle Wu, and Paul Kleinig.
© 2022 John Wiley & Sons Ltd. Published 2022 by John Wiley & Sons Ltd.

in patients with MODY. The test has found no causative mutations in genes causing monogenic diabetes or MODY. However, a change or variation is found in the ABCC8 gene which has been classified as a 'variant of unknown significant (VUS)'. Which of the following advice is correct?

- **A.** The genetic test should be repeated immediately.
- **B.** The result should not be disclosed to patient.
- **C.** The significance of ABCC8 should be reviewed in 5 years.
- **D.** This patient should be treated with a sulphonylurea.

7. A 44-year-old man is diagnosed with early Huntington's disease. Which area of his brain is most likely to be affected?

- **A.** Cerebellum.
- **B.** Hippocampus.
- **C.** Striatum.
- **D.** Thalamus.

8. An 18-year-old woman is admitted to the Acute Medical Unit after a seizure. As you are reviewing her past medical history from the electronic records, you find she has Angelman syndrome due to genomic imprinting.

What defect is seen in disorders of genomic imprinting?

- **A.** DNA methylation.
- **B.** Pleiotropy.
- **C.** RNA methylation.
- **D.** X-linked inactivation.

9. Which of the following occurs in a patient with 47, XXY karyotype?

- **A.** Extra chromosome only from the mother's germ cells.
- **B.** Increased incidence of lens subluxation.
- **C.** Increased incidence of thromboembolism.
- **D.** Reduced incidence of breast cancer.

10. A 54-year-old Caucasian man had stage 5 CKD and received a kidney transplant. His other medical problems include sensorineural hearing impairment, type 1 diabetes, short stature, ischaemic heart disease, and hyperlipidaemia. Further family history reveals several family members had similar conditions and the pedigree is shown below.

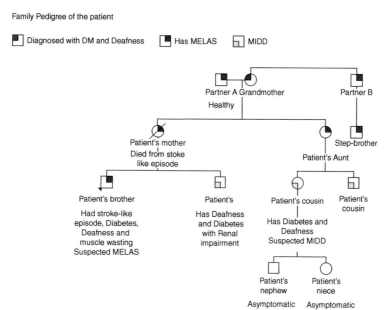

Family Pedigree of the patient

■ Diagnosed with DM and Deafness   ■ Has MELAS   ▢ MIDD

Partner A Grandmother
Healthy

Partner B

Patient's mother
Died from stoke like episode

Step-brother

Patient's Aunt

Patient's brother
Had stroke-like episode, Diabetes, Deafness and muscle wasting Suspected MELAS

Patient's
Has Deafness and Diabetes with Renal impairment

Patient's cousin
Has Diabetes and Deafness Suspected MIDD

Patient's cousin

Patient's nephew
Asymptomatic

Patient's niece
Asymptomatic

What is the inheritance pattern for his conditions?
- **A.** Autosomal dominant inheritance.
- **B.** Maternal inheritance.
- **C.** X-linked dominant inheritance.
- **D.** X-linked recessive inheritance.

11. Which one of the following is a feature of mitochondrially-inherited disorder?
- **A.** Paternal transmission only.
- **B.** Point mutation does not occur in mitochondrial chromosomes.
- **C.** Straightforward genotype-phenotype relationship.
- **D.** The presence of heteroplasmy.

12. Which of the following statements best describes the characteristics of small interfering RNA (siRNA)?
- **A.** siRNA causes base dimerisation.
- **B.** siRNA induces post-transcriptional gene silencing.
- **C.** siRNA interfere with DNA replication.
- **D.** siRNA is single-stranded RNA of 65-70 base pairs in length.

13. A 40-year-old man is evaluated in the neurology clinic because of progressive ataxia. He has no significant past medical history. On neurological examination, he has ophthalmoplegia, prominent vertical and horizontal nystagmus, facial and tongue fasciculations, positive Babinski sign, and ankle and patella clonus. He has a shuffling broad-based gait. There is a family history of ataxia.
What is the most likely hereditary pattern of his condition?
- **A.** Autosomal dominant.
- **B.** Autosomal recessive.
- **C.** Mitochondrial.
- **D.** X-linked recessive.

14. A 35-year-old woman presents with a significant pneumothorax which requires intercostal chest drain. She is known to have epilepsy, angiomyolipomas in both kidneys and in the retroperitoneal space. Her previous chest CT is shown below:

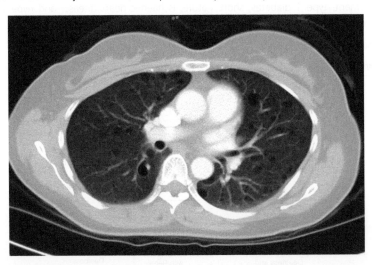

Which of following is the most likely diagnosis?
- **A.** Birt-Hogg-Dube syndrome.
- **B.** Prader–Willi syndrome.
- **C.** Tuberous sclerosis complex.
- **D.** Von Hippel Lindau syndrome.

15. Wilson's disease has a frequency of 1 in 8100 in a particular population. If there is no mutation, random mating, no gene flow, infinite population size, and no selection, what is the carrier rate?

    A. 1 in 45.

    B. 1 in 81.

    C. 1 in 90.

    D. 89 in 90.

QUESTIONS (16–19) REFER TO THE FOLLOWING INFORMATION

For each of the following condition or clinical presentation, select the correct mode of genetic inheritance

    A. Autosomal dominant.

    B. Autosomal recessive.

    C. Codominant.

    D. Complex inheritance.

    E. Genomic imprinting.

    F. Mitochondrial.

    G. X-linked dominant.

    H. X-linked recessive.

16. What is the pattern of inheritance for Gardner syndrome?

17. A 28-year-old woman with spina bifida is planning for in vitro fertilisation (IVF). She wants to know what the pattern of inheritance for spina bifida is.

18. What is the pattern of inheritance for neurofibromatosis 2?

19. A patient has received a lung transplant because of alpha1-antitrypsin deficiency. What is the pattern of inheritance for this condition?

QUESTIONS (20–23) REFER TO THE FOLLOWING INFORMATION

Match the patterns of Inheritance consistent with following pedigrees.

    A. Autosomal dominant.

    B. Autosomal recessive.

    C. Codominant.

    D. Complex inheritance.

    E. Genomic imprinting.

    F. Mitochondrial.

    G. X-linked dominant.

    H. X-linked recessive.

20.

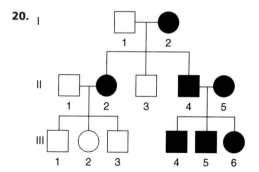

21.

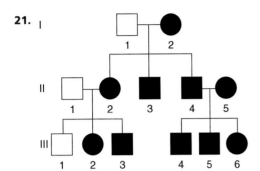

22.

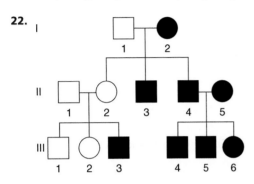

23.

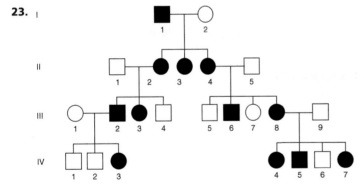

Answers

1. Answer: B

Beta-thalassaemia is an autosomal recessive condition. When two partners each have the recessive gene mutation, the inheritance expression is classically one out of four chance of an affected offspring, two out of four chance of carriers of the recessive gene and one out of four chance of a normal unaffected offspring. Therefore, the probability of a normal (unaffected) child is 0.25. The probability of an offspring who is a carrier of the beta-thalassaemia trait is 0.5.

Taher A, Weatherall D, Cappellini M. Thalassaemia. The Lancet. 2018;391(10116):155–167.
https://www.thelancet.com/journals/lancet/article/PIIS0140-6736(17)31822-6/fulltext

2. Answer: C

Cystic fibrosis is a common life-limiting autosomal recessive genetic disorder. The disease is caused by mutation of a gene that encodes a chloride-conducting transmembrane channel called the cystic fibrosis transmembrane conductance regulator (CFTR), which regulates anion transport and mucociliary clearance in the airways. Functional failure of CFTR results in mucus retention and chronic infection and subsequently in local airway inflammation which is harmful to the lungs. Two types of CFTR modulator have been approved for treatment. These include a potentiator (ivacaftor), which increases CFTR channel opening, and correctors (lumacaftor and tezacaftor), which increase the amount of CFTR protein at the cell surface. Two new, small-molecule CFTR correctors — VX–445 and VX–659 — have shown benefit on combination therapy in treatment of adults with cystic fibrosis with either the Phe508del–Phe508del CFTR mutation or the Phe508del–MF CFTR mutation.

Pancreatic insufficiency is the most common gastrointestinal complication of cystic fibrosis. Approximately 85–90% of patients with cystic fibrosis develop this complication at some point. Pancreatic insufficiency leads to fat malabsorption due to decreased pancreatic enzyme production. As a result, patients may present with steatorrhea, malnutrition, and fat-soluble vitamin deficiencies. However, patients diagnosed late in childhood or in adulthood are more likely to have pancreatic sufficiency and often present with a clinical history of chronic cough and sputum production instead. 10% of patients with cystic fibrosis remain pancreatic sufficient and tend to have a milder disease course.

The development of cystic fibrosis-related diabetes is an increasing problem, occurring in up to 40% of adults, and is associated with poorer survival, particularly in female patients. This disorder is caused by insulin deficiency resulting from the destructive pancreatic disease that ultimately destroys islet cell function.

Cystic fibrosis is inherited in an autosomal recessive fashion, two copies of the abnormal gene, CFTR must be present in an individual for clinical disease to occur. The CFTR gene is located on the long arm of chromosome 7q, band 31.2. The six types of defects that can result from CFTR mutations are:

• Complete absence of CFTR protein synthesis
• Defective protein maturation and early degradation
• Disordered regulation (diminished ATP binding and hydrolysis)
• Defective chloride conductance or channel gating
• Diminished transcription due to promoter or splicing abnormality
• Accelerated channel turnover from the cell surface.

There is strong evidence that *Burkholderia cepacia* complex organisms, *P aeruginosa*, and MRSA can be transmitted from patient to patient. All of these organisms are associated with poor clinical outcomes and substantial effort is now made in cystic fibrosis centres to reduce cross-infection and nosocomial spread.

Chronic sinopulmonary disease is a hallmark of cystic fibrosis. After age 5, panopacification of the sinuses viewed on plain radiography is present in most patients.

Specifically, more than 75% opacification of the maxillary and ethmoid sinuses is considered a hallmark of cystic fibrosis.

Holguin F. Triple CFTR Modulator Therapy for Cystic Fibrosis. New England Journal of Medicine. 2018;379(17):1671–1672.
https://www.nejm.org/doi/10.1056/NEJMe1811996

3. Answer: D

Down's syndrome is the most common chromosomal disorder that is associated with intellectual disability and a characteristic facial appearance. This chromosomal anomaly leads to both structural and functional issues in patients with a wide range of phenotypic variation. Patients with Down's syndrome may have a variety of birth defects. About 60% of patients have ophthalmic manifestations and 50% will have a heart defect. About 5% of patients with Down's syndrome have GI manifestations, including duodenal atresia, Hirschsprung's disease, and coeliac disease.

Individuals with Down's syndrome have an increased risk of developing several complications including GORD, coeliac disease, hypothyroidism, leukaemia, delayed development, and behavioural problems, developing Alzheimer disease at early age.

Trisomy 21 is the cause of approximately 95% of Down's syndrome, with 88% coming from nondisjunction in the maternal gamete and 8% coming from nondisjunction in the paternal gamete. Maternal age is the only factor that has been linked to an increased chance of having a baby with Trisomy 21.

The extra chromosome 21 material that causes Down's syndrome may be due to a Robertsonian translocation. The long arm of chromosome 21 is attached to the long arm of another chromosome, often chromosome 14 [46,XX,t(14;21)] or itself [called an isochromosome, 45,XX,t(21;21)(q10;q10)].

Translocation Down's syndrome can be de novo; that is, not inherited but occurring at the time of an individual's conception or may be inherited from a parent with a balanced translocation. Translocation Down's syndrome is often referred to as familial Down's syndrome. It is the cause of about 4.5% of people with Down's syndrome. It does not show a maternal age effect.

Mosaic Down's syndrome is when some of the cells in the body have a normal karyotype and some cells have trisomy 21, an arrangement called a mosaic (46, XX/47, XX, +21). This can occur when a nondisjunction event during an early cell division leads to a fraction of the cells with trisomy 21. The risk is increased with maternal age. There is considerable variability in the fraction of cells with trisomy 21, both as a whole and tissue-by-tissue. This is the cause of 1–2% of Down's syndromes. Mosaic Down's syndrome may produce less developmental delay, on average, than full trisomy 21.

Rarely, a region of chromosome 21 will undergo a duplication event. This will lead to extra copies of some, but not all, of the genes on chromosome 21 (46, XX, dup(21q)). If the duplicated region has genes that are responsible for Down's syndrome physical and mental characteristics, such individuals will show those characteristics. This cause is very rare, and no rate estimates are possible.

Roizen N, Patterson D. Down's syndrome. The Lancet. 2003;361(9365):1281–1289.
https://psycnet.apa.org/record/2003-03488-004

4. Answer: A

Muscular dystrophy is a group of inherited diseases characterised by weakness and wasting of muscle tissue, with or without the breakdown of nerve tissue. There are 9 types of muscular dystrophy, with each type involving an eventual loss of strength, increasing disability, and possible deformity.

The most well-known of the muscular dystrophies is Duchenne muscular dystrophy (DMD), followed by Becker muscular dystrophy (BMD). DMD is a severe X-linked recessive disorder due to mutations in the very large DMD gene, which encodes the protein dystrophin and is located on X chromosome. It is affected by point mutations, deletions, and duplications of parts of the gene, causing alterations in the reading frame and truncation of the dystrophin protein, which is rapidly degraded.

DMD is a progressive and disabling neuromuscular disease. The mean age of diagnosis is around 4.3 years of age and often is delayed. DMD is diagnosed by genetic testing, biochemical tests, and muscle biopsy. Other typical complications of DMD include scoliosis, heart failure, respiratory insufficiency, fractures of long bones and vertebrae due to osteoporosis, and eventually death. Dystrophin is an important structural protein found in skeletal muscle which connects the cytoskeleton of a muscle fibrer to the extracellular matrix. It is a cytoplasmic protein, and links actin filaments to other structural proteins outside of the cell. Dystrophin is key in maintaining the mechanical stability of skeletal muscle; a lack of it causes these cells to be increasingly fragile and prone to damage. The result of this damage is a steady leak of calcium into the sarcolemma, disrupting signaling pathways and ultimately causing mitochondria to burst. Damaged muscle tissue is progressively replaced by scar tissue and fat.

Cardiac disease is a common manifestation, not necessarily related to the degree of skeletal myopathy; it may be the predominant manifestation with or without any other evidence of muscular disease. Death is usually due to ventricular dysfunction, heart block or malignant arrhythmias. Not only DMD/BMD patients, but also female carriers may present with cardiac involvement. Pathology examination during the late stages of the disease shows cardiomyocytes' hypertrophy, atrophy, and fibrosis. The majority of DMD after the third decade of their age have established cardiomyopathy. Although clinically overt heart failure may be delayed or absent, due to relative physical inactivity. Cardiomyopathy is the leading cause of death in DMD and myocardial damage precedes decline in left ventricular systolic function. Neither the age of onset nor the severity of cardiomyopathy was correlated with the type of mutation.

Improvements in management have changed the natural history of DMD. The use of glucocorticoids and physiotherapy delays the loss of strength and ambulation. Glucocorticoids are the only medication currently available that slows the decline in muscle strength and function in DMD, which in turn reduces the risk of scoliosis and stabilises pulmonary function. Cardiac function might also improve evidenced by slower decline in echocardiographic measures of cardiac dysfunction, early pharmacological therapy for heart failure improves prognosis and survival; and surgery for scoliosis, respiratory physiotherapy, and the use of non-invasive ventilation have enhanced lung capacity. Guidelines and expert opinion strongly urge glucocorticoid therapy in all patients with DMD.

Fox H, Millington L, Mahabeer I, van Ruiten H. Duchenne muscular dystrophy. BMJ. 2020: l7012.
https://www.bmj.com/content/368/bmj.l7012.full

5. Answer: C

Epigenetics is defined as the alterations in the gene expression profile of a cell that are not caused by changes in the DNA sequence. Epigenetic inheritance thus refers to the transmission of certain epigenetic marks to offspring.

Many types of epigenetic processes have been identified such as methylation, acetylation, phosphorylation, ubiquitylation, and sumolyation. DNA methylation is the addition or removal of a methyl group ($CH3$), predominantly where cytosine bases occur consecutively. DNA methylation and demethylation are the most common epigenetic modification and have been observed in pathogenesis of cancer and many other disorders.

Another significant epigenetic process is chromatin modification. Chromatin is the complex of histones and DNA that is tightly bundled to fit into the nucleus. The complex can be modified by substances such as acetyl groups (the process called acetylation), enzymes, microRNAs, and small interfering RNAs. This modification alters chromatin structure to influence gene expression. In general, tightly folded chromatin tends to be shut down, or not expressed, while more open chromatin is functional, or expressed.

Imprinting describes the condition where one of the two alleles of a typical gene pair is silenced by an epigenetic process such as methylation or acetylation. This becomes a problem if the expressed allele is damaged or contains a variant that increases the human's vulnerability to microbes, or other harmful substances.

Alternative splicing leads to changes in gene production but derives from splicing out of different regions of the DNA sequence itself and re-joining it to other sections.

Feinberg A. The Key Role of Epigenetics in Human Disease Prevention and Mitigation. New England Journal of Medicine. 2018;378(14):1323–1334.
https://www.nejm.org/doi/full/10.1056/NEJMra1402513

6. Answer: C

Variant of uncertain significance (VUS) is a variation in a genetic sequence for which the association with disease risk is unclear. According to American College of Medical Genetics and Genomics (ACMG) five-tier classification system, a variant can be classified as:

1. Pathogenic: This variant directly contributes to the development of disease. Some pathogenic variants may not be fully penetrant. Additional evidence is not expected to alter the classification of this variant.
2. Likely pathogenic: There is a high likelihood (>90% certainty) that this variant is disease-causing. Additional evidence is expected to confirm this assertion of pathogenicity, but there is a small chance that new evidence may demonstrate that this variant does not have clinical significance.
3. Uncertain significance: There is not enough information at current time to support a more definitive classification of this variant.
4. Likely benign: This variant is NOT expected to have a major effect on disease; however, the scientific evidence is currently insufficient to prove this conclusively. Additional evidence is expected to confirm this assertion, but we cannot fully rule out the possibility that new evidence may demonstrate that this variant can contribute to disease.
5. Benign: This variant does not cause disease.

In summary, the genetic testing results generally fall into three categories. 'Positive' results usually provide a diagnosis or risk information. 'Negative' results, where no relevant genetic variation is found, can sometimes rule out a diagnosis and need of further assessment. VUS falls in between positive and negative. Driven by methods of next generation sequencing such as whole exome sequencing, the numbers of VUS detection are increasing significantly.

In one study, variant classification and reclassification were evaluated for 1.45 million individuals who received genetic testing from a single testing laboratory over a 10-year period. 6.4% of variants were reclassified in this period. Very few variants initially classified as benign or pathogenic were reclassified to a different clinical category. This indicates that once a variant has reached a definitive classification (benign or pathogenic), it is unlikely that classification will be changed. The overall upgrade rate among all reported VUS was low at 3%. It is difficult to predict with clinical accuracy which variants will be upgraded to pathogenic. The number of patients with VUS will likely continue to rise nationally as: (i) genetic awareness increases leading to more individuals being tested, (ii) disease gene panel adoption rises, (iii) the number of genes included in testing increases, and (iv) the cost of genetic testing decreases. As such, the absolute number of individuals with VUS that are later upgraded to pathogenic will continue to rise. It is the current practice that every VUS should be reviewed every five years if not earlier.

It is generally accepted that VUS should be disclosed to patients with appropriate counselling. A VUS should not be used in clinical decision making. Therefore, it is irrelevant to whether the patient should receive simultaneous pancreas and kidney transplant (SPK) in this case. Generally, SPK is performed in patients with type I diabetes but there are occasionally done in patients with MODY. If VUS is reclassified by a laboratory, the laboratory is generally understood to be responsible for issuing a revised report to the clinician. The process of then getting this information to patients is not always straightforward. Reclassification may occur many years after the original test, it may be a challenge to contact the patient because patients may have out-of-date contact information on file. The heightened uncertainty resulting from a VUS can be greatly distressing for patients.

Mersch J, Brown N, Pirzadeh-Miller S, Mundt E, Cox H, Brown K et al. Prevalence of Variant Reclassification Following Hereditary Cancer Genetic Testing. JAMA. 2018;320(12):1266.
https://jamanetwork.com/journals/jama/fullarticle/2703350

7. Answer: C

Huntington's disease (HD) is a fully penetrant neurodegenerative disease caused by a dominantly inherited CAG trinucleotide repeat expansion in the huntingtin gene on chromosome 4. This results in the production of a mutant huntingtin protein with an abnormally long polyglutamine repeat. Those with greater than 39 CAG repeats are certain to develop the disease, whilst reduced penetrance is seen between 36 and 39 repeats. Anticipation can be seen when the gene is passed down the paternal line, such that a father with a CAG repeat length in the intermediate range may have a child with an expanded pathogenic repeat length. This is because sperm from males shows greater repeat variability and larger repeat sizes than somatic tissues.

HD is characterised by cognitive, motor, and psychiatric disturbance. At the cellular level mutant huntingtin results in neuronal dysfunction and death through several mechanisms, including disruption of proteostasis, transcription, mitochondrial function, and direct toxicity of the mutant protein. Early macroscopic changes are seen in the striatum (which includes the caudate, putamen, and globus pallidus) with involvement of the cortex as the disease progresses.

Diagnosis of HD is based on a confirmed family history or positive genetic test. Prior to testing it is important to inform the patient about HD and its hereditary nature as a positive test has implications both for the patient and his/her family. Predictive genetic testing is done prior to symptom onset in adults who are at risk of inheriting the *Huntingtin* (*HTT*) gene mutation.

There are currently no disease modifying treatments; supportive and symptomatic management is the mainstay of treatment. There has been a large growth in potential therapeutic targets and clinical trials. The most promising of these are the emerging therapies aimed at lowering levels of mutant huntingtin. Antisense oligonucleotide therapy is one such approach with clinical trials currently under way.

McColgan P, Tabrizi S. Huntington's disease: a clinical review. European Journal of Neurology. 2017;25(1):24–34.
https://onlinelibrary.wiley.com/doi/abs/10.1111/ene.13413

8. Answer: A

Angelman syndrome is a complex genetic disorder that primarily affects the nervous system. Clinical features include developmental delay, intellectual disability, severe speech impairment, and problems with movement and balance (ataxia). Most patients have recurrent seizures and microcephaly. Many of the clinical features of Angelman syndrome result from the loss of function of a gene called *UBE3A*.

People normally inherit one copy of the *UBE3A* gene from each parent. Both copies of this gene are active in many of the body's tissues. In certain areas of the brain, however, only the copy inherited from mother (the maternal copy) is active. This parent-specific gene activation is caused by genomic imprinting. If the maternal copy of the *UBE3A* gene is lost, the patient will have no active copies of the gene in some parts of the brain.

Genetic mechanisms that can inactivate or delete the maternal copy of the *UBE3A* gene include chromosome deletion, imprinting error, paternal uniparental disomy, and *UBE3A* mutation. About 70% of Angelman syndrome is caused when a segment of the maternal chromosome 15 containing this gene is deleted. Prader–Willi syndrome is a clinically distinct disorder resulting from paternal deletion of the same 15q11-q13 region. Approximately 3% of Angelman syndrome cases are caused by uniparental disomy, an abnormality in which a person receives both copies of a chromosome from one parent instead of receiving one from each parent. In Angelman syndrome, both copies of chromosome 15 can be received from the father (paternal uniparental disomy). As a result, there are only paternally expressed genes in this region and *UBE3A* is thus not expressed at all in the brain since it is normally only expressed on the maternal-derived chromosome.

Mutations within *UBE3A* have been detected in 10–20% of individuals with Angelman syndrome. *UBE3A* encodes a ubiquitin ligase protein which marks other proteins for degradation, a process known as ubiquitination.

Pleiotropy occurs when one gene influence two or more phenotypic expression seemingly. Such gene is termed a pleiotropic gene. Mutation in a pleiotropic gene may have an effect on several phenotypic expressions simultaneously, due to the gene coding for a product used by a myriad of cells or different targets that have the same signalling function.

Fridman C, Koiffmann C. Genomic imprinting: genetic mechanisms and phenotypic consequences in Prader–Willi and Angelman syndromes. Genetics and Molecular Biology. 2000;23(4):715–724. https://academic.oup.com/molehr/article/3/4/321/989604

9. Answer: C

Klinefelter syndrome (KS) is caused by congenital aneuploidy of the sex chromosomes. 80% of patients have the 47, XXXY karyotype. The remaining 20% have either mosaic 47, XXY/46, XY, supernumerary X chromosome aneuploidy (48, XXY; 49, XXXXY), one or several additional Y chromosomes (e.g. 48, XXYY), or structurally abnormal additional X chromosomes. These numerical chromosome abnormalities are the result of nondisjunction in maternal oogenesis in approximately two-thirds of cases, and in paternal spermatogenesis in the remaining third.

Leading symptoms are signs of testosterone deficiency; very small, firm testes; and infertility. Testosterone replacement corrects symptoms of androgen deficiency but has no positive effect on infertility. However, nowadays patients with KS, including the non-mosaic type, no longer need to be considered irrevocably infertile, because intracytoplasmic sperm injection offers an opportunity for procreation even when there are no spermatozoa in the ejaculate. In a substantial number of azoospermic patients, spermatozoa can be extracted from testicular biopsy samples where pregnancies and livebirths have been achieved.

Almost all organ systems are associated with an elevated risk of morbidity and mortality in KS compared to the male population as a whole. Gynecomastia is common in KS and is associated with a slightly higher incidence of breast cancer than in men with normal karyotype. KS is well-known to cause decreased bone mass, outright fractures, and osteoporosis, affecting morbidity and mortality. Patients with KS suffer from vascular diseases, particularly varicose veins and thromboembolisms, most commonly PE. Central obesity, type 2 diabetes, and metabolic syndrome is often observed. Epilepsy and other neurological and mental disorders occur significantly more frequently in KS patients.

Groth K, Skakkebæk A, Høst C, Gravholt C, Bojesen A. Klinefelter Syndrome—A Clinical Update. The Journal of Clinical Endocrinology & Metabolism. 2013;98(1):20–30. https://academic.oup.com/jcem/article/98/1/20/2823039

10. Answer: B

His clinical features including sensorineural hearing impairment, type 1 diabetes, short stature, ischaemic heart disease, and hyperlipidaemia which are suggestive of mitochondrial disease. The pedigree above shows that females who have the disease pass down these phenotypes to their children but the males who have disease do not pass down to their children. This is typical of a maternal inheritance pattern. This patient has maternally inherited diabetes and deafness (MIDD).

Mitochondria are a double membranous organelle found in most human cells which perform various metabolic activities, but mainly generate adenosine triphosphate (ATP) via the electron transport chain as fuel for cells to carry out their daily activities. Mitochondria consist two types of DNA, extra-chromosomal DNA (mtDNA), which is maternally inherited and nuclear DNA (nDNA). Although only a small percentage of mitochondrial proteins are encoded via mtDNA, mutation in the mtDNA will cause mitochondrial dysfunction and lead to mitochondrial diseases such as mitochondrial encephalopathy, lactic acidosis, and stroke-like episodes (MELAS), MIDD and Kearns-Sayre syndrome (KSS). The dual involvement of the mitochondrial and nuclear genomes results in all possible inheritance patterns – maternal, X linked, autosomal recessive, autosomal dominant, and de novo occurrence.

MIDD and MELAS are maternally inherited mitochondrial diseases. Both MIDD and MELAS are caused mainly by maternally inherited m.3243 A>G mutation in the mitochondrial encoded tRNA leucine (UUA/UUG) gene. MIDD patients are often characterised as having diabetic mellitus and sensorineural hearing loss while MELAS, the more severe form of MIDD, often exhibit the cardinal signs such as lactic acidosis, stroke-like episodes, seizures, and encephalopathy.

Kidney involvement is common in patients with m.3243 A>G mutation, most commonly presenting as focal segmental glomerulosclerosis (FSGS) and tubular diseases mainly affecting the proximal convoluted tubules, distal convoluted tubules, and connecting segments.

Craven L, Alston C, Taylor R, Turnbull D. Recent Advances in Mitochondrial Disease. Annual Review of Genomics and Human Genetics. 2017;18(1):257–275.
https://www.annualreviews.org/doi/full/10.1146/annurev-genom-091416-035426

11. Answer: D

All human cells depend on mitochondrial oxidative phosphorylation to generate energy, which accounts for the remarkable diversity of clinical disorders associated with mitochondrial DNA (mtDNA) mutations.

MtDNA is strictly maternally inherited. Also, in contrast to most nuclear genes, which are present in two copies per cell, each cell can contain hundreds of mitochondria, each with several copies of the mitochondria genome. Thus, mutant mtDNA and normal mtDNA may coexist in varying proportions within the same cell. This is the unique feature of mitochondrial disorder inheritance termed heteroplasmy.

The existence of heteroplasmic mutations leads to another key feature of mitochondrial disorder inheritance called mutational burden, which is the percentage of mutant mtDNA within a cell or tissue. Several factors influence mutational burden. Within an oocyte, some mitochondria can have normal mtDNA while others have mutant mtDNA. The differential distribution of these mitochondria during early divisions of the fertilised oocyte is termed mitotic segregation. As a result of mitotic segregation, the mutational burden from one tissue to another may vary within a single individual. In addition, selection for or against mutant mtDNA can occur during cell divisions. Generally, there is a tendency for selection against mutant mtDNA in rapidly dividing tissues such as blood stem cells, whereas nondividing postmitotic cells such as neurons tend to have a higher mutational burden.

Heteroplasmy, mitotic segregation, and selection account for some of the variability in the clinical expression of mtDNA mutations. An additional factor is the threshold of expression, which is the mutational burden required for signs or symptoms to occur. Mutations present at low mutational burdens generally cause no clinical effects. The specific mutational burden required for symptoms to occur varies among tissues. Those with high energy consumption per gram, such as brain and muscle, tend to manifest symptoms at a lower mutational burden than tissues that are less metabolically active. Putting all these together, there is no straightforward genotype–phenotype relationship.

In addition to the mtDNA-encoded proteins, oxidative phosphorylation requires many proteins encoded in nuclear DNA. Therefore, mitochondrial dysfunction can result from mutations in mtDNA or nuclear DNA. This distinction is complicated by the existence of nuclear genes that control the expression and replication of the mitochondrial genome. For example, autosomal dominant progressive external ophthalmoplegia is associated with multiple mtDNA deletions, implying that a nuclear DNA mutation predisposes to multiple mtDNA deletions. Point mutation does occur in mitochondrial chromosomes.

Schapira A. Mitochondrial diseases. The Lancet. 2012;379(9828):1825–1834.
https://academic.oup.com/molehr/article/3/4/321/989604

12. Answer: B

Small interfering RNA (siRNA), also known as short interfering RNA or silencing RNA, is a class of double-stranded RNA molecules, 20–25 base pairs in length, similar to miRNA.

An RNase III-like enzyme termed Dicer, catalyses production of siRNAs from long dsRNAs and small hairpin RNAs. When formed, siRNAs are bound by a multiprotein component complex termed RISC (RNA induced silencing complex). Within the RISC complex, siRNA strands are separated and the strand with the more stable 5-end is typically integrated to the active RISC complex. The antisense single-stranded siRNA component then guides and aligns the RISC complex on the target mRNA and through the action of catalytic RISC protein the mRNA is cleaved. Therefore, siRNA interferes with the expression of specific genes with complementary nucleotide sequences by degrading mRNA after transcription, preventing translation. The RISC complex can also be directed by a siRNA into the nucleus where it associates with the complementary region of the DNA. Once there the complex recruits the other proteins that modify the structure around the promoter of the gene thus inhibiting transcription.

In summary, siRNA can cause gene silencing through three pathways: mRNA degradation, as described above, translational inhibition and promoter silencing. Base dimerisation is caused by DNA exposure to UV rays causing errors during replication.

siRNA is a potential therapeutic reagent due to its ability to inhibit specific genes in many genetic diseases. siRNAs can be used as tools to study single gene function both in vivo; and in-vitro and are an attractive new class of therapeutics, especially against undruggable targets for the treatment of cancer and other diseases. Patisiran is an example of an approved siRNA therapy for the rare hereditary disease transthyretin-mediated amyloidosis. The siRNA delivery systems are categorised as non-viral and viral delivery systems. The non-viral delivery system includes polymers, lipids, peptides. Effective pharmacological use of siRNA requires 'carriers' that can deliver the siRNA to its intended site of action.

Hu B, Weng Y, Xia X, Liang X, Huang Y. Clinical advances of siRNA therapeutics. The Journal of Gene Medicine. 2019;21(7). https://onlinelibrary.wiley.com/doi/full/10.1002/jgm.3097

13. Answer: A

The most likely diagnosis for this patient is spinocerebellar ataxia (SCA) 3, which is a triplet repeat disorder of autosomal dominant inheritance (chromosome 14, unstable CAG repeat). This group of disorders manifest primarily with ataxia and cerebellar dysfunction, which can be chronic or progressive. There are 29 dominantly inherited SCAs that have been described. The genetic basis for most of these disorders is due to expansion of triplet nucleotide repeats. Most of the triplet expansions affect CAG repeats; in the SCA8 form, an untranslated CTG expansion is involved. There is a great degree of overlap in phenotype including the age of onset, symptoms related to cerebellar and spinocerebellar pathway dysfunction. Cerebellar syndromes with various combinations of oculomotor disorders, dysarthria, dysmetria/kinetic tremor, and ataxic gait are the main manifestations. Findings from neuroimaging studies are relatively nonspecific.

SCA3 is the most common of the autosomal dominant ataxias and has 3 subtypes. Subtype 1 presents with facial dystonia, fasciculations, horizontal and vertical nystagmus, opthalmoparesis especially to vertical gaze, clonus, upgoing plantar reflex, and shuffling gait. Subtype 3 presents in the fifth to seventh decade with dysarthria and extremity ataxia.

Friedreich's ataxia is another triplet repeat hereditary ataxia, however it is accompanied by cardiomyopathy (in 90% of cases). Patients have nystagmus, extremity ataxia, dysarthria, dysmetria, and absence of ankle jerk reflexes with an extensor plantar response. MRI of the spinal cord would show atrophy. It involves the gene frataxin with expanded GAA repeats. Undetectable or very low levels of frataxin mRNA would be present.

de Silva R, Vallortigara J, Greenfield J, Hunt B, Giunti P, Hadjivassiliou M. Diagnosis and management of progressive ataxia in adults. Practical Neurology. 2019;19(3):196–207. https://pn.bmj.com/content/19/3/196.full

14. Answer: C

The CT chest shows multiple thin walled pulmonary cysts suggestive of lymphangioleiomyomatosis. The combination of renal angiomyolipomas, lymphangioleiomyomatosis, and epilepsy are suggestive of tuberous sclerosis complex (TSC).

TSC is a multisystem, autosomal dominant disorder resulting from mutations in one of two genes, *TSC1* (encoding hamartin), or *TSC2* (encoding tuberin). *TSC1* or *TSC2* encodes proteins modulate cell function via the mTOR signalling cascade and serve as key factors in regulating cell growth and proliferation. Though no single feature is diagnostic, there is usually involvement of the skin, lungs, kidneys, and CNS. The characteristic renal lesions are multiple angiomyolipomas which are benign tumours composed of abnormal vessels, immature smooth-muscle cells, and fat cells but which can cause significant haemorrhages. Lungs show lymphangioleiomyomatosis which affects women almost exclusively and is characterised by widespread cystic changes within the lung parenchyma with pneumothorax as a potential complication. The neurologic manifestations include epilepsy and cognitive impairment. CNS lesions may be glioneuronal hamartomas, also called cortical tubers, subependymal giant cell tumours and nodules. Characteristic skin lesions consist of hypopigmented macules (formerly known as ash-leaf spots), adenoma sebaceum, shagreen patch, and ungal fibromas. The mainstay of management of TSC is supportive and treatment of complications. Mammalian target of rapamycin (mTOR) inhibitors such as sirolimus are promising in the treatment of TSC.

Von Hippel Lindau (VHL) syndrome is characterised by multiple renal cysts and renal cell carcinomas of clear cell type, hemangioblastomas in the cerebellum and retina and phaeochromocytomas. The mutation of the VHL gene leads to uncontrolled activation of the transcription factor hypoxia inducible factor (HIF) which is normally central to co-ordinating the cellular responses to hypoxia.

Birt-Hogg-Dube syndrome is characterised by multiple pulmonary cysts, skin lesions called fibrofolliculomas which are benign hamartomatous tumours of hair follicles and multiple renal cell carcinomas which are either chromophobic tumours or a hybrid of chromophobic and oncocytomas.

Prader–Willi syndrome (PWS) is caused by a deletion or disruption of genes in the proximal arm of chromosome 15 or by maternal disomy in the proximal arm of chromosome 15. PWS is characterised by short stature, small hands and feet, central obesity with abnormal body composition (reduced lean tissue and increased fat mass), developmental delay, mild to moderate intellectual disability, characteristic behaviours, and psychological problems. Low levels of growth hormone and sex hormones are common and thyroid function may be impaired. A hypothalamic dysfunction has been implied.

Crino P, Nathanson K, Henske E. The Tuberous Sclerosis Complex. New England Journal of Medicine. 2006;355(13):1345–1356. https://www.nejm.org/doi/full/10.1056/NEJMra055323

15. Answer: A

	A	a
A	AA (normal gene)	Aa (carrier)
a	Aa (carrier)	aa (diseased)

Wilson's disease is an autosomal recessive disease. Patients with an autosomal disease are represented using 'aa' or 'a^2' as shown in the table. In this case, a^2=1/8100 (a=1/90). The sum of frequencies of the dominant and recessive genes equals 1 (A+a=1). As a result, A=1-a = (1 - 1/90) = 89/90. The carrier rate = 2 x A x a = 2 x 89/90 x 1/90. To simplify the calculation, 89/90 approximates to 1. As a result, the carrier rate equals 2 x A x a = 2 x 1 x 1/90 = 1/45.

These calculations assume that the population is at Hardy–Weinberg equilibrium which can be expressed as a^2 + 2Aa + A^2 =1. Hardy–Weinberg principle states that allele and genotype frequencies in a population will remain constant from generation to generation in the absence of other evolutionary influences such as no mutation, random mating, no gene flow, infinite population size, and no natural or sexual selection.

Chang I, Hahn S. The genetics of Wilson disease. Wilson Disease. 2017:19–34. https://www.ncbi.nlm.nih.gov/pmc/articles/PMC5648646/

16. Answer: A

17. Answer: D

18. Answer: A

19. Answer: C

Gardner syndrome is a phenotypic variant of familial adenomatous polyposis. It is an autosomal dominant disease characterised by numerous adenomatous polyps lining the intestinal mucosal surface with a high potential for malignancy. The extracolonic manifestations may include intestinal polyposis, desmoids, osteomas, and epidermoid cysts. Patients with Gardner syndrome may present with osteomas of the mandible and skull, epidermal cysts, or fibromatosis. These manifestations are often found to be asymptomatic but may present with pruritus, inflammation, and rupture.

A genetic connection to the development of Gardner syndrome has been shown within band 5q21, which is associated with the adenomatous polyposis coli (APC) gene, located on chromosome 5 APC a tumour suppressor gene responsible for producing the APC protein that regulates cell growth via appropriate timing in the cell cycle. Gardner syndrome patients suffer from an aberration of this gene which leads to uncontrolled cell growth. In addition to such genetic mutations, a loss of DNA methylation, a mutation of the RAS gene on chromosome 12, a deletion of the colon cancer gene on chromosome 18, as well as, a mutation in P53 gene located on chromosome 17 have also been linked as a possible cause of Gardner syndrome.

Complex inheritance is caused by the interactions of variations in multiple genes and environmental factors. The genes involved may make a person susceptible to the disorder, and the environmental factors may trigger this susceptibility.

The liability to exhibit the phenotype of the complex disorder is determined by both genetic and environmental factors. Only individuals with enough genetic liability (multiple genes) who are in the presence of certain environmental factors will exhibit the phenotype. Complex disorders are often common disorders in the population and include hypertension, diabetes mellitus, asthma, and many birth defects, such as cleft lip +/- cleft palate, and spinal bifida.

Spina bifida is the most common permanently disabling birth defect. Approximately 95% of women who have a spina bifida affected pregnancy have no family history of the condition. About 50% of all neural tube defects could be prevented by taking 0.5 mg of folic acid daily before conception and during the first three months of pregnancy. Fertility is normal in women with spina bifida, while many men with this condition are infertile. A woman who has had one baby with spina bifida is more likely to have subsequent affected pregnancies. There is also an increased chance for spina bifida in any child of a parent who has spina bifida. In both situations, the chance for spina bifida is estimated to be about 3% for each pregnancy, which can be reduced by taking folic acid.

Neurofibromatosis, type 2 (NF2) is a multisystem genetic disorder associated with bilateral vestibular schwannomas, spinal cord schwannomas, meningiomas, gliomas, and juvenile cataracts, with a paucity of cutaneous features, which are seen more consistently in neurofibromatosis type 1. NF2 is inherited as an autosomal dominant pattern, although about 50% of patients with NF2 is due to a new (de novo) gene mutation. The manifestations of NF2 result from mutations in (or, rarely, deletion of) the *NF2* gene, located on the long arm of chromosome 22. The *NF2* gene encodes merlin which is a tumour suppressor.

Alpha 1-antitrypsin deficiency (A1AD) is a genetic disorder that causes defective production of α1-antitrypsin (A1AT), leading to decreased A1AT activity in the blood and lungs, and deposition of excessive abnormal A1AT protein in liver cells. There are several forms and degrees of deficiency, principally depending on whether the sufferer has one or two copies of the affected gene because it is a codominant trait. Severe A1AT deficiency causes panacinar emphysema or COPD in adult life and various liver diseases in a minority of children and adults. With codominant inheritance, two different alleles of a gene can be expressed and determine the phenotypic characteristics of the condition.

 Silverman E, Sandhaus R. Alpha1-Antitrypsin Deficiency. New England Journal of Medicine. 2009;360(26):2749–2757. https://www.nejm.org/doi/full/10.1056/NEJMcp0900449

20. Answer: B

This pedigree shows a pattern of autosomal recessive inheritance. Both parents of an affected person are carriers, and the clinical manifestation of the genetic condition is not typically seen in every generation. The condition can 'skip' a generation. Cystic fibrosis, sickle cell anaemia, Tay–Sachs disease, hereditary haemochromatosis, severe combined immunodeficiency, and autosomal recessive polycystic kidney disease are a few diseases of autosomal recessive inheritance pattern.

21. Answer: A

The pedigree is consistent with autosomal dominant pattern of inheritance. Each affected person has an affected parent. The inherited disease happens in every generation. There is 50% of chance of passing the affected gene from a parent to his/her offspring. You only need one mutated gene to be affected by this type of disease. Some examples of the diseases include autosomal dominant polycystic kidney disease, Huntington's disease, Marfan's syndrome, neurofibromatosis, familial hypercholesterolaemia, hereditary haemorrhagic telangiectasia, and tuberous sclerosis, etc.

22. Answer: H

The pedigree shows an X-linked recessive pattern. Males are more frequently affected since males only need one affected gene on the X chromosome to show phenotype whereas females need two copies of the affected genes on X chromosome to have clinical phenotype of the inherited disease. Affected males are often present in each generation. Haemophilia A, haemophilia B, Duchenne muscular dystrophy are some examples of this pattern of inheritance.

23. Answer: G

This pedigree shows an X-linked dominant pattern of inheritance. Females are more frequently affected. The condition with an X-linked dominant pattern of inheritance can have affected males and females in same generation. Hypophosphataemic rickets and ornithine transcarbamylase (OTC) deficiency, fragile X syndrome, and X-linked dominant porphyria have an X-linked dominant pattern of inheritance.

 Alliance G, Health D. Classic Mendelian Genetics (Patterns of Inheritance) [Internet]. Ncbi.nlm.nih.gov. 2020 [cited 29 March 2020]. Available from: https://www.ncbi.nlm.nih.gov/books/NBK132145/

9 Haematology

Questions

Answers can be found in the Haematology Answers section at the end of this chapter.

1. A 40-year-old woman presents with symptoms of lethargy and pallor. She had diarrhoea 7 days prior to presentation. She has no significant past medical history and does not take regular medications. Her BP is 160/86 mmHg, HR is 85 bpm, SpO2 is 94% on room air, and temperature is 36.5°C. Her baseline creatinine is 65 μmol/L. Her blood film examination shows schistocytes. Stool culture is negative for Shiga toxin-producing *E. Coli* (STEC). Other laboratory results are displayed below.

Tests	Results	Normal values
Haemoglobin	100 g/L	115–55
White blood cell count	5 x 10⁹/L	4–11
Platelet count	78 x 10⁹/L	150–450
Creatinine	200 μmol/L	45–90
Haptoglobin	0.1 g/L	0.3–2.0
LDH	500 U/L	120–250
pH	7.35	7.35–7.45
Bicarbonate	22 mmol/L	22–32 mmol/L
ADAMTS-13	70%	≥68%

She is started on plasma exchange. Which one of the following is the most appropriate next step of management?
- **A.** Cyclophosphamide.
- **B.** Cyclosporin.
- **C.** Eculizumab.
- **D.** Rituximab.

2. A 60-year-old woman presents with pallor and shortness of breath. She is diagnosed with warm-reacting antibody autoimmune haemolytic anaemia (AIHA) for which she is treated with high dose of prednisolone 60mg daily with good response. However, AIHA relapses when the prednisolone dose is tapered to 25mg daily. Her haemoglobin is 65 g/L [115–155], and she is symptomatic. Her type 2 diabetes control is worsening and becomes insulin dependent. Her other comorbidities include hypertension, GORD, and stage 3A CKD.
   Which one of the following is the best management option?
- **A.** Erythropoietin subcutaneous injection.
- **B.** Mycophenolate mofetil 500mg twice a day.
- **C.** Rituximab 375 mg/m² weekly for 4 weeks.
- **D.** Splenectomy after appropriate vaccination.

3. A 66-year-old man with metastatic prostate cancer to the spine, ribs, liver, and lungs presents to the hospital with sudden onset of dyspnoea. He has GORD and osteoarthritis. On examination, HR is 110 bpm in sinus rhythm, BP is 123/59 mmHg, respiratory rate is 24/min, SpO₂ is 90% on room air. CTPA shows bilateral subsegmental pulmonary emboli. ECG and echocardiogram show no evidence of right heart strain.
   Regarding anticoagulation treatment of cancer-related venous thromboembolism (VTE), which one of the following is correct?
- **A.** Oral apixaban is associated with an increased risk of major bleeding compared to subcutaneous dalteparin.
- **B.** Oral apixaban is associated with a higher incidence of recurrent VTE compared to subcutaneous dalteparin.
- **C.** Oral apixaban is non-inferior to subcutaneous dalteparin.
- **D.** Oral apixaban is contraindicated in patients with malignancy related VTE.

How to Pass the FRACP Written Examination, First Edition. Jonathan Gleadle, Jordan Li, Danielle Wu, and Paul Kleinig.
© 2022 John Wiley & Sons Ltd. Published 2022 by John Wiley & Sons Ltd.

4. A 67-year-old man presents with a one-month history of spontaneous bleeding of gums and easy bruising. His other medical history includes smoking-related COPD, type 2 diabetes, and hypertension. He was adopted and his family history is unknown. On examination, extreme pallor of conjunctiva and nail beds is evident. Ecchymotic patches are present on the left lower limb. There is no organomegaly. FBE is shown below. Bone marrow biopsy is consistent with severe aplastic anaemia. Flow cytometry shows the expression of both CD59 and CD55 on RBCs is not reduced.

Tests	Results	Normal values
Hb	76 g/L	135–175
WBC	0.5 x 10^9/L	4–11
Platelet	15 x 10^9/L	150–450

Which one of the following is the most appropriate choice for the initial stage of treatment?
- **A.** Anti-thymocyte globulin followed by cyclosporine.
- **B.** Bone marrow transplantation from an HLA matched donor.
- **C.** Eculizumab intravenous infusion.
- **D.** Oral eltrombopag.

5. The B cell lymphoma 2 (BCL-2) family is an important regulator of the balance between cell survival and cell death. Which of the following best describes the role of BCL-2 proteins?
- **A.** Regulation of cellular growth factors.
- **B.** Regulation of intrinsic, mitochondrial regulated apoptosis.
- **C.** Regulation of mismatch repair recognition.
- **D.** Regulation of the ligand-activated, extrinsic cell death pathway.

6. A 75-year-old man is on long-term treatment with warfarin. He developed a DVT 5 years ago. He was treated with warfarin for 6 months. However, 3 months after stopping warfarin, he developed persistent tachycardia despite taking a β-blocker for his known CCF, hypertension, and CKD. A V/Q scan confirmed multiple PE and he was put on warfarin indefinitely. His most recent INR was 2.0. He will undergo an endoscopy for investigation of epigastric pain and weight loss in one week's time.
The most appropriate management for his anticoagulation is:
- **A.** Bridge with intravenous heparin infusion.
- **B.** Bridge with subcutaneous low molecular weight heparin.
- **C.** Continue current dose of warfarin.
- **D.** Stop warfarin and resume 7 days after endoscopy.

7. A 75-year-old man presents with a 2-month history of weight loss and a low-grade fever. Physical examination shows splenomegaly and palpable lymph nodes in bilateral inguinal regions. He is anaemic with a leucocytosis 56 x10^9 [4-9.5] and has mild thrombocytopaenia. A diagnosis of chronic lymphocytic leukaemia (CLL) is made. The cytogenetic test demonstrates P53 aberration. He has no other medical history apart from osteoarthritis.
The most appropriate initial management is:
- **A.** Chlorambucil.
- **B.** Chlorambucil plus ofatumumab.
- **C.** Ibrutinib.
- **D.** Fludarabine plus cyclophosphamide and rituximab.

8. A 34-year-old woman, G4P1 has a past medical history of 3 spontaneous miscarriages and unprovoked PE, treated with warfarin 1 year ago. She does not take regular medication. Her laboratory results are shown below.

Tests	Results	Normal values
Haemoglobin	135 g/L	115–155
Platelet	160 x 10^9/L	150–450
INR	1.0	0.9–1.3
APTT	70 seconds	24–38
Post-mixing study APTT	70 seconds	24–38

What is the reason for her coagulation study abnormalities?
- **A.** Deficiency in factor V.
- **B.** Deficiency in factor VIII.
- **C.** Deficiency in factor IX.
- **D.** Presence of lupus anticoagulant.

9. Which of the following malignancies is most commonly associated with disseminated intravascular coagulation (DIC) at presentation?
- **A.** Acute lymphoblastic leukaemia.
- **B.** Acute promyelocytic leukaemia.
- **C.** Metastatic ovarian cancer.
- **D.** Metastatic pancreatic cancer.

10. A 49-year-old man is diagnosed with essential thrombocythaemia with a platelet count of 625 x 10^9/L [150-450]. He has no cardiovascular risk factors, and no history of venous or arterial thrombosis. His driver mutation is in the calreticulin (CALR) gene.
   Which of the following treatment strategies is most appropriate?
- **A.** Hydroxyurea alone.
- **B.** Hydroxyurea plus aspirin.
- **C.** Interferon.
- **D.** Observation.

11. A 58-year-old woman presents with fever to the emergency department. She is currently having adjuvant chemotherapy for breast cancer. She has received four, three-weekly cycles of doxorubicin, cyclophosphamide, and 7 days ago received her second dose of weekly paclitaxel. She has been feeling well recently but became hot and sweaty earlier today.
   On examination, temperature is 38.5°C, HR is 90 bpm, and BP is 100/65 mmHg. Her peripherally inserted central catheter (PICC line) insertion site looks clean. The rest of the physical examination is unremarkable. Her liver function and renal function are normal. Her FBE are shown below.

Tests	Results	Normal values
Haemoglobin	105 g/L	115–155
White cell count	1.02 x 10^9/L	4–11
Neutrophils	0.3 x 10^9/L	1.8–7.5
Platelet count	622 x 10^9/L	150–450
Mean corpuscular volume	80 fL	80–100

Which of the following management is most appropriate in addition to an anti-pseudomonal penicillin and beta-lactamase inhibitor?
- **A.** Removal of the PICC line and culture of the tip, antibiotic treatment including glycopeptide.
- **B.** Removal of PICC line and culture of the tip, and two peripheral vein blood cultures.
- **C.** Two sets of blood cultures from the PICC line, two from a peripheral vein, and addition of glycopeptide antibiotic.
- **D.** Two sets of blood cultures from the PICC line, await culture results to guide additional antibiotic treatment.

12. Which of the following immunoglobulins, along with heparin and platelet factor 4, are involved in heparin-induced thrombocytopenia?
- **A.** IgA.
- **B.** IgE.
- **C.** IgG.
- **D.** IgM.

13. A 42-year-old patient presents to her GP with increasing fatigue. She also has a long history of arthritis. Her initial hand X-ray and FBE is shown below.

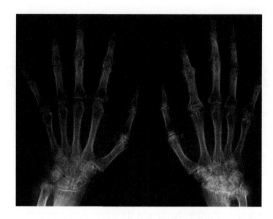

Tests	Results	Normal values
Haemoglobin	86 g/L	125–160
MCV	91 fL	80–98
WBC	7.6 x 10⁹/L	4.00–11.00
Platelets	450 x 10⁹/L	150–450
CRP	35 mg/L	1–8

Which of the following is correct regarding the role of hepcidin in her anaemia ?
  A. Decreased hepcidin level leading to impaired mobilisation of hepatic iron.
  B. Decreased hepcidin level leading to impaired release of iron from macrophages.
  C. Increased hepcidin level leading to a fall in transferrin level.
  D. Increased hepcidin level leading to reduced delivery of iron into the plasma by enterocytes.

14. Which of the following monoclonal antibodies is **LEAST** useful in the treatment of Hodgkin's lymphoma?
  A. Brentuximab vedotin.
  B. Nivolumab.
  C. Pembrolizumab.
  D. Rituximab.

15. Which one of the following statements is true in regard to iron metabolism and storage?
  A. Haem iron and non-haem iron have the same mechanisms of absorption.
  B. Iron is maximally absorbed from the jejunum.
  C. Iron is stored in the cell as free ferrous forms.
  D. Transferrin transports iron in ferric form and delivers it to various tissues.

16. A 27-year-old man is seen in clinic due to a 4-week history of fatigue. He has noticed that he has been bruising more easily. He is very concerned as one of his uncles died from acute leukaemia. He takes a multivitamin daily and protein supplement as part of his gym regimen. On examination, there is no lymphadenopathy or organomegaly. His initial investigations including a blood film are shown below:

Tests	Results	Normal values
Haemoglobin	117 g/L	120–170
WBC	8.0 x 10⁹/L	4.0–11.0
Platelet	45 x 10⁹/L	150–400
INR	1.2	0.9–1.2
APTT	32 seconds	24–38
Creatinine	110 µmol/L	60–110

What is your most appropriate course of action?
A. Arrange a bone marrow biopsy.
B. High dose, pulsed dexamethasone.
C. Intravenous immunoglobulin.
D. No action, watchful waiting.

17. A 72-year-old woman is taking low dose thalidomide for multiple myeloma. She is suffering from severe peripheral neuropathy, constipation, and known to have type 2 diabetes and stage 3 CKD. You are considering a change to lenalidomide. You are discussing with her about the advantage and disadvantage of using lenalidomide.
Which one of the following statements about lenalidomide is correct?
A. It causes haematological toxicity with cytopenia in about 25% of patients.
B. It does not cause peripheral neuropathy.
C. It is not renally cleared so there is no dose adjustment in patients with CKD.
D. It is usually used alone without dexamethasone in patient with diabetes.

18. Which type of monoclonal gammopathy of undetermined significance (MGUS) is associated with an increased rate of progression to multiple myeloma, plasma cell disorder, or other lymphoid disorders and a shorter survival?
A. IgA.
B. IgD.
C. IgG.
D. IgM.

19. A 65-year-old man presents to the emergency department with 3-day history of fever and cough with yellow sputum. He is a current smoker. He has had worsening back pain in the past 3 months and has been taking Ibuprofen every day. He had a fall and landed on his left knee two days ago. On examination, his BP is 105/60 mmHg and temperature is 38 °C. There are crepitations at the right base of the lung. There is tenderness around the left knee. His initial blood test results are shown below. He also has a CXR and plain X-ray of his left knee.

Tests	Results	Normal values
Haemoglobin	93 g/L	135–175
Mean corpuscular volume	90 fL	80–98
White blood cells	8.8 x 10⁹/L	4.0–11.0
Platelets	77 x 10⁹/L	150–400
Creatinine	425 μmol/L	60–110
Calcium	3.20 mmol/L	2.00–2.50
INR	1.5	0.9–1.3

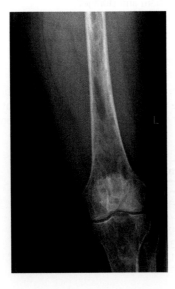
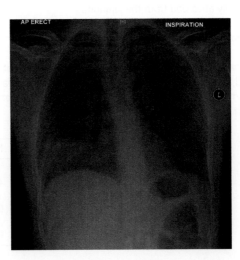

Which investigation would you undertake to make a definitive diagnosis?
   A. Bone marrow biopsy.
   B. Bone scan.
   C. Bronchoalveolar lavage and biopsy.
   D. Kidney biopsy.

20. Ixazomib has been used in the treatment of multiple myeloma, it is classified as a:
   A. Anti-CD38 monoclonal antibody.
   B. Histone deacetylase inhibitor.
   C. Immunomodulatory drug.
   D. Proteasome inhibitor.

21. A 26-year-old woman presents with a two weeks history of right upper quadrant pain and jaundice. She has ascites on examination. She is found to have extensive hepatic vein thrombosis on ultrasound and is started on therapeutic anticoagulation and diuretics. Her beta-hCG is negative. Her liver function tests and symptoms slowly normalise over the subsequent days. She is noted to have the following FBE results:

Tests	Results	Normal values
Haemoglobin	131 g/L	115–155
White cell count	10.25 x 10^9/L	4–11
Platelet count	622 x 10^9/L	150–450
Red blood cells	4.8 x 10^{12}/L	3.5–5.5
Haematocrit	0.42 L/L	0.35–0.45
Mean corpuscular volume	77 fL	80–98

Which of the following tests is most helpful in establishing the diagnosis?
   A. Antiphospholipid antibodies.
   B. Bone marrow biopsy.
   C. Estimation of red-cell mass and plasma-volume.
   D. Flow cytometry of CD55 and CD59 cells.

22. Which of the following statement regarding the cytogenetic abnormalities in non-Hodgkin lymphoma (NHL) is **INCORRECT**?
   A. Burkitt lymphoma results commonly from t(8;14)(q24;q32) translocation or variants leading to overexpression of MYC.
   B. Follicular lymphoma commonly results from t(14;18)(q32;q21) translocation leading to overexpression of BCL-2, which blocks cellular apoptosis.
   C. Mantle cell lymphoma commonly results from t(11;14)(q13;q32) translocation leading to the deregulated expression of cyclin D1.
   D. Peripheral T-cell lymphomas commonly results from t(2;5)(p23;q35) translocation leading to constitutive activation of the ALK tyrosine kinase.

23. A 55-year-old man is diagnosed to have chronic phase chronic myeloid leukaemia with high-risk score. He is started on nilotinib.
   What is the mechanism of action of nilotinib?
   A. Inhibits glutathione reductase.
   B. Inhibits proteasome.
   C. Inhibits programmed death-ligand 1 (PD-L1).
   D. Inhibits tyrosine kinase.

24. A 74-yearr-old woman presents with a 4-month history of gradually increasing fatigue, exertional dyspnoea, and unsteadiness. She has had two falls in the past month. She has noticed numbness and tingling in her hands. On examination, there is no lymphadenopathy or organomegaly. She is pale but is not jaundiced. Neurological examination reveals diminished sensation affecting both feet symmetrically. Both ankle jerks are absent, but the knee jerks are present. Her FBE results and blood film are shown below.

Tests	Results	Normal values
Haemoglobin	85 g/L	115–150
Mean corpuscular volume	115 fl	80–98
WBC	4.1 x 10⁹/L	4.0–11.0
Platelets	155 x 10⁹/L	150–400

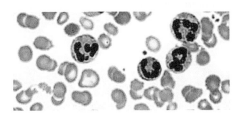

Which one of the following antibodies is most likely to be positive?

A. Anti-dsDNA antibodies.
B. Anti-parietal cell antibodies.
C. Anti-parvovirus B19 antibodies.
D. Anti-thyroglobulin antibodies.

25. A 52-year-old woman has received rituximab, cyclophosphamide, hydroxydaunorubicin, oncovicin, and prednisolone (R-CHOP) therapy for her aggressive mantle cell lymphoma. She is noted to have mild cognitive impairment, dysphasia and dyspraxia while working her up for a stem cell transplant. On lumbar puncture, pressure is normal, there is mild increased protein concentration but normal cell count and glucose level. Her T2-weighted MRI brain shown below:

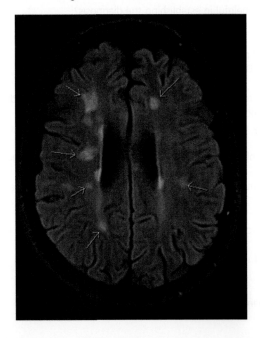

Polymerase chain reaction (PCR) assay of her CSF is most likely to be positive for which virus?

A. BK virus.
B. Herpes simplex.
C. JC virus.
D. Varicella-zoster virus.

26. A 68-year-old retired farmer has polycythaemia vera. He is treated with hydroxyurea 1.5g daily, aspirin 150 mg daily, and venesections for the past 5 years. He develops severe fatigue, weight loss, night sweats, painful leg ulcers, and multiple skin cancers which require surgery with skin graft. His spleen is 20cm on USS which is new. His most recent blood test results are shown below. His bone marrow shows grade 2 fibrosis.

Tests	Results	Normal values
Hb	178 g/L	135–175
Haematocrit	50%	47
WBC	13.7 x 10⁹/L	4–11
Platelet	585 x 10⁹/L	150–450
Creatinine	152 µmol/L	60–110
Bilirubin	30 µmol/L	2–24
LDH	420 IU/L	120–250

Which one of the following is the most appropriate treatment in addition to aspirin and venesection?
  A. A lower dose of hydroxyurea.
  B. Busulphan.
  C. Rituximab.
  D. Ruxolitinib.

27. Which of the following is a significant risk factor for developing chronic graft-versus-host disease (GVHD) in allogeneic haematopoietic stem-cell transplant?
  A. Receiving peripheral-blood stem-cell graft.
  B. Transplant of a male graft to a female recipient.
  C. Transplant of a young graft to a young recipient.
  D. Transplant in a patient with systemic amyloidosis.

28. Which of the following is an indication for exchange transfusion in a patient with sickle cell disease?
  A. Acute chest syndrome.
  B. Acute kidney injury.
  C. Acute pain crisis.
  D. Avascular necrosis.

29. Which one of the following is seen if mobilised peripheral allogenic blood is used as the source for stem cell transplant compared with bone marrow in a patient with acute lymphoid leukaemia?
  A. Faster engraftment.
  B. Less chronic graft versus host disease (GVHD).
  C. Lower patient survival.
  D. Higher rate of relapse.

30. A 38-year-old woman presents with acute right lower limb swelling without recent history of trauma, surgery, or immobility. Ultrasound of the right lower limb confirms a DVT. Her GP had started her on apixaban 2 days ago. There is no family history of DVT, and she is taking no medications.
  What advice would you give to her GP regarding appropriate screening for inherited thrombophilia for this patient?
  A. Screen for inherited thrombophilia now as apixaban has no impact on interpretation of inherited thrombophilia screen.
  B. Screen for inherited thrombophilia once apixaban is ceased after 3 months of treatment.
  C. Stop apixaban for two days, perform the inherited thrombophilia screen then resume apixaban.
  D. There is no indication for screening as there is no family history of DVT.

31. A 40-year-old nurse is admitted to hospital because of melaena. He is on warfarin for a mechanical aortic valve. He was started on cephalexin one week ago because of a skin infection. His INR is 8. Two units of fresh frozen plasma (FFP) are given within two hours. Halfway through the third unit, he develops dyspnoea without fever, chest pain, and cough. His BP is 130/80 mmHg, respiratory rate is 30/min and oxygen saturation is 85% on room air. There are bibasal crepitations. JVP is 3 cm, there is no peripheral oedema and the mechanical valve sounds are normal. His CXR is shown below.

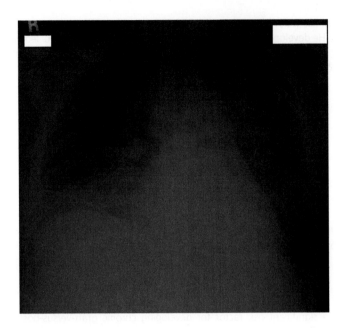

Which one of the following is the most likely diagnosis for this patient?
A. Anaphylaxis.
B. Decompensated heart failure.
C. Disseminated intravascular coagulation.
D. Transfusion-related acute lung injury.

32. A 46-year-old painter presents with a 2-day history of pain, heaviness, and a swollen left arm after painting a ceiling for the prior 10 days. His medical history includes asthma, hypertension, and fatty liver. He is a current smoker. His duplex ultrasound shows left distal subclavian vein thrombosis.

When compared with lower limb DVT, he is more likely to:
A. Have hereditary thrombophilia.
B. Have increased risk of pulmonary embolism.
C. Have recurrence DVT at 12 months.
D. Have underlying occult malignancy.

33. A 22-year-old woman has presented to the emergency department several times with severe epistaxis, which takes a long time to stop bleeding. The patient is well but has noticed that she bruises easily. Her mother also complains of easy and excessive bruising. She is taking vitamin C and B complex but no other medications. Her physical examination is unremarkable. The ENT registrar performs the following tests and asks for a consult.

Tests	Results	Normal values
Hb	135 g/L	115-155
Platelets	200 x 10⁹/L	150–450
INR	1.1	0.9–1.2
APTT	41 seconds	24–38
Thrombin time	16 seconds	12–16
Fibrinogen	2.7 g/L	1.5–4
Factor VIII	45 IU/dL	50–200
D-dimer	<0.5 mg/L	<0.5

Your most likely diagnosis for this patient is:
- **A.** Factor XI deficiency.
- **B.** Factor VIII deficiency.
- **C.** Presence of lupus inhibitor.
- **D.** von Willebrand disease.

34. A 59-year-old Maori woman presents with a 2-month history of weight loss. She developed a severe headache last week and poor vision since yesterday. Her ophthalmologist finds that she has bilateral retinal vein thrombosis, and she is very confused. The ophthalmologist wants her to be reviewed by the medical assessment clinic this afternoon. She is known to have hypertension and type 2 diabetes. On examination, she is afebrile, and her BP is 150/90 mmHg. Cardiovascular and respiratory examinations are unremarkable. Abdominal examination shows hepatosplenomegaly. Her available investigation results are displayed below. Her CT chest and abdomen shows extensive lymphadenopathy including retroperitoneal.

Tests	Results	Normal values
Haemoglobin	87 g/L	115–155
Haptoglobin	3.01 g/L	0.5–2.5
Mean Cell Volume	92 fL	80–98
Reticulocytes	0.6%	0.2–3
Lymphocytes absolute	12.2×10^9/L	1.5–3.5
White Blood Cell Count	16×10^9/L	4–11
Platelet Count	98×10^9/L	150–450
ESR	110 mm/hr	1–20
Creatinine	112 μmol/L	45–90
LDH	263 U/L	120–250
Lactate	1.0 mmol/L	0.2–2.0 mmol/L
IgM	31 g/L	0.5–2.0
Albumin	33 g/L	34–48
Total Protein	96 g/L	60–80 g/L

While awaiting a bone marrow biopsy tomorrow, what is the best management tonight?
- **A.** Anticoagulation with intravenous heparin.
- **B.** Intravenous immune globulin.
- **C.** Intravenous methylprednisolone.
- **D.** Plasma exchange.

35. Protein C acts by:
- **A.** Activating antithrombin III.
- **B.** Activating protein S.
- **C.** Inactivating factor V.
- **D.** Inactivating thrombin.

QUESTIONS (36–39) REFER TO THE FOLLOWING INFORMATION
Match the haematological malignancy with its most likely cytogenetic profile:
- **A.** Complex cytogenetic abnormalities.
- **B.** del(3q).
- **C.** del(9q).
- **D.** Normal karyotype.
- **E.** t(9;22)(q34;q11).
- **F.** t(11;14)(q13q32).
- **G.** t(15;17)(q22;21).
- **H.** Trisomy 12.

36. Acute promyelocytic leukaemia highly responsive to all-trans retinoic acid.

37. Philadelphia chromosome positive chronic myeloid leukaemia.

38. Mantle cell lymphoma.

39. Chronic lymphoid leukaemia.

QUESTIONS (40–45) REFER TO THE FOLLOWING INFORMATION

Match the most likely diagnosis for each of the following clinical presentations and their peripheral blood film examination:

    A. Acute lymphoblastic leukaemia.
    B. Acute myeloid leukaemia.
    C. Atypical haemolytic uremic syndrome.
    D. Beta thalassaemia minor.
    E. Chronic lymphocytic leukaemia.
    F. Chronic myeloid leukaemia.
    G. Hereditary spherocytosis.
    H. Iron deficiency anaemia.
    I. Megaloblastic anaemia.
    J. Multiple myeloma.
    K. Myelodysplastic syndromes.
    L. Sideroblastic anaemia.

40. A 32-year-old woman presents to the emergency department with an 8-hour history of severe right upper quadrant pain. An abdominal ultrasound reveals several mobile gallstones and gallbladder wall thickening which is consistent with acute cholecystitis. The liver is unremarkable but the spleen measures 16 cm. The cholecystitis improves with conservative management. She tells you that her father had a spleen removed and died of infection 2 years later at age of 32. Her investigation results and blood film are displayed below.

Tests	Results	Normal values
Haemoglobin	101 g/L	115–155
Mean corpuscular volume	105 fl	80–98
White blood cells	8.1 x 10⁹/L	4.0–11.0
Platelet count	190 x 10⁹/L	150–400
Reticulocyte count	7%	1–3
Bilirubin	37 µmol/L	2–24
LDH	350 U/L	120–250

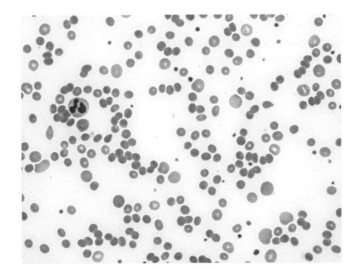

41. An 82-year-old man presents with a 2-month history of gradually increasing tiredness and exertional dyspnoea. He is known to have ischaemic heart disease, severe aortic stenosis, hyperlipidaemia, and stage 3 CKD. His investigation results and blood film are displayed below.

Tests	Results	Normal values
Haemoglobin	100 g/L	135–175
Mean corpuscular volume	76 fl	80–98
White blood cells	8.1 x 10⁹/L	4.0–11.0
Platelet count	190 x 10⁹/L	150–450
Reticulocyte count	4%	1–3
Bilirubin	12 µmol/L	2–24
LDH	200 U/L	120–250

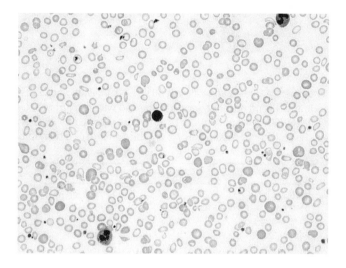

42. A 62-year-old man presents with anorexia, thirst, worsening mid-thoracic back pain. Examination shows tenderness over sternum and mid thoracic spine. There is no lymphadenopathy or organomegaly. Investigation results blood film and CXR are displayed below:

Tests	Results	Normal values
Haemoglobin	100 g/L	135–175
Mean corpuscular volume	90 fL	80–98
White blood cells	8.1 x 10⁹/L	4.0–11.0
Platelets	100 x 10⁹/L	150–400
Creatinine	176 µmol/L	60–110
Calcium	2.60 mmol/L	2.10–2.60
Albumin	20 g/L	34–48
LDH	350 U/L	120–250

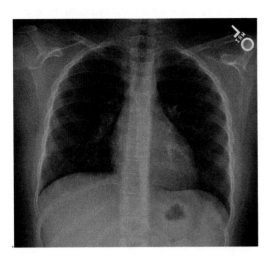
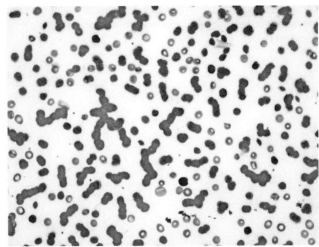

43. A 32-year-old G1P1 woman underwent a Caesarean section at 38 weeks of gestation due to malpresentation. She was found to have hypertension post-surgery. On the second post-operative day she had watery diarrhoea. On the following day, the patient became anuric with hypertension (BP 160/80 mmHg). ADAMTS13 level was reported at 96% and STEC (Shiga toxin-producing *E. coli*) was not present in the stool. Her other investigation results and blood film are displayed below.

Tests	Results	Normal values
Haemoglobin	82 g/L	115–155
Mean corpuscular volume	92 fl	80–98 fl
White blood cells	8.1 x 10^9/L	4.0–11.0
Platelet count	61 x 10^9/L	150–400
Reticulocyte count	7%	1–3
Bilirubin	37 µmol/L	2–24
LDH	1280 U/L	120–250
Creatinine	370 µmol/L	45–90 µmol/L
INR	1.3	0.9–1.3
APTT	32 seconds	24–38
Thrombin time	16 seconds	16–20

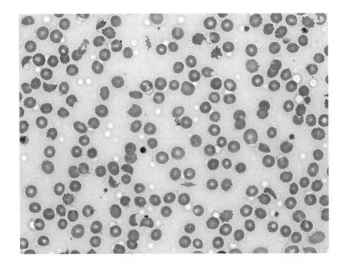

44. A 47-year-old man is brought to emergency department because of fever and chills for 4 hours. His wife reports that he has become fatigued, pale in the last one month, and lost 5 kg of weight. On examination, temperature is 39.5 °C and BP is 100/60 mmHg. There is hepatosplenomegaly, thoracic spine tenderness but no rash or lymphadenopathy. CXR and initial investigation results and blood film are shown below:

Tests	Results	Normal values
Haemoglobin	82 g/L	135–175
Mean corpuscular volume	92 fl	80–98
White blood cells	32.3 x 10⁹/L	4.0–11.0
Platelet count	81 x 10⁹/L	150–400
Reticulocyte count	1%	1–3
Bilirubin	24 μmol/L	2–24
LDH	1280 U/L	120–250
Creatinine	160 μmol/L	60–110
INR	1.8	0.9–1.3
APTT	42 seconds	24–38

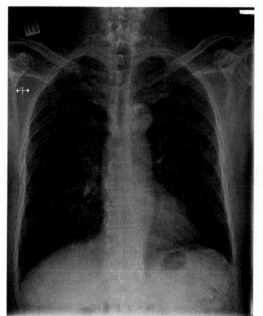

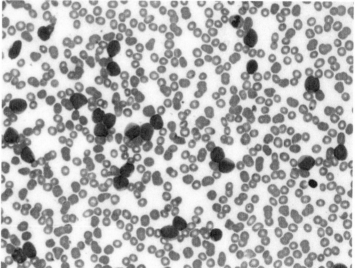

45. A 65-year-old man who presents with a 2-month history of upper abdominal discomfort, anorexia, and two episodes of recent gum bleeds without fever or other bleeding manifestations. He is a chronic smoker with no other comorbidities. Examination reveals moderate hepatosplenomegaly. His initial investigation results and blood film are displayed below.

Tests	Results	Normal values
Haemoglobin	82 g/L	135–175
Mean corpuscular volume	92 fl	80–98
White blood cells	32.5 x 10⁹/L	4.0–11.0
Platelet count	82 x 10⁹/L	150–400
Reticulocyte count	1%	1–3
Bilirubin	24 µmol/L	2–24
LDH	560 U/L	120–250
Creatinine	160 µmol/L	60–110
ESR	102 mm/hr	0–20
APTT	42 seconds	24–38

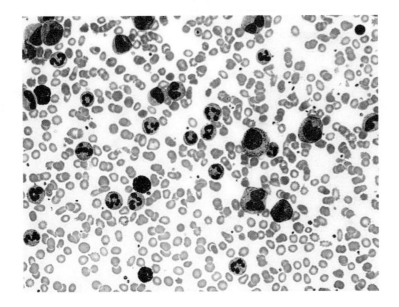

Answers

1. Answer: C

The 2016 International Haemolytic Uraemic Syndrome group classified haemolytic uraemic syndrome (HUS) based on the mechanism of disease into HUS with coexisting diseases or conditions (e.g., malignancy, solid-organ transplantation, haemopoietic stem cell transplantation, autoimmune diseases, medications, malignant hypertension, and pre-existing nephropathy), infection-induced HUS (e.g., Streptococcus pneumoniae-HUS, STEC-HUS, influenza A, H1N1, and HIV), cobalamin C defect-HUS, and atypical HUS.

The patient's clinical presentation and investigations are suggestive of HUS with a typical triad of microangiopathic haemolytic anaemia (MAHA), thrombocytopenia, and AKI. A normal ADAMTS-13 level rules out TTP. The negative stool culture for STEC supports the diagnosis of atypical haemolytic uraemic syndrome (aHUS). During initial presentation, sometimes it is difficult to differentiate typical HUS, TTP from aHUS. Urgent plasma exchange is often indicated until the laboratory test results become available to decide on definitive treatment and can be lifesaving.

Eculizumab is a long-acting humanised monoclonal antibody targeted against complement C5. Eculizumab inhibits the cleavage of C5 into C5a and C5b and hence inhibits deployment of the terminal complement system including the formation of membrane attack complex. Eculizumab is indicated in patients with a diagnosis of aHUS and should be started as soon as the diagnosis of aHUS is confirmed to maximise the renal outcome.

Eculizumab increases the risk of meningococcal and *Neisseria meningitides* infection due to terminal complement pathway blockade and prophylaxis is required for these infections and monitoring of development of complications is important during treatment course. Currently there is insufficient data to suggest the duration of Eculizumab treatment and when it is safe to stop the medication.

	Typical HUS	Atypical HUS	TTP
Diarrhoea	Usually involves diarrhoea (usually bloody)	May or may not involve diarrhoea	Uncommon
MAHA	Yes	Yes	Yes
Thrombocytopenia	Moderate to severe	Moderate to severe	Severe
Epidemic	Yes	No	No
Renal failure	Yes	Yes	Uncommon
Neurologic symptoms	Uncommon	Uncommon	Common
Mechanisms	Shiga-toxin	Alternative pathway complement disorder	AA disintegrin and metalloprotease with thrombospondin type 1 repeats-13 (ADAMTS-13) deficiency
Management	Often resolves with supportive care, with recovery of renal function	May need temporary plasma exchange until diagnosis is clear and then start eculizumab	Urgent plasma exchange

 Fakhouri F, Zuber J, Frémeaux-Bacchi V, Loirat C. Haemolytic uraemic syndrome. The Lancet. 2017;390(10095):681–696. https://www.thelancet.com/journals/lancet/article/PIIS0140-6736(17)30062-4/fulltext

2. Answer: C

Autoimmune haemolytic anaemia (AIHA) is the increased destruction of erythrocytes by anti–erythrocyte autoantibodies. This can occur with or without complement fixation and activation. AIHA can be subdivided into warm- or cold-mediated disease based on the thermal optimum used to detect anti–erythrocyte antibodies. Primary AIHA comprises 50% of cases, while secondary AIHA is usually associated with B-cell malignancies, autoimmune diseases, or medications.

In terms of treatment, if possible, transfusion should be avoided! There is a significant risk for alloantibody formation upon transfusion. Moreover, ongoing haemolysis can be exacerbated by transfusion, since autoantibodies also react with transfused RBCs. The blood product must be compatible with respect to complement-activating alloantibodies present in patient's serum. If possible, the selected product must be negative for the antigens, to which alloantibodies have been identified in the antibody screening. The minimal requirement is that the selected product must be compatible to Rhesus and Kell antigens.

Steroids are effective in the treatment of AIHA and are the treatment of choice. Steroids decrease the production of autoantibodies by B-cells. However, this patient is relapsed with relatively high dose of prednisolone which has caused significant side effects. Therefore, second line treatment should be considered.

With refractory or relapsed AIHA, secondary treatment should be considered in the following situations:

- Requirement of 20 mg of prednisone daily to maintain haemolysis control.
- Clinically significant relapse, haemoglobin <110 g/L or symptomatic anaemia with ongoing evidence of haemolysis.
- Intolerance to a currently effective treatment.

If haemolysis continues but is well compensated after prednisone tapering, starting a second-line treatment may not be necessary. Similarly, Direct Antiglobulin Test (DAT) negativity is not essential with controlled haemolysis. The second line treatment is now rituximab rather than splenectomy. In a meta-analysis of 21 studies, the overall response (OR) and complete response (CR) rates of were 79% and 42%, respectively. The OR was similar regardless of whether it was idiopathic or secondary AIHA (67% vs 72%). In studies with 3 years of follow-up, the relapse rate was 50%; however, most patients responded to rituximab retreatment.

 Go R, Winters J, Kay N. How I treat autoimmune haemolytic anemia. Blood. 2017;129(22):2971–2979. https://ashpublications.org/blood/article-lookup/doi/10.1182/blood-2016-11-693689

3. Answer: C

In patients with malignancy-related VTE, recent guidelines recommend consideration of the use of anti-Xa inhibitors such as oral apixaban. A multinational, randomiseds, open-label, noninferior trial was conducted and found oral apixaban was non-inferior to subcutaneous dalteparin for treatment of VTE in this group of patients. Recurrent VTE was observed in 5.6% in the oral apixaban group and in 7.9% in the dalteparin group. The use of oral apixaban is not associated with an increased risk of major bleeding. Major bleeding happened in 3.8% in the apixaban group and is 4% in the dalteparin group.

 Agnelli G, Becattini C, Meyer G, Muñoz A, Huisman M, Connors J et al. Apixaban for the Treatment of Venous Thrombo-embolism Associated with Cancer. New England Journal of Medicine. 2020;382(17):1599–1607. https://www.nejm.org/doi/pdf/10.1056/NEJMoa1915103

4. Answer: A

Aplastic anaemia (AA) is a rare and heterogeneous disorder. It is defined as pancytopenia with a hypocellular bone marrow in the absence of an abnormal infiltrate or marrow fibrosis. To diagnose AA there must be at least two of the following: haemoglobin <100 g/l, platelet count <50 x 10⁹/l, and neutrophil count <1.5 x 10⁹/l. The majority (70–80%) of cases are idiopathic. Several inherited/genetic disorders are characterised by AA, usually in association with one or more somatic abnormality. AA typically presents in childhood, but this can sometimes be in adulthood.

A fatty bone marrow is the basic diagnostic feature of AA. Accurate diagnosis is required for appropriate and effective management. Idiopathic AA is a diagnosis of exclusion and the diagnostic evaluation must exclude alternative aetiologies of bone marrow failure.

The modified Camitta criteria is used to assess severity. For example, severe AA, marrow cellularity <25%, plus at least 2 of: (i) neutrophils <0.5 x 10⁹/l, (ii) platelets <20 x 10⁹/l (iii) reticulocyte count <20 x 10⁹/l.

Immunosuppressive therapy (IST) is recommended first line therapy for non-severe AA patients requiring treatment, severe or very severe AA patients who lack a matched sibling donor (MSD), and severe or very severe AA patients aged >35–50 years. The current standard first line IST is horse anti-thymocyte globulin (ATG) combined with cyclosporine.

Up-front MSD haematopoietic stem cell transplantation (HSCT) for young and adult patients is the treatment of choice for severe AA, but patients aged between 35–50 years need to be carefully assessed for comorbidities prior to consideration for transplantation. Unrelated donor HSCT in adults should be considered after lack of response to one course of IST. There have been recent improvements in outcomes after alternative donor HSCT for patients who lack a suitably matched donor. There is no place for allogeneic HSCT as first line therapy in patients aged > 60 years.

Haematopoietic growth factors are ineffective in AA. However, eltrombopag, a synthetic mimetic of thrombopoietin, showed activity in patients with refractory AA. Approximately half the patients had robust trilineage improvements in blood counts, which in most cases were durable after discontinuation of the drug. When eltrombopag was added to initial standard IST, it markedly increased the overall response rate to 80% and the complete response rate to 50%, with patients often having rapid haematologic recovery.

All patients with AA should be screened for paroxysmal nocturnal haemoglobinuria (PNH) using flow cytometry on peripheral blood to detect deficiency of glycosylphosphatidyl-inositol (GPI) anchored proteins, such as CD14, CD16 and CD24, as well as fluorescent aerolysin (FLAER) for WBCs, and CD55 and CD59 for RBC analysis. Patients should be screened for PNH at the diagnosis of AA. If persistently negative, test 6-monthly for 2 years and then move to annual testing unless symptoms/signs develop. Small PNH clones can be detected in up to 50% of patients with AA, usually without evidence of haemolysis; large clones are clinically significant and may result in haemolysis as well as increased thrombotic risk. Presence of a small/moderate PNH clone in AA does not directly influence the choice of treatment. Patients with confirmed PNH should be considered for eculizumab treatment.

Young N. Aplastic Anemia. New England Journal of Medicine. 2018;379(17):1643–1656.
https://www.nejm.org/doi/10.1056/NEJMra1413485

5. Answer: B

Ligand-activated (extrinsic) apoptosis, and mitochondrial regulated (intrinsic) apoptosis represent the two main pathways for cellular apoptosis, although there is evidence for some crosstalk between the two systems. Intrinsic apoptosis is activated by internal cellular stimuli representing cellular stress, such as γ-irradiation, cytokines, cellular growth factor withdrawal and DNA damage. Ligand-activated apoptosis requires external binding to transmembrane receptors (for example FasR), to initiate apoptotic pathways. Both pathways result in production of caspases, which results in cleavage of intracellular proteins and cell death.

BCL-2 family proteins can be either pro-apoptotic or anti-apoptotic, and the balance between the two is critical in normal cell development and death. Of particular relevance, different BCL-2 proteins have contrasting roles in the normal development of lymphoid cells, and BCL-2 family proteins are implicated in various lymphoid malignancies. For example, the drug venetoclax mimics the action of BH3–a BCL-2 family protein that has pro-apoptotic activity. Venetoclax has shown some promise in treating chronic lymphoid leukaemia, small lymphocytic lymphoma, and potentially some other lymphoid malignancies.

Campbell K, Tait S. Targeting BCL-2 regulated apoptosis in cancer. Open Biology. 2018;8(5):180002.
https://royalsocietypublishing.org/doi/10.1098/rsob.180002

6. Answer: C

Many patients receive warfarin to minimise their long-term risk of thromboembolism (TE). If a patient needs to undergo a medical procedure/operation, clinicians need to consider the following questions:

1. Does this patient need to stop warfarin?
2. If yes, how soon before the procedure should this patient stop taking wafarin?
3. During the period of not taking wafarin, should the patient receive bridging anticoagulant therapy?
4. After the procedure/operation, when should patient restart warfarin?

Warfarin should not be interrupted for patients undergoing low bleeding-risk procedures (Table 1), particularly those at high risk for TE. Uninterrupted warfarin throughout the periprocedural period is not associated with increased bleeding risk for the listed procedures below, especially when INR is within therapeutic range.

Cataract surgery	Biopsy, superficial and minor
Dermatologic surgery	Minor dental procedures, cleaning
Endoscopy	Endovascular interventions
Percutaneous coronary interventions	Cardiac electrophysiology studies and ablations
Total knee arthroplasty	Arthroscopic surgery

Endoscopy including mucosal biopsy can be performed in patients on warfarin with an INR of 2 to 3. Continuous warfarin can paradoxically reduce periprocedural bleeding relative to interrupted warfarin with heparin bridging. Moreover, warfarin interruption and reinitiation is associated with an increased incidence of stroke. This paradox is due to early depletion of the vitamin K–dependent factors, proteins C and S, creating a hypercoagulable milieu. There are no absolute rules so the risks and benefits should be discussed with the patient before the procedure and an individual decision should be made. If warfarin is stopped, it is safe to restart on the evening of the low bleeding risk procedure.

Bridging anticoagulant therapy is the administration of a short-acting parenteral anticoagulant during the peri-operative period, when the patient is not taking wafarin. The goal is to minimise both the risk of TE events and the risk of bleeding.

When to stop warfarin: Warfarin should be stopped at least 5 days before surgery. About 7% of patients will still have an INR >1.5 after not taking warfarin for 5 days. All patients should have their INR checked on the day of surgery. For patients with an INR of 1.5 to 1.9 on the day prior to surgery, administration of 1 mg of vitamin K will lower the INR to 1.4 in 90% of cases.

Knowledge of a patient's medical history is critical in stratifying peri-procedural TE risk. A history of AF, mechanical heart valve(s), and previous VTE are independent risk factors for peri-procedural thrombotic events. Patients can be risk-stratified based on the anticipated annualised rate of thrombosis or embolisation: <5%, 5% – 10%, or >15% for the respective low, medium, and high-risk groups.

Patients with AF: Low risk is defined as a CHADS2 score of 0 to 2, assuming that the 2 points are not scored for TIA or CVA. Medium risk is a score of 3 or 4. High-risk patients include those with a TIA or CVA within the previous 3 months; a CHADS2 score of 5 or 6 or any patient with a history of rheumatic heart disease. Patients with CHADS2 scores <5 but with a TIA or CVA 3 months ago are high risk.

Patients with a mechanical heart valve: Knowledge of the valve type and location is essential in stratifying the risk of peri-procedural thrombosis. Patients with bileaflet aortic valve prostheses without additional risk factors for stroke or AF are at low risk. Patients with bileaflet valve with additional risk factors for stroke such as AF, age >75, prior CVA (>6 months prior), hypertension, diabetes, or CCF have medium risk. Patients at high risk include those with aortic valve prosthesis with a caged-ball or tilting disc, a mitral valve prosthesis, and those with a mechanical valve with CVA or TIA during the prior 6 months.

Patients with history of VTE: The time that has passed since last VTE is an important factor in stratifying risk for peri-procedural thrombosis. Patients are low risk if they had VTE more than 1 year prior to the procedure. Medium-risk patients are those with VTE events in the preceding 3 to 12 months, those with recurrent VTE, those with active cancer who have received cancer therapy within 6 months, or patients with non-severe thrombophilias such as heterogenous factor V Leiden or prothrombin gene mutation. High-risk patients as those with VTE that has occurred within 3 months or those with severe thrombophilias such as Protein C or S deficiency, antithrombin III deficiency, or antiphospholipid antibody syndrome.

Assessment of procedure-related thrombotic risk: The type of procedure itself conveys peri-procedural thrombotic risk. Heart valve replacement, carotid endarterectomy, or other major vascular surgeries automatically stratify patients in the high-risk category, regardless of underlying medication condition.

Assessment of bleeding risk: Pre-existing bleeding risk factors such as thrombocytopenia and post-procedural bleeding risks should be assessed. Risk factors for increased post-procedural bleeding include: major surgery with extensive tissue injury, procedures involving highly vascularised organs, removal of large colonic polyps, urological procedures, placement of implantable cardioverter-defibrillator/pacemakers, ERCP with sphincterotomy, dilation of strictures, therapy of varices, PEG, EUS with FNA and procedures at sites where minor bleeding would be clinically devastating, such as the brain or spine. Communication with the proceduralist/surgeon regarding the anticipated bleeding risk is vital.

Should the patient receive bridging anticoagulation? Patients considered high risk for peri-procedural thrombosis should receive peri-procedural bridging anticoagulation, while those considered low risk should not. For patients with a moderate peri-procedural risk of thrombosis, the decision should be based on individual and anticipated pre-surgical/procedural thrombotic risks. Bridging anticoagulation should be avoided in patients undergoing procedures with high bleeding risk who are not at high thromboembolic risk.

Selection and pre-operative discontinuation of bridging medication: Unfractionated heparin (UFH) or low molecular weight heparin (LMWH) is the bridging anticoagulants. Evidence supports the use of either intravenous UFH (APTT 1.5 to two times control APTT) or enoxaparin (1 mg/kg BD or 1.5 mg/kg once daily). UFH is preferred over LMWH in patients with CKD stage 4 or 5 due to a more predictable pharmacokinetic profile. Bridging should be started when INR <2 and discontinued 6 hours prior to the procedure. LMWH should be discontinued 24 hours prior to the procedure.

When to restart UHF or LMWH bridge post-procedure: The type of procedure dictates when bridging anticoagulation should resume. In patients who have undergone surgeries that involve high bleeding risk, LMWH should not be resumed until 48–72 hours post-surgery. For those patients undergoing low bleeding risk surgeries, bridging should be resumed 24 hours after the procedure. Enoxaparin administered in one single daily dose, as compared to divided doses, is associated with a greater risk of post-operative bleeding. UFH bridging should resume post-operatively without a bolus dose at 24 hours in low-risk bleeding cases or 48–72 hours in high-risk bleeding cases.

When to restart warfarin: The resumption of warfarin may occur once post-operative haemostasis has been achieved and the patient can resume eating. This most often occurs on the day following surgery, because it takes approximately 5 days for an INR to achieve therapeutic levels.

Novel anticoagulants in the periprocedural period: Novel oral anticoagulants (NOACs) are increasingly used for the treatment of AF and VTE. Patients with AF in large trials did not experience increased TE or bleeding events perioperatively, whether bridged or unbridged – even those undergoing major or urgent surgical procedures. Given their pharmacokinetic similarities to LMWHs, NOACs may potentially offer a safer and simpler periprocedural management strategy than warfarin. In the RE-LY trial, 46% of patients treated with dabigatran were able to have their procedure within 48 h of stopping the drug, compared with only 11% of patients treated with warfarin. Experience is accumulating for the periprocedural use of NOACs. However, further studies and clinical experience are needed. It is unclear if uninterrupted NOAC therapy is appropriate during even low bleeding-risk procedures. It is also unclear how soon after a procedure an NOAC can safely be restarted. Clinical decision about periprocedural use of NOACs may become less challenging as novel reversal agents for NOACs are available now. A recent, nonrandomised cohort study showed that idarucizumab completely reverses the anticoagulant effect of dabigatran within minutes. A conservative strategy that favours less bridging anticoagulation and, therefore, less periprocedural bleeding is recommended when managing periprocedural NOACs.

Rechenmacher S, Fang J. Bridging Anticoagulation. Journal of the American College of Cardiology. 2015;66(12): 1392–1403.https://www.sciencedirect.com/science/article/pii/S0735109715047439?via%3Dihub

7. Answer: C

Chronic lymphocytic leukaemia (CLL) is the most common leukaemia occurring in adults in developed countries and is characterised by the clonal proliferation and accumulation of mature and typically CD5-positive B cells within the blood, bone marrow, lymph nodes, and spleen. Significant advances in understanding the pathogenesis of CLL, especially that more than 80% of patients with newly diagnosed CLL carry a genetic aberration, have led to the development of new prognostic and diagnostic tools and new drugs.

The criteria for initiating treatment rely on the Rai and Binet staging systems and on the presence of CLL symptoms. Most newly diagnosed patients present with asymptomatic, early-stage disease (Rai 0; Binet A); they should be monitored without treatment until disease progression. Initiating treatment early has no benefit but could cause harm. The absolute lymphocyte count should not be used as the sole indicator for treatment. Treatment should be initiated in patients with advanced disease (Rai stage III and IV; Binet stage C) and for patients with symptomatic disease which includes:

- Progressive marrow failure (anaemia or thrombocytopenia or both).
- Massive or progressive or symptomatic splenomegaly or lymphadenopathy.
- Autoimmune anaemia or thrombocytopenia, or both, not responding to corticosteroids.
- B symptoms: unintentional weight loss, fatigue, fevers of more than 38·0 °C for at least 2 weeks without infection, or night sweats. Alternative causes for B symptoms should be ruled out before starting an anti-leukaemic treatment.
- Rapidly progressive lymphocytosis (a lymphocyte doubling time of less than 6 months), when lymphocyte doubling time is used as the sole criteria for treatment initiation, initial blood lymphocyte counts should be more than 30 x 10^9/L

Chemoimmunotherapy with fludarabine, cyclophosphamide, and rituximab (FCR) is the standard treatment for physically fit patients with CLL. For fit patients older than 65 years, obinutuzumab plus chlorambucil (https://www.eviq.org.au/) could be an alternative first-line therapy to decrease potential toxicity. Chlorambucil has long been the standard therapy for elderly patients and patients with comorbidities independent of age. More potent drugs (e.g. fludarabine and alemtuzumab) do not improve survival.

P53 is a gene which is located on the short arm of chromosome 17. Somatic mutations in the P53 gene are one of the most frequent alterations in human cancers, and germline mutations are the underlying cause of Li-Fraumeni syndrome, which predisposes to a wide spectrum of early-onset cancers. P53 mutations are also potential prognostic and predictive markers, as well as targets for pharmacological intervention. CLL patients with a P53 aberration have a very aggressive disease and respond poorly to chemoimmunotherapy. The incidence of P53 aberrations at diagnosis is approximately 5% but increases with disease progression and additional lines of treatment (50%). The outcome for patients with P53 aberration improved with the introduction of ibrutinib, idelalisib, and venetoclax, which all act independently of the P53 pathway. Both ibrutinib alone and idelalisib combined with either rituximab or ofatumumab induce high response rates and promising progression-free survival and overall survival. Despite this progress, the presence of a P53 aberration in the leukaemic clone retains its adverse prognostic effect, and treatment outcomes remain inferior with respect to the quality and duration of response compared with patients who do not have these genetic abnormalities. Cytogenetic tests should be done when active treatment is required.

Hallek M, Shanafelt T, Eichhorst B. Chronic lymphocytic leukaemia. The Lancet. 2018;391(10129):1524–1537. https://www.thelancet.com/journals/lancet/article/PIIS0140-6736(18)30422-7/fulltext

8. Answer: D

If prolonged prothrombin time (PT) and/or APTT is observed, a repeat blood test needs to be done to ensure no sampling errors. Other common causes of prolonged PT and/or APTT include heparin use, anticoagulant use, liver disease, coagulation factor deficiency, and presence of inhibitors, such as lupus anticoagulant or Factor VIII inhibitors.

A mixing study is the next investigation if no other extrinsic causes of prolonged PT and/or APTT are suspected. To perform the test, mix the patient's plasma 1:1 with pooled plasma that contains 100% of the normal factor level. If patients have factor deficiency, the PT and APTT will be normalised after adding normal plasma. However, in patients with inhibitors such as lupus anticoagulant or factor VIII inhibitors, the prolonged PT and APTT will fail to correct.

This patient's mixing study fails to correct the APTT/PT after adding normal pooled plasma. As a result, the prolonged APTT is likely caused by the presence of inhibitors. Antiphospholipid syndrome (APS) is a possible diagnosis given the history of recurrent spontaneous miscarriages and thrombotic complications. APS is associated with thrombosis in the arteries, veins, and/or small vessels. APS can also cause pregnancy-related complications such as recurrent spontaneous miscarriage, stillbirth, preterm delivery, and severe preeclampsia, etc.

The diagnosis criteria of APS require fulfilment of at least one clinical event (i.e., thrombotic or pregnancy-related complications) and at least one laboratory criteria (i.e., antibody blood tests spaced at least three months apart, confirming the presence of lupus anticoagulant, anti-ß2-glycoprotein-1, or anticardiolipin antibody of IgG and/or IgM isotype in serum or plasma.)

In patients with haemophilia A, there is a deficiency in factor VIII. In patients with haemophilia B, there is a deficiency in factor IX. Haemophilia A and B are inherited in an x-linked recessive pattern causing factor deficiencies and lifelong bleeding disorders.

 Chaudhry R, Usama SM, Babiker H. Physiology, Coagulation Pathways [Internet]. Ncbi.nlm.nih.gov. 2020 [cited 13 April 2020]. Available from:
https://www.ncbi.nlm.nih.gov/books/NBK482253/

9. Answer: B

DIC is a state in which the coagulation cascades are excessively activated throughout the circulation, rather than in response to local injury. The resultant over-activity of coagulation results in consumption of factors involved in coagulation, consumption of platelets, elevated fibrin degradation products, prolonged clotting times, and often microangiopathic haemolytic anaemia. This is most often manifested as venous or arterial thrombus formation, or excessive bleeding. Cancer most likely causes hyper activation of the coagulation cascade through cancer procoagulant, cytokines, and treatment of the cancer leading to endothelial injury. Additionally, deranged fibrinolysis leading to excessive hypofibrinogenaemia is a critical step in acute leukaemias. At diagnosis, around 90% of patients with acute promyelocytic leukaemia (APML) meet diagnostic criteria for DIC, as compared to 15–20% of patients with acute lymphoblastic leukaemia, and 7% in solid malignancies, particularly mucin secreting adenocarcinoma. DIC in APML is usually characterised by profound hypofibrinogenaemia and excessive bleeding, whereas DIC in solid malignancy is associated with procoagulants and venous or arterial thrombo-embolism. Non-bacterial thrombotic endocarditis with systemic embolism is a particular feature of mucin-secreting adenocarcinoma with DIC.

 Levi M. Clinical characteristics of disseminated intravascular coagulation in patients with solid and hematological cancers. Thrombosis Research. 2018; 164: S77–S81.
https://www.thrombosisresearch.com/article/S0049-3848(18)30016-1/fulltext

10. Answer: D

Treatment of essential thrombocythaemia (ET) focuses on ensuring freedom from thrombotic and bleeding events. As progression to secondary acute leukaemia is low and prognosis is very good, induction of remission of the disease is not a priority. A bone marrow biopsy is not required if the patient has only thrombocytosis and a driver mutation, e.g., JAK, or CALR, or MPL. A bone marrow biopsy will be performed if the diagnosis is in doubt, e.g., if there is also anaemia, or if blood film shows a leucoerythroblastic blood picture.

Most of the treatment strategies for ET are driven by observational studies quantifying risk of adverse outcomes. However, the use of hydroxyurea in patients at risk of thrombotic events is established by randomised trial data. The three main risk factors taken into consideration for treatment of ET are age, history of thrombotic events, and driver mutation status. Absence of all risk factors constitutes "very low risk' disease, and can be treated with observation alone, or aspirin alone if there are cardiovascular risk factors. Mutation in the Janus kinase 2 (JAK2) or thrombopoetin receptor (MPL) genes, constitutes low risk disease, and can be treated with aspirin alone. Intermediate risk disease is defined by older age (>60 years) without history of thrombosis or JAK2/MPL mutation and can be treated with hydroxyurea and aspirin. High risk disease is defined by a history of thrombosis or older age plus JAK2/MPL mutation and is treated with hydroxyurea plus twice daily aspirin, in the case of arterial thrombosis or hydroxyurea, plus systemic anticoagulation in the case of venous thrombosis. Another important treatment consideration is the avoidance of aspirin in patients with acquired von Willebrand Syndrome, which occurs mostly, but not exclusively, in patients with extremely high platelet counts.

Tefferi A, Vannucchi A, Barbui T. Essential thrombocythemia treatment algorithm 2018. Blood Cancer Journal. 2018;8(1).
https://www.nature.com/articles/s41408-017-0041-8

11. Answer: C

Management of febrile neutropaenia (FN) such in this case requires prompt initiation of antibiotic therapy within one hour of presentation to hospital to minimise risk of complications. Glycopeptide antibiotics should always be administered whenever catheter-related infection (CRI) is suspected. Additional antibiotic regimens differ according to local microbial susceptibility patterns but usually involve administration of a fourth-generation cephalosporin or anti-pseudomonal penicillin plus beta-lactamase inhibitor to provide broad spectrum gram-negative cover. This obviously involves administration of antibiotics prior to knowing the absolute neutrophil count in the majority of cases and relies on the clinician recognising the risk of FN for a particular individual. Reduction of the incidence of FN can be successfully achieved for high-risk groups with administration of granulocyte colony-stimulating factors (G-CSF). The use of preventative antibiotics is more controversial: while this practice decreases the risk of FN, it also makes the emergence of FN with resistant organisms much more likely. Thorough and early work-up is also highly important in guiding future therapy and includes microbiological assessment of any suspected sites of infection.

Risk of morbidity and mortality with FN remains high (up to 10% in hospitalised patients), particularly in patients with acute leukaemia. The risk of FN is also high in older patients, advanced disease, mucositis, poor performance status, dose-dense regimens, and regimens without use of G-CSF. Nadir of neutrophil count typically occurs between 7 and 14 days after administration of chemotherapy but is not predictable.

Patients at low risk for complications can be managed with early outpatient therapy, and their risk can be ascertained by the Multinational Association of Supportive Care in Cancer (MASCC) prognostic index. Blood cultures are positive in around 20% of cases. Historically, gram-negative bacteraemia was found to be the most common cause, but the microbiology of FN is now more diverse, with gram-positives and fungal causes being the more common culprit.

CRI is also an important consideration in any patient undergoing chemotherapy via an indwelling intravenous line. Differential time to positivity (DTTP) is highly sensitive and specific in diagnosing CRI. This involves obtaining two sets of blood cultures at each site and measurement of the difference in time in which the cultures become positive. This method has the benefit of being able to retain lines that are not infected, as well as making informed decisions about risk for the remaining line. Some CRIs (for example those due to coagulase-negative staphylococcus) can be treated with retention of the line, but most require line removal.

Klastersky J, de Naurois J, Rolston K, Rapoport B, Maschmeyer G, Aapro M et al. Management of febrile neutropaenia:
ESMO Clinical Practice Guidelines†. Annals of Oncology. 2016;27(suppl_5). v111–v118.
https://www.esmo.org/Guidelines/Supportive-and-Palliative-Care/Management-of-Febrile-Neutropaenia

12. Answer: C

Heparin-induced thrombocytopenia (HIT) is a prothrombotic adverse reaction that occurs following the administration of unfractionated heparin or low molecular weight heparin and is caused by almost exclusively IgG antibodies to platelet factor 4 (PF4) and heparin. Thrombocytopenia and thrombosis in HIT result from the binding of PF4–heparin–IgG complex to FcγRIIa receptors on the platelet surface. Cross-linking of the receptors then causes intense platelet activation, release of platelet granule content and procoagulant microparticles, thrombin generation, and activation of endothelial cells, neutrophils, and monocytes. Thrombosis could be arterial, venous, or microvascular.

Accurate diagnosis is important and can be lifesaving. Once the condition is suspected, early consultation with a haematology specialist is recommended as delay in diagnosis and appropriate anticoagulant treatment is associated with an initial 6% daily risk of thromboembolism, amputation, and death.

Incidences of HIT are noted more in surgical than medical patients, and rarely in paediatric and obstetric patients, more in patients given unfractionated heparin than low molecular weight heparin, and more in patients given therapeutic dose than prophylactic dose of heparin. Diagnosis of HIT is essential to determine treatment strategies using non-heparin anticoagulants and to avoid unwanted and potential fatal thromboembolic complications.

HIT is a clinicopathological entity and requires good history taking and laboratory testing to confirm the diagnosis. A 4Ts (**t**hrombocytopenia, **t**iming of platelet count fall, **t**hrombosis or other sequalae, other cause of **t**hrombocytopenia) score is recommended to determine the pre-test probability of HIT for all patients suspicious of HIT prior to laboratory testing. If a patient has low probability of HIT on 4Ts score: further testing with an immunoassay or functional assay is not recommended. However, if there are missing or unreliable clinical data, laboratory testing is recommended to exclude HIT. Intermediate or high probability of HIT on 4Ts score and a positive immunoassay result: initial treatment should include discontinuing heparin and considering a non-heparin alternative. Laboratories should provide a rapid, on demand, high sensitivity, IgG selective immunological assay. Positive immunoassay results should be confirmed with functional testing, regardless of 4Ts score.

Heparin and low molecular weight heparin exposure must be ceased in patients with suspected or confirmed HIT. Continued use of heparin, even in low concentrations, has been associated with adverse outcomes in HIT patients. A non-heparin anticoagulant (danaparoid, argatroban, fondaparinux, and bivalirudin) should be used to treat HIT and should be given in therapeutic rather than prophylactic doses. Argatroban is the preferred anticoagulant in the presence of severe renal impairment (creatinine clearance < 30 mL/min). Direct oral anticoagulants can be used in place of warfarin after patients with HIT have responded to alternative parenteral anticoagulants. Patients with isolated HIT should receive therapeutic anticoagulation until platelet levels are > 150 x 10⁹/L. Platelet transfusions are not indicated to treat thrombocytopenia due to HIT in the absence of clinical bleeding. Patients with HIT and thrombosis should receive therapeutic anticoagulation for a minimum of 3 months. Patients with a proven history of HIT should avoid the use of heparin for future procedures.

 Joseph J, Rabbolini D, Enjeti A, Favaloro E, Kopp M, McRae S et al. Diagnosis and management of heparin-induced thrombocytopenia: a consensus statement from the Thrombosis and Haemostasis Society of Australia and New Zealand HIT Writing Group. Medical Journal of Australia. 2019;210(11):509–516.
https://onlinelibrary.wiley.com/doi/abs/10.5694/mja2.50213

13. Answer: D

The hand X-ray shows erosive arthritis affecting bilateral PIP, MCP and wrist joints which is likely due to rheumatoid arthritis or inflammatory arthritis. She has moderate normochromic normocytic anaemia likely secondary to her undiagnosed and untreated rheumatoid arthritis, that is anaemia of chronic disease (ACD).

ACD is the most common cause of anaemia in admitted patients and the second most prevalent cause of anaemia, after iron deficiency anaemia (IDA). The pathophysiology of ACD is multifactorial, including shortened RBC survival, impaired proliferation of erythroid progenitor cells, and abnormal iron metabolism. These mechanisms are immune and/or inflammation driven, but other factors including chronic blood loss, haemolysis, or vitamin deficiencies contribute to ACD. All the abnormalities of iron metabolism observed in ACD can be explained by the effect on hepcidin upregulation.

Hepcidin is a small peptide synthesised by hepatocytes, that inhibits the cellular macrophage efflux of iron and intestinal iron absorption, binding to ferroportin and inducing its internalisation and degradation. Hepcidin synthesis is induced by iron overload, inflammation, and is inhibited by anaemia and hypoxia. It is an acute phase reactant type II. In ACD, the synthesis of hepcidin is up-regulated by increased inflammatory cytokines IL-6 and probably by IL-1. It acts by inhibiting export of iron from the iron-containing cells–duodenal endothelial cells and macrophages. This action is mediated via the effect on ferroportin, whereby hepcidin induces its breakdown/degradation. Ferroportin is the sole iron exporter in iron-containing cells. This is thought to be the main pathogenetic mechanism of ACD. Serum hepcidin is currently being proposed as the most accurate serological marker for the differentiation of ACD and IDA. Patients with mutations in the hepcidin gene have a decreased production of hepcidin, which results in a severe form of juvenile hereditary haemochromatosis. Iron overload occurs in the hepatocytes as intestinal iron absorption and macrophageal iron release continue unhampered in the absence of hepcidin.

ACD is difficult to treat. The recommended approach is the treatment of the underlying disease, which can lead to a major improvement or even resolution of ACD. Currently available treatments (transfusion, iron, and erythropoiesis-stimulating agents) can ameliorate anaemia, but a considerable percentage of non-responders exist.

 Poggiali E, Migone De Amicis M, Motta I. Anemia of chronic disease: A unique defect of iron recycling for many different chronic diseases. European Journal of Internal Medicine. 2014;25(1):12–17.
https://www.ejinme.com/article/S0953–6205(13)00189-1/fulltext

14. Answer: D

Treatment with first-line therapy for Hodgkin's lymphoma results in long-term remission in 75% of cases. Conventional first-line therapy is with combination chemotherapy with or without radiation. Relapsed or refractory disease is treated with salvage chemotherapy followed by autologous stem-cell transplantation (ASCT). The five-year survival of this cohort is reduced to around 50%.

Treatment for relapsed/refractory disease has advanced with monoclonal antibody therapies that can improve long-term response rates significantly. Reed–Sternberg cells almost universally express CD30, which allows anti-CD30 antibody-drug conjugate Brentuximab vedotin (BV) to deliver mono-methyl auristatin E into CD30 expressing cells, inducing apoptosis. BV is indicated for treatment of Hodgkin's lymphoma in the replacement of bleomycin in the "ABVD' regimen, resulting in reduced pulmonary toxicity; relapsed or refractory disease after salvage chemotherapy with or without ASCT; or maintenance therapy after ASCT. Although the studies powering these indications have not been of sufficient duration to show difference in overall survival, the historical evidence would suggest that incorporation of BV into the regimen has resulting in significantly longer survival for patients with relapsed or refractory disease.

Reed–Sternberg cells and cells within their tumour microenvironment, such as benign reactive cells and tumour-associated macrophages are implicated in immune escape, through expression of PD-L1. This can occur as a result of chromosome 9p24.1 amplification, but also due to up-regulation mediated by the EBV. As a consequence, blockade of this pathway with nivolumab and pembrolizumab has also emerged as a treatment strategy in relapsed or refractory disease.

Arulogun S, Hertzberg M, Gandhi M. Recent treatment advances in Hodgkin lymphoma: a concise review. Internal Medicine Journal. 2016;46(12):1364–1369.
https://onlinelibrary.wiley.com/doi/abs/10.1111/imj.13051

15. Answer: D

Iron is an essential metal for oxygen delivery and multiple metabolic cellular processes such as DNA biosynthesis and electron transport. Approximately 10% of dietary iron is absorbed. Iron absorption is the result of complex mechanisms and it occurs predominantly in the duodenum, followed by the proximal jejunum. Absorption of non-haem iron and haem iron is via different non-competitive pathways. Haem iron is an important nutritional source of iron in carnivores that is more readily absorbed than non-haem iron derived from vegetables. Most haem is absorbed in the proximal intestine, and specific proteins such as hephaestin and HCP1, mediate haem uptake by the cells at the luminal brush border membrane of duodenal enterocytes.

Most dietary non-haem iron is ferric iron. This can enter the absorptive cell via the integrin-mobilferrin pathway (IMP). Some dietary iron is reduced in the gut lumen and enters the absorptive cell via the divalent metal transporter-1 (DMT-1/DCT-1/Nramp-2). DMT-1 is the most important transporter of ferrous iron.

Iron is exported from cells to the circulation by FPN1. FPN1 is a multipass protein found in the basolateral membrane of the enterocytes and macrophages. Over-expression of FPN1 is induced by cellular iron, and it is suppressed by hepcidin. Once exported by FPN1, iron needs to be transformed from the ferrous into the ferric form by ferroxidases in order to bind iron to transferrin. Without activity of ferroxidases, FPN1 is internalised and degraded.

Transferrin is the main protein involved in iron transport in plasma. Normally, between 20 and 40% of the binding sites of the protein are occupied by ferric iron. Only ferric iron is transported to the cytoplasm or to mitochondria. Iron is stored within the ferritin molecule to protect the cell from oxidative damage. Free iron is a very toxic producing reactive oxygen species. Each ferritin molecule can sequester up to 4,500 iron atoms. Ferritin also has enzymatic properties, converting ferric to ferrous iron, as iron is internalised and sequestered in the ferritin mineral core. Ferritin is an acute phase reactive protein and small quantities of ferritin are present in serum. Ferritin is elevated in infection, inflammation, and iron overload.

Hepcidin is the key regulator of iron metabolism. Hepatocytes receive multiple signals related to iron balance such as transferrin saturation, erythropoiesis, oxygen level, and infection. They respond by transcriptional regulation of hepcidin expression. Hepcidin is a negative regulator of iron metabolism that represses iron efflux from macrophages, hepatocytes, and enterocytes by its binding to and degrading unique iron export protein ferroportin. Ferroportin degradation leads to cellular iron retention and decreased iron availability.

Waldvogel-Abramowski S, Waeber G, Gassner C, Buser A, Frey B, Favrat B et al. Physiology of Iron Metabolism. Transfusion Medicine and Hemotherapy. 2014;41(3):213–221.
https://www.karger.com/Article/Fulltext/362888

16. Answer: D

Idiopathic thrombocytopenic purpura (ITP) is defined as isolated thrombocytopenia with normal bone marrow and the absence of other causes of thrombocytopenia. ITP is an acquired immune disorder where the thrombocytopenia results from pathologic antiplatelet antibodies, impaired megakaryocytopoiesis, and T cell-mediated destruction of platelets.

In adults, the onset of ITP tends to be insidious, and clinical symptoms include epistaxis, gingival bleeding, petechiae, and easy bruising. Isolated thrombocytopenia on a FBE is the key laboratory finding. Other cell lines are typically normal with normal coagulation studies. The blood smear shows the absence of normal platelets with young, large platelets which are in response to the autoimmune peripheral destruction of platelets. Bone marrow biopsy is most often not necessary in typical cases. Antiplatelet antibody testing is not indicated for the diagnosis of ITP in the majority of patients.

Adults with platelet counts greater than 50,000/mm³ generally do not require treatment. Treatment is indicated for adults with significant mucous membrane bleeding and for individuals with a platelet count less than 30,000/mm³ due to the risk of internal bleeding. Treatment is also indicated for those adults with risk factors for bleeding, such as hypertension and peptic ulcer disease. Glucocorticoids (prednisone 1mg/kg/day for 2–4 weeks) and IVIG are first-line options for ITP. Individuals may require splenectomy or the use of thrombopoietin receptor agonists in refractory cases. Azathioprine may be used as a steroid-sparing agent. Use of anti-RhD immune globulin, cyclosporin, and rituximab has all been reported with good outcomes.

Lambert M, Gernsheimer T. Clinical updates in adult immune thrombocytopenia. Blood. 2017;129(21):2829–2835. https://ashpublications.org/blood/article-lookup/doi/10.1182/blood-2017-03-754119

17. Answer: A

Lenalidomide is an immunomodulatory drug (IMiD) which is derived by modifying the chemical structure of thalidomide to improve its potency and reduce its side effects. Lenalidomide is a 4-amino-glutamyl analogue of thalidomide and has activity against various haematological and solid malignancies. It is approved by for clinical use in myelodysplastic syndromes (MDS) with deletion of chromosome 5q and multiple myeloma. Lenalidomide affects both cellular and humoral limbs of the immune system. It has also been shown to have anti-angiogenic properties. Newer studies demonstrate its effects on signal transduction that can partly explain its selective efficacy in subsets of MDS. Even though the exact molecular targets of lenalidomide are not well known, its activity across a spectrum of neoplastic conditions highlights the possibility of multiple target sites of action.

Lenalidomide is the second generation IMiD. It does not have the high rate of neuropathy seen in thalidomide. The problem with the drug is that it is renally cleared and one therefore needs to dose modify in the elderly and with renal impairment. About 25% of patients develop grade ¾ haematological toxicity with cytopenias. That said, for most patients it is well tolerated in combination with dexamethasone; occasionally one sees disabling tiredness.

Moreau P, Zamagni E, Mateos M. Treatment of patients with multiple myeloma progressing on frontline-therapy with lenalidomide. Blood Cancer Journal. 2019;9(4). https://www.nature.com/articles/s41408-019-0200-1

18. Answer: D

MGUS is defined as the presence of a serum paraprotein/monoclonal protein (M protein) at a concentration ≤ 30 g/L, no monoclonal protein or only modest amounts of monoclonal light chains in the urine, the absence of CRAB features (i.e. hyper**c**alcaemia, **r**enal failure, **a**naemia, and **b**one lesions) that are related to the M protein, ≤ 10% clonal plasma cells in the bone marrow, and no evidence of B-cell lymphoma or other disease known to produce M-protein. MGUS is different from asymptomatic/smouldering plasma cell myeloma where there is presence of monoclonal protein in the serum or urine at myeloma level (> 30 g/L), ≥10% clonal plasma cells in bone marrow, no related organ or tissue impairment, and no myeloma-related symptoms.

MGUS has now been divided into two major subtypes, IgM MGUS and non-IgM MGUS, due to the different rate of malignant progression between these two types.

A cohort study conducted by the Mayo clinic in a cohort of 1384 patients with MGUS, followed up for a median of 34.1 years found patients with IgM MGUS has an increased rate of malignant progression and a shorter survival compared to non-IgM MGUS.

Immunologically, IgM MGUS arises from a CD20+ lymphoplasmacytic cell that has not undergone switch recombination, and is likely to progress to lymphoma, Waldenström macroglobulinaemia, or AL amyloidosis. In contrast, non-IgM MGUS comes from mature plasma cells that have undergone switch combination and is associated with a risk of progression to multiple myeloma and AL amyloidosis. MGUS is a prevalent disorder that has moderate and persistent life-time risks of malignant progression. However, currently there is limited data to suggest that screening or monitoring will improve the outcome of these patients.

Kyle R, Larson D, Therneau T, Dispenzieri A, Kumar S, Cerhan J et al. Long-Term Follow-up of Monoclonal Gammopathy of Undetermined Significance. New England Journal of Medicine. 2018;378(3):241–249. https://www.nejm.org/doi/full/10.1056/NEJMoa1709974

19. Answer: A

Multiple myeloma (MM) is characterised by a proliferation of malignant plasma cells and a subsequent production of monoclonal paraprotein or an immunoglobulin free light chain (FLC). It accounts for approximately 10% of haematologic malignancies. Presenting symptoms of MM tend to vary from patient to patient; patients are asymptomatic in the early stages of MM, and approximately 20% of patients present with mild symptoms such as bone pain and fatigue. Patients with late stage MM typically present with symptoms (**CRAB**) related to end-organ damage which includes:l

- Hyper**C**alcaemia
- **R**enal impairment (AKI or CKD)
- **A**naemia
- **B**ony disease.

This patient has all of these features strongly suggesting a diagnosis of MM. The key investigation is to measure monoclonal protein and serum FLC levels. A monoclonal protein in the serum or urine is a cardinal feature of MM but is seen in only 82% of patients by serum protein electrophoresis. The sensitivity increases to 93% when serum immunofixation is added, and to 97% with the addition of the serum FLC assay. The monoclonal protein type is IgG in approximately 50%, IgA in 20%, FLC only in 20%, IgD in 2%, and IgM in 0.5%. About 1% of MM has no detectable M protein, and is referred to as non-secretory MM.

Bone marrow aspirate and/or bone marrow biopsy are required for the diagnosis of MM, and the diagnosis is confirmed if ≥10% of the cells in the bone marrow are clonal plasma cells in the presence of a myeloma-defining event (CRAB). In October 2014, the International Myeloma Working Group (IMWG) updated MM diagnostic criteria by adding to the classic CRAB features three markers considered to be myeloma-defining events:

- Clonal bone marrow percentage ≥60%, involved/uninvolved serum FLC ratio ≥100, and >1 focal lesion that is ≥5 mm in size.
- Anaemia, which occurs in about 75% of patients, likely contributing fatigue.
- Osteolytic skeletal lesions are detected in approximately 80% of patients, and other common clinical findings at diagnosis include hypercalcaemia and elevated serum creatinine level.

Bone disease should be evaluated at diagnosis in all patients and in accordance with the new IMWG criteria, and using skeletal survey with plain X-rays, low dose CT or 18F-fluorodeoxyglucose PET–CT. However, the exact imaging modality used is determined by availability and resources. Bone scan is not recommended in evaluation of MM. The sensitivity of detecting lesions is less than that of a plain film skeletal survey, as lytic bone lesions are seriously underestimated by bone scans.

Patients can get frequent infections especially pneumonia due to low-normal immunoglobulin level. This patient's clinical features and CXR are consistent with right middle lobe pneumonia. Renal impairment affects 20–40% of new cases of MM. Some cases are reversible if diagnosed and treated early. Renal impairment is associated with a large tumour burden and a poor prognosis. The aetiology of renal impairment is multifactorial and includes:

- cast nephropathy (see figure below)
- interstitial nephritis
- urate nephropathy
- plasma cell infiltration
- hyperviscosity syndrome
- dehydration
- intravenous contrast
- nephrotoxic medications.

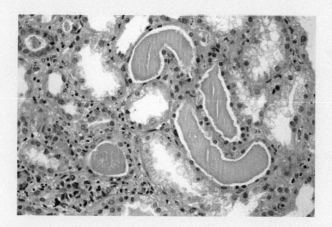

 Kumar S, Rajkumar V, Kyle R, van Duin M, Sonneveld P, Mateos M et al. Multiple myeloma. Nature Reviews Disease Primers. 2017;3(1).
https://www.nature.com/articles/nrdp201746

20. Answer: D

Significant progressions have been made in understanding the biology and treatment of multiple myeloma (MM) in the past two decades. Although MM has no cure, it is highly treatable with many recently approved drugs. Treatment options include chemotherapy, immunosuppression, radiation, autologous stem-cell transplantation, and adjunctive therapy when warranted.

Adjunctive therapy for MM may include radiation that targets areas of pain, impending pathologic fracture, or existing pathologic fracture. Bisphosphonates may be used as prophylactic primary or secondary therapy against skeletal events which include hypercalcaemia, spinal cord compression, pathologic fracture, need for surgery or radiation. Other adjunctive therapies include erythropoietin, corticosteroids, surgical intervention, and plasmapheresis.

There is no one standard of therapy for MM, and treatment is generally selected based on the patient's age, symptoms, functional status, co-morbidities, prior MM treatment, laboratory and cytogenetic test results, and stage of MM.

Current strategies for the treatment of MM involve consecutive stages of therapy:

1. Induction phase: aims to eradicate MM by reducing the size of the cancer as much as possible.
2. Consolidation phase: aims to further diminishes tumour bulk.
3. Maintenance phase: aims for long-term treatment with the goal of keeping residual disease under control and potentially leading to a cure.
4. In transplant eligible patients, they get induction --> transplant --> maintenance.

Proteasome inhibitors (PSIs) and immunomodulatory drugs (IMiDs) are considered the mainstays of MM treatment, but newer and more highly targeted drugs are used as second- or third-line treatment. IMiDs are a group of compounds that are functionally and structurally related to thalidomide. These agents were formulated with increased anticancer and immunologic properties, and their biologic effects include the inhibition of angiogenesis and proinflammatory cytokines, the stimulation of cellular immunity, and the ability to precisely inhibit the growth of tumour cells and induce apoptosis.

Panobinostat, the first oral histone deacetylase inhibitor (HDAC) approved for the treatment of relapsed MM, is indicated for patients with MM who have received at least two prior regimens, including bortezomib and an IMiD; it should be used in combination with bortezomib and dexamethasone.

Daratumumab, is a human CD38-directed monoclonal antibodies used in the treatment of MM. Elotuzumab is a humanised immunoglobulin G1 monoclonal antibodies that specifically targets the protein SLAMF7 which is expressed on myeloma cells independent of cytogenetic abnormalities.

Ixazomib, a PSI indicated in combination with lenalidomide and dexamethasone for the treatment of patients with MM who have received at least one prior therapy. It is the only oral formulation that is considered to be advantageous for patients who prefer an all-oral regimen or do not live near an infusion centre.

Currently used drugs in the treatment of MM
Proteasome inhibitors
Bortezomib
Carfilzomib
Ixazomib
Immunomodulatory drugs
Thalidomide
Lenalidomide
Pomalidomide
Monoclonal antibodies
Daratumumab (anti-CD38)
Elotuzumab (anti-SLAMF7)
Histone deacetylase inhibitor
Panobinostat
Alkylating agents
Melphalan
Cyclophosphamide
Bendamustine
Others
Dexamethasone
Prednisone
Cisplatin
Etoposide
Doxorubicin

Kumar S, Rajkumar V, Kyle R, van Duin M, Sonneveld P, Mateos M et al. Multiple myeloma. Nature Reviews Disease Primers. 2017;3(1).
https://www.nature.com/articles/nrdp201746

21. Answer: C

Myeloproliferative neoplasms (MPNs) are a common cause of Budd–Chiari syndrome in young patients, particularly females. In particular, polycythaemia vera (PV) is a frequent cause of the syndrome. Typically, PV presents with elevated haemoglobin, haematocrit, and mutations to the Janus kinase 2 (JAK2) gene. However, PV can also present with normal haemoglobin and haematocrit, particularly in females, and particularly when iron deficiency is also present. Platelet count can be elevated in any of the MPNs: PV, essential thrombocytosis (ET), and primary myelofibrosis.

Distinguishing between PV and its MPN counterparts has important therapeutic and prognostic implications. Driver mutation status can be helpful in distinguishing MPNs as a patient negative for JAK2 mutations is unlikely to have PV, however, up to 50% of patients with ET and myelofibrosis are also positive for JAK2 mutations. In PV, increase in red cell mass is the important risk factor for thrombosis rather than haemoglobin or red cell concentration. As increased redcell mass is accompanied by plasma expansion, there can be normal haematocrit and haemoglobin values, which can be measured by measuring red-cell mass and plasma volume by nuclear medicine testing. However, these tests are not universally available so an assumption of the diagnosis of PV is reasonable with JAK2 mutation in situations such as these.

Other driver mutations are those encoding calreticulin (CALR) and the thrombopoietin receptor (MPL). These occur very rarely in PV, and more commonly in ET and primary myelofibrosis however, the mutations are not mutually exclusive and not exclusive to a particular MPN. Treatment options for MPNs include chemotherapy, aspirin, hydroxyurea, and in the case of PV, phlebotomy. JAK2 inhibition with ruxolitinib can help symptoms and splenomegaly where hydroxyurea is ineffective, interferon can be considered in some situations.

Spivak J. Myeloproliferative Neoplasms. New England Journal of Medicine. 2017;376(22):2168–2181. https://www.nejm.org/doi/full/10.1056/NEJMra1406186

22. Answer: D

Non-Hodgkin lymphoma (NHL) represents a wide spectrum of illnesses that vary from indolent to aggressive malignancies. They arise from lymphocytes that at different stages of development, and the characteristics of the specific lymphoma subtype reflect those of the originating cell.

Characteristic chromosomal translocations are found to be associated with subtypes of BCell NHL: t(8;14)(q24;q32); Burkitt lymphoma, t(14;18)(q32;q21); follicular lymphoma, and t(11;14)(q13;q32) in mantle cell lymphoma. Only a few recurrent cytogenetic aberrations have been identified in the T cell NHL and the best known is the ALK gene translocation t(2;5)(p23;q35) in anaplastic large cell lymphoma and t(5;9)(q33;q22) in peripheral T cell lymphomas (PTCL).

PTCL is a heterogeneous group of lymphoid malignancies derived from mature post-thymic T cells and natural killer (NK) cells, altogether accounting for around 10% of all NHL in developed countries. Demonstration of T cell clonality, unlike for B cells, cannot be performed by routine immunophenotyping for light chain restriction and requires molecular testing for T cell receptor gene (TCR) rearrangement.

The diagnosis and classification of NHL requires the integration of clinical features in conjunction with the results of morphology, immunophenotype, and cytogenetic study. Although the recurrent chromosomal abnormalities in NHL are not completely sensitive and specific for disease entities, cytogenetic and molecular genetic study is commonly used to aid lymphoma diagnosis and classification. Currently, the main clinical utility is in the employment of interphase Fluorescence In Situ Hybridization (FISH) panels to predict disease aggressiveness to guide therapy, for example identification of double-hit lymphoma, or in prognostication, for example risk-stratification in chronic lymphocytic leukemia. The recent application of high-throughput sequencing to NHL not only advances the understanding of disease pathogenesis and classification but allows the discovery of new drug targets. Coupled with the increasing availability of novel molecular targeted therapeutic agents, the hope for the future is to translate the genetics and genomics information to achieve personalised medicine in NHL.

Armitage J, Gascoyne R, Lunning M, Cavalli F. Non-Hodgkin lymphoma. The Lancet. 2017;390(10091):298–310. https://www.thelancet.com/journals/lancet/article/PIIS0140-6736(16)32407-2/fulltext

23. Answer: D

Chronic myeloid leukaemia (CML), is a myeloproliferative neoplasm which affects both the peripheral blood and the bone marrow. The fusion oncoprotein *BCR-ABL1* defines CML. 90 to 95% of patients with CML have a shortened chromosome 22 because of a reciprocal translocation t (9;22) (q34; q11.2) called the Philadelphia chromosome. The *ABL1* gene encodes a non-receptor tyrosine kinase on chromosome 9 and *BCR* is a breakpoint cluster region on chromosome 22. The translated oncoprotein in most cases is

210 kD and called p210 BCR-ABL1. Alternative splicing results in p190 and p230 BCR-ABL1, which may show different presentations. This oncoprotein acts as a defective constitutively expressed tyrosine kinase. The downstream pathways affected include JAK/STAT, PI3K/AKT, and RAS/MEK; they involve cell growth, cell survival, inhibition of apoptosis, and activation of transcription factors.

CML is classified into three phases.

Chronic phase: The peripheral blood smear shows a leukocytosis due to granulocytes in various stages of maturation. Blast cells are <2% of the WBCs. Bone marrow aspirate and biopsy show hypercellularity with marked granulocytic proliferation significantly increased myelocytes, and significant dysplasia should be absent. Blasts are usually <5%.

Accelerated Phase: The peripheral smear may or may not show increased blasts (10% to 19%). The bone marrow aspirate and biopsy will show similar changes to chronic phase CML with increased blasts (10% to 19%).

Blast Phase: The peripheral smear and/or bone marrow aspirate will show >20% blasts or there will be an extramedullary proliferation of blasts.

There are four first-line treatments for chronic phase CML that are commercially available tyrosine kinase inhibitors (TKIs) which include the first-generation imatinib and second-generation dasatinib, nilotinib, and bosutinib. For chronic phase CML with intermediate- or high-risk score, second-generation TKIs as first-line therapy have an additional benefit over imatinib. Ponatinib, a third-generation TKIs, is a third-line treatment option in chronic phase CML for patients with multiple TKI therapy failures and for patients with *T315I* mutation.

Second- or third-generation TKI therapy should be initiated to reduce CML burden and be considered for early allogeneic hematopoietic stem cell transplant in patients with accelerated or blast phase CML. Omacetaxine is a chemotherapy agent that can be used as an additional treatment in cases refractory to TKI therapy that advanced from chronic phase CML.

Apperley J. Chronic myeloid leukaemia. The Lancet. 2015;385(9976):1447–1459.
https://www.thelancet.com/journals/lancet/article/PIIS0140-6736(13)62120-0/fulltext

24. Answer: B

This patient has moderate macrocytic anaemia, and the blood film shows hypersegmented polymorphonuclear leukocyte. The clinical picture is consistent with pernicious anaemia due to vitamin B_{12} deficiency. Intrinsic factor (IF) antibodies, type 1 and type 2, occur in 50% of patients with pernicious anaemia and are specific for this disorder. They can be used to confirm the diagnosis. Parietal cell antibodies occur in 90% of patients with pernicious anaemia. However, these antibodies are not specific for pernicious anaemia.

B_{12} deficiency is the leading cause of megaloblastic anaemia and though more common in the elderly, can occur at any age. B_{12} absorption requires intact gastric production of IF as well as a functioning cubam receptor for the B_{12}-intrinsic factor complex in the terminal ileum. Impaired IF production can occur in adults due to autoimmune destruction of parietal cells, which secrete IF. Gastrectomy can significantly reduce the production of IF.

Apart from lack of IF, B_{12} deficiency can be caused by folic acid deficiency, altered pH in the small intestine, and lack of absorption of B_{12} complexes in the terminal ileum. B_{12} and folate are intimately connected through their cooperative roles in one-carbon metabolism, and the haematological complications seen with deficiency of either vitamin are indistinguishable. Both are caused by impaired DNA synthesis that results in a prolongation of the S phase of the cell cycle and causes maturation arrest.

B_{12} deficiency may be associated with neurocognitive and neurological consequences. Timely diagnosis and treatment are important as delay can have dire neurological consequences.

The form and dosage of treatment depend on whether the IF-dependent pathway is intact or not. If not intact, intramuscular injection of 1000 μg hydroxocobalamin should be given every other day for 1 to 2 weeks followed by weekly injections for a month and then tapered to once every three months indefinitely. About 10% of each B_{12} dose is retained. The alternative to injected B_{12} is high-dose oral B_{12}. Between 1% and 4% of an oral dose of B_{12} is absorbed passively, even when the intrinsic factor-dependent pathway is abrogated. If the cause of B_{12} deficiency is not known or irreversible, treatment should be lifelong.

Pure red cell aplasia (PRCA) is an uncommon disorder in which maturation arrest occurs in the formation of erythrocytes. Most cases of acute transient PRCA are caused by parvovirus B19 infection. In acute infection IgM parvovirus B19 antibodies are positive.

Green R. Vitamin B_{12} deficiency from the perspective of a practicing hematologist. Blood. 2017;129(19):2603–2611.
http://www.bloodjournal.org/content/129/19/2603.long?sso-checked=true

25. Answer: C

The clinical features and MRI of brain are consistent with progressive multifocal leukoencephalopathy (PML). MRI of the brain shows multiple high intensity signals on T2-weighted sequences affecting widespread subcortical and deep white matter consistent with a demyelinating process.

PML is a progressive demyelinating disease of the central nervous system caused by reactivation of JC virus (JCV) infection. PML usually occurs in immunocompromised patients especially HIV-positive patients. JCV is a ubiquitous polyomavirus infecting 70% or more of the adult population throughout the world, but PML remains a very rare complication of JCV infection in immunocompetent people.

PML occurs almost exclusively in patients with an impaired cellular immune response: 80% of reported PML patients have AIDS, 13% have haematologic malignancies, 5% are transplant recipients, 2% have chronic inflammatory diseases and immunomodulatory therapies.

PML has a rapid clinical course with an extremely poor clinical outcome. Nearly all patients who survive suffer from residual neurologic deficits including hemiparesis, motor aphasia, and visual defects. There is no established therapy for PML, and the treatment is mostly supportive. In cases associated with immunomodulatory agents, the withdrawal of the drug and further elimination by plasma exchange is the most important therapy for immune system recovery. There is evidence that JCV infects the cells through the 5-HT2A serotonin receptor. Mirtazapine, an antidepressant that acts by inhibiting this receptor has been used in treatment of PML.

JCV is a polyomavirus, genetically related to BK virus which can cause BK nephropathy in renal transplant patients. Herpes simplex encephalitis (HSE) is an acute or subacute illness that causes both general and focal signs of cerebral dysfunction. T2-weighted MRI in patient with HSE usually reveals hyperintensity corresponding to oedematous changes in the temporal lobes, inferior frontal lobes, and insula, with a predilection for the medial temporal lobes.

Pavlovic D, Patera A, Nyberg F, Gerber M, Liu M. Progressive multifocal leukoencephalopathy: current treatment options and future perspectives. Therapeutic Advances in Neurological Disorders. 2015;8(6):255–273.
https://journals.sagepub.com/doi/full/10.1177/1756285615602832

26. Answer: D

Polycythaemia vera (PV) is a chronic myeloproliferative neoplasm associated with *JAK2* mutations in almost all cases. PV is associated with reduced survival because of cardiovascular complications and progression to post-PV myelofibrosis or leukaemia.

Major diagnostic criteria are haemoglobin >185 g/l in males or >165 g/l in females, or evidence of an increased red cell mass and a V617F or exon 12 *JAK2* mutation. Minor criteria are bone marrow biopsy showing hypercellularity with panmyelosis, subnormal erythropoietin levels and endogenous erythroid colony growth. To make a diagnosis of PV, fulfilment of both major and one minor criterion or the first major and two minor criteria are required.

A prognostic model for overall survival, has been developed based on age, leucocytosis, and venous thrombosis; it separates patients into 3 groups with median survival of 28, 19, and 11 years. However, risk-adapted therapy in PV is based on an estimate of the likelihood of thrombotic complications and not necessarily on survival and haematologic progression.

The goal of therapy in PV is primarily to reduce the risk of thrombosis without increasing the bleeding tendency and enhancing the intrinsic potential of haematologic progression and, secondarily, to ameliorate symptoms, particularly vasomotor manifestations. No drug is able to cure the disease. Iron supplementation should be avoided.

The mainstay of PV treatment is the correction of abnormal blood viscosity associated with the increased red cell volume. The optimal target of haematocrit is less than 45%.

1. Venesection plus aspirin 100mg daily in low-risk patients.

2. Venesection plus aspirin 100mg twice a day and cytotoxic drugs hydroxyurea 500mg twice a day.

Over time, 10% to 15% of patients on hydroxyurea develop haematologic and extrahaematologic toxicities such as painful leg ulcers, skin cancers, or extensive dermatitis, and fever and thus have to stop the drug or use a suboptimal dose. The second-line therapy for PV includes pegylated IFN-α, busulfan, and ruxolutinib. Busulfan is an alkylating agent that produces haematologic responses in most patients and a decrease of *JAK2* V617F allele burden in some; it must be accurately titrated because of prolonged myelosuppression. There is no firm evidence of an increased leukaemogenic potential of busulfan. However, this patient has had a significant skin cancer burden so busulfan is not the best choice.

This patient's disease control is inadequate. There is evidence of progression to myelofibrosis including constitutional symptoms, increasing splenomegaly, increased LDH. Ruxolitinib, a selective inhibitor of *JAK* 1 and 2 is the best next treatment in this case. In a randomised study, ruxolitinib was compared to best available therapy, in hydroxyurea-resistant or intolerant PV with splenomegaly; treatment with ruxolutinib produced higher rates of haematocrit control (60 vs 20%), ≥ 35% reduction in spleen volume (38 vs 1%) and symptom control (49 vs 5%). It reduces the burden of the V617F mutant *JAK2* allele. However, ruxolutinib therapy showed limited evidence of disease-modifying activity, with complete haematologic remission rate of only 24% and complete molecular remission rate of <2%. In Australia, ruxolitinib is restricted (PBS listed) for use in high risk and intermediate-2 and 1 risk myelofibrosis. The condition must be primary myelofibrosis or post-polycythaemia vera myelofibrosis or post-essential thrombocythaemia myelofibrosis.

 Tefferi A, Vannucchi A, Barbui T. Polycythemia vera treatment algorithm 2018. Blood Cancer Journal. 2018;8(1). https://www.nature.com/articles/s41408-017-0042-7

27. Answer: A

Graft versus host disease (GVHD) is a significant contributor to long-term morbidity and mortality after allogeneic haematopoietic cell transplantation (HCT). Up to 50% of all HCT patients will develop chronic GVHD. Risk factors for acquiring chronic GVHD include:

- Prior acute GVHD
- Increasing HLA disparity between recipient and donor (recipients of unrelated donor marrow have a higher incidence of chronic GVHD)
- The use of non-T cell-depleted bone marrow
- Male recipients of alloimmune female donors
- Older age of recipient or donor
- Recipients of allogeneic peripheral blood stem cells (PBSC) grafts
- Recipients of cord blood grafts
- Recipients of full intensity myeloablative conditioning regimen
- Severe pre-transplant comorbidities
- Diagnosis of chronic myeloid leukaemia

Diagnosis of chronic GVHD is based on NIH consensus criteria. Clinical manifestations of chronic GVHD are the result of a highly complex immune pathology involving both donor B cells and T cells as well as other cells. Steroids are the most widely used first-line therapy for treatment of moderate to severe chronic GVHD with or without the addition of other immunosuppressive agents. If patients fail to respond or have progressive disease with steroid therapy, second-line treatment is required. The response rate to second-line therapy is about 25–50% with no single therapy being better than any other.

 Zeiser R, Blazar B. Pathophysiology of Chronic Graft-versus-Host Disease and Therapeutic Targets. New England Journal of Medicine. 2017;377(26):2565–2579. https://www.nejm.org/doi/full/10.1056/NEJMra1703472

28. Answer: A

Sickle cell disease (SCD) is a common and life-threatening monogenic haematological disorder. Abnormal sickle-shaped erythrocytes disrupt blood flow in small vessels, and this vaso-occlusion leads to distal tissue ischaemia and inflammation, with symptoms defining the acute painful sickle-cell crisis. Repeated sickling and ongoing haemolytic anaemia, even when subclinical, leads to parenchymal injury and chronic organ damage, causing substantial morbidity and premature mortality.

Currently available treatments are limited to transfusions and hydroxyurea, while stem cell transplantation might be a potentially curative therapy. Several new therapeutic options are in development, including gene therapy and gene editing.

The mainstay of treatment for SCD is erythrocyte transfusions, with more than 90% of adults receiving at least one transfusion in their lifetimes. Transfusions are given acutely for immediate benefits, such as increased oxygen-carrying capacity, improved blood flow, prevention of acute vaso-occlusion and reduction of sickle erythropoiesis using the simple transfusion technique. Chronic transfusions help prevent long-term complications by replacing rigid sickled erythrocytes with normal deformable cells and by suppressing formation of sickled erythrocytes, using monthly simple or exchange transfusions.

Exchange transfusions involve removing some of the patient's own blood at the time of transfusion, thereby lowering the percentage of HbS relative to HbA. Exchange transfusions may be used to treat or prevent the occurrence of vaso-occlusive complications such as stroke. Automated exchange transfusions using an apheresis machine have the advantage of being iron neutral, thereby reducing the need for chelation therapy.

Clinical indications for acute simple transfusion include:

- Acute splenic sequestration
- Acute hepatic sequestration

- Transient aplastic crisis
- Symptomatic severe anaemia
- Preoperative preparation.

Clinical indications for acute exchange transfusion include:
- Severe acute chest syndrome
- Acute stroke.

Complications not warranting transfusion include:
- Uncomplicated painful crisis
- Priapism
- AKI
- Asymptomatic anaemia
- Avascular necrosis.

Acute painful crisis, the hallmark clinical feature of SCD, reflects vaso-occlusion and impaired oxygen supply, but also infarction-reperfusion injury. The majority of such events are managed at home with NSAIDs or oral opioid analgesics.

Acute chest syndrome (ACS) is the second most frequent reason for hospitalisations and is a leading cause of mortality in SCD. The initial pulmonary injury is multifactorial, including infection, pulmonary fat embolism, pulmonary infarction, and PE.

Acute ischaemic stroke occurs mainly in childhood, but cerebral haemorrhage occurs primarily in adults. For acute stroke, exchange transfusion should be done promptly, followed by chronic transfusions to prevent stroke recurrence.

Acute anaemia events can occur with acute splenic sequestration crisis, transient red cell aplasia, or increased haemolysis especially following transfusions. Simple transfusion should correct haemoglobin concentrations only to the baseline value, avoiding cardiovascular compromise and hyperviscosity.

Chronic parenchymal damage develops through different mechanisms and almost every organ system can be affected. Complications such as retinopathy, avascular necrosis, neurological decline, leg ulcers, and recurrent priapism are associated with morbidly and impaired quality of life, but CKD and cardiopulmonary disease are the most lethal.

Sickle nephropathy starts in childhood with loss of urine concentrating ability and glomerular hyperfiltration. Frequently, proteinuria develops with glomerulosclerosis, decreased glomerular filtration rate, and eventual ESKD. Pulmonary hypertension and diastolic cardiac dysfunction are responsible for 45% of deaths in adults with SCD.

Ware R, de Montalembert M, Tshilolo L, Abboud M. Sickle cell disease. The Lancet. 2017;390(10091):311–323. https://www.thelancet.com/journals/lancet/article/PIIS0140-6736(17)30193-9/fulltext

29. Answer: A

Peripheral blood stem cell transplant (PBSCT) is the preferred stem cell source compared to bone marrow transplant (BMT) due to quicker engraftment and practicability.

The number of patients receiving allogeneic PBSCT is increasing. Patients with co-morbidities and those 65 years of age and older can be considered for stem cell transplant following the introduction of reduced intensity conditioning (RIC) regimens. PBSCT is also associated with significantly decreased relapse rates in related donors compared to BMT; however, this trend is not seen in unrelated donors.

PBSCT and BMT have non-significant difference in rates of acute graft versus host disease; however, PBSCT is associated with significantly increased rates of chronic graft versus host disease (GVHD). This is associated with substantially reduced quality of life, especially due to long term immunosuppression treatment, often with steroids.

There is no evidence overall that disease-free survival is superior with BMT compared to PBSCT. In one study, patients with acute leukaemia who underwent RIC allogeneic haematopoietic stem cell transplantation were studied to compare the clinical outcomes of peripheral blood (PB) vs bone morrow (BM) as a source of stem cells:
- Cumulative incidence of engraftment defined neutrophil $\geq 0.5 \times 10^9$/L at day 60 was higher in mobilised PB recipients.
- Grade II to IV acute GVHD was higher in mobilised PB recipients.
- Chronic GVHD was significantly higher after peripheral blood grafts.
- Overall survival and leukaemia-free survival were higher in patients transplanted with mobilised PB.
- Risk of leukaemia relapse was lower in mobilised PB recipients.

Savani B, Labopin M, Blaise D, Niederwieser D, Ciceri F, Ganser A et al. Peripheral blood stem cell graft compared to bone marrow after reduced intensity conditioning regimens for acute leukemia: a report from the ALWP of the EBMT. Haematologica. 2015;101(2):256–262.
http://www.haematologica.org/content/early/2015/11/10/haematol.2015.135699

30. Answer: B

Careful selection of patients to screen for inherited thrombophilia is necessary in patients with potential increased risks of VTE. The indications for screening inherited thrombophilia are:

- Thrombosis at a young age (<50 year), especially in association with weak provoking factors (minor surgery, combination oral contraceptives, or immobility) or unprovoked VTE.
- Strong family history of VTE (first-degree family members affected at a young age), recurrent VTE events, especially at a young age.
- VTE in unusual sites such as splanchnic or cerebral veins.

After development of an acute thromboembolic event, it is unnecessary to immediately screen for the inherited thrombophilia since in the acute settings, some of the tests are difficult to interpret, such as protein C, protein S, antithrombin, and lupus anticoagulants can have falsely low results because of acute thrombosis, inflammation, pregnancy, recent miscarriage, and other medical conditions. The presence of anticoagulants can have significant impact on the test results (Table 9.1). Immediate screening for the inherited thrombophilia does not change the management or duration of VTE treatment after an acute event.

In patients with clinically suspected antiphospholipid syndrome (APS), caution needs to be used when deciding whether the presence of antiphospholipid antibodies is clinically significant to make the diagnosis of APS. In patients with confirmed APS, indefinite anticoagulation needs to be considered if no bleeding contraindication due to its potential to cause arterial, venous, microvascular thrombus, and rarely catastrophic APS. In patients with splenic vein or central venous thrombosis, causes like cirrhosis caused by portal vein thrombosis, extrinsic tumour causing compression and thrombosis, paroxysmal nocturnal haemoglobinuria, or myeloproliferative disease need to be excluded.

In patients with inherited thrombophilia on exogenous oestrogen, combined oral contraceptive pills, oestrogen should be stopped to prevent development of VTE.

It is important to determine the duration of anticoagulation therapy based on whether the first event is unprovoked or provoked VTE. Care should be taken when deciding on long-standing anticoagulant treatment based on patients' bleeding risks and benefits of staying on anticoagulant therapy long-term.

Table 9.1   Effects of anticoagulants in thrombophilia tests.

Test	Test method	NOAC- Direct thrombin inhibitor	NOAC-anti Xa	Warfarin
Antithrombin	Xa-based	No effect	Increase	No effect
	IIa-based	Increase	No effect	No effect
Factor V Leiden	Clot-based	Increase	Increase	No effect
Factor VIII	One stage clot	Decrease	Decrease	No effect
Prothrombin G202010A	DNA analysis	No effect	No effect	No effect
Protein C	Chromogenic	No effect	No effect	Decrease
Protein S	Free antigen	No effect	No effect	Decrease
Anticardiolipin Antibodies	Solid phase	No effect	No effect	No effect
Anti-beta2-glycoprotein I	Solid phase	No effect	No effect	No effect
Lupus anticoagulants	APTT, dRVVT	Increase	Increase	Increase or decrease

NOAC: Non-vitamin K antagonist oral anticoagulant

Connors J. Thrombophilia Testing and Venous Thrombosis. New England Journal of Medicine. 2017;377(12):1177–1187. https://www.nejm.org/doi/full/10.1056/NEJMra1700365

31. Answer: D

This patient's presentation and CXR which demonstrated bilateral pulmonary infiltrate are highly suspicious of transfusion-related acute lung injury (TRALI). There is no clinical evidence to suggest decompensated heart failure. Anaphylaxis and DIC will not cause pulmonary infiltrates.

TRALI is characteriseds by sudden onset of acute lung injury after transfusion of blood products. Symptoms and signs (dyspnoea, tachypnoea, frothy sputum, fever, hypotension) of TRALI usually appear within 2 to 6 hours from initiation of transfusion but can occur up to 48 hours after transfusion. Distinguishing TRALI on clinical grounds from other causes of acute lung injury such as cardiac pulmonary oedema, sepsis, trauma, aspiration, or DIC is difficult and requires a high index of clinical suspicion. If suspected, test the donor and recipient serum for human leucocyte antigen (HLA) or human neutrophil antigen (HNA) antibodies and perform an HLA type on the recipient as demonstration of these antibodies supports diagnosis.

TRALI has emerged as the most common serious complication of blood transfusion. It has surpassed haemolytic reactions as the leading cause of transfusion-related mortality in developed countries. Published incidence of TRALI ranges from 0.02% to 0.05% per blood product unit transfused and from 0.08% to 0.16% per patient who receives a transfusion. Although all plasma containing blood products have been implicated, use of FFP, RBCs, and pooled platelets from several donors has a higher risk.

The pathogenesis of TRALI may include: (i) an antibody-mediated reaction between recipient granulocytes and anti-granulocyte antibodies from donors who were sensitiseds during pregnancy (multiparous women) or by previous transfusion. Up to 25% of multiparous women have circulating anti-leukocyte antibodies, (ii) proinflammatory molecules, predominantly lipid products of cell degradation, accumulated during storage of blood product cause lung injury. These two mechanisms may act synergistically to produce acute lung injury.

Management of TRALI is supportive and may include ventilatory support. TRALI has a better short-term prognosis than other causes of acute lung injury; less than 70% of patients with TRALI require mechanical ventilation, and most patients recover within 24 to 48 hours with supportive care.

Cases of suspected TRALI must be reported to the blood bank, and a transfusion reaction work-up should be initiated. In addition to acquiring a posttransfusion blood specimen from the patient, bags from units of blood transfused in the last 6 hours should be returned to the blood bank if possible so that residual donor plasma can be tested without necessitating a time-consuming recall of blood donors. To reduce the risk of antibody-mediated TRALI, donors with a possibility of having HLA or HNA antibodies either because of a history of pregnancy or transfusion are not used for plasma products or apheresis platelets by the Australia Red Cross. In another word, we only use plasma from male donors and apheresis platelets from male or nulliparous women.

Vlaar A, Juffermans N. Transfusion-related acute lung injury: a clinical review. The Lancet. 2013;382(9896): 984–994.
https://www.thelancet.com/journals/lancet/article/PIIS0140-6736(12)62197-7/fulltext

32. Answer: D

Approximately 10% of all cases of deep-vein thrombosis involve the upper extremities (DVT-UE). The incidence of DVT-UE is on the rise especially secondary DVT-UE because of the increased use of central venous catheters and of cardiac pacemakers and defibrillators. Secondary forms are more common than primary forms.

The vessels most often affected by DVT-UE are the subclavian vein (62%), the axillary vein (45%), and the jugular vein (45%), with more than one thrombosis demonstrated in some instances.

Approximately two thirds of patients with primary DVT-UE are young and male; they often report strenuous activity involving force or abduction of the dominant arm before the development of thrombosis, known as the Paget–Schroetter syndrome.

As compared with patients who have thrombosis of a lower extremity, patients with DVT-UE are typically younger, leaner, more likely to have a diagnosis of cancer and less likely to have acquired or hereditary thrombophilia.

In term of complications of DVT, there are less common in the upper extremities than in the lower extremities, include PE (6% for upper extremities vs 15 to 32% for lower extremities), recurrence at 12 months (2 to 5% for upper extremities vs 10% for lower extremities), and the post-thrombotic syndrome (5% for upper extremities vs. up to 56% for lower extremities).

DVT-UE is treated by anticoagulation, with heparin or low molecular weight heparin (LMWH) at first and then with oral anticoagulants. Direct oral anticoagulants are now being increasingly used. The thrombus is often not totally eradicated. Anticoagulation is generally continued as maintenance treatment for 3–6 months. Patients with DVT-UE have a high mortality, though they often die of their underlying diseases rather than of the DVT-UE or its complications.

Upper Extremity Deep Vein Thrombosis – American College of Cardiology [Internet]. American College of Cardiology. 2019 [cited 17 August 2019].
Available from: https://www.acc.org/latest-in-cardiology/articles/2017/11/09/13/30/upper-extremity-deep-vein-thrombosis

33. Answer: D

This patient has presented with prolonged bleeding on several occasions and a family history of bleeding tendency. Her blood tests show a mildly prolonged APTT and low factor VIII level. These features are best explained by von Willebrand disease (VWD).

Von Willebrand factor (VWF) is a large and complex plasma glycoprotein that is essential for normal haemostasis. It is well recognised that deficiency of VWF results in a bleeding disorder that varies in severity according to the degree of deficiency and the specific characteristics of the molecule and which may have features of both primary (involving platelet adhesion) and secondary (involving factor VIII) haemostatic defects.

VWD is one of the few haemostatic disorders characteriseds by both a platelet and coagulation defect because of a defect in VWF, which supports platelet adhesion and serves as a carrier protein for factor VIII (FVIII). VWD is the most common hereditary bleeding disorder. The morbidity in individuals with VWD is variable. Many patients with VWD are asymptomatic. Menorrhagia is a common symptom in females with VWD.

Type 1 VWD is characterised by a partial quantitative decrease of qualitatively normal VWF and FVIII and is inherited as an autosomal dominant trait. Patients with type 1 VWD generally have mild symptoms. Laboratory findings are typically a proportional reduction in VWF activity, VWF antigen, and FVIII.

Type 2 VWD is found in 15–20% of patients, which is a variant of the disease with primarily qualitative defects of VWF. Type 2 VWD can be either autosomal dominant or recessive. Of the five known type 2 VWD subtypes (i.e. 2A, 2B, 2C, 2M, 2N), type 2A VWD is by far the most common. Type 2A VWD is characterised by normal-to-reduced plasma levels of FVIIIc and VWF. Patients with type 2B VWD have a haemostatic defect caused by a qualitatively abnormal VWF and intermittent thrombocytopenia. The abnormal VWF has an increased affinity for platelet glycoprotein Ib. The platelet count may fall further during pregnancy, in association with surgical procedures, or after the administration of desmopressin (1-deamine-8-D-arginine vasopressin, DDAVP). Although some investigators found DDAVP to be clinically useful in persons with type 2B VWD, studies directed at excluding the 2B variant should be completed before DDAVP is used therapeutically.

Type 3 is the most severe form of VWD. In the homozygous patient, type 3 VWD is characteriseds by marked deficiencies of both VWF and FVIIIc in the plasma, the absence of VWF from both platelets and endothelial cells, and a lack of response to DDAVP. Type 3 VWD usually presents as severe bleeding and is inherited as an autosomal recessive trait.

Minor bleeding problems, such as bruising or a brief nosebleed, may not require specific treatment. For more serious bleeding, DDAVP is the treatment of choice. At appropriate doses, DDAVP can cause a 2- to 5-fold increase in plasma VWF and FVIII concentrations in patients with VWD. DDAVP can be used to prepare patients with VWD for surgery.

The presence of a lupus inhibitor is generally associated with a thrombotic, not a bleeding tendency. It does not prolong the bleeding time.

Leebeek F, Eikenboom J. Von Willebrand's Disease. New England Journal of Medicine. 2016;375(21):2067–2080. https://www.nejm.org/doi/full/10.1056/NEJMra1601561

34. Answer: D

This patient's clinical features including organomegaly, anaemia, elevated serum IgM level, lymphadenopathy, are consistent with Waldenström macroglobulinaemia (WM). WM is a B cell clonal disorder characterised by lymphoplasmacytic bone marrow infiltration and monoclonal IgM. WM is more common in men, and Caucasians with a median age of 60–70 years. There are two mutations involved in WM, myeloid differentiation primary response 88 (MYD88) and C-X-C chemokine receptor type 4 (CXCR4).

WM symptoms can be classified into two major categories:

1. Lymphoplasmacytic infiltration symptoms: Lymphadenopathy, hepatosplenomegaly, anaemia, and B-symptoms such as fever, weight loss, fatigue, and night sweats.
2. IgM paraprotein related symptoms: IgM paraprotein can cause various symptoms resulting from systemic amyloidosis, paraprotein depositions in the organs, cryoglobulinemia, peripheral neuropathy and hyperviscosity syndrome.

Hyperviscosity symptoms such as visual impairment, neurologic and cardiovascular compromise commonly occurs when IgM protein levels are above 30g/L. The diagnosis of WM is based on clinicopathologic features. Elevated IgM is present in every patient with WM. Bone marrow examination in WM should demonstrate at least 10% of infiltration by small lymphocytes with lymphoplasmacytic features or lymphoplasmacytic lymphoma. Immuno-phenotype in WM is typically positive for CD19, CD20, CD22, CD25, CD27, CD38, CD79a, FMC7, surface/cytoplasmic IgM, and negative for CD5, CD10, CD11c, CD23, and CD103. These immuno-phenotypic features are useful to differentiate WM from multiple myeloma, mantle cell lymphoma, and chronic lymphocytic leukemia.

This patient has symptoms of hyperviscosity: blurred vision, headache, altered mental state, and bilateral retinal vein thrombosis. Hyperviscosity syndrome secondary to elevated IgM leads to decreased blood flow, compromising microcirculation including the CNS and heart. It is a medical emergency and plasma exchange should be initiated promptly to remove IgM from the serum. Plasma exchange should precede systemic treatment. Systemic treatment regimens include combination therapy utilisings anti-CD20 monoclonal antibodies, nucleoside analogues (fludarabine, cladribine, bendamustine), alkylating agents (cyclophosphamide, chlorambucil), and proteasome inhibitors (bortezomib, carfilzomib).

IVIG can be used if there is a component of haemolytic anaemia, however her LDH is only mildly elevated and haptoglobin is normal. High dose steroids have no role in treatment of hyperviscosity syndrome due to WM. Anticoagulation is ineffective.

Gertz M. Waldenström macroglobulinemia: 2017 update on diagnosis, risk stratification, and management. American Journal of Hematology. 2017;92(2):209–217.
https://onlinelibrary.wiley.com/doi/full/10.1002/ajh.24557

35. Answer: C

Activated protein C along with its cofactor protein S inactivates clotting factors V and VIII. All endothelial cells except those in the cerebral microcirculation produce thrombomodulin. Thrombin which is normally a procoagulant becomes an anticoagulant after binding to thrombomodulin. The thrombin–thrombomodulin complex activates protein C which in the presence of its cofactor protein S inactivates factors V and VIII.

Protein C - an overview | ScienceDirect Topics [Internet]. Sciencedirect.com. 2020 [cited 1 May 2020].
Available from: https://www.sciencedirect.com/topics/medicine-and-dentistry/protein-c

36. Answer: G

37. Answer: E

38. Answer: F

39. Answer: H

Cytogenetic abnormalities play an important role in the diagnosis, management, and prognostication of haematological malignancies. Most of the observed abnormalities occur as translocations, deletions, monosomies, or trisomies. There are some karyotypically normal forms of haematological cancers, which can also provide important information.

The archetypal chromosomal abnormality in cancer is that of the Philadelphia chromosome, which is present in 95% of patients with chronic myeloid leukaemia, and 40% of patients with adult acute lymphoblastic leukaemia. It involves a translocation between chromosomes 9 and 22 [t(9:22)(q34;q11), resulting in the transposition of the *ABL* protooncogene onto the breakpoint cluster region (*BCR*). *ABL* inhibiting tyrosine kinase inhibitors have been used successfully in these malignancies.

In acute myeloid leukaemia (AML), the large array of cytogenetic abnormalities has complicated implications for treatment and prognosis. In acute promyelocytic leukaemia, a translocation results in a fusion protein that disrupts normal myeloid differentiation. If this translocation occurs between chromosome 15 and 17 (15;17)(q22;21), the malignancy typically responds well to all-trans retinoic acid (ATRA), whereas t(11;17)(q23;q21) predicts ATRA resistance. Two abnormalities in AML predict response to cytarabine [t(8;21)(q22;q22) and inv(16)(p13q22)]; these are termed CBF (core-binding factor) leukaemia. These are examples of 'good' risk cytogenetic profiles. Complex abnormalities (more than 3 concurrent chromosomal abnormalities), monosomy of chromosome 5 or 7, and deletion of 3q or 5q are classified as 'poor' risk profiles. Among 'intermediate' risk profiles, normal karyotype deserves special mention. This form of AML is often accompanied by the presence of FMS-like tyrosine kinase 3 (FLT3) internal tandem repeat, for which there are small molecule inhibitors being used currently in clinical trials that appear to have good efficacy.

Cytogenetic abnormalities in the myelodysplastic syndromes (MDS) are used as part of predictive scores, along with percentage of bone marrow blasts, haemoglobin, platelets and absolute neutrophil count. Y monosomy, and del(11q) are 'very good'; normal karyotype, 5q or 20q deletions or double abnormalities including del(5q) are 'good'; monosomy 7, inv(3)/t(3q)/del(3q) or 3 abnormalities are 'poor'; greater than 3 abnormalities is 'very poor'. Treatment related AML/MDS has two distinct cytogenetic profiles which correlate with the causative agent and prognosis. Radiation or alkylating agent related disease often presents as refractory anaemia with excess blasts and a complex cytogenetic profile, progressing to AML and has poor prognosis. Topoisomerase II-inhibitor related AML usually presents without preceding MDS and usually has balanced translocation of 11q23 or 21q22 – these usually respond to treatment as per de novo AML.

Multiple cytogenetic abnormalities are observed in acute lymphoid leukaemias (ALL), mostly involving immunoglobulin or T-cell receptor genes. Of clinical significance are translocations involving chromosome 8q24 and genes coding immunoglobulin light chains or heavy chains in Burkitt lymphoma. Also important is the detection of the Philadelphia chromosome in around 30% of adult ALL, which predicts poor prognosis, but good response to tyrosine kinase inhibitors and subsequent stem-cell transplant.

B-cell lymphomas have translocations involving 14q32. In mantle cell lymphoma the *BCL1* gene encoding cyclin D1, which together with a cyclin-dependent kinase is involved in cell-cycle regulation, is disrupted by t(11;14)(q13;32). Anaplastic large cell lymphoma exhibiting a fusion protein of anaplastic lymphoma kinase and nucleophosmin, have a better prognosis than those without this translocation, this protein is created by t(2;5)(p23;q35). Chronic lymphoid leukaemia can arise as a result of trisomy 12 or t(13;19)(q32;13.1).

Recently, advances in research utilising fluorescence in situ hybridisation (FISH) have identified cytogenetic abnormalities in multiple myeloma that have traditionally not been observed using traditional cytogenetic methods. For example, hyperdiploid myeloma is associated with better prognosis, whereas chromosome 13 deletion is associated with shorter prognosis, and poor response to chemotherapy.

Ohyashiki K, Kuroda M, Ohyashiki J. Chromosomes and Chromosomal Instability in Human Cancer. In: Coleman W, Tsongalis G, ed. by. New York, NY.: Humana Press; 2017. p. 241–262.
https://link.springer.com/chapter/10.1007/978–1-59745-458-2_15

40. Answer: G

This patient's history is strongly suggestive of hereditary spherocytosis, which is associated with increased haemolysis and subsequent raised risk of gallstones, as seen here. Spherocytosis is caused by inherited defects in the membrane of RBCs that reduce cell deformability. This leads to cells being removed by the spleen, which causes progressive splenic enlargement.

Disease is mild in 20–30% of patients. As in this case, hereditary spherocytosis can present later in life. However, 60–70% of patients have more severe anaemia and splenomegaly, which leads to presentation in childhood.

Hereditary spherocytosis is most commonly associated with dominant inheritance (75%). Mutations of genes encoding ankyrin, spectrin or Band 3 red cell proteins account for most cases.

The diagnosis of hereditary spherocytosis is usually made on clinical grounds, based upon the presence of **spherocytes on blood film**. Several tests are available for identifying individuals with hereditary spherocytosis:

- Osmotic fragility testing
- Ektacytometry
- Acidified glycerol lysis test (AGLT)
- Cryohaemolysis test
- Eosin-5-maleimide binding test (EMA binding test)

Elective splenectomy is often required in severe cases, but patients with mild hereditary spherocytosis may require no intervention at all.

41. Answer: H

This patient has microcytic anaemia based on the FBE. Heyde syndrome is a triad of aortic stenosis (AS), an acquired coagulopathy and anaemia due to bleeding from intestinal angiodysplasia (IA). IA and AS are chronic degenerative diseases that are often asymptomatic, with a higher prevalence in the population than is clinically apparent. The incidence of both conditions increases with age. Many studies suggest that there is an increased prevalence of IA in AS and vice versa. Severe AS may cause type 2 acquired von Willebrand's disease. This involves loss of the large multimers, which are required to maintain haemostasis in high flow conditions, such as occur in angiodysplastic arteriovenous malformations. Treatment options include localisation of angiodysplastic bleeding points with cauterisation, but this is associated with a high recurrence rate. Aortic valve replacement has been shown to improve the haematological abnormalities, and this is paralleled by clinical improvements. Valve replacement should be considered in most cases, particularly in those in whom the AS is symptomatic.

The blood smear for patient with iron deficiency shows *hypochromic (pale, relatively colourless) and small red blood cells (normal lymphocyte for comparison purposes is seen in the smear), may also show poikilocytosis (variation in shape) and anisocytosis (variation in size). Target cells* may also be seen.

42. Answer: J

This patient has clinical features of CRAB. Therefore, the clinical diagnosis is multiple myeloma.

- Hyper **C**alcaemia
- **R**enal impairment (AKI or CKD)
- **A**naemia
- **B**ony disease.

The blood film examination is usually normal except for *rouleaux* on blood film. Rouleaux are linear aggregates of red blood cells that form in the presence of increased plasma proteins.

43. Answer: C

Atypical haemolytic uraemic syndrome (aHUS) is a rare disorder characterised by thrombocytopaenia, evidence of microangiopathic haemolytic anaemia, AKI. ADAMTS13, also known as von Willebrand factor-cleaving protease levels are normal and STEC (Shiga toxin-producing E. coli) is not present in the stool. The precipitants for aHUS include complement regulation deficits, inflammation, drugs, cancer, pregnancy, preeclampsia, and infections. The pathogenesis involves activation of complement via the alternative pathway leading to a thrombotic microangiopathy with end-organ involvement predominantly affecting the renal and neurological systems. Early diagnosis of aHUS is challenging often mimicking other diseases that occur during pregnancy or postpartum such as preeclampsia, acute fatty liver of pregnancy, haemolysis, elevated liver enzymes, and low platelet count (HELLP) syndrome, and TTP.

Blood smear usually shows microangiopathic haemolytic anaemia with *schistocytes, helmet cells, red cell fragmentation* and thrombocytopenia.

Terminal complement inhibitors have emerged as an effective therapy for aHUS. Eculizumab is a humanised recombinant mono-clonal antibody that inhibits the terminal pathway of complement activation by blocking the activation of complement protein C5. Eculizumab has been shown to control haemolysis and to lead to improvements in renal function.

44. Answer: B

This patient's clinical presentation, hepatosplenomegaly, and initial FBE are suggestive of acute myeloid leukemia (AML). AML presents with signs and symptoms resulting from bone marrow failure, organ infiltration with leukaemic cells, or both. The time course is variable. It can present with acute symptoms that develop over a few days to 1–2 weeks.

Symptoms of bone marrow failure are related to anaemia, neutropenia, and thrombocytopenia. The common symptoms of anaemia are fatigue, exertional dyspnoea, and dizziness. Patients with AML often have decreased neutrophil levels despite an increased total WBC count. Patients generally present with fever, which may occur with or without specific documentation of an infection. This patient's CXR is normal. Patients may present with bleeding gums and multiple ecchymoses. Due to thrombocyto-penia, coagulopathy may result from DIC.

Alternatively, disease manifestations may be the result of organ infiltration with leukaemic cells. The most common sites of infiltration include the spleen, liver, gums, and skin. Patients with gum infiltration often present to their dentist first. Gingivitis due to neutropenia can cause swollen gums, and thrombocytopenia can cause the gums to bleed. Patients with a high leukaemic cell burden may present with bone pain caused by increased pressure in the bone marrow.

Patients with markedly elevated WBC counts can present with symptoms of leukostasis (i.e. respiratory distress and altered mental status). Leukostasis is a medical emergency that calls for immediate intervention.

The RBC is usually relatively normal. Large, sometimes hypogranular platelets can be seen. Peripheral blood film examination will detect *blasts* in most patients, although it can be difficult to distinguish among leukemia subtypes. In most patients, AML and acute lymphoblastic leukaemia (ALL) can be distinguished on morphologic grounds. The *blasts from patients with AML are larger, with more abundant cytoplasm and more prominent, often multiple nucleoli. The definitive diagnosis depends on the presence of Auer rods, which are linear bundles of myeloid-containing granules* (present in 50% of those with AML), or demonstration of at least 3% granulated precursors in AML, usually visible on Wright stain and confirmed by staining with either myeloperoxidase or Sudan black B.

45. Answer: F

The clinical manifestations of chronic myelogenous leukaemia (CML) are insidious and nonspecific such as fatigue and weight loss. Patients often have symptoms related to enlargement of the spleen, liver, or both. The peripheral blood smear in patients with CML shows a ***typical leukoerythroblastic blood picture, with the presence of precursor cells of the myeloid lineage. In addition, basophilia, eosinophilia, and thrombocytosis can be seen*** as seen in this case. All of the guidelines recommend the tyrosine kinase inhibitors (TKIs) imatinib, nilotinib, or dasatinib as first-line treatment for CML. The selection of first-line TKI therapy should be based on the patient's risk score, ability to tolerate therapy, comorbid conditions, and the adverse effect profile of the TKI.

 Bain B. Diagnosis from the Blood Smear. New England Journal of Medicine. 2005;353(5):498–507.
https://www.nejm.org/doi/full/10.1056/NEJMra043442

10 Immunology and Allergy

Questions

Answers can be found in the Immunology and Answers section at the end of this chapter.

1. A 72-year-old woman, who has a history of ischaemic heart disease, CCF, type 2 diabetes, hypertension, and chronic back pain, develops massive tongue swelling at midnight. There is no accompanying urticaria, wheeze, or dizziness. She has not eaten any unusual foods and she is a current smoker. She has documented penicillin and Kiwi fruit allergy which result in a rash. She has taken aspirin, clopidogrel, metformin, linagliptin, atenolol, perindopril, ibuprofen, and tramadol for the past 5 years. She has never had tongue swelling before.

Which of the following is most likely to be responsible for her tongue swelling?
- **A.** Atenolol.
- **B.** Ibuprofen.
- **C.** Idiopathic anaphylaxis.
- **D.** Perindopril.

2. Adrenaline is the first-line treatment for anaphylaxis. Regarding the safe use of adrenaline autoinjector, which one of the following statements is **INCORRECT**?
- **A.** When a patient is suspected to be experiencing anaphylaxis, adrenaline should be given as soon as possible.
- **B.** If the patient responds to the adrenaline and appears to be stable, there is no need for hospital assessment.
- **C.** Adrenaline can be used to treat anaphylaxis in patients with a history of ischaemic heart disease.
- **D.** Patients with a high concentration of serum IgE but no history of anaphylaxis should not carry an adrenaline autoinjector.

3. A 65-year-old patient reports a previous allergic reaction to amoxicillin. In which of the following scenarios would it be safest to rechallenge?
- **A.** Acute generalised exanthematous pustulosis (AGEP) 8 years ago.
- **B.** Drug reaction with eosinophilia and systemic symptoms (DRESS) 10 years ago.
- **C.** Hypotensive anaphylaxis 12 years ago.
- **D.** Stevens–Johnson syndrome 3 years ago.

4. Which of the following complement fragments is a biomarker for antibody-mediated rejection in renal transplants?
- **A.** C3.
- **B.** C4.
- **C.** C4d.
- **D.** C1 esterase inhibitor.

5. Which of the following cells is primarily responsible for the secretion of soluble antibodies?
- **A.** Cytotoxic T lymphocytes.
- **B.** Memory B cells.
- **C.** Plasma cells.
- **D.** T helper cells.

How to Pass the FRACP Written Examination, First Edition. Jonathan Gleadle, Jordan Li, Danielle Wu, and Paul Kleinig.
© 2022 John Wiley & Sons Ltd. Published 2022 by John Wiley & Sons Ltd.

6. A 30-year-old woman has a past medical history of recurrent sinusitis, bronchitis, pneumonia, and granulomatous lesions in the lungs. Which one of the following is consistent with a diagnosis of common variable immunodeficiency (CVID)?
   A. Elevated serum levels of IgM.
   B. Low serum levels of IgG.
   C. Normal serum levels of IgG.
   D. Normal response to vaccinations.

7. A 56-year-old woman with a past medical history of intravenous drug use and hepatitis C infection presents with lethargy, arthralgia, muscle weakness, burning sensation in the lower extremities, and bilateral lower limb rash, as shown in the figure. She also has AKI with a creatinine level of 170 µmol/L [45-90] and an eGFR of 35ml/min/1.73m². Urinalysis shows significant proteinuria and microscopic haematuria. A 24-hour urine collection shows 1.5g/24 hours proteinuria. Her BP is 125/70 mmHg, HR 87 bpm, and temperature 36 °C. What is the most likely cause of her lower limb rash?

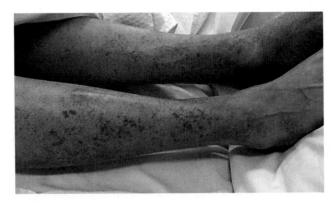

   A. Cryoglobulinaemia.
   B. IgA nephropathy.
   C. Polyarteritis nodosa.
   D. Post-streptococcal glomerulonephritis.

8. A 42-year-old man with a past medical history of mild allergic rhinitis and a family history of atopy presented to his GP after an episode of widespread urticaria with light-headedness and wheeze which developed whilst rock-climbing. The symptoms resolved on rest. Prior to rock-climbing he had had lunch at a regional hotel which included a focaccia with seafood, he had also consumed a glass of white wine, and required ibuprofen for a headache. Further history revealed similar episodes of lesser severity in the past, always when exercising, and soon after eating. Further testing shows significantly elevated levels of IgE to Omega-5 gliadin.
   Which of the following factors is **LEAST LIKELY** to have contributed to the episode?
   A. Alcohol ingestion.
   B. Non-steroidal anti-inflammatory drug use.
   C. Strenuous exercise.
   D. Sulfites in wine.

9. An 18-year-old woman presents to the emergency department with acute severe abdominal pain, nausea, and vomiting. She has had recurrent abdominal pain that lasts 2 to 5 days from 8 years of age. She has extensive investigations previously that have included ultrasound abdomen, CT abdomen and pelvis, MRCP, upper and lower endoscopy, capsule endoscopy, and laparoscopic exploration without finding any obvious abdominal pathology. Her past medical history includes swelling of the face and airway, requiring intubation three times and fresh-frozen plasma infusion for laryngeal swelling. She reports a family history of 'sudden or unexplained death'. She also suffers from anxiety and depression due to fear of recurrence of attacks, an inability to exercise, and many missed days of school.
   Which one of the following biologic mediators is likely to cause her symptoms?
   A. Bradykinin.
   B. C3a.
   C. Histamine.
   D. Tumor necrosis factor.

10. A 48-year-old man is referred due to abdominal pain, weight loss, jaundice, and lethargy. His blood test results are shown below. IgG and IgG4 levels are found to be elevated in the serum. Abdominal CT scan reveals swelling of the pancreatic head, both kidneys, and retroperitoneal fibrosis. Histological examination by endoscopic ultrasonography-guided fine-needle aspiration revealed lymphoplasmacytic sclerosing pancreatitis and IgG4-positive plasma cells.

Tests	Results	Normal values
Bilirubin	75 umol/L	2–24
ALP	200 U/L	30–110
GGT	135 U/L	9–48
ALT	50 U/L	0–5
AST	45 U/L	0–45
Creatinine	150 µmol/L	60–110

What is the most appropriate treatment at this stage?
  A. ACE inhibitor.
  B. Glucocorticoid.
  C. Mycophenolate.
  D. Rituximab.

11. A 50-year-old man is incidentally diagnosed with tertiary syphilis after surgical repair of a saccular ascending aortic aneurysm. He is otherwise clinically well with no regular antihistamine use. He has a label of "penicillin allergy" on his drug chart which he reports he has had since childhood. His mother is still alive and reports that she was advised that her son should never receive penicillin after experiencing a rash with penicillin exposure after an upper respiratory tract infection. She cannot remember the rash, or how it developed, but can recall that her son was otherwise well at the time.

Which of the following management strategies is most appropriate?
  A. Doxycycline therapy.
  B. Intravenous vancomycin.
  C. Penicillin skin testing followed by challenge.
  D. Penicillin desensitisation.

12. Several COVID-19 RNA vaccines have been developed. When compared with a traditional inactive vaccine, which one of the following is correct regarding RNA vaccines?
  A. The RNA strand in the vaccine does not elicit any unintended immune reaction.
  B. The RNA strand in the vaccine integrates itself into the host genome and increases antigen production.
  C. RNA vaccines are faster and cheaper to produce than traditional vaccines.
  D. There are other RNA vaccines approved for human use with few side effects.

13. A 45-year-old woman was brought into the emergency department by ambulance after an episode of anaphylaxis after drinking alcohol with friends. She has self-administered adrenaline after experiencing symptoms of flushing, urticaria, shortness of breath, tightness in the throat and chest, nausea, vomiting, and abdominal cramps. She is allergic to penicillin, cephalexin, gentamicin, prednisolone, eggs, and flu-vaccinations. She reports previous anaphylactic reactions after exertion and emotional events. The basal tryptase level is 25 ng/ml [≤ 20] and the tryptase level after the anaphylactic event is 39 ng/ml. Tryptase immunohistochemistry analysis of the skin shows clustering of mast cells. Mutation of which gene has been linked to this condition?
  A. *C1INH*.
  B. *BCR-ABL1*.
  C. *KIT*.
  D. *KRAS*.

14. A 32-year-old woman presents with urosepsis. After receiving a dose of intravenous ceftriaxone, her systolic BP falls from 170 mmHg to 90 mmHg. She has a known penicillin allergy resulting in a rash. Hypotension caused by anaphylaxis is suspected. Serum tryptase level is checked.

Which one of the following is correct when interpreting tryptase levels?
  A. Normal tryptase level 2 hours after an anaphylactic event excludes anaphylaxis.
  B. Peak tryptase levels occur at two hours after an anaphylactic event.
  C. Tryptase is more useful in food-related anaphylaxis than medication-related anaphylaxis.
  D. Tryptase level may be significantly elevated in patient with sepsis.

15. Toll like receptors function in which one of the following ways?
 A. Activation of immunoglobulin chain switching.
 B. Activation of the complement pathway.
 C. Regulation of B cell activation by antigen binding.
 D. Recognition of pathogens by the innate immune system.

QUESTIONS (16–20) REFER TO THE FOLLOWING INFORMATION

Match the immune cell and the correct statement:
 A. Follicular dendritic cell.
 B. Helper T cell.
 C. Cytotoxic T cell.
 D. Macrophages.
 E. Mature myeloid-derived dendritic cell.
 F. Naïve mature B cell.
 G. Natural killer cell.
 H. Regulatory T cell.

Questions:

16. Expresses CD3, CD25 and FoxP3.

17. Is the main source of interleukin-1.

18. Is the main source of interleukin-2.

19. Expresses IgD and IgM on the cell surface.

20. Expresses MHC Class II, CD80/88 and secretes IL-12.

QUESTIONS (21–26) REFER TO THE FOLLOWING INFORMATION

Match vaccine characteristics and selection with the following immunisations against infectious disease
 A. BCG (Bacillus Calmette-Guerin) vaccine.
 B. Hepatitis B vaccine.
 C. Hepatitis C vaccine.
 D. *Haemophilus influenzae* type B (Hib) vaccine.
 E. Influenza vaccine.
 F. Monovalent varicella vaccine.
 G. Pneumococcal vaccine.
 H. Tetanus vaccine.

Questions:

21. Which vaccine is contraindicated in a liver transplant recipient but also should not be given to a healthy individual who has received this vaccine before?

22. Which vaccine is the first recombinant antigen vaccine approved for human use?

23. Which vaccine is a polysaccharide vaccine?

24. Which vaccine is a conjugated vaccine?

25. Which one is a toxoid vaccine?

26. A 45-year-old man had his spleen removed after the motor vehicle accident. Apart from quadrivalent (ACWY) meningococcal conjugate vaccine, meningococcal B recombinant vaccine, what are the other **THREE** vaccines you would recommend?

QUESTIONS (27–30) REFER TO THE FOLLOWING INFORMATION

Match the neurological clinical presentation to the autoantibody most likely to be associated with it:

A. Amphiphysin.

B. Ma2.

C. Neuro-oncological ventral antigen 1 (NOVA 1).

D. *N*-methyl-D-aspartate receptor (NMDA-R).

E. P/Q type voltage-gated calcium channel (P/Q VGCC).

F. Hu (type 1 antineuronal nuclear antibody).

G. Voltage-gated potassium channels (VGKC).

H. Yo (cerebellar degeneration-related protein 2).

Questions:

27. A 72-year-old life-long smoker presents with limb weakness that worsens with activity. CXR shows a large right hilar mass.

28. A 47-year-old woman presents with breathlessness and is found to have a large pleural effusion, drainage shows adenocarcinoma which is positive for oestrogen and progesterone receptors. Whilst being investigated she reports unsteadiness and examination shows intention tremor, dysarthria, and ataxia.

29. A 68-year-old woman presents with slowed movements and is found to have stiffness of the axial muscles and limbs. Examination also shows a large right-sided breast mass.

30. A 27-year-old woman presents with uncharacteristic personality changes including paranoia and hallucinations, progressing to profound drowsiness. CT scanning shows a large heterogeneous pelvic mass with internal calcification.

Answers

1. Answer: D

Angioedema is reported to occur in 0.1–0.2% of patients who take ACE inhibitors. ACE inhibitors are usually given long term and patients can develop angioedema at any time during therapy, as seen in this case. ACE inhibitor induced angioedema is thought to result from defective degradation of vasoactive peptides: bradykinin, des-Arg9-BK (a metabolite of bradykinin), and substance P.

Risk factors for developing angioedema are age greater than 65 years, asthma and allergy, COPD, and rheumatoid arthritis. Furthermore, the use of calcium channel blockers and NSAIDs is associated with a higher risk.

The incidence of angioedema in patients receiving angiotensin receptor blockers (ARBs) is lower than in patients receiving ACE inhibitors. The incidence of angioedema in patients switched to an ARB following ACE inhibitor induced angioedema has been described mainly in case reports and case series, with an incidence ranging from 10% to 50%. The switch must be clinically necessary, and the risk must be discussed with the patient.

Treatment is to maintain the airway and discontinue ACE inhibitors. Other treatment can be trialled including: ecallantide, which inhibits bradykinin, and icatibant which prevents the binding of bradykinin to the receptor. Treatment with C1 inhibitor by fresh frozen plasma or as a C1 inhibitor concentrate could also be tried.

Terreehorst I, Reitsma S, Cohn D. Current Treatment of Angioedema Induced by ACE Inhibitors. Current Treatment Options in Allergy. 2019;6(1):18–26.
https://link.springer.com/article/10.1007/s40521-019-0203-y

2. Answer: B

Anaphylaxis is a severe, life threatening systemic reaction that can affect all ages. The clinical syndrome may involve multiple target organs, including skin, respiratory, gastrointestinal, and cardiovascular systems. The severity of previous reactions does not predict the severity of subsequent reactions. Intramuscular adrenaline is the first line treatment for anaphylaxis. Adrenaline (e.g., EpiPen®) is approved for use in Australia and New Zealand for the emergency treatment of anaphylaxis. Early use of adrenaline in anaphylaxis is associated with improved outcomes.

An ambulance should be called immediately after giving an adrenaline autoinjector to take the person to hospital, so they can remain under medical observation until symptoms have resolved. There are no absolute contraindications for use of an adrenaline autoinjector in a person who is experiencing anaphylaxis even in patient with known ischaemic heart disease or unstable angina. Further adrenaline doses may be given if there is no response five minutes after giving the previous dose. Any patient with a history of anaphylactic reaction should carry an adrenaline autoinjector. There is no indication for patients with a high concentration of serum IgE but no history of anaphylaxis to carry an adrenaline autoinjector.

Fromer L. Prevention of Anaphylaxis: The Role of the Epinephrine Auto-Injector. The American Journal of Medicine [Internet]. 2016 [cited 10 July 2020];129(12):1244–1250.
Available from: https://www.sciencedirect.com/science/article/pii/S0002934316307951

3. Answer: C

Drug allergy is immunologically mediated drug hypersensitivity reactions. These may be either IgE–mediated (immediate) or non–IgE-mediated (delayed) hypersensitivity reactions. A drug allergy is not a drug side effect or drug toxicity.

Immediate drug allergic reactions are typically IgE-mediated and occur within minutes to hours after the last drug administration. Symptoms include urticaria, angioedema, rhinitis, conjunctivitis, bronchospasm, or anaphylaxis and anaphylactic shock. Delayed-onset drug allergic reactions occur days to weeks after drug administration and are associated with a T cell dependent immune mechanism. Most delayed-onset reactions are uncomplicated cutaneous manifestations such as maculopapular exanthemas and delayed urticaria. However, delayed-onset reactions also include severe cutaneous adverse reactions (SCARs) that may be life-threatening, such as Stevens–Johnson syndrome, toxic epidermal necrolysis, and drug reaction with eosinophilia and systemic symptoms syndrome (DRESS).

Penicillin allergy is the most commonly reported drug allergy. About 90% of patients with self-reported penicillin allergy are actually able to tolerate penicillins after undergoing evaluation for penicillin allergy. Because most patients have subsequent negative allergy challenge test and tolerate penicillins, this reduces unnecessary exposure to broader-spectrum antibiotics. Overall, clinically significant IgE-mediated or T lymphocyte–mediated penicillin hypersensitivity is uncommon (<5%). Moreover, the rate of IgE-mediated penicillin allergies is decreasing, potentially due to a decreased use of parenteral penicillins, and because severe anaphylactic reactions to oral amoxicillin are rare. IgE-mediated penicillin allergy wanes over time, with 80% of patients becoming tolerant after a decade. Cross-reactivity between penicillin and cephalosporin drugs occurs in about 2% of cases, less than the 8% reported previously.

Direct amoxicillin challenge is appropriate for patients with low-risk allergy histories. Moderate-risk patients can be evaluated with penicillin skin testing, which carries a negative predictive value that exceeds 95% and approaches 100% when combined with an amoxicillin challenge. High risk patients who have a history of anaphylaxis, respiratory distress, rashes, gastrointestinal symptoms, or unknown index symptoms, can have allergy challenge test or desensitisation on a case by case basis and under the clinician's direct monitoring within an appropriate resuscitation facility.

Delayed-onset adverse drug reactions mediated by T cells are primarily cutaneous and cannot result in acute anaphylaxis. Specific allergy testing or rechallenge is inappropriate for patients with any of the following histories: Stevens–Johnson syndrome, toxic epidermal necrolysis, haemolytic anaemia, nephritis, hepatitis, or oral and/or skin blisters associated with or attributed to previous drug use. These patients should continue to avoid the specific drug or class of drugs implicated and the risk presented by rechallenge is too great. Furthermore, patients with reactions mediated by IgG or T cells cannot be desensitised but can be blunted with corticosteroids.

Classical desensitisation protocols are designed to treat Type 1 (IgE–mediated) mast cell reactions. Drug desensitisation can be described as induction of drug tolerance without an adverse reaction. In other words, it is controlled anaphylaxis – that is, the drug is administered at a concentration and rate that will cause drug-specific IgE-armed mast cells to degranulate at lower rates that do not precipitate a systemic reaction. Serial doses of medication are gradually increased (usually doubled) for each administration (often at 15- to 20-minute intervals), and the number of IgE receptors on the mast cells are suppressed, which deceases the sensitivity of the mast cell to the point where a full dose of drug can be safely given. This defines a clinically tolerant state to the continued administration of the drug with little risk of a significant mast cell–mediated reaction during the course of therapy. It is critical to note that this procedure does not eliminate the IgE-mediated drug sensitivity; rather, it desensitises the individual to allow them to receive the therapeutic course safely. Once desensitised, the patient usually does not react to administration of the drug for the duration of therapy. Once therapy is completed, the desensitised state will only last for up to four half-lives ($T\frac{1}{2}$) of the drug. After that, sensitivity is assumed to have returned, and future therapeutic courses will require repeated desensitisation protocols.

Blumenthal K, Peter J, Trubiano J, Phillips E. Antibiotic allergy. The Lancet. 2019;393(10167):183–198. https://www.thelancet.com/journals/lancet/article/PIIS0140-6736(18)32218-9/fulltext

4. Answer: C

Antibody-mediated rejection (ABMR) adversely affects long-term renal allograft survival. Diagnosis of ABMR is based on histological changes in the transplant renal biopsy. Histological features of ABMR include capillary endothelial swelling, arteriolar fibrinoid necrosis, and fibrin thrombi in glomerular capillaries. Severe vasculitis, glomerulitis with neutrophils in the glomerular capillary and peritubular capillaries (PTCs), fibrin thrombi, fibrinoid necrosis, and interstitial haemorrhage are more commonly seen with ABMR compared with T cell-mediated rejection. Rarely, ABMR may present only with evidence of acute tubular necrosis (ATN). The presence of linear staining for C4d along the PTCs, a degradation product of the complement pathway that binds covalently to the endothelium, is highly suggestive of ABMR.

Stites E, Renner B, Laskowski J, Le Quintrec M, You Z, Freed B et al. Complement fragments are biomarkers of antibody-mediated endothelial injury. Molecular Immunology. 2020; 118: 142–152. https://pubmed.ncbi.nlm.nih.gov/31884386/

5. Answer: C

In adaptive immunity, naïve memory B cells can be stimulated directly by soluble antigens or by co-stimulation with T cells. This response is also mediated by a number of co-stimulatory receptors and cytokines. In response, these B cells undergo clonal proliferation, and maturation to immunoblasts to lymphoplasmacytoid cells to plasma cells which are responsible for secreting large quantities of antibodies. This process takes several days to unfold. T cell dependent B cell stimulation tends to produce more versatile and robust immune response, whereas T cell independent responses are more rapid. Memory B cells are latent long-lived immune cells which retain the memory of previous antigen exposure and subsequent immune activation in a highly selective fashion, and on re-challenge to a particular antigenic stimulus, rapidly differentiate into plasma cells.

Klimov V. From Basic to Clinical Immunology. Springer, Cham; 2019, pp. 161–216 https://link.springer.com/book/10.1007/978-3-030-03323-1#toc

6. Answer: B

This patient's clinical presentation is consistent with common variable immunodeficiency (CVID), which is the most frequent clinically symptomatic primary immunodeficiency. CVID is an autoimmune disease which can occur in children, adolescence, and adults. CVID can affect both males and females equally and affects around 1 in 25,000 to 1 in 50,000 individuals. Due to the low awareness of the condition among health care professionals and variable presentations, the diagnosis of CVID is often delayed. B cells in patients with CVID fail to differentiate, leading to low immunoglobulin levels, specially IgG and IgA, and sometimes IgM. Due to low levels of immunoglobulins, patients often present with recurrence of infections, especially sinopulmonary, ear, and gastrointestinal infections and some patients have granulomas in the lungs, liver, and other organs. Patients may also have splenomegaly, lymphadenopathy, and poor response to vaccines. In some patients with CVID, there are genetic causes (<10%) and in others it is associated with autoimmune diseases and malignancies, such as gastric cancer and lymphoma.

Diagnosis of CVID can be made if the patient is over 4 years of age and meets the following criteria:

1. Consistent clinical features (infections, autoimmunity, granulomatous disease, and lymphadenopathy).
2. Marked decrease of IgG, IgA and/or IgM levels.
3. Poor response to vaccines (and/or absent isohaemaglutinins).
4. Secondary causes of hypogammaglobulinaemia have been excluded.

Treatment of CVID consists of either IVIG or subcutaneous immunoglobulins (SCIg), prophylaxis and treatment of infections, surveillance for autoimmune diseases and malignancy.

 Ghafoor A, Joseph S. Making a Diagnosis of Common Variable Immunodeficiency: A Review. Cureus. 2020. https://www.cureus.com/articles/26170-making-a-diagnosis-of-common-variable-immunodeficiency-a-review

 Primary immunodeficiencies (PID) Clinical Update [Internet]. Allergy.org.au. 2020 [cited 7 June 2020]. Available from: https://www.allergy.org.au/images/stories/pospapers/ASCIA_HP_Clinical_Update_PID_2017.pdf

7. Answer: A

The patient's presenting symptoms and a background history of hepatitis C infection suggest the possibility of underlying cryoglobulinaemia. IgA nephropathy can also be associated with lower limb vasculitic rashes (Henoch–Schönlein purpura) and nephritic syndrome, however patients typically also present with hypertension. Patients sometimes also report symptoms of respiratory tract infection, diarrhoea, or vomiting prior to developing IgA nephropathy. In postinfectious glomerulonephritis, glomerulonephritis typically does not happen until three weeks after the initial infection. In contrast, IgA nephropathyn may present with "synpharyngitic glomerulonephritis"–pharyngitis and glomerulonephritis around the same time.

Cryoglobulinaemia is defined as the presence of cryoglobulins in a patient's serum that precipitate at low temperatures (less than 37 °C and dissolve upon warming). Hepatitis C is often associated with mixed Type II/III cryoglobulinaemia, a mixture of a monoclonal IgM (or IgG or IgA) with rheumatoid factor activity and polyclonal immunoglobulins. Other causes of mixed Type II/III cryoglobulinaemia include connective tissue disease and B-cell non-Hodgkin's lymphoma. Type I cryoglobulinaemia is associated with clonal haematological diseases, such as B-cell lineage malignancy, including multiple myeloma, Waldenström macroglobulinemia, or chronic lymphocytic leukaemia, or monoclonal gammopathy of undetermined significance (MGUS). Treatment strategies of cryoglobulinaemia depend on the underlying causes.

For treatment of infectious mixed cryoglobulinaemia associated with hepatitis C in patients with severe diseases (cutaneous ulcers, glomerulonephritis, and progressive/debilitating peripheral neuropathy), consider using Rituximab plus corticosteroids or cyclophosphamide plus corticosteroids based on the patient's profile. In life-threatening mixed cryoglobulinaemia cases (patients with symptoms of rapidly progressive glomerulonephritis, gastrointestinal ischaemia, CNS involvement, or pulmonary haemorrhage), consider treating the disease with pulse corticosteroids, plasma exchange, rituximab, or other immunosuppressants. Treatment of hepatitis C with antiviral medications is important in patients with infectious mixed cryoglobulinaemia.

 Muchtar E, Magen H, Gertz M. How I treat cryoglobulinemia. Blood. 2016;129(3):289–298. http://www.bloodjournal.org/content/129/3/289.long?sso-checked=true

8. Answer: D

Food-dependent, exercise-induced anaphylaxis (FDEIA), is a less common form of anaphylaxis where various augmenting factors are required to clinically manifest significant symptoms. By definition, exercise is required to be the proximate trigger for the symptoms, and symptoms usually resolve with rest, however, episodes can carry high risk of morbidity, and fatalities have occurred. The initial allergen is usually a food, most commonly wheat components in Western populations, and wheat or shellfish in Asian populations, usually ingested within 4 hours of exercise. Often, co-factors are required in addition to the allergen and exercise in order to manifest symptoms, and the most frequently encountered are NSAIDs and alcohol – both of which could conceivably increase gastric permeability to the antigen, as well as lowering the activation threshold of peripheral mast cells. Other potentially triggering factors include high temperature, infection, sleep deprivation, and a range of less common factors.

Diagnosis of FDEIA can be made by the characteristic clinical history in the absence of other diagnoses, and evidence of specific IgE to the foodstuff implicated, either by skin testing or food-specific assays. Serum tryptase levels should be measured when asymptomatic to rule out systemic mast cell disorders. Avoidance of the culprit food before exercise is the most important part of managing FDEIA, however other measures are also advised: exercising with an adrenaline autoinjector, exercising with someone who can use an autoinjector, exercising with a mobile phone, advice to cease exertion on symptoms, and avoiding augmenting factors prior to exercise. Data about pharmacological measures aimed at preventing FDEIA are lacking, however, cromolyn sodium, misoprostol and omalizumab have been used for this purpose.

 Feldweg A. Food-Dependent, Exercise-Induced Anaphylaxis: Diagnosis and Management in the Outpatient Setting. The Journal of Allergy and Clinical Immunology: In Practice [Internet]. 2017 [cited 14 July 2020];5(2):283–288. Available from: https://www.sciencedirect.com/science/article/abs/pii/S2213219816305803?via%3Dihub

9. Answer: A

The patient's history, clinical features, and family history are highly suspicious of the diagnosis of hereditary angioedema (HAE). HAE is a rare autosomal dominant condition causing recurrent episodes of swelling in cutaneous and submucosal tissues, most commonly in the limbs, face, intestinal tract, airway, and infrequently the genitalia. It is estimated to affect 1 in 50,000 people. To diagnose the condition acutely requires a high index of suspicion since the diagnosis is often delayed.

HAE is caused by C1 inhibitor (C1-INH) deficiency and/or dysfunction. Cl-INH is a protease inhibitor in the serpin superfamily. Minor trauma, dental procedure, surgery, infection, menstruation, alcohol, emotional stress may trigger angioedema. Sometimes no obvious trigger is identified. During an acute attack of HAE, plasma proteolytic cascades are activated, and several vasoactive substances are released. Studies have shown that bradykinin is the predominant mediator of enhanced vascular permeability. The most severe symptom of HAE is potentially life-threatening airway obstruction. In patients with intestinal tract involvement, typical symptoms are nausea, vomiting, and abdominal pain. There may also be a history of extensive investigations or unnecessary surgeries without any obvious abdominal pathology identified. HAE is not associated with urticaria or pruritis. However, about one-third of patients develop a non-itchy rash, erythema marginatum, during an attack. Symptoms of HAE typically start in childhood and worsen during puberty, up to an attack every 1 to 2 weeks.

There are three types of HAE. Mutations in the SERPING1 gene cause HAE type I and type II. Mutations in the F12 gene are associated with some cases of HAE type III to increase coagulation factor XII by increasing bradykinin which leads to inflammation. All family members of an index patient need to be tested. If clinical suspicion of HAE is low, C4 alone is an adequate screening test. If clinical suspicion is high measure C4 and C1 esterase inhibitor level and function.

Three types of HAE:
- HAE Type 1 (85% of cases): caused by deficiency and low function of C1-INH. The most common type.
- HAE Type 2 (15% of cases): caused by low C1-INH function. C1-INH level is normal. Phenotypically indistinguishable from HAE type 1.
- HAE Type 3: symptoms are similar to HAE Type 1 and 2. Caused by mutations in factor XII. It occurs very rarely.

Patients with HAE do not respond to antihistamines, adrenaline, and corticosteroids. ACE inhibitors are contraindicated since they block bradykinin metabolism and can exacerbate HAE attacks. Exogenous oestrogens are known to increase the severity of the disease and should be avoided.

Medications for management of acute attacks include Icatibant (a bradykinin B2 receptor antagonist), plasma-derived C1-INH, including intravenous (IV) and recently available subcutaneous formulation of Berinert and Cinryze. Short term prophylaxis is required to prepare patients with HAE for elective dental, surgical procedures, or known triggers, IV Berinert is administered 1 to 6 hours before the procedure. Berinert should be readily available after operation in case of acute attacks. If Berinert is not available, increased doses of danazol (an attenuated androgen with unclear mechanism of action) for a few days before and after the procedure may be used. Danazol and tranexamic acid have been used for long-term prophylaxis. A clear sick day plan should be given to the patient and well documented in case of emergency.

 Busse P, Christiansen S. Hereditary Angioedema. New England Journal of Medicine. 2020;382(12):1136–1148.
https://www.nejm.org/doi/full/10.1056/NEJMra1808012

10. Answer: B

This patient has a diagnosis of IgG4-related type I autoimmune pancreatitis. IgG4-related disease (IgG4-RD) is a relatively new and rare disease entity that is still under-recognised. It is a chronic relapsing–remitting inflammatory disease. Its diagnosis is often delayed due to heterogenous symptoms and presentations. Common features include tumour-like swelling around the organs, which is indolent. However, without treatment it can progress to fibrosis and cause organ damage. Major presentations include type 1 autoimmune pancreatitis, salivary gland disease, orbital disease, and retroperitoneal fibrosis. Patients may have elevated plasma IgG and IgG4 levels, but the gold standard for diagnosis is based on histology findings including lymphoplasmacytic infiltrates rich in IgG4-positive plasma cells, storiform fibrosis, and obliterative phlebitis.

IgG4-RD is usually responsive to steroid treatment. However, relapses are frequently observed during steroid tapering. Steroid-sparing agents may be required in patients who have relapses and as maintenance therapy. Rituximab has been shown to be effective as induction and relapse treatment. Levels of IgG4 are not reliable for assessing response to treatment and can rebound above normal in up to 70% patients after withdrawal of glucocorticoid treatment. Currently there are no shared international classification, diagnostic criteria, and there are lack of evidence-based treatment guidelines, activity, and damage indices. Further studies and international trials are required to formulates diagnostic and treatment guidelines.

 Iaccarino L, Talarico R, Scirè C, Amoura Z, Burmester G, Doria A et al. IgG4-related diseases: state of the art on clinical practice guidelines. RMD Open. 2019;4(Suppl 1): e000787.
https://www.ncbi.nlm.nih.gov/pmc/articles/PMC6341179/

11. Answer: C

Penicillin allergy is common, and penicillins remain common causes of adverse drug reactions, including anaphylaxis, and severe delayed hypersensitivity reactions. Consequently, there is understandable caution around administering penicillin antibiotics to patients labelled as penicillin allergic. However, up to 90% of patients labelled as allergic to penicillin can safely receive penicillin drugs. Penicillins remains the drug of choice for multiple infections, including syphilis and methicillin-sensitive *Staphylococcus aureus*. Additionally, the use of penicillin in hospitalised patients reduces exposure to fluoroquinolones, vancomycin, and clindamycin. Patients with a penicillin-allergy label are reported to have higher rates of surgical-site infections, longer hospital admissions, higher readmission rates and increased rates of MRSA, VRE, and *Clostridium difficile*. Treatment of patients with penicillin allergy label also appears to be more costly.

Consequently, de-labelling penicillin allergic patients is a highly useful strategy, and in cases where penicillin treatment is imperative for clinical success, it is a foundational part of treatment. For low-risk histories, where the purported allergy includes a history of non-allergic symptoms attributed to allergy (such as nausea or diarrhoea), oral challenge in a primary care setting is reasonable. For moderate risk histories such as isolated rash, or unknown reaction, skin testing and drug challenge is warranted – desensitisation is often useful if tests are positive, but penicillin therapy is desirable. For a history of anaphylaxis, desensitisation may be required in urgent settings, and skin testing and drug challenge may still be warranted. For delayed severe reactions such as organ dysfunction or severe cutaneous reactions, delayed testing is required, and exposure to the culprit drug should be avoided unless further testing is negative. There is some research to suggest that oral challenge without skin testing is safe in both low and medium risk histories in children, but this has not been replicated in adults.

 Castells M, Khan D, Phillips E. Penicillin Allergy. New England Journal of Medicine. 2019;381(24):2338–2351.
https://www.nejm.org/doi/full/10.1056/NEJMra1807761

12. Answer: C

RNA vaccines offer some advantages over DNA vaccines and traditional vaccines in terms of production, administration, and safety.

An RNA vaccine consists of an mRNA strand that codes for a disease-specific antigen. Once the mRNA strand in the vaccine is inside the body's cells, the cells use the genetic information to produce the antigen. This antigen is then displayed on the cell surface, where it is recognised by the immune system and generates immune protection.

RNA does not integrate itself into the host genome and there is no alteration in host genome. The RNA strand in the vaccine is degraded once the protein is made.

RNA vaccines can be faster and cheaper to produce than traditional vaccines. Production of RNA vaccines is laboratory based, and the process could be standardised and scaled, allowing quick responses to large outbreaks, never-before-seen, fast-spreading viruses such as SARS-CoV-2. It bypasses the challenges of producing pure viral proteins. However, the mRNA strand in the vaccine may cause an unintended immune reaction. Delivering the mRNA strand effectively to cells is challenging since free RNA in the body is quickly degraded. To help achieve delivery, the RNA strand is incorporated into a larger molecule to help stabilise it and/or packaged into particles or liposomes.

Pardi N, Hogan M, Porter F, Weissman D. mRNA vaccines — a new era in vaccinology. Nature Reviews Drug Discovery. 2018;17(4):261–279.
https://www.nature.com/articles/nrd.2017.243#citeas

13. Answer: C

The above symptoms and elevated tryptase level after the anaphylactic event are suggestive of systemic mastocytosis. The basal tryptase level is ≥ 20 ng/ml, the tryptase level after the anaphylactic event increases by ≥ 20% of the basal tryptase level plus 2 ng/ml above the basal level, which fulfil the minor criteria of diagnosis of systemic mastocytosis. A 'gain-of-function' mutation in KIT [most commonly in codon 816 (D816V), where a valine is substituted for an aspartate] is found in over 90% of patients with systemic mastocytosis. KRAS mutations are linked to pancreatic, colon, lung cancer, and leukaemia. The presence of BCR-ABL1 mutation is linked to chronic myeloid leukaemia, acute lymphoblastic leukaemia, acute myelogenous leukaemia, and mixed-phenotype acute leukaemia. C1INH (SERPING1) gene mutation is associated with hereditary angioedema which may be associated with anaphylactic reaction, swellings of the skin and mucosal surfaces, gastrointestinal tract, and larynx. Patients with hereditary angioedema do not usually have urticaria. The diagnosis of systemic mastocytosis is based on the presence of one major and one minor or three minor criteria established by the WHO. The major criterion is multifocal clustering of mast cells (>15 mast cells per cluster) detected in in bone marrow and/or other extracutaneous organs, and confirmed by tryptase immunohistochemistry or KIT immunohistochemical analysis. Minor criteria include abnormal morphologic features of mast cells (e.g. spindle shapes with cytoplasmic projections and sometimes bilobed and multilobed nuclei), the presence of the KIT D816V mutation, expression of CD2 or CD25 on mast cells, and an increased basal serum tryptase level (≥20 ng/ml). Emergency treatment with intramuscular adrenaline injection at a dose of 0.3mg of 1:1000 solution in adults is recommended in patients with acute anaphylaxis. Antihistamines are used to treat or prevent skin and gastrointestinal symptoms. Emotional stress, physical stress, medications, food, insect bites (Hymenoptera venom), exercise, and alcohol have all been described to cause mast cell degranulation in patients with systemic mastocytosis.

Theoharides T, Valent P, Akin C. Mast Cells, Mastocytosis, and Related Disorders. New England Journal of Medicine. 2015;373(2):163–172.
https://pubmed.ncbi.nlm.nih.gov/26154789/

14. Answer: B

Anaphylaxis is an IgE-mediated type I hypersensitivity reaction. Identifying anaphylaxis is critical because further episodes and deaths can be prevented by recognising the likely causes. Hence, appropriate avoidance strategies, immunotherapy, provision of an adrenaline autoinjector, and an action plan can be provided to the patient.

Anaphylaxis is a clinical diagnosis. Measurement of mast cell tryptase may be useful in cases where the diagnosis of anaphylaxis is uncertain. Tryptase is more useful in insect venom and medication-related anaphylaxis compared to food-related anaphylaxis. Peak levels occur within 1–2 hours, with a serum half-life in vivo of approximately 2 h. Single measurement of tryptase has low sensitivity because the peak may be missed or occur within the normal range. Serial measurements (presentation, 2 and 24 h later and then on discharge) improve sensitivity by up to 75%. An elevated tryptase level at 2 h, comparative to baseline/24h level, is strongly suggestive of systemic mast cell degranulation with release of inflammatory mediators into the circulation.

However, not all anaphylactic reactions are associated with a rise in tryptase levels. The sensitivity of tryptase can be increased if the percentage difference between the baseline and peak concentration is considered, regardless of whether or not the peak concentration is outside the reference range. A persistently raised tryptase level occurs in mastocytosis, which can present with headache, diarrhoea, urticaria, angioedema, hypotension, and shock. A number of triggers can lead to significant mediator release in mastocytosis, such as stings, stress, drugs (aspirin, opioids, muscle relaxants, antibiotics), and radiographic contrast media. It is important to follow an elevated result with a convalescent sample to rule out this diagnosis.

Beck SC, Biomarkers in Human Anaphylaxis: A Critical Appraisal of Current Evidence and Perspectives. Front. Immunol. 2019;10: 494.
https://pubmed.ncbi.nlm.nih.gov/31024519/

15. Answer: D

Toll-like receptors (TLRs) are a class of pattern recognition receptors (PRRs) that initiate the innate immune response by sensing conserved molecular patterns for early immune recognition of a pathogen. They are single, membrane-spanning, non-catalytic receptors that recognises structurally conserved molecules derived from microbes and subsequently activate immune cells. Lipopolysaccharide (LPS) which is the primary endotoxin found in gram negative bacteria, is considered to be the prototypical 'pathogen-associated molecular pattern' and TLR4 functions as an LPS sensing receptor. Molecules broadly shared by pathogens, known as pathogen-associated molecular patterns (PAMPs), and the host endogenous damage-associated molecular pattern molecules (DAMPs), include double-stranded RNA, DNA, peptidoglycan, and lipopeptides can be recognised by TLR. Ten TLRs have been identified in humans (TLR1–TLR10).

TLRs stimulate apoptosis of infected cells. It stops its protein synthesis, limit the infection, and down-regulate the immune response as in dendric cells during the sepsis. TLRs play an important role in the pathogenesis of many diseases such as SLE, rheumatoid arthritis and cancers.

El-Zayat, S.R., Sibaii, H. & Mannaa, F.A. Toll-like receptors activation, signaling, and targeting: an overview. Bull Natl Res Cent 43, 187 (2019).
https://link.springer.com/article/10.1186/s42269-019-0227-2

16. Answer: H

Regulatory T cells (Tregs) are critical to the maintenance of immune cell homeostasis. Natural Tregs are CD4+, CD25+ T cells which develop, and emigrate from the thymus to perform their key role in immune homeostasis. Adaptive Tregs are non-regulatory CD4+ T cells which acquire CD25 (IL-2R alpha) expression outside of the thymus, and are typically induced by inflammation and disease processes, such as autoimmunity and cancer. FoxP3 expression is unique to Tregs.

17. Answer: D

Macrophages perform the following functions: (i) phagocytosis, (ii) antigen presentation, and (iii) cytokine production. Macrophages produce several cytokines, the most important of which are interleukin-1 (IL-1) and tumour necrosis factor (TNF). IL-1 activates a wide variety of target cells including T and B lymphocytes, neutrophils, epithelial cells, and fibroblasts, to grow, differentiate or synthesise specific proteins. For example, IL-1 stimulates T-lymphocytes to differentiate and produce IL2. IL-1 also acts on the hypothalamus to cause fever associated with infections and other inflammatory reactions. In recent years, a recombinant form of human IL-1 receptor antagonist (e.g., Anakinra) has been used in the treatment of inflammatory disorders such as rheumatoid arthritis. This class of drug neutralises the activity of IL-1 and reduces the inflammatory response.

18. Answer: B

Interleukin-2 (IL-2) is produced by helper T lymphocytes and stimulates both helper and cytotoxic T lymphocytes to grow. Resting helper T lymphocytes are stimulated by antigens or other stimulators to produce IL-2 and to form IL-2 receptors on their surface, thereby acquiring the capacity to respond to IL-2. Interaction of IL-2 with its receptor stimulates DNA synthesis. IL-2 also acts synergistically with IL-4 to stimulate the growth of B cells. Antibodies to the IL-2 receptor are in routine clinical use in solid organ transplantation to reduce the incidence of rejection (e.g. Basiliximab which is a chimeric mouse–human monoclonal antibody to the α chain (CD25) of the IL-2 receptor of T cells).

19. Answer: F

Immature B cells are very sensitive to antigen binding, so if they bind self-antigens in the bone marrow, they die. B cells that do not bind self-antigens express d chain and membrane IgD with their IgM around the time they leave the marrow and become mature naïve (resting) B cells. Membrane markers for mature naïve B cell include CD45R, CD19, CD21, CD40, IgM, and IgD.

20. Answer: E

Dendritic cells (DC) are classified into two different functional states, 'mature' and 'immature'. These are distinguished by many features, but the ability to activate antigen-specific naïve T cells in secondary lymphoid organs is the hallmark of mature DC. DC maturation is triggered by tissue homeostasis disturbances, detected by the recognition of pathogen-associated molecular patterns (PAMP) or damage-associated molecular patterns (DAMP). Maturation turns on metabolic, cellular, and gene transcription programs allowing DC to migrate from peripheral tissues to T-dependent areas in secondary lymphoid organs, where T lymphocyte-activating antigen presentation may occur. Mature dendritic cells express high levels of MHC Class II and CD80/88.

 Patente T, Pinho M, Oliveira A, Evangelista G, Bergami-Santos P, Barbuto J. Human Dendritic Cells: Their Heterogeneity and Clinical Application Potential in Cancer Immunotherapy. Frontiers in Immunology. 2019;9. https://pubmed.ncbi.nlm.nih.gov/30719026/

21. Answer: A

BCG vaccination does not prevent the transmission of TB infection to an individual. The direct effect of the vaccine is to limit the spread of primary infection in an infected individual. BCG is a live vaccine; therefore, it is contraindicated in transplant recipients. BCG revaccination is not recommended, regardless of tuberculin skin test reaction as it can cause severe reaction.

Live, attenuated vaccines contain laboratory-weakened versions of the original pathogenic agent. Therefore, these vaccines produce a strong cellular and antibody responses and typically produce long-term immunity with only one to two doses of vaccine. Many of the first vaccines that were produced consisted of live attenuated vaccines, such as measles, mumps, and chickenpox, yellow fever, rabies and BCG.

Inactivated vaccines such as influenza vaccine are produced by destroying a pathogenic agent with chemicals, heat, or radiation. This inactivation of the microorganism makes the vaccine more stable. These vaccines do not require refrigeration and is easy for transport. However, these vaccines produce weaker immune responses therefore booster shots are usually required to maintain immunity.

22. Answer: B

A recombinant vaccine is a vaccine produced through recombinant DNA technology. This involves inserting the DNA encoding an antigen (such as a bacterial surface protein) that stimulates an immune response into bacterial or mammalian cells, expressing the antigen in these cells and then purifying it from them. Hepatitis B vaccine is the first approved recombinant vaccine.

23. Answer: G

Polysaccharide vaccines are a unique type of inactivated subunit vaccine composed of long chains of sugar molecules that make up the surface capsule of certain bacteria. There are two main pure polysaccharide vaccines: pneumococcal vaccine and *Salmonella typhi* vaccine.

24. Answer: D

Conjugate vaccines as exemplified by the *Haemophilus influenzae* type B (Hib) and *Meningococcal* ACWY vaccine are a special type of subunit vaccine. In a conjugate vaccine, antigens or toxoids from a microbe are linked to polysaccharides from the outer surface of that microbe to stimulate immunity. Protection from the conjugate vaccines lasts longer than that from the polysaccharide vaccine. Conjugate vaccines generate long term memory cells allowing rapid boosting of immunity with booster doses up to many years later. Polysaccharide vaccines do not generate long term memory cells, there is nothing to boost when the same vaccine is received again years later. Repeat polysaccharide vaccine doses generate fewer circulating antibodies than previous doses. Conjugate vaccines are more expensive than polysaccharide vaccines.

25. Answer: H

Toxoid vaccines as exemplified by the diphtheria and tetanus vaccines are produced by inactivating bacterial toxins with formalin. These toxoids stimulate an immune response against the bacterial toxins.

26. Answer: D, E and G

Patients with asplenia or functional asplenia are at a life-long increased risk of bacterial overwhelming post-splenectomy infection (OPSI) due to *Streptococcus pneumoniae, Neisseria meningitidis (meningococcus), and Haemophilus influenzae.* Splenectomy is the most common cause of asplenia and the most frequent reasons for splenectomy are trauma, haematological disorders, malignancies, and incidental trauma at the time of intra-abdominal surgery. The following vaccines should be given post splenectomy:

- 13 valent pneumococcal conjugate vaccine (13vPCV)
- Quadrivalent (ACWY) meningococcal conjugate vaccine (4vMenCV)
- Meningococcal B recombinant vaccine (4CMenB)
- Haemophilus influenzae type b conjugate vaccine (Hib).
  Annual influenza vaccination is recommended as the prevention of influenza may reduce the risk of secondary bacterial infection.

 The Australian Immunisation Handbook [Internet]. Australian Government Department of Health, Canberra. 2018 [cited 13 July 2020]. Available from: https://immunisationhandbook.health.gov.au/

27. Answer: E

28. Answer: H

29. Answer: A

30. Answer: D

In a normally functioning immune system, autoimmune attacks are avoided by systematic self-immune tolerance. In paraneoplastic autoimmune conditions, it is hypothesiseds that antigens present during tumour development share similarities to 'self" antigens triggering an immune response. Neurological autoimmune conditions are a commonly observed phenomenon in a number of neoplastic conditions, both benign and malignant.

Small cell lung cancer is capable of triggering a wide range of neurological autoimmune conditions including: Lambert-Eaton myasthenic syndrome (associated with antibodies to voltage-gated calcium channels); retinopathy; neuromuscular excitability syndromes presenting with myotonia (associated with antibodies to voltage gated potassium channels); paraneoplastic encephalomyelitis (associated with anti-Hu antibodies); and occasionally opsoclonus-myoclonus-ataxia syndrome. Breast cancer is associated with paraneoplastic stiff-person syndrome and amphiphysin antibodies, paraneoplastic cerebellar degeneration due to anti-Yo antibodies, and sometimes paraneoplastic retinopathy and opsoclonus-myoclonus-ataxia. Thymoma can cause myasthenia gravis with acetylcholine receptor antibodies, paraneoplastic hyperexcitability with VGKC channels, and paraneoplastic autoimmune encephalitis with leucine-rich glioma inactivated protein 1 antibodies. One of the most common and troubling syndromes is paraneoplastic autoimmune encephalitis caused by antibodies to NMDA-R in the setting of teratoma, which frequently occurs in younger patients.

 Geng G, Yu Xiuyi, Jiang J, Yu X. Aetiology and pathogenesis of paraneoplastic autoimmune disorders. *Autoimmunity Rev*. 2020; 19(1) https://www.sciencedirect.com/science/article/pii/S1568997219302320

11 Infectious Disease

Questions

Answers can be found in the Infectious Disease Answers section at the end of this chapter.

1. A 75-year-old woman is admitted to hospital because of severe sepsis due to left lower leg cellulitis on the background of poorly controlled type 2 diabetes, stage 4 CKD, and peripheral vascular disease. She receives intravenous vancomycin, ciprofloxacin, and metronidazole. On day 5, she develops watery diarrhoea, abdominal pain, and low-grade fever. Faecal *C. difficile* toxin test is positive.

Which of the following is correct regarding the pathophysiology of this condition?
- **A.** This condition is caused by aggregation of *C. difficile* on the bowel lumen and forming pseudomembranes.
- **B.** This condition is caused by *C. difficile* exotoxin which induces necrosis of the mucosa.
- **C.** This condition is caused by invasion of *C. difficile* into the mucosa and forming pseudomembranes.
- **D.** This condition is not caused by *C. difficile* infection because the patient is receiving intravenous vancomycin and metronidazole.

2. A 65-year-old woman presents to hospital with abdominal pain and fever. Three months ago, she underwent a hemicolectomy for early stage bowel cancer in Japan. Her post-operative course was complicated by an anastomotic leak requiring ICU admission and return to theatre for peritoneal washout and re-anastomosis. On her current admission, CT shows a 6 cm collection in the right iliac fossa, and her blood cultures grow *Candida auris*.

Which of the following antifungals is most appropriate while awaiting sensitivity testing?
- **A.** Amphotericin B.
- **B.** Anidulafungin.
- **C.** Fluconazole.
- **D.** Griseofulvin.

3. Caspofungin is an antifungal agent used in the treatment of invasive aspergillosis, candidiasis, and candidaemia. Which one of the following describes its mechanism of action?
- **A.** Deposit in newly formed keratin and disrupt microtubule structure.
- **B.** Inhibit cytochrome P450 dependent 14 α-demethylation.
- **C.** Inhibit ergosterol synthesis by inhibiting squalene epoxidase.
- **D.** Inhibit the synthesis of β (1–3)-D-glucan.

4. A 22-year-old woman presents with iron deficiency anaemia. In the same consult, she asks you about screening for chlamydia. On further questioning, you ascertain that she is in a new relationship, has had several male sexual partners over the last few years, with infrequent condom use. She and her partner do not have a history of sexually transmitted disease.

Which of the following statements is most correct?
- **A.** Her sexual history means that screening is unnecessary.
- **B.** Screening and treatment of *Chlamydia trachomatis* is unnecessary in the absence of symptoms.
- **C.** Screening and treatment of *Chlamydia trachomatis* is recommended.
- **D.** Screening and treatment of *Chlamydia trachomatis* reduces the likelihood of HIV infection.

5. Which one of the following descriptions regarding COVID-19 infection is correct?
- **A.** Lymphopenia is a risk factor for developing ARDS.
- **B.** The reproductive number (R0) of severe acute respiratory syndrome coronavirus 2 (SARS-CoV-2) is 1.
- **C.** The sensitivity of current diagnostic PCR test for COVID-19 infection is about 97%.
- **D.** The virus that causes COVID-19 infection is a single-stranded DNA virus.

How to Pass the FRACP Written Examination, First Edition. Jonathan Gleadle, Jordan Li, Danielle Wu, and Paul Kleinig.
© 2022 John Wiley & Sons Ltd. Published 2022 by John Wiley & Sons Ltd.

6. Regarding the prevention of carbapenemase-producing Enterobacterales (CPE) in the healthcare setting, which one of the following statements is **INCORRECT**?

    A. CPE screen is not required for all health care workers who have come into contact with a patient who was positive for CPE, but was not isolated initially.

    B. High level resistance in CPE can be due to combinations of efflux pumps, β-lactamases production, and mutational alteration of porins.

    C. If a patient has a history of CPE carriage, followed by two negative screening test results, patient's isolation should be discontinued.

    D. While determining their CPE colonisation status, pre-emptive isolation in a single room of at-risk patients is used as a strategy to control CPE transmission.

7. A 40-year-old man returns from Thailand 5 days ago. He presents to the emergency department with fever, severe myalgia, arthralgia, and a headache. He has previously had dengue fever, and this is suspected again. On examination, he is alert and orientated, BP is 120/70 mmHg, HR 90 bpm, and oxygen saturation 96% on room air. Investigation results are displayed below.

Tests	Results	Normal values
Haemoglobin	150 g/L	135–175
Haematocrit	0.65 L/L	0.4–0.5
White Blood Cell Count	3.1×10^9/L	4–11
Platelet Count	35×10^9/L	150–450
C-reactive protein	30 mg/L	0–8
Sodium	133 mmol/L	135–145
Potassium	3.7 mmol/L	3.5–5.2
Creatinine	80 μmol/L	60–110
INR	1.1	0.9–1.3
APTT	38 seconds	24–38
D-dimer	0.80 mg/L	<0.50

What is the most appropriate treatment?

    A. High dose intravenous methylprednisolone.

    B. Intravenous Ringer's solution.

    C. Platelet transfusion.

    D. Supportive therapy and regular NSAIDs.

8. A 48-year-old man was diagnosed with HIV after presenting with *Pneumocystis* pneumonia which was successfully treated with trimethoprim/sulfamethoxazole. He was commenced on highly active antiretroviral therapy (HAART) 3 weeks ago. He presents to the emergency department today with cough, fever and CXR reveals bilateral lung infiltrates. He has mild neutrophilia; CRP is 30 mg/L [0-8]. His CD4 count was 50 cells/mm³ but is now 150 cells/mm³. His viral load is 900 copies/ml compared to 320,000 copies/ml before treatment.

What is the most likely diagnosis?

    A. Aspergillosis pulmonary infection.

    B. Immune reconstitution inflammatory syndrome (IRIS).

    C. Mycobacterium avium complex (MAC) pulmonary infection.

    D. Recurrent Pneumocystis pneumonia.

9. A 25-year-old man is going to Amsterdam for holiday and asks for pre-exposure HIV prophylaxis as he needs to take a short course of prednisolone almost every two months for the exacerbation of asthma. He is on salbutamol inhaler and regular Seretide puffer but no other medications. He is bisexual and inconsistently uses condoms. He is planning to have sexual intercourse, but he worries that he is immunosuppressed due to the periodic high-dose prednisolone. Your advice is:

    A. For prophylaxis because he inconsistently uses condoms.

    B. For prophylaxis because he may be immunocompromised due to intermittent high-dose prednisolone use.

    C. Not for prophylaxis because it will increase resistance due to potential poor adherence.

    D. Not for prophylaxis because there is no randomised control trial demonstrating the efficacy of HIV prophylaxis.

10. A 28-year-old woman presented 4 weeks ago with a sore throat, rash, and low-grade fever after returning from Thailand. She had unprotected sex. Her HIV screening test was positive, but her confirmation test was negative. She complains of fatigue, but other symptoms have resolved. Her investigations results show mild lymphocytopenia She has normal liver and renal function. Her hepatitis B and C serology are all negative. She is very concerned that she may have HIV infection.

The next most appropriate step in this patient's care would be to:
- **A.** Arrange a HIV nucleic acid test.
- **B.** Reassure the patient as the confirmation test is negative.
- **C.** Repeat the screening test in 3 months.
- **D.** Retest only if she has new exposures or risk factors.

11. A 28-year-old man presents to the emergency department with human bite wounds on his right hand after a clenched-fist fight in a pub. He had splenectomy 6 years ago due to trauma. He takes no medications.

What is the appropriate management?
- **A.** Arrange a CT scan for the right hand involving the metacarpophalangeal joint (MCP).
- **B.** Give oral prophylactic antibiotics.
- **C.** Perform a primary wound closure.
- **D.** Take a culture of the bite wounds.

12. Human T-lymphotropic virus 1 (HTLV-1) is associated with:
- **A.** Adult T-cell lymphoma.
- **B.** Hodgkin's lymphoma.
- **C.** Marginal zone lymphoma.
- **D.** Primary central nervous system lymphoma.

13. An 80-year-old woman was admitted to the intensive care unit (ICU) due to septic shock secondary to urosepsis and possible aspiration pneumonia. She has COPD, type 2 diabetes, AF, and chronic back pain. She spent 72 hours in the ICU before being discharged to the ward. She has moved wards on several occasions. You have reviewed her. She is feeling better and her vital signs are stable. She has an indwelling urinary catheter (IDC), a central line, and a peripheral intravenous line. You just been told that the patient next to her bed has returned a positive VRE screen.

What is the most important risk factor for the development of a healthcare-associated infection in this patient?
- **A.** The exposure to a patient who is VRE positive.
- **B.** The fact that she is bed bound and cannot cough properly.
- **C.** The length of hospital stay and the number of times that she moves wards.
- **D.** The presence of an IDC and a central line.

14. With regard to influenza vaccine, which one of the following statements is **INCORRECT**?
- **A.** High-dose influenza vaccine has higher seroconversion rate than standard-dose vaccine in elderly (>65 years) people.
- **B.** Influenza vaccine has 50%–60% efficacy against influenza A and 70% efficacy against influenza B.
- **C.** Influenza vaccination becomes effective 3–5 days after intramuscular administration.
- **D.** Influenza vaccination can be given to pregnant women safely in the first trimester.

15. Which of the following organisms is usually resistant to cephalosporins?
- **A.** *Klebsiella spp.*
- **B.** *Listeria monocytogenes.*
- **C.** *Proteus mirabilis.*
- **D.** *Streptococcus pyogenes.*

16. A 42-year-old woman presents to the emergency department with a 24-hour history of fever and malaise. She is a nature photographer and has returned from a trip to Madagascar chasing lemurs 5 days ago. She was in rural Madagascar for two weeks.

On presentation, she looks extremely unwell and is hypotensive with a BP of 75/40 mmHg, HR of 85 bpm, respiratory rate of 35/min, and a temperature of 39.7°C. She is not jaundiced but is mildly confused and irritable, neurological examination is otherwise normal. Cardiorespiratory and abdominal examinations are normal. She is not pregnant.

She is given a fluid bolus, broad-spectrum antibiotics, and remains unwell. While resuscitating the patient you are called by the laboratory to inform you that light microscopy on thick and thin films show abundant parasitised red cells that are not enlarged.

Which of the following is the most appropriate treatment?
  A. Artemether.
  B. Artesunate.
  C. Atovaquone/proguanil.
  D. Quinidine.

17. A 68-year-old man with type 2 diabetes, harmful alcohol use, and stage 3 CKD presents with a one-month history of dyspnoea, productive cough, arthritis, and fever. He travelled to Northern Queensland during the wet season 1 month prior to presentation. He has not responded to oral amoxycillin given 1 week prior to presentation. His temperature is 38°C, BP 90/70 mm Hg, respiratory rate 30/min, HR 128 bpm, and weight 75 kg. On examination, bronchial breath sounds, crackles are heard on the left side of his chest, and splenomegaly is noted. His right knee is swollen. Two sets of blood cultures are positive for *Burkholderia pseudomallei*. CXR is showed below.

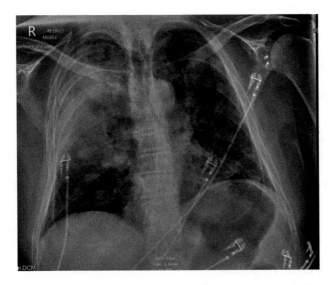

What is the mainstay of treatment for this condition?
  A. IV Ceftriaxone.
  B. IV Ceftazidime -and oral Trimethoprim/sulfamethoxazole.
  C. IV Gentamicin.
  D. IV Vancomycin.

18. A 60-year-old woman has stage 4 CKD with baseline serum creatinine 180 μmol/L [45-90] due to obstructive uropathy. She has bilateral ureteric stents and has had several episodes of urosepsis for which the urine culture was positive for *Proteus mirabilis*. Her urologist wants to start her on long-term methenamine Hippurate (Hiprex) for prophylaxis of recurrent urosepsis. Your advice is:
  A. Commence oral sodium bicarbonate to alkalinise the urine before starting Hiprex.
  B. Hiprex is ineffective in this patient because of growth of *Proteus mirabilis*.
  C. The dose of Hiprex should be reduced because of her stage 4 CKD.
  D. This oral antibiotic is bactericidal and is well absorbed with high urine concentration.

19. A 50-year-old man presents with an unsteady gait, personality change, psychosis, confusion, and memory loss. On examination, his GCS is 14 (confused), he has an ataxic gait, a positive Romberg's sign, and reduced deep and proprioceptive sensation. His serum rapid plasma reagin (RPR) is positive and CSF shows an elevated white cell count, an elevated protein level, and a positive CSF Venereal Disease Research Laboratory (VDRL) results. His HIV serology is negative.
  Which one of the following antibiotics is preferred for treatment of the condition?
  A. Ceftriaxone.
  B. Doxycycline.
  C. Penicillin.
  D. Tetracycline.

20. A 76-year-old woman who lives in a nursing home is admitted to an Acute Medical Unit because of a 2-day history of watery diarrhoea and dehydration. Her stool test is positive for norovirus. Her two roommates have just been sent to the emergency department because of severe vomiting but no diarrhoea.

   Which one of the following statements is correct?
   - **A.** Alcohol-based hand sanitisers are effective at killing norovirus so it should be available at the room for hand hygiene.
   - **B.** All cases of norovirus infection are notifiable.
   - **C.** Her two roommates- should be tested for norovirus in their vomitus despite no diarrhoea.
   - **D.** Infection period is from the day of symptoms until the day they recover.

21. A 32-year-old woman is admitted with pyrexia of unknown origin (PUO) for investigation. She has no significant past medical history apart from mild asthma in childhood. After careful history from her and her family, physical examination, and initial investigations, you suspect that she may have factitious fever.

   Which one of the following tests will be most helpful to distinguish PUO from factitious fever?
   - **A.** CT chest, abdomen, and pelvis.
   - **B.** Erythrocyte sedimentation rate (ESR).
   - **C.** Serum procalcitonin level.
   - **D.** Trial of empirical steroid treatment.

22. Q fever is caused by which one of the following organisms?
   - **A.** *Borrelia burgdorferi.*
   - **B.** *Brucella abortus.*
   - **C.** *Coxiella burnetii.*
   - **D.** *Rickettsia australis.*

23. Which one of the following parasites can perpetuate its infection through an autoinfection cycle?
   - **A.** Ascariasis.
   - **B.** Enterobiasis.
   - **C.** Hookworm.
   - **D.** Strongyloides.

24. Regarding the treatment of pulmonary TB, which one of the following statements is correct?
   - **A.** A 6-month course of isoniazid and pyrazinamide therapy should cure drug-susceptible TB with less than 5% chance of relapse.
   - **B.** Addition of fluoroquinolone to the standard treatment regimen shortens treatment duration.
   - **C.** Daily administration of treatment has better outcomes than twice-weekly treatment.
   - **D.** Rifampicin-resistant TB is the most common form of drug-resistant TB.

25. Which toxin produced by microorganisms activates large numbers of T lymphocytes?
   - **A.** Aspergillus aflatoxin.
   - **B.** Botulinum toxin.
   - **C.** Staphylococcal toxin.
   - **D.** Vibrio cholera toxin.

26. A heart transplant patient needs to travel to Southeast Asia, which of the following vaccines is contraindicated?
   - **A.** Meningococcal conjugate.
   - **B.** Pertussis.
   - **C.** Rabies.
   - **D.** Yellow fever.

27. Acute vertebral osteomyelitis is most commonly caused by which of the following pathogens?
   - **A.** *Escherichia coli.*
   - **B.** *Proteus mirabilis.*
   - **C.** *Staphylococcus aureus.*
   - **D.** *Streptococcus pyogenes.*

28. Which one of the following regarding Zika virus infection is correct?
  A. Zika virus belongs to mosquito-borne group of DNA flaviviruses.
  B. Zika virus can be detected in the blood but not in urine.
  C. Zika virus infection can be associated with Guillain-Barré syndrome.
  D. Zika virus infection is not transmitted via sexual transmission.

29. A 78-year-old woman is diagnosed with herpes zoster ophthalmicus. Her other medical history included myelodysplastic syndrome and type 2 diabetes. Which one of the following statements about her treatment is correct?
  A. Aciclovir can be used in patients with myelodysplastic syndrome.
  B. Aciclovir reduces the incidence or severity of post-herpetic neuralgia is effective in treating post-herpetic neuralgia.
  C. Famciclovir is more effective than aciclovir, leading to a shorter duration of symptoms.
  D. Topical steroid eye drops should be initiated as soon as herpes zoster ophthalmicus is suspected.

30. An 18-year-old college student presents to the emergency department as her classmate has been diagnosed with meningitis caused by meningococcus group A. They are living in the same house, studying for examinations and they have unprotected sex regularly.
  What action would you recommend for this patient?
  A. Immunisation with meningococcal vaccine (types A, B, C, W and Y).
  B. Single dose intramuscular ceftriaxone 250 mg.
  C. Single dose intramuscular ceftriaxone 250 mg plus immunisation with meningococcal vaccine.
  D. Single dose oral ciprofloxacin plus immunisation with meningococcal vaccine.

QUESTIONS (31-38) REFER TO THE FOLLOWING INFORMATION
Match the following anti-bacterial agents with their primary mechanism of action:
  A. Inhibiting DNA topoisomerase.
  B. Competition with the A site on the 50S ribosomal subunit.
  C. Direct disruption of the cell membrane.
  D. Inhibition of DNA-dependent RNA-polymerase.
  E. Inhibition of translocation of tRNA at the 50S ribosomal subunit.
  F. Disruption of dihydrofolate reductase.
  G. Inhibition of de novo folate biosynthesis.
  H. Binds penicillin binding protein to inhibit cell wall synthesis.

Questions:

31. Meropenem.

32. Ciprofloxacin.

33. Trimethoprim.

34. Erythromycin.

35. Rifampicin.

36. Colistin.

37. Sulfamethoxazole.

38. Doxycycline.

QUESTIONS (39-42) REFER TO THE FOLLOWING INFORMATION
What is the most frequent molecular mechanism by which each of the following bacteria acquires its associated anti-microbial resistance phenotype?
  A. Chemical alteration of the antibiotic.
  B. Destruction of the antibiotic.

C. Disruption to cellular entry via decreased permeability.

D. Efflux of the antibiotic.

E. Point mutations in genes encoding the target.

F. Enzymatic alterations of the binding site.

G. Replacement of the original antibiotic target by creation of a new target.

H. Global cell adaptation to antibiotic effects.

Questions

39. Vancomycin-resistant *Enterococcus faecium* (VRE).

40. Aminoglycoside-resistant *Escherichia coli*.

41. Extended spectrum beta-lactamase producing (ESBL) *Enterobacteriaceae*.

42. *Staphylococcus aureus* with intermediate sensitivity to vancomycin.

QUESTIONS (43–46) REFER TO THE FOLLOWING INFORMATION

Match each of the following antiviral actions with the drug it best describes:

A. Adefovir.

B. Entecavir.

C. Famciclovir.

D. Oseltamivir.

E. Raltegravir.

F. Ritonavir

G. Tenofovir.

H. Zidovudine.

Questions

43. A guanosine analogue phosphorylated within virally infected cells into a triphosphate that then incorporates into viral DNA, halting the replication process.

44. A guanosine derivative phosphorylated within virally infected cells to a triphosphate that inhibits DNA polymerase.

45. Inhibition of viral protease.

46. Inhibition of viral neuraminidase.

QUESTIONS (47–50) REFER TO THE FOLLOWING INFORMATION

Match each of the HIV-associated cancers with the virus most commonly implicated in its causation:

A. Endogenous retrovirus.

B. Epstein-Barr virus.

C. Human herpesvirus 6.

D. Human herpesvirus 8.

E. Human papillomavirus.

F. Human T-lymphocyte virus.

G. Parvovirus B19.

H. Polyomavirus.

Questions

47. Kaposi's sarcoma.

48. Merkel cell carcinoma.

49. Primary central nervous system lymphoma.

50. Squamous cell anal cancer.

Answers

1. Answer: B

Clostridium difficile infection (CDI) is defined by the presence of diarrhoea and either a stool test positive for *C. difficile* toxins or detection of toxigenic *C. difficile*, or colonoscopic or histopathologic proven pseudomembranous colitis. CDI is increasing at an alarming rate. *C. difficile* produces exotoxin that induces necrosis of the superficial mucosa leading to pseudomembrane formation. The bacteria do not invade the mucosa.

There is no evidence to support using metronidazole or oral vancomycin prophylactically to patients without diarrhoea and/or signs of CDI who are receiving antimicrobial therapy for an underlying infection. Every patient who is taking any antimicrobial increases the risk for CDI, and for patients with established *C. difficile* infection, antimicrobial exposure increases the likelihood of future relapse. The use of vancomycin or metronidazole may increase the patient's risk for CDI and use of vancomycin has the potential to promote the development of vancomycin resistance in other bacteria.

Practice guidelines recommend **NOT** testing for CDI if there is no diarrhoea and **NOT** repeating testing within 7 days during the same episode of diarrhoea. Although there is an epidemiologic association between proton pump inhibitors (PPIs) and CDI, the evidence suggests that PPIs do not need to be discontinued to prevent CDI. PPIs should be continued or discontinued as appropriate.

Oral metronidazole is recommended for the first line treatment for mild to moderate CDI. The second line and for severe cases treatment is oral vancomycin. The recurrence rate after a single episode of CDI is 15%, typically within the first 3 months. The recommendation is to give oral vancomycin for the first recurrence of CDI using a tapered and pulsed regimen. The alternative is to treat with fidaxomicin for 10 days. Faecal transplant should be considered in patients with multiple recurrences. For patients who get treated for CDI but continue to require systemic antibiotics, the recommendation is to stop CDI therapy at the end of the 10-day course but consider an empiric continuation in high-risk patients, this may include vancomycin 125 mg daily or fidaxomicin 200 mg daily. Current guidelines do not recommend the use of probiotics for primary prevention. Lactobacillus and Saccharomyces species have been purported as potentially beneficial for preventing recurrence.

McDonald L, Gerding D, Johnson S, et al. Clinical Practice Guidelines for Clostridium difficile Infection in Adults and Children: 2017 Update by the Infectious Diseases Society of America (IDSA) and Society for Healthcare Epidemiology of America (SHEA). Clinical Infectious Diseases. 2018;66(7): e1-e48.
https://academic.oup.com/cid/article/66/7/e1/4855916

2. Answer: B

C. auris is an emerging strain of candida which has caused severe infection in sporadic cases world-wide. Initially reported following its isolation from external ear discharge from a patient in Japan. There are four clades (genetically distinct variations) of *C. auris*. The simultaneous detection of *C. auris* on multiple continents, the clonality of isolates from different regions, and the various geographic resistance mechanisms suggest independent clonal expansion and evolution. Common factors such as the use of broad-spectrum antibiotics, and antifungals, in immunocompromised patients, might have promoted the emergence of *C auris* in different geographic locations. The clinical importance of *C. auris* is that it has high levels of anti-fungal resistance and is transmitted via inert media for long periods of time. *C. auris* is resistant to azole antifungals in up to 90% of cases and to amphotericin in up to 30% of cases. However, at present only around 5% of cases have significant resistance to echinocandins, such as caspofungin, micafungin, or anidulafungin.

Currently, the standard of care for a patient with *C. auris* infection requires echinocandin treatment, isolation with daily disinfection of the patient's surroundings, and notification to local public health authorities. Echinocandin should be used initially while awaiting antifungal susceptibility results, and monitoring for response. Chlorine bleach is commonly used for environmental disinfection, and patient disinfection with chlorhexidine or povidone-iodine is also employed although the efficacy of such strategies has not been determined. Mortality rates of *C. auris* infections are high, between 30–60%. For patients at high risk of colonisation, such as those who have had an overnight stay in an overseas healthcare institution within the last 12 months, screening for *Candida auris*, along with preemptive isolation pending the result, is recommended.

Ong C, Chen S, Clark J, Halliday C, Kidd S, Marriott D et al. Diagnosis, management and prevention of Candida auris in hospitals: position statement of the Australasian Society for Infectious Diseases. Internal Medicine Journal. 2019;49(10):1229–1243.
https://onlinelibrary.wiley.com/doi/abs/10.1111/imj.14612

Bradley S. What Is Known About Candida auris. JAMA. 2019;322(15):1510.
https://jamanetwork.com/journals/jama/article-abstract/2749798

3. Answer: D
There are four main classes of antifungals: polyenes, pyrimidine analogues, azoles, and echinocandins:

- **Polyenes** (amphotericin B): Bind to cell membrane ergosterol, forming artificial pores which permit potassium efflux and cell death and indicated for many invasive fungal infections. Common side effects include renal toxicity (including AKI in 30%), infusion reactions, electrolyte disturbances, and hepatotoxicity. Polyenes have few drug–drug interactions but have the potential for additive nephrotoxicity especially in combination with immunosuppressants, i.e., tacrolimus.

- **Pyrimidine analogues** (5-fluorocytosine): Binds to fungal cytosine permease, which imports it into the cell, where cytosine deaminase converts it to fluorouracil which impairs nucleic acid synthesis. It is mainly indicated for pathogenic yeasts, with broader use inhibited by quick resistance development. The two main side effects are bone marrow suppression and liver toxicity. There are few drug–drug interactions, but drugs which reduce renal clearance may predispose to flucytosine toxicity.

- **Azoles** (imidazoles: clotrimazole, ketoconazole, miconazole, and triazoles: fluconazole, itraconazole, voriconazole, posaconazole, isavuconazole) Inhibit C14-α–sterol demethylase, which leads to the accumulation of sterol precursors and reduction of ergosterol. Different azoles have different indications, importantly *Candidiasis* (fluconazole, itraconazole, voriconazole, posaconazole), *Cryptococcosis* (fluconazole, itraconazole), invasive *Aspergillosis* (voriconazole, isavuconazole), and *Mucormycosis* (isavuconazole). Azoles are generally well tolerated, but require liver function monitoring due to risk of hepatotoxicity (31% with voriconazole), ECG monitoring due to QT prolonging effects (except isavuconazole which is QT shortening) and comprehensive drug–drug interaction monitoring due to many interactions as inhibitors of CYP450 as well as variable affinity or CYP2C19 CYP3A4 and CYP2C9. Unique side effects of voriconazole include photosensitivity, reversible photopsia, and bone marrow toxicity.

- **Echinocandins** (capsofungin, micafungin, anidulafungin) inhibit fungal cell well polysaccharide β −1,3 glucan synthesis, which results in fungicidal activity, and for *Aspergillus spp* inhibition at the hyphal tip which is fungistatic. Echinocandins are indicated for the empiric treatment and prevention of invasive fungal infections, especially *Candida spp*. Echinocandins are generally very well tolerated and have minimal drug–drug interactions. Uniquely, Caspofungin uses the OATP–1B1 transporter, and requires dose reduction when used with other drugs which use this transporter i.e., rifampin, phenytoin, and dexamethasone.

Kullberg B, Arendrup M. Invasive Candidiasis. New England Journal of Medicine. 2015;373(15):1445–1456. https://www.nejm.org/doi/full/10.1056/NEJMra1315399?url_ver=Z39.88-2003&rfr_id=ori:rid:crossref.org&rfr_dat=cr_pub%3dpubmed

4. Answer: C
Sexually transmitted chlamydial infection in females is typically asymptomatic and occurs most commonly in sexually active females between the ages of 15 and 24. As an important cause of infertility, ectopic pregnancy, and pelvic inflammatory disease (PID), annual screening is recommended in sexually active women under 25 years of age, and older women with other risk factors. Other risk factors include new or multiple sex partners, partner with a sexually transmitted disease (STD), comorbid STD, commercial sex work, or incarceration. Although cervicitis due to chlamydial infection increases HIV susceptibility and shedding, it is unclear whether screening and treatment decreases this risk. Screening however does appear to reduce risk of PID.

Positive screening necessitates treatment with azithromycin or doxycycline, as well as counselling on ongoing risk reduction, and screening for gonorrhoea, HIV, and syphilis. Additionally, women with *Chlamydia trachomatis* infection are at risk for rapid re-infection after treatment and should be retested in three months. A negative test in an at-risk individual should lead to rescreening within one year if still at risk.

Wiesenfeld H. Screening for Chlamydia trachomatis Infections in Women. New England Journal of Medicine. 2017;376(8):765–773. https://www.nejm.org/doi/full/10.1056/NEJMcp1412935

5. Answer: A
Severe acute respiratory syndrome coronavirus 2 (SARS-CoV-2) is a novel RNA virus that causes coronavirus disease 2019 (COVID-19), with highly variable clinical severity and fatality rate of 1–3 %. Currently the gold standard diagnostic RT-qPCR test detects RNA expression of the open reading frame of the 1ab gene of SARS-CoV-2 from nasopharyngeal swab samples but has only approximately 70% sensitivity.

R0 refers to the average number of people that one infected patient goes on to infect in a group that has no immunity. R0 is used to predict how far and how fast a disease will spread, and the number can also inform policy decisions about how to contain an outbreak and can decline with measures such as social distancing. Studies suggest the R0 for COVID-19 is 2.2 to 5.7 unless public health measures are instituted.

Presentations of COVID-19 have ranged from asymptomatic/mild symptoms to severe respiratory failure and mortality. Common symptoms include fever (98%), cough (76%), myalgia/fatigue (44%), and shortness of breath.

Risk factors associated with ARDS and death in patients with COVID-19 include:

- Older age
- High fever (>39°C)
- Comorbidities (e.g., hypertension, diabetes, COPD, CCF, ESKD, immunocompromised)
- Neutrophilia
- Lymphocytopenia
- Elevated end-organ–related indices (e.g., AST, LDH, and urea)
- Elevated inflammation-related indices (CRP and serum ferritin)
- Elevated coagulation function related indicators (prothrombin time and D-dimer).

The median incubation period is estimated to be 5.1 days. 97.5% of patients who develop symptoms do so within 11.5 days of infection. Transmission is believed to occur via respiratory droplets from coughing and sneezing. Asymptomatic patients are still able to transmit infection.

Gandhi R, Lynch J, del Rio C. Mild or Moderate Covid-19. New England Journal of Medicine. 2020.
https://www.nejm.org/doi/full/10.1056/NEJMcp2009249

6. Answer: C

Infections with carbapenemase-producing Enterobacterales (CPE) are increasing in Australian and New Zealand healthcare settings. Infections with CPE are difficult to treat because few, and in some cases no, antibiotics remain effective against them, due to their extensive resistance patterns. They are associated with high morbidity, mortality, and health care costs.

Carbapenemases are β-lactamases that hydrolyse carbapenems, and other β-lactams. The most frequently occurring species of Enterobacterales which are found to produce carbapenemases, are *Klebsiella pneumoniae* and *Escherichia coli*. CPE displays various resistance profiles, depending on the type of genetic elements they harbour and the type of carbapenemases they produce. It may be chromosomally encoded or more commonly, plasmid mediated.

Besides carbapenemase production, carbapenem resistance may also be caused by combinations of efflux pumps, production of other β-lactamases, and mutational alterations of porins. Carbapenem resistant organisms can be highly resistant to a diverse range of antibiotics due to these mechanisms, along with carriage of genes that confer specific resistance to other classes of antibiotics such as fluoroquinolones and colistin.

A number of risk factors have been identified for carriage of CPE, particularly overseas healthcare exposure, with an overnight stay within the past 12 months, and being a direct inpatient contact (e.g., sharing the same room for 24 hours) of a patient with CPE colonisation. A number of other risk factors for CPE colonisation amongst hospitalised patients have been identified, such as receipt of a broad-spectrum antibiotic, renal failure, and receipt of cancer chemotherapy. If a patient has a history of CPE carriage, isolation should be continued indefinitely regardless the following screening test results.

Pre-emptive isolation of patients considered at risk of CPE colonisation is a strategy employed to minimise the risk of healthcare transmission of CPE. Patients pre-emptively isolated are then screened for CPE and remain isolated until the criteria for not having CPE carriage are met, typically using a faecal sample or rectal swab tested for the presence of CPE.

Screening of healthcare workers is generally not recommended, as proper infection control practices by healthcare workers with CPE should significantly mitigate the risk of transmission to patients.

Magiorakos A, Burns K, Rodríguez Baño J, et al. Infection prevention and control measures and tools for the prevention of entry of carbapenem-resistant Enterobacteriaceae into healthcare settings: guidance from the European Centre for Disease Prevention and Control. Antimicrobial Resistance & Infection Control. 2017;6(1).
https://aricjournal.biomedcentral.com/articles/10.1186/s13756-017-0259-z

Carbapenemase-Producing Enterobacteriacaea (CPE) Guide [Internet]. Australian Commission on Safety and Quality in Health Care. 2019 [cited 12 May 2020]. Available from:
https://www.safetyandquality.gov.au/our-work/healthcare-associated-infection/cpe-guide

7. Answer: B

This patient has clinical features of severe dengue haemorrhagic fever and leakage syndrome. He has had a previous infection and the secondary infection increases the risk of severity. A large, infected cell mass results in elevated concentrations of acute-phase response proteins, cytokines, and chemokines; generation of immune complexes; and consumption of complement. The host immunologic response is thought to create a physiological environment in tissues that promotes capillary permeability. However, the exact mechanisms are unclear. Loss of essential coagulation proteins may cause coagulopathy.

Dengue is the most common arthropod-borne viral infection in humans, caused by one of four serotypes of the dengue virus, a member of the Flavivirus genus. It is the leading cause of acute febrile illness in return travellers from Asia and South America. It is transmitted by mosquitoes of the genus Aedes. Dengue fever is typically a self-limiting disease, with a mortality rate of less than 1%. A small percentage of persons who have previously been infected by one dengue serotype develop bleeding and endothelial leak upon infection with another dengue serotype. This syndrome is termed 'dengue haemorrhagic fever.' The mortality rate for untreated dengue haemorrhagic fever approaches 50%; but with supportive treatment mortality is 2%–5%.

The incubation period is 3–14 days (average, 4–7 days). If the onset of symptoms is >14 days after the patient departs from an endemic area, then dengue is unlikely. Classic dengue fever symptoms include sudden onset of fever; chills; and severe headache, back and extremities pain which is called 'breakbone'. WHO guidelines classify symptomatic dengue infection into three categories: probable dengue, dengue with warning signs, and severe dengue.

The minimal criteria for the diagnosis of dengue haemorrhagic fever are as follows:
- Fever.
- Haemorrhagic manifestations such as haemoconcentration, thrombocytopenia, petechiae and purpura, bleeding at venepuncture sites, nasal or gingival bleeding, melaena, haematemesis, and menorrhagia).
- Circulatory failure, such as signs of vascular permeability (hypoproteinaemia, effusions).
- Hepatomegaly.

As the symptoms of dengue fever are nonspecific, laboratory investigation is important to make the diagnosis and the diagnostic criteria include one or more of the following:
- Isolation of the dengue virus from serum, plasma, leukocytes, or autopsy samples.
- Demonstration of a fourfold or greater change in reciprocal IgG or IgM antibody titres to one or more dengue virus antigens in paired serum samples.
- Demonstration of dengue virus antigen in autopsy tissue via immunohistochemistry or immunofluorescence or in serum samples via enzyme immunoassay.
- Detection of viral genomic sequences in autopsy tissue, serum, or cerebrospinal fluid samples via PCR.

Haemorrhagic laboratory abnormalities may include:
- Positive FOBT
- Hypoproteinaemia
- Prolonged prothrombin time
- Prolonged activated partial thromboplastin time
- Decreased fibrinogen
- Increased amount of fibrin split products.

There is no effective antiviral treatment for dengue infection currently. The main treatment remains supportive including:
- The presence of any warning sign indicates the need for hospitalisation and close observation.
- Careful fluid management in patients with inadequate oral intake is essential.
- Prompt fluid resuscitation to restore plasma volume, followed by ongoing fluid therapy to support the circulation to maintain critical organ perfusion is imperative to reduce mortality rates due to dengue haemorrhagic fever and dengue shock syndrome. Isotonic crystalloid solutions are the first choice and isotonic colloid solutions should be reserved for patients presenting with profound shock or those who do not have a response to initial crystalloid therapy.
- Platelet concentrates, FFP and cryoprecipitate may be needed depending on the presence of coagulopathy. However, there is no evidence that prophylactic platelet transfusions are helpful.
- High dose of steroid has been shown to have no benefit in a prospective double-blinded RCT.
- NSAIDs are contraindicated in patients with suspected or confirmed dengue fever despite severe muscular and skeletal pain. It exposes patients to risks of further bleeding complications and renal impairment.

 Simmons C, Farrar J, van Vinh Chau N, Wills B. Dengue. New England Journal of Medicine. 2012;366(15):1423–1432. https://www.nejm.org/doi/full/10.1056/NEJMra1110265

8. Answer: B
Immune reconstitution inflammatory syndrome (IRIS) is a paradoxical clinical worsening of a known infectious condition or the appearance of a new infections condition after initiating highly active antiretroviral therapy (HAART) in HIV-infected patients.

Pre-existing infections in individuals with IRIS may have been previously diagnosed and treated or they may be subclinical and unmasked by the host's regained immunity to specific infectious or non-infectious antigens to mount an inflammatory response.

The pathogenesis of IRIS involves a combination of: (i) underlying antigenic burden, (ii) degree of immune restoration following HAART, and (iii) host genetic susceptibility. Following HAART an increase in memory CD4+ cells is observed possibly as a result of redistribution from peripheral lymphoid tissue. This CD4+ phenotype is primed to recognise previous antigenic stimuli, and thus may be responsible for manifestations of IRIS seen soon after HAART initiation.

Diagnosis of IRIS remains a challenge. There is no definitive test available to establish an IRIS diagnosis. The major criteria for diagnosis include:

- Atypical presentation of 'opportunistic infections (OI) or tumours' in patients responding to HAART.
- Decrease in plasma HIV RNA level by at least 1 $\log_{10}$copies/mL.

Minor criteria include:

- Increased blood CD4+ T-cell count after HAART.
- Increase in immune response specific to the relevant pathogen.

Approximately 20% of patients initiating HAART will develop IRIS. Risk factors identified for the developments of IRIS include:

- Male sex
- Younger age
- Lower CD4+ T-cell count at HAART initiation
- Higher HIV RNA at HAART initiation
- Lower CD4+ T-cell percentage at HAART initiation
- Lower CD4+:CD8+ ratio at HAART initiation
- More rapid initial fall in HIV RNA on HAART
- Antiretroviral naïve at time of OI diagnosis
- Shorter interval between OI therapy initiation and HAART initiation.

If immune function improves rapidly following the commencement of HAART, systemic or local inflammatory reactions may occur at the site or sites of the pre-existing infection. Spontaneous resolution of the infection disease is common without specific antimicrobial therapy especially if the pre-existing infection is effectively treated. It is paramount important to continue HAART. However, long-term sequelae and fatal outcomes may rarely occur, particularly when neurologic structures are involved.

 Wilkinson R, Walker N, Scriven J, Meintjes G. Immune reconstitution inflammatory syndrome in HIV-infected patients. HIV/AIDS–Research and Palliative Care. 2015;2015(7):49–64.
https://www.dovepress.com/immune-reconstitution-inflammatory-syndrome-in-hiv-infected-patients-peer-reviewed-fulltext-article-HIV

9. Answer: A

HIV is still a disease of disparities and significant global burden despite advances in HIV research and treatment. About 2 million people worldwide are newly infected with HIV each year.

There are several randomised control trials which have demonstrated the efficacy of HIV prophylaxis by using the combination of antiretroviral regimen and tenofovir disoproxil fumarate (TDF)/emtricitabine, taken as a single pill once daily. It is also cost effective. Understanding risk factors that place patients at a high risk of HIV infection and individualised approach to discussing and prescribing pre-exposure prophylaxis (PrEP) are key. A combination of behavioural risk reduction counselling, STD surveillance and HIV PrEP can decrease HIV transmission risk.

There are theoretical concerns of risk compensation (increased unsafe sex among PrEP users that may undermine prevention efforts) for prescribing PrEP. However, several of the major PrEP trials did not demonstrate risk compensation. There was no increase in STDs from baseline. The risk of drug resistance was low if the patient subsequently became HIV positive.

 Riddell J, Amico K, Mayer K. HIV Preexposure Prophylaxis. JAMA. 2018;319(12):1261.
https://jamanetwork.com/journals/jama/article-abstract/2676116

10. Answer: A

This patient has risk factors and a clinical presentation suggestive of an acute HIV infection. The screening test for HIV is an antigen (p24)/antibody immunoassay that detects HIV-1 and HIV-2 antibodies and HIV-1 p24 antigen to test for established HIV-1 and HIV-2 infection and for acute HIV-1 infection, respectively. No further testing is required for specimens that are non-reactive on the initial immunoassay. However, if there is a possibility of very early infection leading to a non-reactive initial screening test, such as when recent HIV exposure is suspected or reported, then an HIV-1 nucleic acid test (NAT) should be conducted or repeat test in 4–6 weeks.

If the screening test is positive, it should be tested with an FDA-approved supplemental antibody immunoassay (confirmation test) that differentiates HIV-1 antibodies from HIV-2 antibodies. Positive results on the screening test and the HIV-1/HIV-2 antibody differentiation immunoassay should be interpreted as positive for HIV-1 antibodies, HIV-2 antibodies, or HIV antibodies, untypeable (undifferentiated).

If the screening test is positive but confirmation test is negative, patients should be offered HIV-1 NAT:

- A positive HIV-1 NAT result and negative confirmation test indicates laboratory evidence of acute HIV-1 infection.
- A negative HIV-1 NAT result and negative confirmation test indicates an HIV-1 false-positive result on the initial immunoassay screening test.
- A negative HIV-1 NAT result and repeatedly HIV-2 indeterminate or HIV indeterminate antibody differentiation immunoassay result should be referred for testing with a different validated supplemental HIV-2 test (antibody test or NAT) or repeat the algorithm in 2 to 4 weeks, starting with an antigen/antibody immunoassay.

Bernard M. B, S. Michele O, Laura G. W, Berry B, Barbara G. W, Kelly E. W et al. Laboratory testing for the diagnosis of HIV infection: updated recommendations [Internet]. Centers for Disease Control and Prevention. 2014 [cited 12 January 2020].
Available from: https://stacks.cdc.gov/view/cdc/23447

11. Answer: B

Approximately 10–15% of human bite wounds become infected. Patients with a prior splenectomy, the presence of a prosthetic valve or joint, chronic liver disease, and immunosuppression have an increased risk of infection or sequelae. Routine culture of all human bite wounds is unnecessary because it demonstrates no growth in >80% of cases, and rarely alters first-line therapy. Cultures of human bite wounds are usually polymicrobial with aerobes and anaerobes equally represented. Beta-lactamase production occurs frequently. Commonly isolated aerobes include *Eikenella corrodens, Staphylococcus, Streptococcus*, and *Corynebacterium* species. Do not close hand wounds, puncture wounds, infected wounds, or wounds more than 12 hours old. Allow such wounds to heal by secondary intention. Antibiotic prophylaxis is recommended in these patients. X-ray of the hand is indicated in all patients with closed fist injuries, to reveal fractures in particular MCP joint, foreign bodies, or air within a joint. Current recommendations specify the use of amoxicillin/clavulanate or ampicillin/sulbactam in patients with an infected human bite wound. Cephalexin, which is commonly used for skin and soft-tissue infections, is ineffective against *E. corrodens*, an important pathogen in infected human bites.

Barrett J, Revis D. Human bites [Internet]. Medscape. 2020 [cited 12 January 2020].
Available from: https://emedicine.medscape.com/article/218901-overview

12. Answer: A

Human T-cell lymphotropic virus type 1 (HTLV-1) is a human retrovirus that causes a lifelong infection. Although the majority of HTLV-1 carriers remain asymptomatic, HTLV-1 is the aetiologic agent of adult T-cell leukemia/lymphoma (ATL), a rapidly progressing clonal malignancy of CD4+ T lymphocytes. HTLV-1 infection is also associated with inflammatory syndromes such as myelopathy/tropical spastic paraparesis, uveitis and opportunistic infections including Strongyloides stercoralis hyperinfection. The virus can be transmitted from mother to child, through sexual contact, and through contaminated blood products. There are an estimated 5 million to 20 million HTLV-1 infected individuals worldwide; their lifetime risk of developing ATL is 3–5%, and high HTLV-1 proviral loads have been shown to be an independent risk factor. Indigenous Australian residents of central Australia have the highest HTLV-1 prevalence in the world; exceeding 50% for adults in some remote communities surveyed. Recent advances in the treatment of ATL are the introduction of treatment targeted against CC chemokine receptor 4 (CCR4), which is abundantly expressed on most ATL cells, and allogeneic haemopoietic stem-cell transplantation for aggressive ATL. Promising outcomes are also reported with early intervention for indolent ATL with interferon α and zidovudine.

Schierhout G, McGregor S, Gessain A, Einsiedel L, Martinello M, Kaldor J. Association between HTLV-1 infection and adverse health outcomes: a systematic review and meta-analysis of epidemiological studies. The Lancet Infectious Diseases. 2020;20(1):133–143.
https://www.thelancet.com/journals/laninf/article/PIIS1473-3099(19)30402-5/fulltext

13. Answer: D

Healthcare-associated infections (HCAIs) are infections that occur while receiving health care, developed in a hospital or other health care facility that first appear 48 hours or more after hospital admission, or within 30 days after having received health care. Acute care settings do present more risk to patients because of the volume of patients and the interventions that take place.

Study data suggests the presence of 83,096 HCAIs per year in Australia, comprising 71,186 UTIs, 4902 Clostridium difficile infections, 3946 surgical site infections, 1962 respiratory tract infections in acute stroke patients, and 1100 hospital-onset Staphylococcus aureus bacteraemia. This is a very large underestimate given the lack of or incomplete data on common infections such as pneumonia, gastroenterological and bloodstream infections, thus potentially missing up to 50%–60% of infections. If that is the case, the incidence of HCAIs in Australia may be closer to 165,000 per year.

All the answers listed are risk factors for HCAIs, but the presence of an invasive indwelling device and the degree of underlying illness are the greatest risk factors for the development of infection in any patient, regardless of their age.

Every health care worker is responsible for infection control care – it is a fundamental and integral part of patient care and an important patient safety issue. The key message is to remove any invasive indwelling device that is not required.

 Zingg W, Holmes A, Dettenkofer M, Goetting T, Secci F, Clack L et al. Hospital organisation, management, and structure for prevention of health-care-associated infection: a systematic review and expert consensus. The Lancet Infectious Diseases. 2015;15(2):212–224.
https://www.thelancet.com/journals/laninf/article/PIIS1473-3099(14)70854-0/fulltext

14. Answer: C

Influenza, one of the most common infectious diseases, is a highly contagious airborne disease that occurs in seasonal epidemics and manifests as an acute febrile illness with respiratory and systemic symptoms, ranging from mild fatigue to respiratory failure and death.

Influenza vaccine provides reasonable protection against immunised strains. The vaccination becomes effective 10–14 days after administration. Influenza vaccine has had 50%–60% efficacy against infection with influenza A viruses and 70% efficacy against influenza B viruses.

Influenza vaccination in Australia is recommended for everyone aged 65 years and over, all pregnant women (any trimester), all Aboriginal and Torres Strait Islander children aged 6 months up to 5 years of age, all Aboriginal and Torres Strait Islander people 15 years of age and over, people 6 months of age or older with the following underlying chronic medical conditions: cardiac disease, chronic respiratory conditions including severe asthma, other chronic illnesses requiring regular medical follow up or hospitalisation in the previous year, for example diabetes, CKD, chronic metabolic disease and haemoglobinopathies, chronic neurological conditions that may impact on respiratory function including multiple sclerosis, spinal cord injuries, seizure disorders and other neuromuscular disorders, people with impaired immunity, including HIV infection, malignancy, and chronic steroid use. Very similar recommendations and funding rules apply in New Zealand.

The Communicable Diseases Network Australia (CDNA) recommends influenza vaccine be administered during pregnancy (all trimesters) and prompt treatment with a neuraminidase inhibitor (i.e. within 2 days of symptom onset) if influenza occurs during pregnancy.

Vaccination may provide less protection against influenza in patients older than 65 years. In order to improve the immunogenicity of influenza virus vaccine in elderly adults, a high-dose trivalent inactivated influenza vaccine was developed. In a multicentre, randomiseds, double-blind controlled trial involving elderly adults (≥65 years), those who received the high-dose vaccine exhibited a statistically significantly higher seroconversion rate than those who received the standard-dose vaccine. The high-dose vaccine met superiority criteria for both strains of influenza A, and non-inferiority criteria were met for influenza B strains.

 Seasonal Influenza Infection CDNA National Guidelines for Public Health Units [Internet]. 2019 [cited 18 August 2019]. Available from: https://www1.health.gov.au/internet/main/publishing.nsf/Content/3D622AEAE44DDEB2CA257BF0001ED884/$File/influenza-infection-2019.pdf

15. Answer: B

Listeria monocytogenes is a small gram-positive facultative intracellular bacillus that is ubiquitous in nature. The primary mode of human transmission is via consumption of contaminated food products, especially unpasteurised dairy meats, and vegetables. Vertical transmission can also occur, transplacental in nature or during delivery. Overt disease is relatively rare but the mortality secondary to infection is high, with rates recorded up to 17%. This is, in part, due to Listeria's ability to evade the immune system by hijacking the actin polymerisation propulsion system and spread from cell to cell without entering the extracellular environment.

Listeria can cause meningoencephalitis, sepsis, and gastroenteritis. Infection in pregnancy can lead to premature birth or foetal death. Immunosuppressed and elderly patients, patients with poorly controlled diabetes, pregnant women, and newborns of infected mothers are typically affected by *L monocytogenes*.

Listeria monocytogenes is intrinsically resistant to cephalosporins, mainly due to modified penicillin binding proteins with poor affinity to cephalosporins, but also including multidrug resistance transporters, and cell envelope proteins with a detoxification function.

As Listeria is always resistant to cephalosporins, ampicillin is the treatment of choice.

 Buckley N, *Australian Medicines Handbook 2019*. Adelaide, SA: AUSTRALIAN MEDICINES Handbook Pty Ltd; 2019. https://resources.amh.net.au/subscribers/tables/organism_susceptibility_cephalosporins.pdf

16. Answer: B

The vast majority of malarial infections arising in sub-Saharan Africa are a result of *Plasmodium falciparum*. *P falciparum* causes severe malarial infections through the sequestration of mature parasites in medium and small vessels, leading to end-organ damage. In children, cerebral malaria, and severe haemolytic anaemia are common manifestations, whereas adults frequently experience acute tubular necrosis and acute respiratory distress syndrome. Additionally, children have extremely high risk of concomitant bacterial infection with sepsis, often with non-typhoidal *Salmonella*. Severe *Plasmodium vivax* malaria is less common and is not observed frequently in returned travellers, although high mortality rates from vivax malaria are locally observed (for example in West Papua). Vivax and falciparum malaria occur with similar frequency in south and south-east Asia, and vivax malaria is more common in the Americas. Incubation periods are typically 10–14 days for *P falciparum* and 2–3 weeks for *P vivax*, however some individual strains have considerably longer incubation periods (up to 6 months).

Treatment of severe malaria involves rapid intravenous administration of artesunate, which has shown to be superior to quinidine and artemether. Early organ support such as ventilation and dialysis is recommended. Reversal of severe anaemia is warranted, although optimal thresholds and strategies have not been defined. Fluid resuscitation must be performed cautiously due to the increased risk of pulmonary oedema. Artemisinin-based combination therapy (ACT) is recommended once the patient is able to swallow.

Treatment of uncomplicated malaria involves understanding of the local resistance patterns and the strain identified. *P vivax* infections are typically treated with chloroquine, except if the strain is from Indonesia or Oceania, where ACT is used. ACT is first-line therapy for uncomplicated *P. falciparum* malaria, and atovaquone–proguanil is an alternative, particularly if ACT treatment has failed. Artemisinin–resistant *P falciparum* is a significant issue in south-east Asia, and several new combinations and drugs are being evaluated for efficacy in this setting.

 Ashley E, Pyae Phyo A, Woodrow C. Malaria. The Lancet. 2018;391(10130):1608–1621. https://www.thelancet.com/journals/lancet/article/PIIS0140-6736(18)30324-6/fulltext

17. Answer: B

Melioidosis is caused by the bacterium *Burkholderia pseudomallei*, an aerobic, oxidase positive, Gram negative bacillus. *Burkholderia pseudomallei* is endemic in northern Australia, with cases most commonly occurring during the wet season in patients with diabetes, hazardous alcohol use, and CKD. Pneumonia is the most common presentation, and the majority of patients have bacteraemia. Infection may involve almost any organ, such as the skin and soft tissues, genitourinary system, liver, spleen, kidneys, prostate, bone, and joints. CNS involvement is rare but has a higher mortality.

A high index of suspicion for melioidosis is required to diagnose the disease, especially in individuals who have travelled to Northern, tropical Australia, or from other endemic regions. Chronic infection has also been described in individuals who had distant travel history to the endemic areas.

Treatment of melioidosis consists of an intensive phase with intravenous antibiotics followed by a prolonged eradication phase with oral antibiotics. Recommended intensive phase treatment includes intravenous ceftazidime (2 g, 6 hourly) or intravenous meropenem (1 g, 8 hourly; 2 g, 8 hourly if neurological involvement) for at least 14 days. In patients with neurological, bone or joint, genitourinary, skin and soft tissue infections, oral Trimethoprim/sulfamethoxazole (TMP-SMX 320/1600 mg) (≥60 kg: orally 12-hourly 40–60 kg: 240/1200 mg orally 12-hourly) is added to the intensive regimen. Folic acid 5 mg daily is given to patients receiving TMP-SMX. For septic arthritis or deep-seated collection, the recommended intensive phase treatment with the above intravenous regimen is 4 weeks with eradication phase oral antibiotics up to 3 months. If there is evidence of pneumonia with lymphadenopathy, ICU admission should be considered.

TMP-SMX remains the treatment of choice for oral eradication therapy. For people who cannot tolerate TMP-SMX, oral doxycycline 100 mg bd or oral amoxicillin-clavulanate are appropriate alternatives. Duration of eradication is usually for 3 months following the intensive intravenous antibiotics treatment.

People who are immunosuppressed and at risk of acquiring melioidosis are advised to wear gardening gloves and footwear when coming into contact with soil in endemic regions.

 Smith S, Hanson J, Currie B. Melioidosis: An Australian Perspective. Tropical Medicine and Infectious Disease. 2018;3(1):27. https://www.mdpi.com/2414-6366/3/1/27/htm

18. Answer: B

Methenamine Hippurate (Hiprex) has no intrinsic antibacterial activity and it is not an antibiotic. However, it is hydrolysed in the urine, when urine pH is <5.5, to form ammonia and formaldehyde. Formaldehyde is bactericidal to almost all pathogens and lacks bacterial resistance, in another word it is a urinary antiseptic. Hiprex has a relatively limited side-effect profile and is often been used for recurrent UTI prophylaxis. It is active against *E. coli* and to a lesser extent, other bacilli. However, the clinical evidence is weak, but studies suggest that it is more effective at reducing recurrent UTIs at 12 months compared with placebo. It is not indicated for treatment of established UTI.

Hiprex is given orally and is well absorbed. It excretes into the urine in high concentration. For maximum effect, it is common practice to use oral acidifying agents such as ascorbic acid, pure cranberry juice, grape juice, or ammonium chloride concurrently to reduce urinary pH to 5.5 or less.

Hiprex is not effective against urea splitting organisms such as Proteus, which promotes an alkaline urine, which makes it difficult to achieve the urine pH necessary to produce sufficient formaldehyde concentrations. Hiprex is useless if the pH is higher than 6. It takes time for methenamine to convert to formaldehyde. If a patient has an indwelling catheter, continuous bladder drainage will not allow time for formaldehyde production in the bladder sufficient to provide a clinical benefit.

When methenamine converts to formaldehyde it also releases ammonia molecules. Therefore, it should generally be avoided in patients with severe hepatic dysfunction. Hiprex is also contraindicated in renal impairment and dehydration. Concomitant methenamine and sulfonamides use should be avoided because some sulfonamides can form an insoluble precipitate with formaldehyde in the urine. Methenamine use in patients with gout may increase urate crystal formation in the urine.

 Urinary tract infection (recurrent): antimicrobial prescribing [Internet]. National Institute for Health and Care Excellence. 2020 [cited 14 October 2019].
Available from: https://www.nice.org.uk/guidance/ng112/resources/urinary-tract-infection-recurrent-antimicrobial-prescribing-pdf-66141595059397

19. Answer: C

This patient's presenting features are consistent with a diagnosis of neurosyphilis. Syphilis is a multisystem chronic infection caused by treponema pallidum, a spirochaete bacterium. Neurosyphilis has varied presentations. Neurosyphilis affects the nervous system, including meninges, brain parenchyma, and the spinal cord. It can cause psychiatric disorders such as depression, mania, psychosis, personality changes, delirium, and dementia.

Syphilis progresses into four stages if untreated as primary, secondary, latent, and tertiary stages. Primary syphilis is characterised by a typical painless syphilitic ulcer called chancre seen at the inoculation region, lasting for 2–3 weeks. Secondary syphilis appears weeks or months later and lymphadenopathy, gastrointestinal abnormalities, and CNS alterations are seen. At the end of the latent period, tertiary syphilis develops in 25% of the untreated patients and is seen 1–30 years after primary infection. This inflammatory disease progresses slowly as neurosyphilis or gummatous syphilis.

Diagnosis of the condition requires a high index of suspicion and depends on clinical recognition. The diagnosis of neurosyphilis is based on serum and CSF serologic tests. The blood and CSF serologic tests are classified as nontreponemal (tests using VDRL and RPR techniques) or treponemal (tests using fluorescent treponemal–antibody absorption [FTA-ABS' and related techniques]. CSF pleocytosis (an increase in CSF WBC count), mildly elevated protein levels are found in patients with neurosyphilis. However, CSF pleocytosis is less specific for diagnosing neurosyphilis in patients who have HIV-related meningitis. Serum venereal disease research laboratory (VDRL) and rapid plasma reagin (RPR) are reactive in almost all cases of neurosyphilis during and after the secondary stage of syphilis but can be negative in late neurosyphilis because of reducing titres over time, especially after treatment. The CSF VDRL test is specific for neurosyphilis but is only 70% sensitive. In patients with a possible false negative CSF VDRL results when the clinical features suggest a diagnosis of neurosyphilis, CSF treponemal test can be used to confirm the diagnosis.

There are five types of neurosyphilis, including asymptomatic neurosyphilis, meningeal neurosyphilis (occurs between the first few weeks to the first few years of getting syphilis; presenting symptoms and signs include headache, neck stiffness, nausea, vomiting), meningovascular neurosyphilis (symptoms similar to meningeal neurosyphilis plus strokes), general paresis (can occur 3 to 30 years after syphilis infection and patients may also have mood and personality changes), and tabes dorsalis (can occur 5 to 50 years after initial syphilis infection; patients present with ataxic gait, prominent Romberg's sign, lancinating pains in legs and trunk, impaired deep and proprioceptive sensation, Charcot joints due to a slow demyelination process of the neural tracts in the dorsal columns of the spinal cord), Argyll Robertson pupils, paraparesis with leg areflexia, and sphincter dysfunction. Patients with untreated neurosyphilis, meningovascular syphilis, general paresis, or tabes dorsalis usually have long-term sequalae of the disease.

Patients with HIV/AIDS are at higher risk of having neurosyphilis and it is important to screen for co-infection of HIV and syphilis. Penicillin is the preferred antibiotics for treatment of neurosyphilis. If patients have hypersensitivities to penicillin, skin testing and desensitisation are recommended. Limited evidence suggests that ceftriaxone, or doxycycline is effective in the treatment of neurosyphilis.

Ropper A. Neurosyphilis. New England Journal of Medicine. 2019;381(14):1358–1363.
https://www.nejm.org/doi/full/10.1056/NEJMra1906228

20. Answer: C

Norovirus, an RNA virus, is a leading cause of acute gastroenteritis across all age groups, from infants to the elderly. Although most cases of norovirus infection are self-limiting, dehydration is the most common complication, which often leads to hospitalisations, and even deaths. Infants and children under 2 years, adults aged 65 years or older, and people who are immunocompromised, are at higher risk for severe norovirus illness.

Norovirus is frequently implicated in hospital ward and nursing home outbreaks. These closed-space outbreaks can present both a logistic challenge in terms of eradicating the source and a financial burden to health care. Within hospitals or nursing homes, person-to-person transmission is the primary mode of transmission and can occur between both patients and staff. Therefore, handwashing with soap and water is the first line of defence against norovirus. Alcohol-based hand sanitisers are generally NOT effective at killing norovirus. To ensure that norovirus is removed from hands, thorough handwashing with soap and water for at least 20 seconds is important. Alcohol-based hand sanitisers can be used in addition to handwashing, but not as a substitute for washing with soap and water.

Incubation period is usually 24–48 hours. Norovirus can be found in the faeces and vomit of infected people from the day they start to feel ill and up to 2 weeks after they recover. Stool is the preferred clinical specimen to detect norovirus, and specimens should be collected in a closed container within 48–72 h of the onset of symptoms but the virus can also be detected in vomitus and rectal swabs. Highly sensitive real-time reverse transcription-polymerase chain reaction (RT-qPCR) assays to detect norovirus RNA are the gold standard for the detection and typing of norovirus. There are no proven antiviral therapies for patients with norovirus illness.

Individual cases of norovirus are not notifiable; however, outbreaks are reportable in all states in Australia, so if you suspect a norovirus outbreak, notify your local health department. There is no vaccine available for prevention of norovirus infection at this stage.

Robilotti E, Deresinski S, Pinsky B. Norovirus. Clinical Microbiology Reviews. 2015;28(1):134–164.
https://cmr.asm.org/content/28/1/134.long

21. Answer: B

The classical definition of pyrexia of unknown origin (PUO) is a persistent fever above 38.3°C that evades diagnosis for at least 3 weeks, including 1 week of investigation in hospital. With the development of advanced diagnostic techniques and shortened length of hospital stay, a week of hospitalisation is no longer required. PUO can be classified into five groups: classical, nosocomial, neutropenic, HIV-related, and elderly patient group, each requiring different investigative strategies.

The diagnostic approach to a patient with PUO should be methodical. A thorough history and comprehensive examination of the patient is essential. Investigations should be conducted to confirm or rule out the most likely diagnosis/diagnoses, based on the history and examination findings. Investigation should proceed through at least two stages, baseline tests followed by more specific tests. Early blanket testing for all possible aetiologies is inappropriate. A baseline set of investigations includes FBE with a differential cell count, renal function, electrolytes, LFTs, TFTs, CRP, and ESR, at least two blood cultures (while not receiving antibiotics) and a HIV test. A CXR, ultrasound of the abdomen and a urine dipstick should also be performed. The ESR is helpful in distinguishing real disease from a factitious fever. Whole body CT scan is not helpful in confirming factitious fever; however, PET-CT testing may be helpful in the patient's early diagnostic journey when there are no localising clues in the history or examination. Empirical antimicrobial or steroid trials should not be performed in the workup of PUO.

Procalcitonin is a biomarker that exhibits greater specificity than other proinflammatory markers (e.g., cytokines) in identifying patients with sepsis and can be used in the rapid diagnosis of bacterial infection, especially for use in hospital emergency departments and ICUs. Currently, there is no role for procalcitonin measurement in the workup of PUO. Despite investigations, in approximately 50% of cases the underlying cause remain unknown. If the cause for PUO is found, it can be considered in four categories: infective (17–35%), inflammatory (24–36%), neoplastic (10–20%) and miscellaneous (3–15%).

Fernandez C, Beeching N. Pyrexia of unknown origin. Clinical Medicine. 2018;18(2):170–174.
https://www.rcpjournals.org/content/clinmedicine/18/2/170

22. Answer: C

In Australia, Q fever is the most commonly reported zoonotic disease. Cases occur throughout Australia, with higher rates occurring in northern New South Wales and southern Queensland. Q fever often presents as an undifferentiated febrile illness associated with headache, extreme fatigue, drenching sweats, weight loss, arthralgia, and myalgia, and abnormal LFTs. It is caused by the bacteria *Coxiella burnetii,* an obligate gram-negative intracellular bacterium. The bacteria affect sheep, goats, cattle, dogs, cats, birds, rodents, and ticks. Infected animals shed this bacterium in birth products, faeces, milk, and urine. Humans get Q fever through inhalation of contaminated droplets released by infected animals and drinking raw milk. People at high risk for this infection are farmers, sheep and dairy workers, and veterinarians. It usually takes about 20 days after exposure to the bacteria for symptoms to occur. Q fever is diagnosed with a blood antibody test. The main treatment for the disease is with antibiotics. For acute Q fever, doxycycline is recommended. For chronic Q fever, a combination of doxycycline and hydroxychloroquine is often used long term.

Lyme disease is caused by infection with the bacteria *Borrelia burgdorferi.* There is little evidence that locally acquired Lyme disease occurs in Australia. There is a continuing risk of Lyme disease for overseas travellers. *Rickettsia australis* causes tick typhus, spotted fever. Brucellosis is an infection caused by the bacterium *Brucella.* It can be transmitted to humans from some animals such as cows, sheep, goats, and pigs. While this disease is common in many parts of the world, it is very rare in Australia. Cases usually result from contact with feral pigs or from consuming unpasteurised dairy products while overseas.

Eastwood K, Graves S, Massey P, Bosward K, van den Berg D, Hutchinson P. Q fever: A rural disease with potential urban consequences. Australian Journal of General Practice. 2018;47(3):112–116.
https://www1.racgp.org.au/ajgp/2018/march/q-fever

23. Answer: D

An unusual feature of Strongyloides is its capacity to mature inside the gastrointestinal tract of infected individuals and later on penetrate the skin, causing a cycle called autoinfection. This may perpetuate the infection through the host's lifetime.

Strongyloides stercoralis adults may be either parasitic or free-living. Parasitic adults are exclusively female; there are no parasitic males. Very thin-shelled, embryonated eggs release rhabditiform larvae, which develop into infective-stage filariform larvae. Free-living adult males and females live in the soil and reproduce sexually.

In autoinfection, first-stage larvae transform into infective larvae while they are in the intestine or on the skin of the perianal region; these larvae penetrate the wall of the intestine or the perianal skin. Some eventually develop into adults in the small intestine after a migration. The occurrence of autoinfection is the main reason strongyloidiasis is such a serious disease. Infection is life-long since adult worms are replaced by young worms and the infection does not end when the original crop of adults die. Worm numbers can rise incrementally to produce severe disease, known as the hyperinfection syndrome. Autoinfection also accounts for the persistence of this infection in patients who no longer live in endemic areas.

S. stercoralis is more prevalent in tropical regions of the world, including tropical Australia. Rural and remote regions of Australia, including Queensland, Northern Territory, Western Australia, north of South Australia, and northern areas of New South Wales are the endemic area. Australia's Indigenous communities have high prevalence of strongyloidiasis as do immigrants from other endemic countries, travellers to these countries and military personnel who have spent time in endemic regions.

Strongyloidiasis is usually symptomatic but most signs and symptoms are non-specific. The exception is with larva currens, a rapidly moving urticarial linear rash that marks the passage of an autoinfective larvae through the skin. This is pathognomonic of strongyloidiasis. The other non-specific signs and symptoms include gastrointestinal symptoms such as abdominal pain, nausea, diarrhoea, weight loss; respiratory symptoms such as cough, haemoptysis; cutaneous such as dermatitis, swelling, itching, urticaria and general malaise.

Diagnosis is made by stool testing for ova and parasites or by stool antigen or serologic antibody testing. Ivermectin is the first-line therapy.

Miller A, Smith M, Judd J, Speare R. Strongyloides stercoralis: Systematic Review of Barriers to Controlling Strongyloidiasis for Australian Indigenous Communities. PLoS Neglected Tropical Diseases. 2014;8(9): e3141.
https://journals.plos.org/plosntds/article?id=10.1371/journal.pntd.0003141

24. Answer: C

TB is an airborne infectious disease caused by organisms of the *Mycobacterium tuberculosis* complex. TB remains the leading cause of death from an infectious disease among adults worldwide.

Patients at increased risk of TB in Australia and New Zealand include:

- Aboriginal and Torres Strait Islanders
- Elderly patients
- Patients from high TB-burden countries, such as sub-Saharan Africa, India, China, and other Asian countries
- Healthcare workers who have been working in high burden countries
- Immunocompromised states including HIV infection (risk of TB reactivation is 10% per annum although this is substantially reduced with antiretroviral therapy)
- Medication-related such as chemotherapy & post-transplant immunosuppressants

For pan-sensitive TB, the first line treatment consists of four drugs (isoniazid, rifampicin, pyrazinamide, and ethambutol) given for a total of 2 months followed by two drugs (isoniazid and rifampicin) given for an additional 4 months. Daily administration of therapy results in improved treatment outcomes compared with thrice-weekly treatment. All patients diagnosed with TB should be given daily treatment with fixed-dose combinations. Although high dose rifampicin shows early promise for treatment shortening, randomised controlled trials with the fluoroquinolones did not show a treatment-shortening benefit. Isoniazid-resistant forms of TB are the most common forms of drug-resistant TB in the world. Rifampicin non-resistant TB (with retained susceptibility to isoniazid) is increasing. There are several new and repurposed drugs that WHO recommend for drug-resistant TB, which include bedaquiline, delamanid, pretomanid, linezolid, sutezolid, and clofazimine.

Furin J, Cox H, Pai M. Tuberculosis. The Lancet. 2019;393(10181):1642–1656.
https://www.thelancet.com/journals/lancet/article/PIIS0140-6736(19)30308-3/fulltext

25. Answer: C

S. aureus exotoxins cause disease because they are superantigens. Superantigens are molecules that are able to activate large numbers of T cells, often up to 20% of all T cells at one time (compared with 0.001% by a normal antigen), resulting in massive cytokine and chemokines release from both T cells and antigen-presenting cell (APCs).

In typical T cell recognition, an antigen is taken up by APCs, processed, expressed on the cell surface in complex with class II MHC in a groove formed by the alpha and beta chains of class II MHC, and recognised by an antigen-specific T cell receptor. By contrast, superantigens do not require processing by APCs but instead interact directly with the invariant region of the class II MHC molecule. The superantigen-MHC complex then interacts with the T cell receptor at the variable (V) part of the beta chain. Thus, all T cells with a recognised V beta region are stimulated. Activated T cells then release interleukin (IL)-1, IL-2, tumour necrosis factor (TNF)-alpha and TNF-beta, and interferon (IFN)-gamma in large amounts, resulting in staphylococcal toxic shock syndrome (TSS).

Clinical features of TSS include high fever, rash, late desquamation of the palms of the hands and feet, hypotension, and multi-organ failure. TSS is divided into menstrual and non-menstrual TSS. Menstrual TSS is associated with tampon usage in women colonised vaginally by superantigen-producing *S. aureus* and usually occurs within 2 days after the initiation of menstruation or within 2 days after completion of menstruation. Non-menstrual TSS occurs as a complication of *S. aureus* infections after surgical procedures, burns or post-influenza pneumonia.

Botulinum toxin is a neurotoxic protein produced by the bacterium *Clostridium botulinum*. It blocks the release of the neurotransmitter acetylcholine from axon endings at the neuromuscular junction and thus causes flaccid paralysis. Aflatoxins are mycotoxins produced by aspergillus fungi and can occur in foods (including wheat, soybeans, and peanuts). It has been associated with the development of hepatocellular carcinoma likely due to high rates of p53 mutation. Following ganglioside mediated binding to enterocytes, components of the *Vibrio cholera* toxin catalyses the ADP-ribosylation of a GTP-binding protein, leading to persistent activation of adenylate cyclase. The increase of cAMP in the intestinal mucosa leads to increased chloride secretion and decreased sodium absorption, producing the massive fluid and electrolyte losing diarrhoea characteristic of cholera.

Chan B, Maurice P. Staphylococcal Toxic Shock Syndrome. New England Journal of Medicine. 2013;369(9):852–852.
https://www.nejm.org/doi/full/10.1056/NEJMicm1213758

26. Answer: D
Vaccination recommendations for adult transplant recipients include:

Routine Vaccinations	
Influenza	Annual
Pneumococcal	Recommended; booster after 5 years
Tetanus/diphtheria	Recommended; booster every 10 years
Pertussis	Recommended in combination with Tetanus/ Diphtheria once
Human Papilloma virus	Recommended when indicated
Measles/mumps/rubella (MMR)	**Contraindicated**
Varicella	**Contraindicated**
Varicella zoster	**Contraindicated**

Travel-related Vaccinations	
Hepatitis A	Recommended when indicated
Hepatitis B	Recommended when indicated
Meningococcal conjugate	Recommended when indicated
Inactivated polio	Recommended when indicated
Rabies	Recommended when indicated
Japanese encephalitis	Recommended when indicated
Cholera vaccine	Recommended when indicated
Typhim Vi™	Recommended when indicated
S. Typhi	**Contraindicated**
Oral polio	**Contraindicated (including family members)**
Bacillus Calmette–Guérin (BCG)	**Contraindicated**
Yellow Fever	**Contraindicated**

The contraindicated vaccines often contain live organisms. Vaccination does not appear to promote rejection. Vaccination recommendations for travel destination/country can be found at the following websites.

Table. Recommended vaccines for people before and after a solid organ transplant | The Australian Immunisation Handbook [Internet]. Australian Immunisation Handbook. 2020 [cited 16 May 2020].
Available from: https://immunisationhandbook.health.gov.au/resources/handbook-tables/
table-recommended-vaccines-for-people-before-and-after-a-solid-organ

Destinations | Travelers' Health | CDC [Internet]. Wwwnc.cdc.gov. 2020 [cited 16 May 2020].
Available from: https://wwwnc.cdc.gov/travel/destinations/list/

27. Answer: C
Vertebral osteomyelitis is most frequently of the haematogenous type and generally involves the lower dorsal or lumbar spine; involvement of the cervical spine is very rare. The disease usually presents in adults as acute back pain or worsening back pain and fever. An arterial route is believed to be the most likely route of infection. This is because the segmental arteries supplying the vertebrae generally bifurcate to supply both adjacent bony segments and the disease involves two adjacent vertebrae and subsequently their intervertebral disc. In some patients, inflammation of the disc occurs before vertebral infection. In patients with recurrent UTIs, retrograde spread of infection through the venous pelvic and paravertebral plexus has been suggested as a possible mechanism of dissemination.

Plain X-rays are usually normal at presentation, but abnormalities on MRI are early clues to the diagnosis and appear within days; later, narrowing of the disc space, mottled destruction of adjacent vertebral plateaus, and anterior bridging are observed.

Vertebral osteomyelitis is generally caused by *Staphylococcus aureus* (39%) followed by *Escherichia coli*, *Streptococcus pyogenes*, and *Pseudomonas aeruginosa*. The key message is that needle biopsy under CT guidance is essential and the diagnostic procedure of choice because many organisms can cause vertebral osteomyelitis. In addition to aerobic and anaerobic bacterial cultures, the samples should be sent for fungal and mycobacterial culture as well as for histology. If the first set of cultures is negative, an open surgical biopsy should be considered before therapy is started.

Lew D, Waldvogel F. Osteomyelitis. The Lancet. 2004;364(9431):369-379.
https://www.thelancet.com/journals/lancet/article/PIIS0140-6736(04)16727-5/fulltext

28. Answer: C

Zika virus is part of the mosquito-borne group of RNA flaviviruses. It is mainly transmitted by Aedes aegypti mosquitoes, which also transmit dengue virus, chikungunya, and yellow fever virus. Zika virus infection might be responsible for false positive dengue virus infection. Zika virus can be sexually transmitted. Blood transfusion and perinatal transmission also occur. Prevention for transfusion-transmitted infection can be achieved via nucleic acid testing of blood donations or pathogen inactivation in the donor blood. Patients develop antibody post Zika infection which provides life-long protection against reinfection.

Acute phase diagnosis relies on detection of Zika virus RNA. Blood and urine are the samples of choice. The virus can be detected only briefly in plasma or serum during acute illness. Zika RNA can be detected in the urine within the first week after symptom onset and expands the window of detection.

Approximately 80% of patients infected with Zika virus are asymptomatic. Zika virus can infect human embryonic cortical neural progenitor cells causing cell death leading to microcephaly. The pathogenesis of Zika virus-associated Guillain-Barré syndrome is still unknown: direct neuropathogenic mechanisms, hyperacute immune response, immune dysregulation, and molecular mimicry against nervous antigens are all hypotheses.

 Baud D, Gubler D, Schaub B, Lanteri M, Musso D. An update on Zika virus infection. The Lancet. 2017;390(10107): 2099-2109.
https://www.thelancet.com/journals/lancet/article/PIIS0140-6736(17)31450-2/fulltext

29. Answer: A

Herpes zoster is a viral infection that occurs with reactivation of the varicella-zoster virus (VZV). More than 95% of immuno competent individuals aged 50 years or older are seropositive for VZV. It is usually a self-limited infection with rash, and pain but it can lead to postherpetic neuralgia, which can be severe and incapacitating.

Ophthalmic manifestations of herpes zoster infection include conjunctivitis, scleritis, episcleritis, keratitis iridocyclitis, retinitis, choroiditis, optic neuritis, optic atrophy, lid retraction, and ptosis. The risk for ophthalmic complications in patients with herpes zoster does not correlate with age, sex, or severity of the rash.

Risk factors for developing herpes zoster include:

- Age, VZV-specific immunity, and cell-mediated immunity generally declines with age
- Immunosuppression (e.g., by HIV infection or AIDS)
- Immunosuppressive therapy
- Immune reconstitution inflammatory syndrome
- Acute lymphocytic leukaemia and other cancers.

Oral aciclovir has been shown to shorten the duration of rash, severity of pain, as well as to reduce the incidence and severity of herpes zoster ophthalmicus complications. However, such benefits have only been confirmed in patients treated within 72 hours of the onset of rash. Although these agents may be helpful as long as new lesions are being formed, they are not likely to be of use in patients with lesions that have crusted.

While aciclovir can reduce the pain during the acute phase, it has no demonstrated effect on reducing the incidence or severity of post-herpetic neuralgia. Both famciclovir and valaciclovir have been shown to be as effective as aciclovir in the treatment of herpes zoster and to reduce complications. Famciclovir is a prodrug that is metabolised to an active metabolite, penciclovir. Aciclovir is not haematotoxic and can be used in patients with myelodysplastic syndrome.

Topical steroids alone do not reactivate the virus but may exacerbate spontaneous recurrences. In addition, while steroid eye drops may be beneficial for specific complications of herpes zoster ophthalmicus such as keratitis, ophthalmologic consultation is mandatory prior to initiating ocular steroid therapy.

 Cohen J. Herpes Zoster. New England Journal of Medicine. 2013;369(3):255–263.
https://www.nejm.org/doi/10.1056/NEJMcp1302674

30. Answer: C

Once a case of meningococcal disease is confirmed, Public health follow-up focuses on identifying the subset of 'higher-risk' contacts who require information and clearance antibiotics and vaccination in some instances. Other lower-risk contacts groups may be given information only.

Higher-risk contacts include:

- Household or household-like contacts: of a case are those who lived in the same house (or dormitory-type room) or were having an equivalent degree of contact with the case in the 7 days prior to the onset of the case's symptoms until completion of 24 hours of appropriate antibiotic treatment.

- Intimate kissing and sexual contacts: in the 7 days prior to the onset of the case's symptoms until completion of 24 hours of appropriate antibiotic treatment.
- Child-care: to be considered a higher-risk contact, children and staff in childcare should have an equivalent degree of contact with the case as a household contact.
- Passengers: seated immediately adjacent to the case during long distance travel (>8 hours duration) by aeroplane, train, bus, or another vehicle.
- Healthcare workers who have had unprotected close exposure of their airway to large particle respiratory droplets of a case during airway management (e.g., suctioning, intubation), or mouth to mouth resuscitation up until the case has had 24 hours of appropriate antibiotic treatment.

Household and other higher risk contacts of a case will need clearance antibiotics, vaccination, and information. The main rationale for clearance antibiotics is to eliminate meningococci from any carrier within the network of contacts close to each case, thereby reducing the risk of further transmission of what may be a more virulent strain of the organism within the social network and preventing further cases of invasive disease. Clearance antibiotics given to household contacts is approximately 89% effective in preventing secondary cases.

The current (April 2019) Therapeutic Guidelines lists ciprofloxacin, ceftriaxone, and rifampicin as suitable agents. Ciprofloxacin is the preferred agent for adults and children. Rifampicin needs a two-day course. Ceftriaxone should be used in pregnant woman, or if pregnancy status is uncertain. Ceftriaxone is the preferred agent for rural and remote communities, especially in indigenous communities because compliance is likely to be good and it is readily available. A single dose of 250 mg intramuscular ceftriaxone is very effective (97%) in eradicating pharyngeal meningococci from carriers and more effective than oral rifampicin 600 mg twice a day for 2 days (75–81%).

Due to the prolonged risk of secondary cases in household settings or close contact, vaccination is indicated for unimmunised household and sexual/close contacts of cases of confirmed vaccine-preventable invasive meningococcal disease. Vaccination should be offered to these contacts as soon as the serogroup is confirmed, and within 4 weeks of onset of disease in the index case. This should include tetravalent meningococcal polysaccharide vaccines (4vMenPVs) providing protection against serogroups A, C, W_{135} and Y. and MegB providing protection against serogroups B.

 Meningococcal disease control guidelines [Internet]. NSW Government Health. 2019 [cited 12 May 2020]. Available from: https://www.health.nsw.gov.au/Infectious/controlguideline/Pages/meningococcal-disease.aspx

31. Answer: H
The cell wall of bacteria consists of a layer of peptidoglycan polymer. In gram-positive bacteria this is in the form of a polymer of up to 40 layers, and in gram-negative bacteria is only a single layer thick. Meropenem is a beta-lactam antibiotic, and as with other beta-lactam antibiotics such as cephalosporins and penicillins, carbapenems act by inhibiting synthesis of the cell wall. This is achieved by binding penicillin-binding proteins, which in turn inhibits the insertion of the peptidoglycan building blocks into the cell wall.

32. Answer: A
DNA gyrase is a form of topoisomerase enzyme that is found in prokaryotic organisms. It allows for 'detangling' of DNA by producing a negative supercoil of DNA which is an important step in DNA replication for bacteria. Quinolone antibiotics are specific inhibitors of this bacterial topoisomerase.

33. Answer: F
As folate is required for bacterial DNA synthesis, folate reduction is an important target for antibacterial drugs. Inhibition of dihydrofolate reductase can obviously have significant side effects when utilised as a therapeutic strategy, however. Trimethoprim is significantly more active as an inhibitor of bacterial dihydrofolate reductase as opposed to the human enzyme, making it a useful antibacterial antibiotic. The opposite is true of methotrexate, which is largely inactive against bacterial dihydrofolate reductase, and highly active against human dihydrofolate reductase.

34. Answer: E
One of the major mechanisms of action of antibiotics is inhibition of protein synthesis through inhibition of the bacterial ribosome. This process takes advantage of the differences in the structure of the ribosome between eukaryotic and prokaryotic cells. Bacterial ribosomes consist of a 50S subunit and a 30S subunit, whereas mammalian subunits are 60S and 40S. Macrolides, chloramphenicol and clindamycin inhibit the transpeptidation and translocation of RNA at the ribosome. Aminoglycosides inhibit codon elongation in the ribosomal unit. Linezolid and quinipristin/dalfopristin are other antibiotics that also target the bacterial ribosome.

35. Answer: D

Another enzyme that has significant differences between mammalian and bacterial type is RNA-polymerase. Rifampicin (as well as rifaximin and rifabutin) have high specificity for binding and inhibiting the bacterial form of this enzyme. A mammalian analogue for this drug's mechanism is cytarabine which inhibits alpha-DNA polymerase, whereas acyclovir inhibits the herpes virus version of DNA polymerase.

36. Answer: C

Colistin is a polymixin antibiotic that contains lipophilic and hydrophilic groups, which causes direct damage to the cell membrane. It is suggested that this occurs through a detergent-like process.

37. Answer: G

Sulfonamides contain an inactive structural analogue of p-aminobenzoic acid, which is used by most species to synthesise folate. Sulfonamides such as sulfamethoxazole can as a result lead to impaired DNA synthesis, and subsequently impair bacterial growth and replication.

38. Answer: B

Tetracycline antibiotics also act on the 50S ribosomal subunit. This occurs through competitive binding for the A site for tRNA binding, inhibiting the initiation of protein synthesis.

Ritter J, Flower R, Henderson G, Loke Y, MacEwan D, Rang H. Basic principles of antimicrobial chemotherapy. Rang and Dale's pharmacology. Edinburgh, Elsevier; 2019.
https://www.elsevierhealth.com.au/rang-dales-pharmacology-9780702074486.html

39. Answer: G

40. Answer: F

41. Answer: B

42. Answer: H

Bacteria have significant genetic plasticity which has evolved over millions of years in response to diverse environments, including sharing a niche with other antimicrobial producing organisms. It is hardly surprising therefore that disease causing bacteria can rapidly adapt to the changing environment of antimicrobial therapy. Bacteria can use mutation in their own genes (chromosomal modifications) to achieve this but can also acquire foreign DNA through horizontal gene transfer (plasmid-based transformation).

The resultant changes have downstream effects that have significant implications for ongoing strategies to mitigate antimicrobial resistance. Broadly speaking, mechanisms of antimicrobial resistance can be classified into four major categories: modification of the antimicrobial molecule; preventing the molecule from reaching the target; modification of the target site and resistance due to global cell adaptive processes. Antimicrobial resistance strategies are not mutually exclusive and extensively drug resistant bacteria have usually acquired more than one resistance mechanism. Similarly, there are multiple ways in which bacteria can become resistant to a particular antibiotic.

Modification of the antibiotic molecule can be achieved either by destruction of the molecule, or by chemical alteration, both of which can render the drug ineffective. Bacterial production of β-lactamase is a typical example of a cellular process by which the drug is destroyed. More than 1000 different β-lactamases have been described, which are capable of destroying β-lactam antibiotics to varying degrees. Modification of antibiotics can also be achieved by acetylation, phosphorylation, and adenylation, and this is the major mechanism by which gram-negative bacteria become resistant to aminoglycosides such as gentamicin. This process has also been noted to confer resistance to chloramphenicol, streptogramins and lincosamides.

Prevention of transport to the drug's target can be achieved by altering the bacterial cell's permeability to the drug, or by active efflux of the drug from the cell. Permeability changes are mostly achieved through alteration of the structure of porins, which allow substances to penetrate the outer layer of gram-negative organisms. This accounts for much innate resistance to antibiotics – for example, innate resistance to β-lactams, fluoroquinolones, and tetracyclines. It can also account for some acquired resistance, *Enterobacteraciae* and *Pseudomonas* being capable of shifting porin expression to exclude some antibiotics. More commonly, upregulation of efflux pumps can cause resistance, and quite extensive resistance to seemingly unrelated antibiotics. Efflux pumps can impart tetracycline-resistance to gram-negative bacteria and macrolide-resistance to *Streptococci*. There are some efflux pumps capable of using multiple antibiotics as a substrate, such as those of the resistance nodulation division family, which in some gram-negative bacteria has been observed to confer resistance to tetracyclines, chloramphenicol, some β-lactams, novobiocin, fusidic acid and fluoroquinolones.

Modification of the target site can be achieved by target protection, target alteration, or complete bypass of the target site. Target protection can confer low-grade fluoroquinolone resistance to gram-negative bacteria, and tetracycline resistance to a wide variety of bacteria. Target mutation is important in rifampin resistance and is a major contributor to fluoroquinolone resistance. Methylation of part of the 50S ribosomal subunit can result in therapeutic failure of macrolides and lincosamides. MRSA and VRE both involve complete replacement of the antibiotic's intended target with a biologically active substitute, both of which allow cell wall synthesis to continue in the presence of antibiotics that normally inhibit this process.

More recently, it has been recognised that exposure to particular antibiotics can induce multi-step, complicated intracellular processes that can result in clinical failure. This is thought to be a reasonable explanation for treatment failure with daptomycin in some gram-positive infections, and treatment failure with vancomycin for *S. aureus* with seemingly sensitive or intermediate mean inhibitory concentrations *in vitro;*.

 Munita J, Arias C. Mechanisms of Antibiotic Resistance. Microbiology Spectrum. 2016;4(2). https://www.asmscience.org/content/journal/microbiolspec/10.1128/microbiolspec.VMBF-0016-2015

43. Answer: B

44. Answer: C

45. Answer: F

46. Answer: D

Viruses are small, obligate intracellular organisms that require the use of host cell nuclear apparatus in order to replicate and reassemble, such that they can leave the infected cell (shed) and consequently infect other cells and other organisms. Most antiviral drugs subvert this process by deactivating the DNA replication, or other enzymatic reactions required for viral replication.

Reverse transcriptase is used by retroviruses (and some non-retroviruses such as HBV) including HIV to convert viral RNA into DNA, which is then incorporated into genome of the virally infected cell, which allows the virus to use host mechanisms for replication. Reverse transcriptase inhibitors subvert this process by halting one of the steps involved. Nucleoside analogue reverse transcriptase inhibitors (NRTIs) and nucleotide reverse transcriptase inhibitors (NtRTIs) are both analogues of naturally occurring deoxynucleotides incorporated into a growing chain of viral DNA. However, as they do not share exactly the same structure as naturally occurring deoxynucleotides, their incorporation results in termination of the growing chain, as the next deoxynucleotide cannot attach, and therefore disruption of viral replication. To become active, both NRTIs and NtRTIs require phosphorylation by cellular kinases, NRTIs into active triphosphate form, NtRTIs into phosphonate-diphosphonate state. Zidovudine is the prototype NRTI and is a thymidine analogue; didanosine is an adenosine analogue NRTI; lamivudine and emtricitabine are cytosine analogue NRTIs; abacavir and entecavir are guanosine analogue NRTIs; tenofovir and adefovir are guanosine analogue NtRTIs. Non-nucleotide reverse transcriptase inhibitors bind to the reverse transcriptase enzyme itself near the catalytic site, which de-activates the enzyme: examples are efavirenz and nevirapine.

After incorporation into the host genome, viral DNA is converted into biologically inert polyproteins by mRNA. Virus-specific proteases are required to cleave these polyproteins into viral proteins. Protease inhibitors block this step by targeting the proteases specific to each virus. Darunavir, ritonavir and lopinavir are examples of HIV-1 protease inhibitors; boceprevir, grazoprevir and telaprevir are examples of HCV protease inhibitors.

Antivirals for the herpesvirus group (including CMV, HSV, varicella zoster) most commonly target viral DNA polymerase, required to replicate identical DNA strands from a single original DNA molecule. Acyclovir, valaciclovir, and famciclovir are initially phosphorylated by viral kinases and subsequently phosphorylated to triphosphate form by cellular kinases in order to become the active molecule. Ganciclovir and valganciclovir use the same process, but the viral kinase required to phosphorylate the drug is more specific to CMV. Cidofovir is a DNA polymerase inhibitor as well as potentially having other antiviral actions.

Neuraminidase is a transmembrane protein present on the influenza virus. Influenza enters the host cell via the viral haemagglutinin binding to sialic residues on the host cell membrane, the complex is then endocytosed. Neuraminidase allows viral disassembly of the viral structure, by severing the bonds between the particle coat in the sialic acid, which then allows viral RNA to enter the host nucleus. Neuraminidase inhibitors oseltamivir and zanamivir inhibit this enzyme.

Other clinically important anti-viral medications work by inhibiting HIV integrase (raltegravir), inhibiting HCV RNA polymerase (sofosbuvir) and antagonising chemokine receptor 5 (maraviroc). Antiviral medications commonly have a diverse and potentially severe side-effect profile, and significant potential for interaction with other medications, making judicious prescription and monitoring integral to patient care.

Ritter J, Flower R, Henderson G, Loke Y, MacEwan D, Rang H. The vascular system. Rang & Dale's Pharmacology. Edinburgh: Elsevier; 2019.
https://www.elsevierhealth.com.au/rang-dales-pharmacology-9780702074486.html

47. Answer: D

48. Answer: H

49. Answer: B

50. Answer: E

Since the AIDS was first observed, certain cancers were associated with the syndrome, and became AIDS-defining illnesses. Initially observations that certain cancers, for example Kaposi's sarcoma, occurred in clusters gave rise to the theory that certain cancers observed with AIDS were caused by secondary viral infections, and that AIDS allowed these infections to become oncogenic. The arrival of anti-retroviral therapy (ART) cut the incidence of AIDS-defining cancer significantly. However, as life expectancy with HIV/AIDS continues to improve, and subsequently the total population of HIV infected patients ages and grows in number, these cancers are now seen across a spectrum of CD4 counts, and other cancers that are not typically AIDS-defining become more prevalent. Indeed, in many western countries, cancer is now the leading cause of death in HIV-infected patients.

Kaposi's sarcoma is a multicentric tumour characterised by proliferation of spindle-cells of endothelial origin, and typically presents as an ulcerated lesion or lesions on the lower extremities. Treatment is with anti-retroviral therapy, but metastatic or unresponsive disease can be treated with local therapy or systemic chemotherapy. Kaposi's sarcoma is caused by Kaposi's sarcoma-associated herpesvirus (KSHV) otherwise known as human herpesvirus 8. KSHV infection usually does not cause Kaposi's sarcoma in immune-competent individuals, but sporadic cases of relatively indolent disease are observed in elderly men in Mediterranean regions. In HIV-infected individuals, incidence of the virus is much higher in men who have sex with men and individuals in sub-Saharan Africa. Risk of Kaposi's sarcoma is inversely proportional to CD4 count, but risk in HIV infected individuals with normal CD4 count is still substantially elevated. KSHV also causes primary effusion lymphoma and KSHV multicentric Castleman's disease.

HIV-associated lymphomas are often associated with EBV infected lymphocytes, presenting as Hodgkin's lymphoma, plasmablastic lymphoma, or primary CNS lymphoma. Some cases of diffuse large-B-cell lymphoma are EBV positive, but the majority are not, and this is also true of HIV-associated Burkitt's lymphoma. Lymphoma is often the presenting pathology in HIV infection, which argues for universal HIV screening at diagnosis of Hodgkin's lymphoma or aggressive B-cell lymphoma. Treatment of HIV-associated lymphoma now has survival rates approaching that of lymphoma not associated with HIV infection. As a result of the aggressive nature of the disease and effective available treatment regimes, rapid and definitive tissue diagnosis is of great value. This can present some difficulty in the case of CNS lymphoma, where imaging characteristics can overlap with cerebral toxoplasmosis, and stereotactic biopsy is often needed. However, certain MRI and FDG-PET characteristics, in combination with high EBV viral load in CSF, can be diagnostic, where biopsy is not possible.

HIV-infected patients have significantly elevated risk for a number of other cancers. HPV-associated cancers are good examples; cervical carcinoma, and anal squamous cell carcinoma are all far more prevalent in HIV-infected individuals. Additionally, a good proportion of head and neck cancer and oropharyngeal cancer in HIV-infected patients is HPV related. Merkel-cell carcinoma is a rare neuroendocrine cancer of the skin associated with Merkel-cell polyomavirus and is much more common in HIV-infected patients and is occasionally seen in solid organ transplant recipients. Lung cancer and hepatocellular carcinoma also have high incidence in HIV-infected patients.

Yarchoan R, Uldrick T. HIV-Associated Cancers and Related Diseases. New England Journal of Medicine. 2018;378(11):1029–1041.
https://www.nejm.org/doi/full/10.1056/NEJMra1615896

12 Medical Obstetrics

Questions

Answers can be found in the Medical Obstetrics Answers section at the end of this chapter.

1. A 38-year-old woman has antiphospholipid syndrome, with two previous miscarriages and known lupus anticoagulant and anticardiolipin antibodies positivity. She is 12 weeks pregnant.
Which of the following therapeutic strategies would you recommend?
A. Aspirin 150 mg a day.
B. Aspirin 150 mg a day and prophylactic dose of low molecular weight heparin.
C. Prophylactic dose of low molecular weight heparin.
D. Rivaroxaban.

2. A 19-year-old woman has asthma that has required four episodes of hospitalisation over the past 2 years. She is 14 weeks pregnant.
Which one of the following statements is correct?
A. Asthma control usually improves during pregnancy.
B. In acute asthma, drug therapy should be given as for a non-pregnant patient.
C. Long acting β2-agonists should be avoided during pregnancy.
D. Steroid medication should be avoided during pregnancy.

3. A 30-year-old woman is 7 weeks pregnant and is vomiting frequently and unable to tolerate food. She has not responded to prochlorperazine or metoclopramide but manages to keep herself hydrated.
Which of the following treatments should be administered?
A. Diazepam.
B. Intravenous 5% dextrose.
C. Prednisolone.
D. Pyridoxine plus doxylamine.

4. A 31-year-old woman is in the 23rd week of her third pregnancy. She has chronic hypertension but has not always taken her prescribed antihypertensive medication. She had hypertension during her previous pregnancies but did not tolerate labetalol because of dizziness. Her BP is 150/90 mmHg. Which of the following should be instituted?
A. No treatment unless proteinuria present.
B. Treatment with ACE inhibitor.
C. Treatment with methyldopa.
D. Treatment with metoprolol.

5. A 34-year-old woman has known hypothyroidism and takes 100 mcg of thyroxine a day. She has become pregnant and wants to know what she should do about her treatment.
Which one of the following statements is correct?
A. During pregnancy there is usually an increase in TSH levels.
B. Her thyroxine dose should be decreased by 25%.
C. Her thyroxine dose should be increased by 25%.
D. The foetus produces T3 and T4 during early pregnancy.

How to Pass the FRACP Written Examination, First Edition. Jonathan Gleadle, Jordan Li, Danielle Wu, and Paul Kleinig.
© 2022 John Wiley & Sons Ltd. Published 2022 by John Wiley & Sons Ltd.

6. Which one of the following investigations is predictive for the development of preeclampsia?
   A. Reduced levels of beta-human chorionic gonadotrophin (beta-hCG).
   B. Reduced levels of placental growth factor (PlGF).
   C. Reduced levels of soluble fms-like tyrosine kinase 1 (sFlt-1).
   D. Reduced levels of uric acid.

7. A 20-year-old women is 13 weeks pregnant. In her only previous pregnancy, she developed preeclampsia and underwent an early Caesarean section because of proteinuria and hypertension. Which of the following measures would you advise?
   A. Aspirin 150mg per day.
   B. Fish Oil supplements.
   C. Folic acid 5mg per day.
   D. Magnesium sulphate 4g per day.

8. Which one of the following features is consistent with the diagnostic criteria of preeclampsia?
   A. A blood pressure of 158/102mmHg at 16 weeks gestation.
   B. Serum creatinine 82 μmol/L [45-80].
   C. Severe right upper quadrant pain and ALT 245 U/L [0-30].
   D. Urate 0.53 mmol/L [0.15-0.35].

9. A 30-year-old woman with renal failure due to lupus nephritis received a living donor kidney transplant from her husband. Her creatinine is stable at 110 μmol/L [45-90], urine albumin creatinine ratio (ACR) is 4.5 mg/mmol [<2.5], and BP is 110/70 mmHg. Her medications included tacrolimus, mycophenolate mofetil, prednisolone, trimethoprim-sulfamethoxazole, and irbesartan. At 12 months post-transplant, she is determined to start a family.
   Which one of the following medications is safe to continue while attempting pregnancy?
   A. Irbesartan.
   B. Mycophenolate.
   C. Prednisolone.
   D. Trimethoprim-sulfamethoxazole.

10. A 32-year-old woman is 39 weeks pregnant and presents to hospital in early labour and has a BP of 130/75 mmHg. She feels breathless when walking quickly. A FBE is normal except for a platelet count of 110 x 10⁹/L [150-450] and a haemoglobin of 110 g/L [115-155]. A D-dimer test is 1.5 mg /L [<0.5 mg/L].
   Which of the following diagnoses is most likely?
   A. Gestational thrombocytopenia.
   B. Haemolytic uremic syndrome.
   C. Idiopathic thrombocytopenic purpura (ITP).
   D. Pulmonary embolus.

Answers

1. Answer: B

The antiphospholipid syndrome (APS) is a systemic autoimmune disease defined by thrombotic or obstetric events in patients with persistent antiphospholipid antibodies. Thrombotic APS is characterised by venous, arterial, or microvascular thrombosis. Patients with catastrophic APS can present with thrombosis involving multiple organs. APS should be considered in patients presenting with thrombosis at a young age, with an unusual site or recurrent thrombosis, with late pregnancy loss, with early or severe preeclampsia, or with the haemolysis, elevated liver enzymes, low platelet count (HELLP) syndrome.

Obstetric APS is characterised by foetal loss after 10 weeks gestation, recurrent early miscarriages, intrauterine growth restriction, or severe preeclampsia. Patients have persistent antiphospholipid antibodies (lupus anticoagulant, anticardiolipin antibodies, or anti-β2GPI antibodies). The current strategy for the prevention of pregnancy complications in patients with obstetric APS, based on low-quality evidence, is low-dose aspirin and prophylactic dose heparin. Direct oral anticoagulants appear less effective than warfarin for the prevention of thrombosis in high-risk patients with APS. Warfarin is contraindicated during pregnancy. Low-dose aspirin and therapeutic-dose heparin should be given during pregnancy in women with thrombotic APS, regardless of the pregnancy history. Antiphospholipid-antibody positive patients without a history of thrombosis should usually receive a prophylactic dose of low-molecular-weight heparin for at least 6 weeks postpartum, given the increased risk of thrombosis during this period. Long-term antithrombotic therapy is usually not advised for women who have a history of obstetric APS but no other risk factors for thrombosis.

Garcia D, Erkan D. Diagnosis and Management of the Antiphospholipid Syndrome. New England Journal of Medicine. 2018;378(21):2010–2021.
https://www.nejm.org/doi/full/10.1056/NEJMra1705454

McLintock C, Brighton T, Chunilal S, Dekker G, McDonnell N, McRAE S et al. Recommendations for the prevention of pregnancy-associated venous thromboembolism. Australian and New Zealand Journal of Obstetrics and Gynaecology. 2011;52(1):3–13.
https://obgyn.onlinelibrary.wiley.com/doi/abs/10.1111/j.1479-828X.2011.01357.x

2. Answer: B

The natural history of asthma during pregnancy is extremely variable. A quarter of pregnant women show an overall improvement but a third deteriorate. 11–18% of pregnant women with asthma will have at least one emergency department visit for acute asthma and of these two-thirds will require hospitalisation. If symptoms do worsen this is most likely in the second and third trimesters, with a peak in the sixth month.

In general, the medicines used to treat asthma are safe in pregnancy. A large population-based case-control study found no increased risk of major congenital malformations in children of women receiving asthma treatment in the year before or during pregnancy. Women with asthma should be advised of the importance and safety of continuing their asthma medications during pregnancy to ensure good asthma control. Short-acting β2 agonists, long-acting β2 agonists and inhaled corticosteroids (ICS) should be used as normal during pregnancy. A severe asthma exacerbation will be of greater harm to the foetus than the ICS. Prescribe steroid tablets as normal when indicated during pregnancy for women with severe asthma. Steroid tablets should never be withheld because of pregnancy and women should be advised that the benefits of treatment with oral steroids outweigh the risks. Some pregnant women stop their ICS due to the risk of cleft palate/ lip with steroids in the first trimester, but the ICS have a localised effect and are at a low dose, so the risk is low.

Drug therapy should be given as for a non-pregnant patient with acute asthma, including nebulised β2 agonists and early administration of steroid tablets. In severe cases, intravenous β2 agonists, aminophylline or intravenous bolus magnesium sulphate can be used as indicated. In pregnant patients with acute asthma, deliver high-flow oxygen immediately to maintain saturation 94–98%. Acute severe asthma in pregnancy is an emergency and should be treated vigorously in hospital. Use prostaglandin F2α with extreme caution in women with asthma because of the risk of inducing bronchoconstriction. Women with asthma can breastfeed and use asthma medications as normal during lactation.

Australian Asthma Handbook [Internet]. Asthmahandbook.org.au. 2020 [cited 22 February 2020].
Available from: https://www.asthmahandbook.org.au/populations/pregnant-women

3. Answer: D

Nausea and vomiting affect 75% of pregnant women. Hyperemesis gravidarum (HG) is a common complication of early pregnancy (1–3% of pregnancies) and is diagnosed when there is protracted nausea and vomiting in pregnancy that leads to more than 5% pregnancy weight loss, dehydration, and electrolyte imbalance.

Initial management of nausea and vomiting in pregnancy (NVP) is in the community with oral antiemetics. Antihistamine (H_1 receptor antagonists) and phenothiazine anti-emetics are safe and efficacious, and they should be prescribed when required for NVP and HG. Pyridoxine is a water-soluble vitamin, inhibits H_1 receptor, acts indirectly on vestibular system, some inhibition of muscarinic receptors to decrease stimulation of vomiting centre. It is more effective when used in combination with doxylamine or dicyclomine.

Ondansetron is effective and can be used. However, there is a concern due to a small increase in the risk of cleft palate and cleft lip. Patients should counselled about this risk if it is prescribed.

Corticosteroids' antiemetic effect is on the chemoreceptor trigger zone in the brainstem. It improves sense of well-being, appetite, and increased weight gain in HG patients. There is a possible increased risk of oral clefts when used < 10 week's gestation, but data are weak. It is restricted to refractory cases.

Benzodiazepines such as diazepam are thought to be helpful in HG, presumably through alleviating psychosomatic symptoms such as anxiety. However, the safety of these medications in pregnancy is still controversial with some studies demonstrating a positive association between neonatal exposure to diazepam and prematurity and low birth weight.

Inpatient management should be considered if there is at least one of the following: continued nausea and vomiting and inability to keep down oral antiemetics, or associated with ketonuria and/or weight loss (greater than 5% of body weight), despite oral antiemetics; confirmed or suspected comorbidity (such as urinary tract infection and inability to tolerate oral antibiotics). An index of nausea and vomiting such as the Pregnancy–Unique Quantification of Emesis (PUQE) score can be used to classify the severity of NVP.

Correction of significant dehydration and electrolyte abnormalities is clearly important and may require intravenous fluids. Most women admitted to hospital with HG are hyponatraemic, hypochloraemic, hypokalaemic, and ketotic, so normal saline and appropriate potassium chloride should usually be administered. Furthermore, Dextrose containing solutions might precipitate Wernicke's encephalopathy in thiamine deficient individuals. Dextrose infusions are inappropriate unless sodium levels are normal, and thiamine has been administered. Urea, creatinine, and electrolyte levels should be checked daily in women requiring intravenous fluids. Thiamine should be given to all women admitted with prolonged vomiting.

In general, patient should have oral intake as tolerated. Iron tablets should be held. If an antiemetic is ineffective at maximal dose, discontinue before commencing an alternative agent. If an antiemetic is partially effective, optimise dosage and timing, and only add additional agents after maximal doses of the first agent have been trialled.

The Management of Nausea and Vomiting of Pregnancy and Hyperemesis Gravidarum, 2016. Royal College of Obstetricians and Gynaecologists. Rcog.org.uk. (2020). [online] Available at: https://www.rcog.org.uk/globalassets/documents/guidelines/green-top-guidelines/gtg69-hyperemesis.pdf

4. Answer: C

Hypertension in pregnancy affects 10% of pregnant women. This includes women with chronic hypertension and women with hypertension related to pregnancy (gestational hypertension and preeclampsia). Untreated hypertension can lead to adverse events for both the woman and her baby, including increased risk of stroke, lower birth weight, and baby requiring neonatal intensive care. Preeclampsia is new onset hypertension (>140 mmHg systolic or >90 mmHg diastolic) after 20 weeks of pregnancy and new-onset proteinuria (urine protein : creatinine ratio ≥30 mg/mmol, or albumin : creatinine ratio ≥8 mg/mmol, or ≥1 g/L [2+] on dipstick testing) and other maternal organ dysfunction, such as renal, liver, neurological, or haematological involvement or complications, or uteroplacental dysfunction (e.g., foetal growth restriction, abnormal umbilical artery Doppler waveform analysis, or stillbirth).

Pregnant women with chronic hypertension should be advised about weight management, exercise, healthy eating, and lowering dietary salt. Existing antihypertensive treatment should be continued if safe in pregnancy (ACE inhibitors and metoprolol are NOT), or switch to an alternative treatment, unless blood pressures are consistently <110/70 mmHg. Antihypertensive treatment should be offered to pregnant women with chronic hypertension if they have sustained BP ≥140/90 mmHg and aim for a target of 135/85 mmHg. Labetalol, nifedipine or methyldopa are the preferred agents. Pregnant women with chronic hypertension should be offered aspirin 75–150 mg once daily from 12 weeks of pregnancy and placental growth factor (PlGF)-based testing may help rule out the development of preeclampsia between 20 weeks and 35 weeks of pregnancy.

Hypertension during pregnancy predisposes women to hypertension in the future and an increased likelihood of hypertensive disorders of pregnancy in future pregnancies and of long-term hypertension and cardiovascular disease in later life.

Webster, K., Fishburn, S., Maresh, M., Findlay, S. and Chappell, L., 2019. Diagnosis and management of hypertension in pregnancy: summary of updated NICE guidance. BMJ, p.l5119. https://www.bmj.com/content/366/bmj.l5119

5. Answer: C

During pregnancy, the thyroid gland undergoes hyperplasia and increased vascularity. The increase in beta-human chorionic gonadotrophin (β-HCG) in the first trimester can directly stimulate the TSH receptor as β-HCG has structural similarities to TSH. This leads to increased free T3 and T4 which suppresses TSH secretion and a serum TSH below 0.1 mIU/L is present in 5% of women by the 11th week of pregnancy. The TSH subsequently normalises as β-HCG falls in the second and third trimesters. The foetal thyroid starts functioning from 10 weeks gestation but does not fully mature until the third trimester and foetal requirements are met by maternal thyroxine.

Pregnant and lactating women have an increased iodine due to increased thyroid hormone production, increased renal iodine excretion and foetal iodine requirements.

For women with hypothyroidism, TSH should be optimised before conception. Thyroid deficiency in pregnancy is associated with an increased risk of premature birth, low birth weight and miscarriage. After conception, an increase in thyroxine as soon as possible is recommended to normalise the TSH concentration. This will usually require an increase in the thyroxine dose of 20–30%. Serum TSH should be monitored every four weeks in the first trimester and then six to eight weekly and maintained in the appropriate pregnancy ranges. Postpartum, the thyroxine dose should be reduced to the preconception dose, assuming the woman was euthyroid on that dose and thyroid function checked 4–6 weeks after their dose has been reduced.

A new diagnosis of overt hypothyroidism should lead to immediate thyroxine replacement and testing for thyroid autoantibodies, such as antithyroid peroxidase antibodies (anti-TPO), antithyroglobulin antibodies (TgAb), thyrotropin receptor antibodies (TRAb) (if there is a history of treated Graves' disease). The usual starting dose of thyroxine is at least 50 micrograms per day with maintenance between 100 and 150 micrograms per day titrated to achieve TSH suppression.

 Smith A, Eccles-Smith J, D'Emden M, Lust K. Thyroid disorders in pregnancy and postpartum. Australian Prescriber. 2017;40(6):214–219.
https://www.nps.org.au/australian-prescriber/articles/thyroid-disorders-in-pregnancy-and-postpartum

6. Answer: B

Preeclampsia affects between 2% and 8% of pregnancies and remains a leading cause of maternal and perinatal mortality and morbidity worldwide. Although the pathogenesis of preeclampsia is not completely understood, altered levels of angiogenic factors appear to play a role. Mammalian placental development requires extensive angiogenesis to establish a suitable vascular network to supply oxygen and nutrients to the foetus. A variety of proangiogenic (VEGF, PlGF) and antiangiogenic factors (sFlt-1) are produced by the developing placenta, and the balance among these factors is important for normal placentation. Increased production of antiangiogenic factors disturbs this balance and is associated with the systemic endothelial dysfunction characteristic of preeclampsia.

Elevated levels of soluble fms-like tyrosine kinase 1 (sFlt-1; an inhibitor of vascular endothelial growth factor) and reduced levels of placental growth factor (PlGF), or combined give an increased sFlt-1:PlGF ratio occurs both in women with established preeclampsia and in women before the development of preeclampsia. In women between 24–37 weeks of gestation who present with a clinical suspicion of preeclampsia a lowered sFlt-1: PlGF ratio <38) has been reported to have a negative predictive value of 99%. Recent trials have also suggested that the availability of PlGF test results substantially reduced the time to clinical confirmation of preeclampsia was associated with a lower incidence of maternal adverse outcomes.

High total hCG concentration in early pregnancy is associated with an increased risk of preeclampsia but lacks sufficient sensitivity or specificity and is not used clinically. Although hyperuricaemia is common in women with preeclampsia, it is not useful for predicting which women will develop preeclampsia.

 Duhig K, Myers J, Seed P, Sparkes J, Lowe J, Hunter R et al. Placental growth factor testing to assess women with suspected pre-eclampsia: a multicentre, pragmatic, stepped-wedge cluster-randomised controlled trial. The Lancet. 2019;393(10183):1807–1818.
https://www.thelancet.com/journals/lancet/article/PIIS0140-6736(18)33212-4/fulltext

 Mol B, Roberts C, Thangaratinam S, Magee L, de Groot C, Hofmeyr G. Pre-eclampsia. The Lancet. 2016;387(10022): 999–1011.
https://www.thelancet.com/journals/lancet/article/PIIS0140-6736(15)00070-7/fulltext

7. Answer: A

Aspirin has been shown to reduce the incidence of preeclampsia in high risk individuals. A recent trial showed preeclampsia-occurred in 1.6% of the aspirin group, as compared with 4.3% in the placebo group (odds ratio: 0.38). Most guidelines recommend aspirin therapy beginning at 12 weeks of gestation in patients who are considered to be at high risk for preeclampsia. Neither fish oil nor folic acid supplementation has reduced the incidence of preeclampsia in clinical trials.

Risks for the development of preeclampsia include previous pregnancy with preeclampsia, especially early onset and with an adverse outcome, multi-foetal pregnancies, chronic hypertension, diabetes, CKD, and autoimmune diseases.

Magnesium sulphate has not been shown to reduce the incidence of preeclampsia but is the treatment of choice in the management of eclampsia and is used in many units for prevention of eclampsia in patients with severe preeclampsia. Treatment should be commenced with magnesium sulphate given as a 4 g loading dose (diluted in normal saline over 15–20 minutes) followed by an infusion of (1–2 g/hr, diluted in normal saline). Magnesium sulphate by infusion should continue for 24 hours after the last seizure. Serum magnesium levels do not need to be measured routinely unless renal function is compromised. Magnesium sulphate is excreted via the kidneys and extreme caution should be used in women with oliguria or renal impairment. Serum magnesium concentration should be closely monitored in this situation.

Rolnik D, Wright D, Poon L, O'Gorman N, Syngelaki A, de Paco Matallana C et al. Aspirin versus Placebo in Pregnancies at High Risk for Preterm Preeclampsia. New England Journal of Medicine. 2017;377(7):613–622.
https://www.nejm.org/doi/full/10.1056/NEJMoa1704559

8. Answer: C

Preeclampsia is a multi-system disorder unique to human pregnancy characterised by hypertension and involvement of one or more other organ systems and/or the foetus. A diagnosis of preeclampsia can be made when hypertension arises after 20 weeks gestation accompanied by one or more of the following signs of organ involvement:

- Renal involvement indicated by significant proteinuria, creatinine > 90 µmol/L or oliguria: <80mL/4 hr
- Haematological involvement indicated by thrombocytopenia <100,000 /µL; Haemolysis indicated by schistocytes or red cell fragments on blood film, raised bilirubin, raised LDH >600 U/L, decreased haptoglobin or DIC.
- Liver involvement with raised serum transaminases, severe epigastric and/or right upper quadrant pain.
- Neurological involvement with convulsions (eclampsia), hyperreflexia with sustained clonus, persistent, new headache, persistent visual disturbances (photopsia, scotomata, cortical blindness, posterior reversible encephalopathy syndrome, retinal vasospasm)
- Stroke
- Pulmonary oedema
- Foetal growth restriction (FGR).

Preeclampsia is rare before 20 weeks gestation; usually associated with a predisposing factor such as hydatidiform mole, multiple pregnancy, foetal triploidy, severe renal disease, or antiphospholipid syndrome.

Hyperuricaemia is a common but not diagnostic feature of preeclampsia. HELLP syndrome occurs in a subset of women with severe preeclampsia with haemolysis, raised liver enzymes (transaminases), and low platelets.

Gestational hypertension is new onset of hypertension after 20 weeks gestation without any maternal or foetal features of preeclampsia, followed by return of BP to normal within 3 months after delivery. Chronic hypertension is a BP ≥ 140 mmHg systolic and/or 90 mmHg diastolic confirmed before pregnancy or before 20 weeks gestation. Pre-existing hypertension is a strong risk factor for preeclampsia.

Lowe S, Bowyer L, Lust K, McMahon L, Morton M, North R et al. Guideline for the Management of Hypertensive Disorders of Pregnancy [Internet]. Society of Obstetric Medicine of Australia and New Zealand; 2014 [cited 15 February 2020].
Available from: https://ranzcog.edu.au/RANZCOG_SITE/media/RANZCOG-MEDIA/Women%27s%20Health/SOMANZ-Hypertension-Pregnancy-Guideline-April-2014.pdf?ext=.pdf

9. Answer: C

Fertility and sexual function improve after kidney transplantation and by 6 months, the hypothalamic-pituitary-gonadal axis is restored to normal. Recipients of childbearing age should use contraception if pregnancy is not desired. Guidelines recommend delaying pregnancy until one year after renal transplantation. Predictors of good maternal and foetal outcomes include a younger maternal age, stable allograft function with serum creatinine <130 µmol/L with no recent episodes of rejection, proteinuria <0.5 g/day, and normal or well controlled hypertension.

Medications should be reviewed prior to attempting pregnancy. The Federal Drug Administration (FDA) grants letter grades of medications which may be used (grades A, B, and C) and drugs considered unsafe (grades D and X).

The calcineurin inhibitors, cyclosporine and tacrolimus have been linked to foetal growth retardation and preterm delivery, but are generally felt to be safe, however, mycophenolate is a teratogen and should be substituted with azathioprine at least 6 weeks before attempting pregnancy. Mammalian target of rapamycin (mTOR) inhibitors are not safe and should be avoided. Prednisolone, especially low dose is considered safe in pregnancy.

ACE inhibitors (ACEis) and angiotensin-receptor blockers (ARBs) are known teratogenic agents and contraindicated in pregnancy. Agents such as labetalol, methyldopa, and the calcium channel antagonists are first-line choices for treatment of hypertension prior to and during pregnancy.

Both components of trimethoprim-sulfamethoxazole, cross the placenta in humans. There are no controlled data in human pregnancy. Retrospective epidemiologic studies suggest an association between first trimester exposure to this drug with an increased risk of congenital malformations, particularly neural tube defects, cardiovascular abnormalities, and urinary tract defects. This patient is 12 months post-transplant. The risk of *Pneumocystis jiroveci* pneumonia is low, therefore trimethoprim-sulfamethoxazole should be stopped.

Cabiddu G, Spotti D, Gernone G, Santoro D, Moroni G, Gregorini G et al. A best-practice position statement on pregnancy after kidney transplantation: focusing on the unsolved questions. The Kidney and Pregnancy Study Group of the Italian Society of Nephrology. Journal of Nephrology. 2018;31(5):665–681.
https://link.springer.com/article/10.1007/s40620-018-0499-x

10. Answer: A

In women with uncomplicated pregnancies, platelet counts decline in the first trimester and continue throughout pregnancy, with the nadir occurring around delivery, when 10% of women have platelet counts of less than 150×10^9/L. At around 7 weeks after delivery, platelet counts recover to the level of platelet counts in non-pregnant women. The mechanism of this gestational thrombocytopenia may include the increased plasma volume that occurs during pregnancy and pooling by the spleen which increases in size by 50% during pregnancy.

It is important to be aware of the physiological changes that occur in pregnancy and the altered reference ranges for commonly requested laboratory tests. Important changes include reductions in the levels of creatinine, sodium, albumin, and haemoglobin. Haemoglobin concentration decreases in the first trimester, then remains relatively constant until returning to pre-pregnancy values approximately 4 months postpartum. The concentration of TSH normally decreases during the first trimester of pregnancy during which there is maximal cross-stimulation of the TSH receptor by beta-HCG. The TSH concentration then returns to its pre-pregnancy level in the second trimester and then rises slightly in the third. Mild breathlessness is very common in normal pregnancy.

Troponin levels and CRP are not altered in pregnancy, but D-dimer levels rise steadily during pregnancy. D-dimer levels are above the non-pregnancy threshold in up to a half of women in first trimester, 2/3 in second trimester and virtually all women in the third trimester and are markedly elevated during labour, decreasing rapidly during the first 3 days post-delivery and usually normalising by 4 weeks. Therefore, D-dimer levels are not usually a helpful diagnostic test during pregnancy.

Reese J, Peck J, Deschamps D, McIntosh J, Knudtson E, Terrell D et al. Platelet Counts during Pregnancy. New England Journal of Medicine. 2018;379(1):32–43.
https://www.nejm.org/doi/full/10.1056/NEJMoa1802897

Morton A, Teasdale S. Review article: Investigations and the pregnant woman in the emergency department - part 1: Laboratory investigations. Emergency Medicine Australasia. 2018;30(5):600–609.
https://onlinelibrary.wiley.com/doi/abs/10.1111/1742-6723.12957

13 Medical Oncology

Questions

Answers can be found in the Medical Oncology Answers section at the end of this chapter.

1. Which of the following treatment strategies has the best evidence for improving overall survival in the setting of metastatic renal cell cancer with progression on sunitinib?
   A. Bevacizumab plus interferon therapy
   B. Everolimus
   C. Nivolumab
   D. Sorafenib.

2. Which statement best describes the use of bevacizumab in cancer?
   A. It activates vascular endothelial growth factor (VEGF) in angiogenesis.
   B. The most frequent adverse effect is hypotension.
   C. Clinical improvements are minor due to multiple pathways involved in tumour angiogenesis.
   D. It is an anti-platelet-derived growth factor (PDGF) antibody generated in rats.

3. Which of the following statements best describes the risk of cancer diagnosis in women with *BRCA1* and *BRCA2* gene mutations?
   A. *BRCA1* carriers have a much higher cumulative lifetime risk of breast cancer than *BRCA2* carriers.
   B. *BRCA1* carriers have a much higher cumulative lifetime risk of ovarian cancer than *BRCA2* carriers.
   C. *BRCA1* carriers have a lower cumulative incidence of contralateral breast cancer by 20 years after initial breast cancer diagnosis.
   D. Cumulative risk of breast cancer diagnosis peaks earlier in *BRCA2* carriers than *BRCA1* carriers.

4. Which of the following molecular targets has been most useful in the development of chimeric antigen receptor T-cells (CAR T) for the treatment of lymphocytic malignancies?
   A. BCL-2.
   B. Carbonic anhydrase 9.
   C. CD19.
   D. CD20.

5. All of the following are correct in the new national cervical screening program **EXCEPT**:
   A. Cervical Screening Test screens for the presence of HPV.
   B. First Cervical Screening Test is two years from their last normal Pap Test.
   C. HPV-vaccinated women should be screened for cervical cancer.
   D. The interval between routine Cervical Screening Tests in immunosuppressed women is two years.

6. A 62-year-old woman is going to start carboplatin-based combination chemotherapy for ovarian cancer. Which is the most appropriate prophylactic antiemetic regimens?
   A. Intravenous NK1 receptor antagonist, fosaprepitant.
   B. Intravenous metoclopramide and granisetron transdermal patch.
   C. Oral dexamethasone, ondansetron and NK1 receptor antagonist, aprepitant.
   D. Oral dexamethasone and NK1 receptor antagonist, aprepitant.

How to Pass the FRACP Written Examination, First Edition. Jonathan Gleadle, Jordan Li, Danielle Wu, and Paul Kleinig.
© 2022 John Wiley & Sons Ltd. Published 2022 by John Wiley & Sons Ltd.

7. A 67-year-old retired nurse presents with peripheral oedema. She has nephrotic range proteinuria (4 g/day). Kidney biopsy showed membranous nephropathy but PLA2R antibody is negative. CXR and CT chest reveal a 2.5 cm spiculated lesion in the left upper lobe. Biopsy confirms an adenocarcinoma. PET scan demonstrates no uptake apart from the primary lung lesion. She underwent a lobectomy which was uncomplicated. Her proteinuria is now 1 g/day.

What is the best next step in management?

    A. Cisplatin-based chemotherapy.
    B. Erlotinib therapy.
    C. Radiation therapy.
    D. Surveillance chest imaging periodically.

8. Isocitrate dehydrogenase (IDH) mutations are commonly seen in which of the following tumours?

    A. Gliomas.
    B. Prostate cancer.
    C. Breast cancer.
    D. Renal cell carcinoma.

9. A 45-year-old woman presents with diplopia and headache. Her history is significant for metastatic breast cancer diagnosed 6 years prior, treated with multiple lines of chemotherapy, and resection of a solitary frontal lobe metastasis 3 years prior. She is currently not having any anti-cancer treatment. On examination she has mild weakness of her right temporalis muscle and her right eye is displaced laterally and inferiorly and will not adduct. Additionally, she is noted to have a mild weakness in left foot dorsiflexion with altered sensation over the dorsum of the left foot. CT of the brain is normal.

Which single test has the highest likelihood of diagnosing the causative pathology?

    A. CSF cytology for malignant cells.
    B. MRI of the brain and spinal cord.
    C. Peripheral nerve biopsy.
    D. Varicella zoster PCR on CSF.

10. A patient has a strong family history of colorectal cancer and has wondered if they might have Lynch syndrome. Which one of the following is true of Lynch syndrome?

    A. It has an autosomal recessive pattern of inheritance.
    B. There is a lifetime risk of colorectal cancer of 25%.
    C. It is usually due to mutations in P53.
    D. It is the commonest hereditary colorectal cancer predisposition syndrome.

11. A 39-year-old man presents with weight loss, night sweats and fevers. Examination is suspicious for the impression of a paraumbilical mass, and there is mild bipedal pitting oedema. Basic blood tests are unremarkable; an axial slice of a portal venous phase CT with oral contrast is shown below:

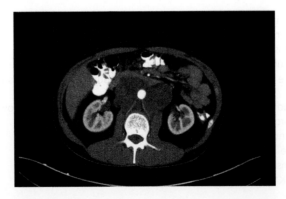

Which of the following serum tumour markers would be most useful in furthering diagnosis?

    A. Alpha-fetoprotein (α-FP).
    B. CA 19.9.
    C. Carcinoembryonic antigen (CEA).
    D. Prostate specific antigen (PSA).

12. A 48-year-old man with metastatic melanoma presents with acute back pain. The pain started yesterday in the midline of the mid-thoracic spine. There is no radiation of the pain, no limb weakness, no limb numbness and no bowel or bladder dysfunction. His metastatic disease is known to include liver, lung, and spinal metastases. Neurological examination of the lower limbs and rectal examination is normal. He is tender over the mid thoracic vertebrae in the midline.

Which is the most appropriate next investigation?
  - **A.** CT scanning of the thoracic spine.
  - **B.** MTI of the whole spine.
  - **C.** Plain x-ray of the thoraco-lumbar spine.
  - **D.** Whole body isotopic bone scan.

13. Which of the following IS **NOT** an advantage of multiparametric MRI-guided prostate biopsy over transrectal ultrasound (TRUS) biopsy in the diagnosis of prostate cancer?
  - **A.** Higher detection of apical and anterior tumours.
  - **B.** Higher detection of clinically relevant cancer.
  - **C.** Higher detection of low-grade tumours.
  - **D.** Safe decrease in the number of patients who need a biopsy.

14. A patient is diagnosed with advanced adenocarcinoma of the lung. Which of the following driver mutations has the **LEAST** relevance in guiding treatment decisions?
  - **A.** *ALK.*
  - **B.** *EGFR.*
  - **C.** *KRAS.*
  - **D.** *ROS1.*

15. The incidence of which of the following cancers is most strongly associated with obesity:
  - **A.** Adenocarcinoma of the oesophagus.
  - **B.** Colorectal adenocarcinoma.
  - **C.** Ovarian cancer.
  - **D.** Pancreatic adenocarcinoma.

16. A 48-year-old man is diagnosed with metastatic melanoma with bone and brain metastases. He is about to start therapy with nivolumab.

Which of the following immune related adverse events (irAEs) are most likely to occur as a result of his therapy?
  - **A.** Colitis.
  - **B.** Hypophysitis.
  - **C.** Pneumonitis.
  - **D.** Thyroid disease.

17. Which of the following statements best describes the role of programmed death ligand 1 (PD-L1), in dampening an adaptive immune response?
  - **A.** Down-regulation of antigen presentation to cytotoxic T cells.
  - **B.** Inhibiting antibody release by B-cells towards a specific antigen.
  - **C.** Inducing Interleukin-10 production by regulatory T cells thus dampening a T cell response to a particular antigen stimulus.
  - **D.** Transmission of an inhibitory signal to antigen-specific and naïve T cells, dampening the cytotoxic response.

18. Which one of the following is a risk factor for prostate cancer?
  - **A.** Benign prostatic hyperplasia.
  - **B.** *BRCA1* gene mutation.
  - **C.** Previous vasectomy.
  - **D.** *PSA* gene mutation.

19. An 80-year-old man is admitted to the ward with an infective exacerbation of COPD. This is on the background of two previous exacerbations this year, ongoing smoking (30/day) and two coronary artery stents inserted following an acute myocardial infarction 2 months ago. He is currently on aspirin, clopidogrel, atorvastatin, perindopril, budesonide plus formoterol fumarate dehydrate and salbutamol inhalers.

You note that on a previous admission last year his PSA was 16 ng/mL [< 3.25 ng/mL] and repeat PSA was 16.5 ng/mL. The urology team recommended a prostate MRI which showed one PIRADS 2 lesion in the peripheral zone, anterior aspect.

What is the most appropriate next step in caring for him?
- **A.** Digital rectal exam (DRE).
- **B.** Prostate biopsies.
- **C.** Prostate ultrasound.
- **D.** Surveillance PSAs.

20. What is the role of chemotherapy in concurrent chemoradiotherapy (CCRT) in the treatment of locally advanced head and neck cancer?
- **A.** Acts as a radiosensitiser.
- **B.** Eliminates micrometastases.
- **C.** Enhances immunogenic cell death.
- **D.** Reduces radiation toxicity.

21. Which one of the following techniques is used in radiotherapy for a patient with stage IB non-small cell lung cancer with severe COPD to counteract the effect of tumour motion due to breathing?
- **A.** Gating.
- **B.** Modulation.
- **C.** Shunting.
- **D.** Stereotactic.

22. Risk factors for primary epithelial ovarian cancer include which of the following?
- **A.** Early menopause.
- **B.** Multiple pregnancies.
- **C.** Nulliparity.
- **D.** Prolonged oral contraceptive use.

23. A 49-year-old man from Southeast Asia presents with generalized lymphadenopathy. He is known to have G6PD deficiency. A diagnosis of stage 4 diffuse large B-cell lymphoma was made after a lymph node biopsy and CT scan. His other investigation results are shown below. He is about to start chemotherapy with R-CHOP in standard dose.

Tests	Results	Normal values
Haemoglobin	98 g/L	135–175
WBC	29 x 10^9/L	4–12
Platelets	356 x 10^9/L	150–450
Creatinine	136 µmol/L	60–110
LDH	3256 U/L	120–250

Which option would you consider most appropriate before the chemotherapy?
- **A.** Intravenous normal saline.
- **B.** Intravenous normal saline and allopurinol.
- **C.** Intravenous normal saline and rasburicase.
- **D.** Intravenous normal saline and rasburicase plus urinary alkalinisation.

24. Which one of the followings is **NOT** a characteristic of an ideal tumour marker?
- **A.** Correction with tumour volume.
- **B.** Long half-life in blood circulation.
- **C.** Long lead-time.
- **D.** Minimal post-translational modifications.

QUESTIONS (25–30) **REFER TO THE FOLLOWING INFORMATION**

Match the adverse event with the chemotherapeutic agent most likely to cause it

- **A.** Doxorubicin.
- **B.** Oxaliplatin.
- **C.** Fluorouracil.
- **D.** Cisplatin.
- **E.** Bleomycin.
- **F.** Cyclophosphamide.
- **G.** Ifosphamide.
- **H.** Intrathecal methotrexate.

Questions

25. Encephalopathy

26. Myocardial ischaemia

27. Acute symptomatic neuropathy

28. Aseptic meningitis

29. Acute kidney injury

30. Delayed cardiomyopathy

QUESTIONS (31–38) **REFER TO THE FOLLOWING INFORMATION**

Match the targeted molecular agent with its best indication in advanced cancer:

- **A.** Clear cell renal cell carcinoma.
- **B.** Hepatocellular carcinoma.
- **C.** ALK positive non-small cell lung carcinoma.
- **D.** Oestrogen receptor positive, HER2 negative breast cancer.
- **E.** EGFR mutation positive non-small cell lung cancer.
- **F.** BRAF positive melanoma.
- **G.** BCR-ABL positive chronic myeloid leukaemia.
- **H.** HER2 positive breast cancer.

Questions

31. Palbociclib

32. Dasatinib

33. Osimertinib

34. Brigatinib

35. Dabrafenib

36. Pazopanib

37. Lapatanib

38. Regorafenib

Answers

1. Answer: C

Systemic treatment strategies for metastatic renal cell cancer (mRCC) are generally defined by the molecular subtypes, prognostic risk criteria score, burden of disease, and the presence or absence of symptoms.

Systemic treatment options include cytokines, anti-vascular endothelial growth factor (VEGF), anti-mammalian target of rapamycin (mTOR), multi-target anti-VEGF agents, and more recently, checkpoint inhibitors.

All options given above have been approved as systemic therapies for mRCC as they confer a significant improvement in progression-free survival (PFS). However, only cabozantinib and nivolumab have been found to demonstrate significantly improved overall survival (OS).

Lalani A, McGregor B, Albiges L, Choueiri T, Motzer R, Powles T et al. Systemic Treatment of Metastatic Clear Cell Renal Cell Carcinoma in 2018: Current Paradigms, Use of Immunotherapy, and Future Directions. European Urology. 2019;75(1):100–110.
https://www.europeanurology.com/article/S0302–2838(18)30751–6/fulltext

Motzer R, Escudier B, McDermott D, George S, Hammers H, Srinivas S et al. Nivolumab versus Everolimus in Advanced Renal–Cell Carcinoma. New England Journal of Medicine. 2015;373(19):1803–1813.
https://www.nejm.org/doi/full/10.1056/NEJMoa1510665

2. Answer: C

Angiogenesis is a critical step in the proliferation, growth, and metastatic potential of cancer cells. Without angiogenesis, tumour growth would be limited to around 1–2 mm^3 and would lack metastatic potential via haematogenous spread. Angiogenesis occurs because of a complex relationship between cancer cells, the surrounding microenvironment, and distant sites.

Four main mechanisms are described allowing angiogenesis to occur. Firstly, sprouting angiogenesis occurs when the basement membrane protecting endothelial cells is compromised, triggering proliferative, migratory, and invasive potential of specialised endothelial cells allowing branching growth of existing blood vessels. Secondly, chemokines, cytokines, and growth factors secreted by tumour cells and surrounding stromal cells leads to distant activation of MMP9 and subsequently Kit which allows migration and homing of endothelial progenitor cells. Thirdly, some tumour cells can de-differentiate to adopt multiple cellular phenotypes, including endothelial properties, allowing for a creation of a vasculogenic-like network that mimics an embryonic vascular plexus. Finally, shear stress in the absence of VEGF can allow larger vessels to split into multiple smaller functional vessels as a result of remodelling of endothelial cells without the need for endothelial cell proliferation, in a process called intussusceptive microvascular growth.

These processes are heavily influenced by the production of proangiogenic molecules by tumour cells themselves, but the interaction with surrounding immune cells, the extra-cellular matrix and interaction with vascular components such as platelets and pericytes are all important. There are a raft of important signalling pathways involved in these processes, many of which are activated by hypoxia, the most integral being VEGF, C-X-C chemokine receptor type 4, stromal derived factor-1, and platelet derived growth factor (PDGF), as well as inflammatory cytokines.

The complexity of this system has important clinical implications, the first of which is that targeting of a single angiogenic pathway is unlikely to result in a substantial anti-tumour response. Bevacizumab is a recombinant humaniseds monoclonal antibody that blocks angiogenesis by inhibiting VEGF A. The 'zu' substem indicates that it is a humanised antibody, i.e. it is an antibody generated from non-human species whose protein sequences have been modified to increase their similarity to antibody variants produced naturally in humans. Bevacizumab is largely used in combination with other agents where there is an additive anti-tumour effect. Although side effects of bevacizumab are generally mild, occasional life-threatening events have been observed, including venous thromboembolism and severe bleeding. Tyrosine kinase inhibitors against multiple targets within this system have shown greater efficacy as monotherapy in various cancers – examples include sorafenib, sunitinib, and pazopanib.

Rajabi M, Mousa S. The Role of Angiogenesis in Cancer Treatment. Biomedicines. 2017;5(4):34.
https://pubmed.ncbi.nlm.nih.gov/28635679/

Zuazo-Gaztelu I, Casanovas O. Unravelling the Role of Angiogenesis in Cancer Ecosystems. Frontiers in Oncology.2018;8.
https://www.ncbi.nlm.nih.gov/pubmed/30013950

3. Answer B:

BRCA 1 and 2 are tumour suppressor genes that repair DNA damage to prevent tumour development. Mutations in these genes predispose to development of several malignancies, particularly for breast and ovarian cancers. Although most breast and ovarian cancers are sporadic, approximately 7% of breast cancer and 15% of ovarian cancer cases are caused by variants in the breast cancer susceptibility gene 1 (*BRCA1*) or 2 (*BRCA2*) genes and are also associated with lethal prostate cancer. Risk assessment incorporating personal and family history is vital in assigning risk and significance of any variations in the *BRCA* genes. This is particularly important in providing accurate guidance for women at high risk who may be considering risk-reducing bilateral salpingo-oophorectomy or mastectomy.

Registry data suggest that lifetime risk of breast cancer diagnosis is roughly equal in carriers of either mutation at around 70%. However, earlier diagnosis occurs more frequently in *BRCA1* carriers, with a cumulative risk of 25% by the age of 40, compared to 13% for *BRCA2* carriers. Contralateral breast cancer diagnosis at 20 years after initial diagnosis of breast cancer is also more frequent in *BRCA1* than *BRCA2* carriers (40% vs. 26%). Lifetime incidence of ovarian cancer is more common in *BRCA1* carriers (44% vs. 17%).

Interestingly, *BRCA1/2* gene mutation carrier status has a predominantly positive association with survival in ovarian cancer [hazard ratio (HR) for death 0.76]. *BRCA1* appears to be associated with worse survival in breast cancer (HR 1.50), but *BRCA2* mutation is not associated with worse survival in breast cancer.

Zhong Q, Peng H, Zhao X, Zhang L, Hwang W. Effects of BRCA1- and BRCA2-Related Mutations on Ovarian and Breast Cancer Survival: A Meta-analysis. Clinical Cancer Research. 2015;21(1):211–220.
https://clincancerres.aacrjournals.org/content/21/1/211.long

Kuchenbaecker K, Hopper J, Barnes D, Phillips K, Mooij T, Roos-Blom M et al. Risks of Breast, Ovarian, and Contralateral Breast Cancer for BRCA1 and BRCA2 Mutation Carriers. JAMA. 2017;317(23):2402.
https://jamanetwork.com/journals/jama/fullarticle/2632503

4. Answer: C

Chimeric antigen receptor (CAR) T-cells therapy uses engineered synthetic receptors on T-lymphocytes to augment the immune response toward cancer cells. This is achieved through specificity of the receptor towards a particular tumour antigen, without the need for traditional HLA-derived antigen presentation. The major issue with this form of therapy is that 'tumour' antigens are almost always also 'self' antigens and treatment toxicity can occur. Anti-CD19 T-cell therapy has thus been the most successful and best tolerated CAR T-cells therapy, with response rates of up to 90% in adult, B-cell acute lymphoblastic leukaemia. CD19 is a biomarker for normal and neoplastic B cells, as well as follicular dendritic cells. CD19 functions in establishing intrinsic B cell signalling thresholds through modulating both B cell receptor-dependent and independent signalling. Predictably, B-cell aplasia and hypogammaglobulinaemia requiring intravenous immunoglobulin supplementation is the most common adverse effect of this therapy, with minor clinical significance. However, life-threatening and severe cytokine-release syndrome is not uncommon and is treated with the anti-IL-6 antibody, tocilizumab. Neurological toxicity is also observed with anti-CD19 CAR T-cells therapy. Theoretically, other targets for CAR T-cell exist on many solid tumours and haematological malignancies, and development is ongoing, limited by potential toxicity.

June C, Sadelain M. Chimeric Antigen Receptor Therapy. New England Journal of Medicine. 2018;379(1):64–73.
https://www.nejm.org/doi/full/10.1056/NEJMra1706169

5. Answer: D

Australia and New Zealand have the lowest rates of cervical cancer in the world due to the success of the National Cervical Screening Program over the last 25 years. Recent changes to the program were based on the latest available evidence on the development and prevention of cervical cancer. It focuses on HPV testing as it better identifies women at risk of pre-cancerous changes and cervical cancer.

The new changes are summarised below:
- A Cervical Screening Test is used instead of a Pap Test.
- The recommended screening age is between 25–74.
- The interval between routine tests is 5 years and 3 years for immunocompromised women.
- Women should have their first Cervical Screening Test two years from their last Pap Test.

- Cervical Screening Test screens for the presence of HPV, and if found, performing a reflex liquid-based cytology (LBC) test on the same sample to check for abnormal cervical cells.
- HPV-vaccinated women need cervical screening, because the current HPV vaccine only protects against two HPV types (16 and 18) that cause about 70% of cervical cancers.

Implementing the changes to the National Cervical Screening Program: A guide for clinicians. [Internet]. Family Planning NSW. 2020 [cited 9 January 2020].
Available from: https://www.fpnsw.org.au/sites/default/files/assets/Cervical_Screening_Clinician_Guide_151217.pdf

6. Answer: C

The control of chemotherapy-induced nausea and vomiting (CINV) is an important issue for patients undergoing chemotherapy. The objective of antiemetic therapy is the complete prevention of CINV, and this should be achievable in the majority of patients.

The emetogenicity of chemotherapy agents is used as a framework for defining antiemetic treatment guidelines. A four-level classification of intravenous chemotherapy agents has been used: high (emetic risk >90%), moderate (30–90%), low (10–30%), and minimal (<10%). For combination regimens, the emetic level is determined by identifying the most emetic agent in the combination and then assessing the relative contribution of the other agents.

Carboplatin AUC <4 is classified as having moderate emetogenicity by NCCN (2018) MASCC/ESMO (2016) and ASCO (2017) Antiemetic Guidelines. An NK1 receptor antagonist, a 5HT3 receptor antagonist in combination with dexamethasone are recommended for primary prophylaxis of carboplatin-induced nausea and vomiting.

Navari R, Aapro M. Antiemetic Prophylaxis for Chemotherapy-Induced Nausea and Vomiting. New England Journal of Medicine. 2016;374(14):1356–1367.
https://www.nejm.org/doi/full/10.1056/NEJMra1515442

7. Answer: D

Management of lung cancer involves a multidisciplinary approach from physicians, surgeons, and oncologists. This patient has stage IA non-small cell lung cancer (NSCLC). It is designated 'A' because the cancer is less than 3 cm. The membranous nephropathy may be related to NSCLC as a paraneoplastic syndrome.

Lobectomy is the gold standard treatment approach for patients with stage IA NSCLC with no medical contraindications. For patients with stage I NSCLC who are high-risk candidates for surgery, sublobar resections or other minimally invasive techniques may be considered over no therapy. Similarly, stereotactic body radiation therapy (SBRT) is a valid alternative to inoperable early stage peripheral NSCLC. The use of adjuvant radiotherapy or chemotherapy for completely resected stage I NSCLC has been found to be detrimental and is not recommended. The use of tyrosine kinase inhibitors, erlotinib, has proven benefit in patients harbouring EGFR mutation tumours and is not the standard treatment in the adjuvant setting. Patient should receive periodic surveillance chest imaging to detect recurrent disease or a second primary lung cancer early enough to allow for an intervention which would result in an improved long-term survival.

The use of adjuvant chemotherapy using contemporary platinum-based regimen for stage II NSCLC is recommended and has shown mortality benefit. It has also been noted to increase survival rates for a subset of patients with stage IB NSCLC.

There is no evidence that the presence of paraneoplastic syndrome should alter the management plan for NSCLC. Paraneoplastic syndrome usually improves after the definitive treatment for lung cancer, such as in this case.

Jones G, Baldwin D. Recent advances in the management of lung cancer. Clinical Medicine. 2018;18(Suppl 2):s41–s46.
https://www.ncbi.nlm.nih.gov/pubmed/29700092

McDonald F, De Waele M, Hendriks L, Faivre-Finn C, Dingemans A, Van Schil P. Management of stage I and II nonsmall cell lung cancer. European Respiratory Journal. 2016;49(1):1600764.
https://erj.ersjournals.com/content/49/1/1600764

8. Answer: A

IDH enzymes catalyse isocitrate into alpha-ketoglutarate as part of the citric acid cycle. A mutation in either *IDH1* or *IDH2* results in an accumulation of the oncometabolite, 2-hydroxyglutarate (2-HG). 2-HG can inhibit enzymatic function of many alpha-ketoglutarate dependent dioxygenases, including histone and DNA demethylases, causing widespread changes in histone and DNA methylation and potentially promoting tumorigenesis. Approximately 20% of patients with acute myeloid leukaemia (AML) have an *IDH* mutation and up to 70% of gliomas and 25% of cholangiocarcinomas have an *IDH* mutation. The role of IDH inhibitors is developing and patients with relapsed or refractory AML can be treated with the IDH1 inhibitor ivosidenib.

 Fujii T et al. Targeting isocitrate dehydrogenase (IDH) in cancer. Discovery Medicine. 2016; 21(117):373–80.
http://www.discoverymedicine.com/Takeo-Fujii/2016/05/targeting-isocitrate-dehydrogenase-idh-in-cancer/

9. Answer: B

The most likely diagnosis for this patient is leptomeningeal carcinomatosis. This process involves metastatic disease infiltrating the meninges surrounding the CNS, and is most frequently seen in aggressive haematological malignancies, breast cancer, lung cancer, and melanoma. The clinical presentation can be due to hydrocephalus, cerebral oedema, or nerve root infiltration. The most common symptom is headache, followed by nausea, seizure, and focal neurological deficits, which are attributable to a nerve root infiltration, these are usually sub-acute in onset, and fluctuating.

Diagnosis of leptomeningeal disease can be challenging, but MRI of the brain and spine has a sensitivity of around 75%, with findings of linear meningeal enhancement or as obvious nodules within the meninges. MRI needs to be performed prior to lumbar puncture as leptomeningeal enhancement because of lumbar puncture is a commonly observed phenomenon. CSF cytology has poorer sensitivity but approaches 75% with repeat lumbar puncture. CSF lymphocytosis, high opening pressure, high protein, and low glucose are suggestive, but not particularly sensitive or specific. CT with contrast can usually identify only bulky leptomeningeal nodules.

Prognosis of leptomeningeal carcinomatosis is generally poor, and patients with poor risk disease benefit most from a symptomatic approach – radiotherapy to bulky symptomatic areas and corticosteroids are the most commonly used treatments in this setting. In good risk patients, control of increased intracranial pressure (if present) is the highest priority, often with ventriculoperitoneal (VP) shunting, which unfortunately often precludes further intrathecal cytotoxic chemotherapy. Selecting therapy directed at decreasing disease burden within the CNS depends on histology and mutation status. ALK or EGFR mutated lung cancers can be treated with tyrosine kinase inhibitors, and melanoma may response to combined immunotherapy. Intrathecal chemotherapy may be used (for example high-dose methotrexate) and probably prolongs survival in good risk candidates, although studies are small. Prior to administering intrathecal chemotherapy, some authors recommend identifying areas of poor CSF flow and irradiating them to improve circulation of chemotherapy.

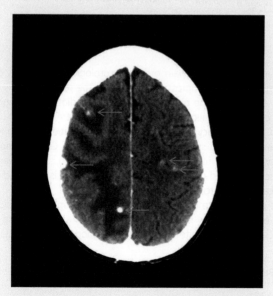

Axial section of computed tomography scan of the brain above the lateral ventricles showing enhancing leptomeningeal nodules (red arrows) in a patient with breast cancer. Note the significant vasogenic oedema within the right hemisphere.

 Freres P, Gennigens C, Martin D, Jerusalem G. Leptomeningeal carcinomatosis from solid tumours: a systematic review of the literature. Belgian Journal of Medical Oncology, 2017; 11(6):259–64.
https://www.ariez.nl/wp-content/uploads/2018/08/259–264.pdf

10. Answer: D

Lynch Syndrome (LS) or hereditary nonpolyposis colorectal cancer (HNPCC), is the most common form of hereditary colorectal cancer predisposition syndrome, representing 2% to 4% of all colorectal neoplasms. LS is an autosomal dominant genetic syndrome that also predisposes individuals to multiple cancer types. The known cancers associated with LS include colorectal, ovarian, endometrial, stomach, urinary tract, hepatobiliary tract, pancreas, small bowel, transitional cell carcinoma of the ureter or renal pelvis, cholangiocarcinoma, sebaceous gland tumours, keratoacanthomas, and brain tumour (usually glioblastoma) but is not limited to these cancers. There is a lifetime risk of colorectal cancer approaching 80%.

Screening for mismatch repair (MMR) deficiency is recommended in Australia to identify LS-related cancers. The mismatch repair genes MLH1, MSH2, MSH6 or PMS2 or a deletion in EPCAM affecting MSH2 function cause the hereditary cancer predisposition of LS.

Samadder N, Baffy N, Giridhar K, Couch F, Riegert-Johnson D. Hereditary Cancer Syndromes—A Primer on Diagnosis and Management, Part 2: Gastrointestinal Cancer Syndromes. Mayo Clinic Proceedings. 2019;94(6):1099–1116.
https://www.ncbi.nlm.nih.gov/pubmed/31171120

11. Answer: A

Investigation of cancer of unknown primary (CUP) is carried out in an attempt to identify particular subgroups of patients who will benefit from a treatment regime targeted towards a specific underlying cancer type. Thorough history taking and examination are the crucial first steps in this process, as clinical information that would otherwise be missed can be integral in making a diagnosis. Depending on the clinical situation, investigations such as CT scan to assess extent of disease and the most favourable biopsy site, and mammography in women are almost always of value; endoscopy/colonoscopy might be appropriate and the role of PET scanning is emerging. Core biopsy of the presumed cancer with analysis of representative immunohistochemical staining is usually required. Most tumour markers are of limited diagnostic utility in diagnosing CUP, but there are exceptions: AFP and β-HCG in midline masses suspicious of extragonadal germ cell tumour as in this case; PSA in widespread sclerotic bony metastases; and also AFP in liver-predominant disease in patients at risk for hepatocellular carcinoma. Also emerging is the role of cancer genome sequencing.

Qaseem A, Usman N, Jayaraj J, Janapala R, Kashif T. Cancer of Unknown Primary: A Review on Clinical Guidelines in the Development and Targeted Management of Patients with the Unknown Primary Site. Cureus. 2019;
https://www.ncbi.nlm.nih.gov/pmc/articles/PMC6820325/

12. Answer: B

This patient presents with potential metastatic spinal cord compression. Back pain or new neurological lower limb deficit in a patient with known bony metastases necessitates rapid exclusion of cord compression by tumour. The reason for this is that the earlier in the course of cord compression that treatment with dexamethasone plus either surgery or radiotherapy is initiated, the better the outcome. Some protocols for investigation of cord compression allow urgent CT imaging where MRI is unavailable, or where there is no known history of bony metastasis. The diagnostic accuracy of different imaging modalities for diagnosing cord compression is well studied – MRI is the superior test, with sensitivity and specificity approaching 100%, CT by comparison has a sensitivity of only 66%, bone scan has very limited sensitivity, and plain films are generally only useful in cases of vertebral collapse, which only occurs in around 22% of cases of metastatic spinal cord compression. Whole spine MRI is preferred as up to a third of patients have a second level of compression anatomically distant to the symptomatic level.

Treatment of metastatic cord compression should comprise of immediate glucocorticoids administration, and consideration of either radiotherapy or surgery followed by radiotherapy - all of which show benefits in relieving pain and improving functional outcomes. Surgery is indicated for those with good functional status, a single site of compression, good prognosis otherwise, with relatively radioresistant tumours.

Lawton A, Lee K, Cheville A, Ferrone M, Rades D, Balboni T et al. Assessment and Management of Patients with Metastatic Spinal Cord Compression: A Multidisciplinary Review. Journal of Clinical Oncology. 2019;37(1):61–71.
https://ascopubs.org/doi/abs/10.1200/JCO.2018.78.1211

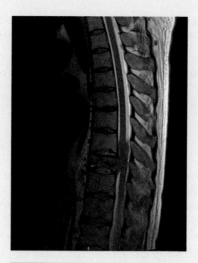
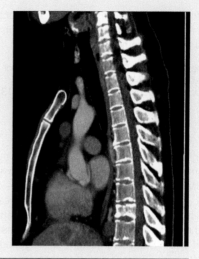

MRI (T2 weighted sagittal image) and CT (mediastinal window, sagittal image) of the same patient two days apart showing the relative insensitivity of CT for detecting cord compression. CT shows the sclerotic metastasis with crush fracture of the 9th thoracic vertebra but misses the displacement of the spinal cord by epidural soft tissue extension of tumour.

13. Answer: C

Transrectal ultrasound (TRUS) biopsy of the prostate uses a sextant approach to identify the prostate, and systematically biopsy areas of the prostate in a representative approach. MRI-guided prostate biopsy is able to first identify lesions within the prostate that are of higher malignant potential and focus the biopsy to these lesions. MRI-guided biopsy has been established in patient groups who remain at high risk after a negative TRUS biopsy and diagnoses clinically relevant apical and anterior tumours that the systematic biopsy can miss. In biopsy naïve patients, MRI-guided biopsy has a higher rate of clinically relevant tumour diagnosis than TRUS biopsy. In contrast, TRUS biopsy picks up more low-grade tumours, the relevance of which is uncertain, and may be patient specific. As a consequence, some systems advocate TRUS biopsy first and MRI-guided biopsy where this has failed, some systems advocate MRI-guided biopsy and acceptance of the lower sensitivity for low-grade tumours.

Lebastchi A, Pinto P. The role of multiparametric MRI in biopsy-naive prostate cancer. Nature Reviews Urology. 2019;16(5):276–277.
https://www.nature.com/articles/s41585-019-0173-7

14. Answer: C

The treatment of advanced lung cancer is a rapidly evolving one. The most frequently encountered driver mutation in non-squamous non-small cell lung cancer (NSCLC) is in the *KRAS* gene, present in up to 25% of cases. Unfortunately, attempts to directly target *KRAS*, for example with tyrosine kinase inhibitors (TKIs), have not been successful to date. It has been hypothesised that *KRAS* mutation may be predictive of response to immune checkpoint inhibitors.

Mutations in *ALK*, *ROS* or *EGFR* predict efficacy to targeted therapy that exceeds traditional platinum-based chemotherapy. Driver mutations in either *ALK* or *ROS* predict response to crizotinib, however resistance mechanisms develop relatively early, and pre-treated patients can be sequentially treated with ceritinib or alectinib. Additionally, alectinib has shown superiority in untreated patients with ALK mutation compared to crizotinib. *EGFR* mutations can also be targeted with TKIs, with studies establishing the role of erlotinib or gefitinib in this setting. The occurrence of secondary *EGFR* mutations leads to disease progression in many patients after around 9 months of treatment. Osimertinib is an irreversible TKI to the most common of these release mutations and has shown good efficacy in treating these patients. Additionally, osimertinib as first-line therapy may improve overall survival compared first-line gefitinib or erlotinib. Other driver mutations in non-squamous NSCLC include *BRAF*, *RET*, *HER2*, *MET* and *NTRK* mutations, and research is ongoing in how to best target these.

Reck M, Rabe K. Precision Diagnosis and Treatment for Advanced Non–Small-Cell Lung Cancer. New England Journal of Medicine. 2017;377(9):849–861.
https://www.nejm.org/doi/full/10.1056/NEJMra1703413

15. Answer: A

There is increasing recognition that obesity plays a role in both the incident risk of cancer and the risk of poor outcomes. For the most part, excess incident risk attributable to obesity is modest, with risk ratios in the range of 1.1–1.8 for most cancers, compared to those with normal BMI. By contrast, adenocarcinoma of the oesophagus and uterine cancer are associated with well over a doubling of relative risk. Evidence for adverse association between obesity and survival is less well established but suggested by reasonably strong data linking lower BMI to longer survival at diagnosis of breast cancer. The mechanisms by which this association is thought to occur is through impacts of obesity on cellular metabolism, in particular the impact of alterations in sex hormone metabolism, insulin, and insulin like growth factor signalling, and adipokine pathways.

Cancer incidence (relative risk RR per 5kg/m² increase):

	MALES	FEMALES
Oesophageal adenocarcinoma	1.52	1.51
Colon cancer	1.24	1.09
Ovarian cancer	–	1.03
Pancreatic adenocarcinoma	–	1.12

Lauby-Secretan B, Scoccianti C, Loomis D, Grosse Y, Bianchini F, Straif K. Body Fatness and Cancer — Viewpoint of the IARC Working Group. New England Journal of Medicine. 2016;375(8):794–798.
https://www.nejm.org/doi/full/10.1056/NEJMsr1606602

Lohman AE, Goodwin PJ, Chlebowski RT, et.al. Association of obesity-related metabolic disruptions with cancer risk and outcome. J Clin Oncol 2016; 34:4249–4255.
https://ascopubs.org/doi/full/10.1200/JCO.2016.69.6187

16. Answer: D

Antibodies blocking the anti-programmed cell death 1 (anti-PD-1) receptor on T cells or its ligand (anti-PD-L1) are increasingly being used in the treatment of cancer. Blockade of this system allows immune destruction of tumour cells. As these ligands are also present in normal tissues to prevent immune-mediated cell death, a number of immune related adverse events (irAEs) are caused by monoclonal antibodies targeting this immune checkpoint. Most trials supporting the benefit of this therapy are open-label and adverse events are clinician reported which gives significant risk of bias expected to, perhaps, underestimate the frequency and severity of irAEs. However, meta-analysis of these trials shows that thyroid disease is the irAE with the highest absolute and relative risk, with an odds ratio of around 7 compared to other active treatment. Hepatitis, pneumonitis, hypophysitis, and colitis have odds ratios of between 2 and 4. In total, more than 10% of patients receiving either nivolumab or ipilimumab will experience grade 3 or 4 toxicity.

Emerging evidence suggests that immune activation symptoms of myalgia, arthralgia, and arthritis may be more common than the typically presented irAEs, but that these are under-reported in early studies. Pneumonitis is the irAE with the highest likelihood of severe morbidity and mortality, but colitis, hepatitis and hypophysitis can all be life-threatening. Myocarditis, although rare, has a very high fatality rate. Combinations of anti-CTLA-4 antibody and an anti-PD-1 antibody increase the rate and severity of irAEs. Theoretically, by conserving PD-2 signalling, anti-PD-L1 drugs (avelumab, atezolizumab) may result in fewer and less severe irAEs (particularly with regards to pneumonitis), but this has not been conclusively demonstrated. Pneumonitis is far more frequently observed in patient with lung cancer. Pre-existing autoimmune disease is the patient related factor that confers the highest the individual risk of irAE.

Treatment of irAEs requires exclusion of alternate diagnosis, and often involves high dose glucocorticoids in the first instance, with a long taper over months. Colitis and pneumonitis can be steroid-refractory, and frequently require infliximab for resolution, and pneumonitis can be responsive to cyclophosphamide. Decision to re-challenge with immunotherapy after irAE should be specific to the individual but is not recommended in many neurological irAEs.

Martins F, Sofiya L, Sykiotis G, Lamine F, Maillard M, Fraga M et al. Adverse effects of immune-checkpoint inhibitors: epidemiology, management and surveillance. Nature Reviews Clinical Oncology. 2019;16(9):563–580.
https://www.nature.com/articles/s41571-019-0218-0

17. Answer: D

PD-L1 plays an important role in inhibiting adaptive immunity through down-regulating T-cell response to antigenic stimuli. This allows for evasion of T-cell induced apoptosis for cells that are presenting foreign antigens. This is particularly important in immune privileged tissues such as placenta, testis, and anterior chamber of the eye, but is present in other tissues as well, which prevents T-cell mediated autoimmunity. In this setting PD-L1 binds to programmed death 1 (PD-1) on antigen naïve T-cells which inhibits their proliferation and differentiation. Additionally, the PD-L1/PD-1 interaction also plays an important role in decreasing the amount of T-cell mediated tissue destruction in chronic infection, which is upregulated as a response to persistent antigen presentation: a process called immune exhaustion. In cancer this process is commandeered by the tumour in order to escape immune-mediated destruction. PD-L1 being up-regulated on tumour cells, which in turn leads to up-regulation of PD-1 on tumour infiltrating T-cells, leading to persistent immune evasion. Additionally, PD-1 expression on T-cells is also regulated by the hypoxia-inducible factor-1α, suggesting interplay between angiogenesis and immune evasion.Given this interaction in cancer, anti-PD-1 and anti-PD-L1 antibodies are useful therapy in a number of cancers. However, immune side-effects, while uncommon, can be very serious, and include immune-mediated thyroid disease, colitis, pneumonitis, and hypophysitis.

Kythreotou A, Siddique A, Mauri F, Bower M, Pinato D. PD-L1. Journal of Clinical Pathology. 2017;71(3):189–194.
https://jcp.bmj.com/content/71/3/189

18. Answer: B

Prostate cancer is the most commonly diagnosed cancer among males in Australia. The following factors may raise a man's risk of developing prostate cancer:

- *Age*. The risk of prostate cancer increases with age, especially after age 50. More than 80% of prostate cancers are diagnosed in men age 65 or older.
- *Ethnicity*. Black men have a higher risk of prostate cancer than white Caucasian men. They are also more likely to develop prostate cancer at an earlier age and to have more aggressive tumours.
- *Family history*. Prostate cancer may be familial in approximately 20% of cases. Familial prostate cancer develops as a result of a combination of shared genes and shared environmental or lifestyle factors.
- *BRCA1 and/or BRCA2 genes*. This mutation is the most commonly associated with an increased risk of breast and ovarian cancers in women. However, men with this mutation also have an increased risk of developing breast cancer and a more aggressive form of prostate cancer. Mutations in the *BRCA1* and *BRCA2* genes are thought to cause only a small percentage of familial prostate cancers. Men who have *BRCA1* or *BRCA2* mutations should consider screening for prostate cancer at an earlier age.
- *Smoking*. Smoking may have an effect on both the risk of developing prostate cancer and its prognosis once a diagnosis is established.

However, the relationship between prostatitis and prostate cancer remains unclear. The available data from case-control studies, cohort studies, and meta-analyses suggest a significant but modest increase (approximately 1.5- to 2-fold) in the risk of prostate cancer in men with prostatitis, but the data is generally of a low quality. A prior vasectomy does not increase the risk of prostate cancer. There is also no evidence that benign prostatic hyperplasia is associated with a higher risk of prostate cancer.

Attard G, Parker C, Eeles R, Schröder F, Tomlins S, Tannock I et al. Prostate cancer. The Lancet. 2016;387(10013):70–82.
https://www.thelancet.com/journals/lancet/article/PIIS0140-6736(14)61947-4/fulltext

19. Answer: D

It is important to rule out prostate cancer in this patient. However, this is complicated by the MRI result as well as his significant co-morbidities.

Prostate MRI has become an increasingly common adjunctive procedure in the detection of prostate cancer. It is the most commonly used in patients with an increasing PSA and/or previously negative biopsies. MRI lesions are reported through the Prostate Imaging-Reporting and Data System (PIRADS). This system was first established in 2012 and then refined in 2015 and there are several studies that confirm the PIRADS system improves the diagnostic accuracy of MRI. The PIRADS classification is as follows:

PI-RADS classfication (5-point Likert-type scale)	
PI-RADS 1	Very low (clinically significant cancer is highly unlikely to be present)
PI-RADS 2	Low (clinically significant cancer is unlikely to be present)
PI-RADS 3	Intermediate (the presence of clinically significant cancer is equivocal)
PI-RADS 4	High (clinically significant cancer is likely to be present)
PI-RADS 5	Very high (clinically significant cancer is highly likely to be present)

In the PIRADS system, clinically significant cancer is defined as Gleason score ≥7 (including 3 + 4 with prominent but not predominant Gleason 4 component), and/or volume ≥0.5 cc, and/or extra prostatic extension. Studies demonstrate that the percentage of men with clinically significant cancer was highest among participants with a PI-RADS version 2 score of 5 (83%), followed by those with a score of 4 (60%) and those with a score of 3 (12%). Conversely, the percentage of men without cancer was highest among participants with a PI-RADS version2 score of 3 (67%), followed by those with a score of 4 (31%) and those with a score of 5 (6%). As such the scoring system allows greater identification of clinically significant cancers whilst also reducing the rate of diagnosis of clinically insignificant cancers, hence reducing overtreatment rates.

MRI also enhances the accuracy of prostate biopsies. Ultrasound guided systematic biopsies miss approximately 21–28% of prostate cancer and under-grade 14–17%.

This patient's significant co-morbidities and PIRADS score make biopsies an inappropriate choice. He is not fit enough to undergo biopsies and his PIRADS score suggests clinically significant cancer is unlikely to be present. A DRE and a prostate ultrasound will provide no further information. The MRI has already located and classified the lesion. Hence, surveillance PSA testing is the most appropriate option as it will monitor his disease progression and, should there be a significant change, allow appropriate referral for treatment.

Litwin MS. The diagnosis and treatment of prostate cancer: A Review. JAMA. 2017;317(24):2532–2542.
https://www.ncbi.nlm.nih.gov/pubmed/28655021

20. Answer: A

Radiotherapy is used to treat cancers and can be used alone or in combination with chemotherapy, surgery, or both. Palliative radiotherapy is often used to reduce pain or mass effect from primary tumours or metastases such as spinal cord compression. Radiation can be delivered from outside the patient, known as external-beam radiation therapy (EBRT), or by implanting radioactive sources in cavities or tissues (brachytherapy), or through systemic administration of radiopharmaceutical agents.

Clinical trials demonstrated that concurrent use of systemic chemotherapy and radiotherapy can increase local control and, in some situations, survival. Combined chemotherapy and radiotherapy have also provided an opportunity to preserve organs that otherwise would have been surgically removed, such as the larynx and bladder. Chemotherapeutic agents act as radiosensitisers, causing potential damage by forming DNA adducts and cell cycle arrest in G2 phase. The addition of chemotherapy has increased the risk or severity of treatment side effects, such as dermatitis, diarrhoea, and haematologic toxicity.

Preclinical studies have suggested that localised irradiation has immunomodulatory effects that may enhance tumour recognition. There is evidence that radiotherapy as a complement to immunotherapy increases the efficacy. More recently, it was observed that delivery of radiation in combination with antibodies against cytotoxic T-lymphocyte–associated antigen 4 (CTLA-4) resulted in regression of unirradiated tumours (known as an abscopal response). The underlying mechanisms by which radiotherapy enhances immune recognition and may complement immunotherapy are complex. Radiation induced injury and killing of tumour cells result in immunogenic modulation and immunogenic cell death.

Citrin D. Recent Developments in Radiotherapy. New England Journal of Medicine. 2017;377(11):1065–1075.
https://www.nejm.org/doi/10.1056/NEJMra1608986

21. Answer: A

Accurately tracking tumour position is critically important when maximisings radiation dose to the tumour and limiting normal tissue exposure. In certain locations in the body such as the lungs, stomach, and liver, tumours can move as the patient breathes. In the past, this movement has confounded the ability to precisely map the tumour location and to accurately deliver radiation therapy.

Gating is a system that tracks a patient's normal respiratory cycle with an infrared camera and chest/abdomen marker. The system is coordinated to only deliver radiation when the tumour is in the treatment field. This is to prevent unnecessary radiation exposure to normal structures. Lung cancer lesions move with respiration especially in patient with severe COPD. If this variation is great, four dimensional CT can be used to obtain a series of CT scans at different phases of the respiratory cycle. The information can help define the motion of the tumour, which can then be targeted with respiratory gating. This involves tracking the patient's respiratory cycle, commonly using surface markers and delivering treatment at specific phases of the cycle.

Ahmad S, Duke S, Jena R, Williams M, Burnet N. Advances in radiotherapy. BMJ. 2012;345(dec04 1): e7765–e7765. https://www.bmj.com/content/345/bmj.e7765

22. Answer: C

Ovarian cancer is the fourth commonest cause of female cancer death in the developed world. Primary cancers include epithelial ovarian carcinoma (70% of all ovarian cancers) which is the commonest cause of gynaecological cancer-associated death and mostly originate from the fallopian tubes. Epidemiological studies have shown that the risk of ovarian cancer is reduced by states of anovulation, such as pregnancy or the use of oral contraception; or through tubal ligation-reduced reflux of menstrual products onto the ovary.

Parity is an important risk factor. Multiple pregnancies offer an increasingly protective effect. The risk for epithelial ovarian cancer is increased in women who have not had children and those with early menarche or late menopause. Women who have been pregnant have a 50% decreased risk for ovarian cancer compared with nulliparous women. Oral contraceptive use significantly decreases the risk for ovarian cancer. Family history plays an important role in the risk of developing ovarian cancer. The lifetime risk for developing ovarian cancer is 1.6% in the general population. This is 7% when two relatives are affected. 5–10% of cases of ovarian cancer occur in an individual with a family history of the disease. Hereditary epithelial ovarian cancer occurs at a younger age (approximately 10 years younger) than nonhereditary epithelial ovarian cancer, but the prognosis may be somewhat better. Supraphysiological ovarian stimulation for treating infertility has been implicated, but not proven, to increase the risk of ovarian cancers.

Success in screening for ovarian cancer requires sufficiently sensitive and specific test to detect curable cancer. Attempts to screen the general population with measurement of serum CA-125 concentration, transvaginal ultrasound, or both have not yet provided convincing evidence that early-stage, curable ovarian cancer can be detected in sufficient numbers, without an excessive number of non-malignant lesions precipitating unnecessary surgery. Unlike cervical cancer, ovarian cancer does not have a detectable pre-invasive phase. However, women at very high risk of developing ovarian cancer (e.g. those with deleterious germline BRCA mutations) in whom the risk of developing ovarian cancer is 55–60%, may consider annual pelvic ultrasound screening and risk-reducing salpingo-oophorectomy.

Jayson G, Kohn E, Kitchener H, Ledermann J. Ovarian cancer. The Lancet. 2014;384(9951):1376–1388. https://www.thelancet.com/journals/lancet/article/PIIS0140-6736(13)62146-7/fulltext

23. Answer: B

This patient is at high risk of developing tumour lysis syndrome (TLS) which is a constellation of metabolic abnormalities resulting from either spontaneous or chemotherapy-induced tumour cell death. It is the most commonly seen in patients with non-Hodgkin's lymphoma (NHL), particularly Burkitt-type lymphoma, and other haematologic malignancies, such as acute lymphocytic leukaemia (ALL) and acute myeloid leukaemia (AML). TLS has also been described with solid malignancies especially with large tumour burden and metastatic disease. The characteristic findings include hyperuricemia, hyperkalaemia, hyperphosphataemia, and hypocalcaemia. These electrolyte and metabolic disturbances can progress to toxic effects, including renal failure, cardiac arrhythmias, seizures, and death due to multi-organ failure.

Laboratory TLS (LTLS) is defined as two or more of the following abnormalities within 3 days before or 7 days after the initiation of chemotherapy: 1) 25% decrease from baseline in serum calcium, and/or 2) 25% increase from baseline in the serum urate, potassium, or phosphorous. Clinical TLS (CTLS) is confirmed when LTLS is accompanied by one or more clinical manifestations such as cardiac arrhythmia, death, seizure, or AKI with an elevated serum creatinine, 1.5 times above the upper limit of normal. Additionally, this definition of CTLS assumes that the clinical manifestations are not caused directly by the therapeutic agent and patient has received volume expansion and prophylaxis with a hypouricaemic agent.

Prevention of TLS begins with recognition of risk factors and close laboratory and clinical monitoring. A high-dose intravenous crystalloid fluid (IVT) up to 3 L/day is recommended for all patients and is ***essential*** for those with higher TLS risk. The target urine output is 2 mL/kg/h. Urine alkalinisation (increasing urine pH from 5 to 7) can increase the solubility of uric acid by 10-fold. However, urinary alkalinisation decreases calcium–phosphate solubility, thereby exacerbating its precipitation and deposition. Furthermore, if urinary alkalinisation results in rising serum pH, free calcium may bind albumin more avidly and further exacerbate hypocalcaemia. Thus, urinary alkalinisation is **NOT** recommended in the prevention/management of TLS.

Allopurinol is converted in vivo to oxypurinol and as a xanthine analogue acts as a competitive inhibitor of xanthine oxidase and blocks the conversion of purines to uric acid. This prevents hyperuricaemia but does not treat pre-existing hyperuricaemia. Furthermore, because oxypurinol also inhibits the conversion of xanthine to uric acid, serum and urine xanthine levels may rise and precipitate xanthine crystal deposition in the renal tubules and xanthine-induced obstructive nephropathy. Allopurinol is recommended for prophylaxis in patients with low and intermediate risk of developing TLS. Febuxostat is a novel xanthine oxidase inhibitor lacking the hypersensitivity profile of allopurinol. Because it is metaboliseds to inactive metabolites by the liver, adjustment for reduced GFR is not necessary. It has been used as an alternative to allopurinol in TLS prophylaxis for patients with allopurinol hypersensitivity or severe renal dysfunction. However, recent data have shown its chronic usage is associated with increased cardiovascular and all-cause mortality. Rasburicase catalyses the conversion of uric acid to allantoin, carbon dioxide, and hydrogen peroxide. Allantoin is 10-fold more soluble than uric acid and is readily excreted. Rasburicase should be used for prophylaxis in patients at high risk of developing TLS. Rasburicase does not require dosing adjustment for GFR and is not known to have any known clinically relevant drug–drug interactions. Patients with glucose 6-phosphate dehydrogenase (G6PD) deficiency can develop significant methemoglobinaemia and haemolysis due to oxidative stress triggered by hydrogen peroxide. Accordingly, patients should have G6PD status tested prior to starting rasburicase.

G6PD deficiency is the most common enzyme deficiency in humans, affecting 400 million people worldwide. It has a high prevalence in African, Asian, and Mediterranean descent. It is inherited as an X-linked recessive disorder. G6PD deficiency is polymorphic, with more than 300 variants.

Many patients with G6PD deficiency are asymptomatic. G6PD deficiency can present as neonatal hyperbilirubinaemia. Patients with this disorder can experience episodes of brisk haemolysis after ingesting fava beans or being exposed to certain infections or drugs (see below). Less commonly, they may have chronic haemolysis. Most patients with G6PD deficiency do not need treatment. However, they should be educated to avoid drugs and chemicals that can cause oxidant stress, notably:

1. Oxidant drugs: antimalarial drugs primaquine, chloroquine, pamaquine, and pentaquine
2. Nalidixic acid, ciprofloxacin, niridazole, norfloxacin, chloramphenicol, phenazopyridine, and vitamin K analogues
3. Sulfonamides: sulfanilamide, sulfamethoxypyridazine, sulfacetamide, sulfadimidine, sulfapyridine, sulfamerazine, and sulfamethoxazole
4. NSAIDs and nitrofurantoin

Edean A, Shirali A. Tumor lysis syndrome [Internet]. Asn-online.org. 2020 [cited 7 May 2020]. Available from: https://www.asn-online.org/education/distancelearning/curricula/onco/Chapter4.pdf

24. Answer: B

Tumour markers play an important role in all aspects of cancer care including screening, early detection, diagnostic confirmation, prognosis, prediction of therapeutic response, and monitoring disease and recurrence.

Tumour markers are substances/molecules that are present in, or produced by, a tumour itself or produced by host in response to a tumour (altered quantitatively or qualitatively in precancerous or cancerous conditions), which can be used to differentiate a tumour from normal tissue, or to determine the presence of a tumour based on measurements in blood, body fluid or secretions.

In clinical practice, tumour marker usually refers to a molecule that can be detected in plasma or other body fluids. Tumour markers include a variety of substances such as cell surface antigens and glycoproteins, cytoplasmic proteins, enzymes, hormones, metabolites, oncofetal antigens, receptors, oncogenes and their products (mutations/translations).

Genetic alteration in a tumour cell affects directly or indirectly the gene expression pattern of the tumour cell or the surrounding tissue. These genetic alterations can be reflected at various levels, from viral genomic incorporation to genetic defects, forming the molecular basis of tumour markers.

The important characteristics of an ideal tumour marker are:
- Highly specific to a given tumour type
- Provide a lead-time over clinical diagnosis

- High sensitivity and specificity for cancerous growth
- Correlate reliably with the tumour burden
- Accurately reflect any tumour progression or regression
- Short half-life allowing frequent serial measurements
- The test used for detection should be cheap and reliable.

In reality, a perfect tumour marker does not exist.

Screening a large population for occult tumours by using a tumour marker and thereby enabling early therapeutic intervention is not currently advisable because no tumour marker is 100% specific, and many tumour markers may be elevated in benign conditions. The use of a particular tumour marker may change depending upon the clinical scenario, ranging from initial presentation to differential diagnosis to recurrence. Tumour markers cannot be used as primary modalities for the diagnosis of cancer because of the lack of sufficiently high specificity and sensitivity. It should not be used as 'fishing test' in the investigation of pyrexia of unknown origin (PUO) or weight lost. Their current main utility is to support the diagnosis or in follow-up of patients being treated for malignancy. Tumour marker levels, in certain situations, reflect tumour burden in the body and hence can be used in staging, prognostication, or prediction of response to therapy. Monitoring disease, perhaps, constitutes the most common clinical use of serum tumour markers. Multiple tumour markers may associate with individual malignancy; vice versa, individual tumour markers may be associated with various malignancies. Thus, the use of multiple markers based on the combination pattern for the selected malignancy will improve sensitivity and specificity of the detection.

Lindblom A. Regular review: Tumour markers in malignancies. BMJ. 2000;320(7232):424–427.
https://www.bmj.com/content/320/7232/424

25. Answer: G

Ifosfamide is an alkylating agent often used in sarcoma and lymphoma. It is commonly associated with encephalopathy, with a prevalence of between 10–30%. The most commonly accepted mechanism for this complication is through CNS accumulation of chloracetaldehyde, one of its metabolites. Cessation of the drug and correction of metabolic abnormalities are the most important steps in treatment; however, methylene blue is commonly used as treatment. Acute encephalopathy is exceedingly rare and only seen with high dose methotrexate.

Ajithkumar T, Parkinson C, Shamshad F, Murray P. Ifosfamide Encephalopathy. Clinical Oncology. 2007;19(2):108–114.
https://www.clinicaloncologyonline.net/article/S0936–6555(06)00417-1/fulltext

26. Answer: C

Cardiac toxicity due to fluorouracil is the most commonly experienced as anginal chest pain during infusion or bolus administration and represents myocardial ischaemia with or without necrosis. The most likely mechanism for this is through coronary vasospasm, although metabolites of the fluorouracil are cardiotoxic, and may directly contribute to cardiac ischaemia. Immediate management is cessation of the drug, and further investigations for underlying coronary disease are reasonable where the fluorouracil is felt critical to the patient's management. If symptomatic coronary disease is found and treated angiographically in this context, re-challenge is reasonable, if no coronary disease is found, re-challenge is only likely to cause further myocardial damage.

Kanduri J, More L, Godishala A, Asnani A. Fluoropyrimidine-Associated Cardiotoxicity. Cardiology Clinics. 2019; 37(4):399–405.
https://www.sciencedirect.com/science/article/abs/pii/S0733865119300530?via%3Dihub

27. Answer: B

Peripheral neuropathy is common in chemotherapeutic agents, and most common in platinum containing agents. Oxaliplatin causes symptoms of peripheral neuropathy acutely in over 80% of cases, and severity of acute neuropathic symptoms correlates with chronic neuropathy. The mechanism of acute symptoms is thought to be through neuronal disinhibition as a result of the effects on voltage-gated calcium-dependant sodium channels. Cisplatin and carboplatin also cause neuropathy but are less likely to cause acute symptoms. Chronic sensory neuropathy, which has profound impacts on quality of life, is common with both cisplatin and oxaliplatin, and is dose dependent. Consequently, regular monitoring of peripheral nerve function is of critical importance during treatment. Chronic neuropathy is most likely due to long term effects of platinum deposition in dorsal root ganglion cells. Cisplatin is the most ototoxic of the platinum-based chemotherapeutic agents. Taxanes, thalidomide, eribulin, nitrosureas, and vinca alkaloids are also associated with neuropathy.

Ewertz M, Qvortrup C, Eckhoff L. Chemotherapy-induced peripheral neuropathy in patients treated with taxanes and platinum derivatives. Acta Oncologica. 2015;54(5):587–591.
https://www.tandfonline.com/doi/full/10.3109/0284186X.2014.995775

28. Answer: H

Methotrexate causes a range of neurotoxicities including those already mentioned in previous answers, but intrathecal administration also brings a range of potential complications. Aseptic meningitis, with headache, nuchal rigidity, fever, and vomiting occurs in around 10%, although microfiltration of methotrexate has decreased its incidence. It can be distinguished from iatrogenic bacterial meningitis by the history; typically occurring within two to four hours of injection as opposed to days for bacterial aetiology. Corticosteroids may be useful for management or prevention. Intrathecal methotrexate can also cause encephalopathy, myelopathy, radiculopathy, non-cardiogenic pulmonary oedema, and seizures.

Valcovici M, Andrica F, Serban C, Dragan S. Cardiotoxicity of anthracycline therapy: current perspectives. Archives of Medical Science. 2016; 2:428–435.
https://www.archivesofmedicalscience.com/Cardiotoxicity-of-anthracycline-therapy-current-perspectives,53483,0,2.html

29. Answer: D

Prior to protocol development involving aggressive pre-hydration, cisplatin caused AKI in more than 50% of cases. As nephrotoxicity is dose-dependent and relative to pre-existing renal dysfunction, dose-adjustment decreases likelihood of AKI. As a result, significant AKI probably now only occurs in around 5% of patients on cisplatin chemotherapy – estimates differ based on protocols, dose exposure and patient factors. Other agents implicated include pemetrexed, methotrexate, anthracyclines, and gemcitabine which can cause a thrombotic microangiopathy.

Crona D, Faso A, Nishijima T, McGraw K, Galsky M, Milowsky M. A Systematic Review of Strategies to Prevent Cisplatin-Induced Nephrotoxicity. The Oncologist. 2017;22(5):609–619.
https://theoncologist.onlinelibrary.wiley.com/doi/full/10.1634/theoncologist.2016-0319

30. Answer: A

Anthracycline-related late cardiomyopathy is a major problem associated with cancer survivorship, with clinical diagnosis of heart failure often occurring many years after treatment for cancer. Risk is higher in females, children and the elderly – risk also greater with higher dosage, pre-existing heart failure and co-administration of other cardiotoxic medications such as taxanes, cyclophosphamide, and trastuzumab. Decreasing lifetime anthracycline exposure, and the use of liposomal preparations seem to reduce risk of cardiomyopathy. The use of cardioprotective medications such as beta-blockers, aldosterone antagonists, and ACE inhibitors as prophylaxis has shown early promise in surrogate markers, but the long lag-time for developing symptomatic late cardiomyopathy means that meaningful clinical end-points have not been achieved in clinical trials.

Valcovici M, Andrica F, Serban C, Dragan S. Cardiotoxicity of anthracycline therapy: current perspectives. Archives of Medical Science. 2016; 2:428–435.
https://www.termedia.pl/Cardiotoxicity-of-anthracycline-therapy-current-perspectives,19,27374,1,1.html

31. Answer: D

Palbociclib is an inhibitor of cyclin-dependent kinases CDK4 and CDK6, which have an important role in regulation of the cell cycle. In combination with an aromatase inhibitor, palbociclib has been shown to have progression-free survival benefit in first line therapy for ER positive, HER2 negative, post-menopausal advanced breast cancer versus aromatase inhibitor alone, at the expense of higher haematologic toxicity. Similar benefits are seen in combination with fulvestrant for disease progressive on initial hormone therapy. Another CDK4/6 inhibitor, ribociclib or abemiciclib, has also been shown to have similar efficacy.

 Finn R, Martin M, Rugo H, Jones S, Im S, Gelmon K et al. Palbociclib and Letrozole in Advanced Breast Cancer. New England Journal of Medicine. 2016;375(20):1925–1936.
https://www.nejm.org/doi/full/10.1056/NEJMoa1607303

32. Answer: G

Dasatinib is a multikinase inhibitor with main actions against BCR-Abl –the dominant protein product of the Philadelphia chromosome, and the Src kinase family. It is approved for the treatment of patients with chronic myeloid leukaemia (CML) in chronic, accelerated, or blast phase with resistance or intolerance to imatinib, or for treatment-naïve chronic phase CML, or for those with Philadelphia chromosome-positive acute lymphoblastic leukaemia who are intolerant or resistant to other treatment.

 Breccia M, Salaroli A, Molica M, Alimena G. Systematic review of dasatinib in chronic myeloid leukemia. OncoTargets and Therapy. 2013;2013(6):257–65.
https://www.dovepress.com/systematic-review-of-dasatinib-in-chronic-myeloid-leukemia-peer-reviewed-article-OTT

33. Answer: E

Osimertinib is a third generation tyrosine kinase inhibitor (TKI) indicated in the treatment of EGFR mutation positive non-small cell lung cancer. Osimertinib selectively inhibits both the sensitising and T790M resistance mutations in EGFR in this setting and has shown efficacy in TKI pre-treated patients whose cancer harbours this mutation. Additionally, in comparison to standard TKI in the first line setting, osimertinib is superior to first generation TKIs with regard to progression-free survival, with overall survival data awaited. Other EGFR TKIs include gefitinib, erlotinib, and afatinib.

 Soria J, Ohe Y, Vansteenkiste J, Reungwetwattana T, Chewaskulyong B, Lee K et al. Osimertinib in Untreated EGFR-Mutated Advanced Non–Small-Cell Lung Cancer. New England Journal of Medicine. 2018;378(2):113–125.
https://www.nejm.org/doi/full/10.1056/NEJMoa1713137

34. Answer: C

Brigatinib is a next generation anaplastic lymphoma kinase (ALK) inhibitor with a broad range of activities both against ALK and ROS mutations. Brigatinib has increased progression free survival in a trial comparing its efficacy to crizotinib, a first generation ALK inhibitor. Given its CNS penetration, brigatinib performed particularly well in patients with intracranial metastases. Alectinib and ceritinib are other examples of ALK inhibitors.

 Camidge D, Kim H, Ahn M, Yang J, Han J, Lee J et al. Brigatinib versus Crizotinib in ALK-Positive Non–Small-Cell Lung Cancer. New England Journal of Medicine. 2018;379(21):2027–2039.
https://www.nejm.org/doi/full/10.1056/NEJMoa1810171

35. Answer: F

Dabrafenib is a BRAF kinase inhibitor that has shown good outcomes compared with dacarbazine as initial therapy, for BRAF mutated melanoma. However, dabrafenib in combination with a MEK inhibitor as first-line therapy has been shown to be even more efficacious. Vemurafenib is another BRAF inhibitor, which also has better results combined with a MEK inhibitor.

 Hauschild A, Grob J, Demidov L, Jouary T, Gutzmer R, Millward M et al. Dabrafenib in BRAF-mutated metastatic melanoma: a multicentre, open-label, phase 3 randomised controlled trial. The Lancet. 2012;380(9839):358–365.
https://www.thelancet.com/journals/lancet/article/PIIS0140-6736(12)60868-X/fulltext

36. Answer: A

Pazopanib is a multi-kinase inhibitor with actions against multiple angiogenic pathways, as well as the c-KIT pathway. Sunitinib and pazopanib are both reasonable first line options in clear cell variant renal cell carcinoma, with either good risk disease, or in intermediate/poor risk disease where immunotherapy is unavailable. In a head-to-head trial there was little difference between the two agents in primary outcomes, but better quality of life with pazopanib. Cabozatinib has not been compared with pazopanib but seems to have better progression-free survival compared to sunitinib, without a benefit on overall survival. Pazopanib may also be used in soft tissue sarcoma.

 Motzer R, Hutson T, Cella D, Reeves J, Hawkins R, Guo J et al. Pazopanib versus Sunitinib in Metastatic Renal-Cell Carcinoma. New England Journal of Medicine. 2013;369(8):722–731.
https://www.nejm.org/doi/full/10.1056/NEJMoa1303989

37. Answer: H

Lapatinib inhibits both EGFR and HER2 and is indicated in HER2 positive breast cancer as second- or third-line treatment in combination with either trastuzumab or capecitabine. With multiple active agents in HER2 positive disease, selecting agents can become complicated, and the long prognosis with breast cancer means that multiple agents are likely to be used over the span of the disease process. With HER2 positive disease, continuing trastuzumab despite progression on trastuzumab seems reasonable, whereas other agents are likely to require cessation on progression of disease.

 Geyer C, Forster J, Lindquist D, Chan S, Romieu C, Pienkowski T et al. Lapatinib plus Capecitabine for HER2-Positive Advanced Breast Cancer. New England Journal of Medicine. 2006;355(26):2733–2743.
https://www.nejm.org/doi/full/10.1056/NEJMoa064320

38. Answer: B

Regorafenib is an anti-angiogenic TKI with most activity on VEGF pathways. It is the only systemic treatment that has been shown to provide survival benefit in hepatocellular carcinoma among patients who progressed on sorafenib first line treatment. Further studies are under way with regorafenib in combination with other systemic or immunotherapy agents. Regorafenib is also used to manage metastatic colorectal cancer or gastrointestinal stromal tumours (GIST).

 Bruix J, Qin S, Merle P, Granito A, Huang Y, Bodoky G et al. Regorafenib for patients with hepatocellular carcinoma who progressed on sorafenib treatment (RESORCE): a randomised, double-blind, placebo-controlled, phase 3 trial. The Lancet. 2017;389(10064):56–66.
https://www.thelancet.com/journals/lancet/article/PIIS0140-6736(16)32453-9/fulltext

14 Mental Health

Questions

Answers can be found in the Mental Health Answers section at the end of this chapter.

1. A 43-year-old woman is taken to the emergency department by her ex-husband when he finds that she had taken 26 temazepam tablets and 15 paracetamol tablets. She and her husband recently separated. She has a past medical history of schizophrenia but is not been on any treatment for the past 10 years, and has a recent diagnosis of thyroid cancer. Her father died of suicide. She is drowsy but vital signs are stable. This is her first presentation of this nature.

Which one of the following is most strongly associated with completed suicide?
- **A.** Family history of suicide.
- **B.** Female sex.
- **C.** History of schizophrenia.
- **D.** Recent cancer diagnosis.

2. A 35-year-old woman (G1P0) is 8-weeks pregnant. She has a medical history of bipolar disorder for 8 years and her mood disorder has been stable on valproate and lithium. Her other regular medications include folic acid 5 mg daily and iron tablet 1 tablet daily.

Which one of the following statements is true in terms of the treatment of bipolar disease during pregnancy?
- **A.** Carbamazepine is the preferred option during pregnancy for patients with severe bipolar disorder.
- **B.** Lithium is the preferred mood stabiliser for pregnant women in the second trimester with severe bipolar disorder.
- **C.** Valproate can be safely used in women planning for pregnancy.
- **D.** Valproate should be continued since there is no evidence to suggest it causes foetal congenital abnormality.

3. A 27-year-old woman is admitted to the Acute Medical Unit because of community acquired pneumonia and treated with intravenous penicillin and azithromycin. She is known to have schizophrenia which is treated with clozapine 100 mg in the morning and 300 mg at night for the last 12 months and is on monthly monitoring. The home team has held the clozapine for 5 days because of the concern of sepsis. Her pneumonia is improving, WBC is normal, but her symptoms of schizophrenia are worsening. After discussion with the on-call psychiatric team, it has been decided to resume clozapine.

What is the appropriate action at this point?
- **A.** Resume clozapine 200 mg twice a day.
- **B.** Give a loading dose of 600 mg clozapine and then resume previous dose.
- **C.** Start on clozapine 12.5 mg daily and titrate dose up.
- **D.** Start on clozapine 100 mg daily and titrate dose up.

4. A 35-year-old school teacher is brought to emergency department by her partner with an ongoing history of episodes of torticollis, blepharospasm, right hand weakness, and loss of sensation in her left foot. She experiences an episode at least once a month. Examination findings are non-contributory. An extensive workup including MRI of the head was unremarkable. She has not attended work in the past 6 months because of these symptoms and her partner is concerned. She denies any mood disturbance or psychotic symptoms.

What is the most likely diagnosis?
- **A.** Conversion disorder.
- **B.** Factitious disorder.
- **C.** Illness anxiety disorder.
- **D.** Multiple sclerosis.

How to Pass the FRACP Written Examination, First Edition. Jonathan Gleadle, Jordan Li, Danielle Wu, and Paul Kleinig.
© 2022 John Wiley & Sons Ltd. Published 2022 by John Wiley & Sons Ltd.

5. Which of the following statements is correct regarding depression in older adults?
   A. Clinical response rates with antidepressant are similar to those in younger adults.
   B. Cognitive behavioural therapy is not an effective treatment.
   C. Lithium augmentation is not effective in older adults.
   D. Two-year mortality rates are less than 10%.

6. A 25-year-old man has recently separated from his girlfriend and complains of symptoms of depressed mood. His mother has brought him to the emergency department. On further questioning, he can work, and reports no symptoms of sleep disturbance, anhedonia, hopelessness, lack of energy, poor concentration, appetite change, psychomotor retardation, or thoughts of harming himself or other people. His medical history includes poorly controlled type 1 diabetes, hypertension, and previous anxiety disorder. There are no concerns from the family regarding his social interactions. What is the appropriate first-line treatment for his depression?
   A. Duloxetine.
   B. Mirtazapine.
   C. Psychotherapy.
   D. Sertraline.

7. Which of the following statement best describes the clinical utility of electroconvulsive therapy (ECT) in the treatment of catatonia?
   A. ECT is a useful treatment for catatonia regardless of the cause.
   B. ECT is only effective if the catatonia is in the context of major depression, as opposed to other psychiatric or medical causes.
   C. ECT is reserved for treatment of catatonia only when the absorption of psychotropic medications is impaired.
   D. ECT should only be considered if an extensive trial of multiple medications for the underlying psychiatric illness has been undertaken.

8. An over-worked physician in the emergency department during the COVID-19 pandemic presents after self-harm, having consumed a bottle of vodka and a variety of 'pain killing' tablets.
   Which one of the following suggests the greatest risk for future suicide in this doctor?
   A. Alcohol misuse.
   B. Choice of medications taken.
   C. Combination of medications taken.
   D. Female sex.

9. Which of the following treatments for neuroleptic malignant syndrome has the highest risk of adverse outcomes in the case of misdiagnosis with serotonin syndrome ?
   A. Amantadine.
   B. Bromocriptine.
   C. Dantrolene.
   D. Lorazepam.

10. A 23-year-old man presents with his parents who report a 5-week history of strange behaviour. Over this period, they report their son has repeatedly voiced the concern that the police are after him, although he is adamant that he has never committed a crime. Over this time, they have also found it more difficult to understand and maintain conversation with him. Upon further questioning, prior to this period, they had noticed that their son was more withdrawn and over the past 6 months, has stopped playing tennis, something which he previously enjoyed; and he has been unable to leave the house over this period, resulting in him losing his job as a painter. On mental state examination, he appears dishevelled and agitated; he struggles to maintain conversation and is fixated on the belief that the police are going to arrest and torture him.
   Based on this scenario, this patient meets the criteria for which diagnosis?
   A. Depression with psychotic features.
   B. Schizoaffective disorder.
   C. Schizophreniform disorder.
   D. Schizophrenia.

11. Which of the following antidepressants poses the greatest risk of a life-threatening adverse event when it is ceased, and a second antidepressant is started immediately?
- **A.** Fluvoxamine.
- **B.** Fluoxetine.
- **C.** Duloxetine.
- **D.** Mirtazapine.

12. A 28-year-old man is brought into the emergency department by his close friend because he has not eaten any food for the past two days. He is known to have major depression but has not been taking medications for the last two weeks due to the COVID-19 lockdown and isolation. His vital signs are normal. He has no other medical history. On examination, he is alert, orientated and appears calm. During the interview, he tells you his very detailed plan to kill his ex-girlfriend's boyfriend. He says that all his problems are caused by the broken-down relationship with his ex-girlfriend. You want to admit him and tell him that you will need to inform the intended victim of his detailed plan. You think there is a significant risk he will act on the threat. He refuses admission and ask you not to contact anyone else at all. He insists that you, as his current treating doctor, have a duty of confidentially. You go out to ask for senior advice. When you return 5 minutes later, he has absconded.
What appropriate action you should take?
- **A.** Contact patient's close friend and ask him to persuade the patient to abandon the plan.
- **B.** Notify patient's psychiatrist and ask him to see the patient as early as possible.
- **C.** Notify the police and the intended victim of your patient's statement.
- **D.** Respect the confidentiality request from your patient and provide him with an antidepressant if he returns to the emergency department.

QUESTIONS (13–20) REFER TO THE FOLLOWING INFORMATION

The following descriptors are used in the framing of psychiatric problems. Match each clinical scenario to the best or most likely descriptor for the phenomenon:
- **A.** Looseness of association.
- **B.** Derealisation.
- **C.** Thought broadcasting.
- **D.** Word salad.
- **E.** Thought blocking.
- **F.** Grandiose delusion.
- **G.** Flight of ideas.
- **H.** Idea of reference.
- **I.** Hallucination.
- **J.** Echolalia.

13. A 32-year-old man reports that he is fearful of being targeted by the police. When asked for evidence of this, he reports that, whilst walking down the street, he saw two policemen talking, and one of them said 'Yes I am' to his colleague, which confirmed his suspicions.

14. While interviewing a patient with severely depressed mood, you note that the individual has very little to say, often repeating words that you have just used over and over.

15. You are interviewing a patient with elevated mood and he reports that he is about to win the lottery. When questioned about this, he reports that he can control all the numbers as they are the second coming of Christ.

16. Categorise the following content of a patient's speech, which is of normal rate and cadence: 'I mean, how can anyone say that the Mormons control it? When I go to the shops there is nothing there that I love. Wednesdays are not often open to me in any event. The other time I went sailing it was grassy.'

17. Categorise the following content of a patient's speech: 'Blagless on a burpday. Smolder, augur, noff. Edgeling have nockins.'

18. You notice that a patient is becoming more and more suspicious of you as the interview progresses. When you comment on this and ask about why this might be the case, the patient reports that 'You don't have to ask me – you already know what I'm thinking.'

19. Categorise the following content of a patient's speech, which flows rapidly: 'There is nothing so satisfying as a good egg. When I go birdwatching, I will always find a rare one. Steak is excellent bloody, 'just scare it with the pan' I say. I sometimes get frightened when I'm looking for gold.'

20. You interview a patient with low mood, and obvious psychomotor retardation. You observe that he sometimes stops mid-sentence for several seconds seemingly unable to articulate his ideas.

QUESTIONS (21–23) REFER TO THE FOLLOWING INFORMATION

Match each of the following antidepressants with their predominant mechanism of action:
- **A.** Inhibition of monoamine oxidase.
- **B.** Inhibition of noradrenaline reuptake.
- **C.** Inhibition of serotonin reuptake.
- **D.** Inhibition of serotonin and noradrenaline reuptake.
- **E.** Monoamine receptor antagonist.
- **F.** N-methyl-D-aspartate receptor antagonist.
- **G.** Noradrenaline receptor agonist.
- **H.** Serotonin receptor agonist.

21. A 65-year-old man is taking **mirtazapine** for depression and weight loss.

22. A 65-year-old woman is taking **duloxetine** for major depression and fibromyalgia.

23. A 60-year-old veteran is taking **phenelzine** for his depression clinically characterised as 'atypical,' 'nonendogenous,' or 'neurotic.'

QUESTIONS (24–29) REFER TO THE FOLLOWING INFORMATION

Match each of the following adverse effects with the psychotropic medication it is most commonly caused by:
- **A.** Carbamazepine.
- **B.** Sertraline.
- **C.** Sodium valproate.
- **D.** Mirtazapine.
- **E.** Lithium.
- **F.** Haloperidol.
- **G.** Olanzapine.
- **H.** Ziprasidone.

24. Obesity.

25. Diabetes insipidus.

26. Delayed ejaculation.

27. QT prolongation.

28. Stevens–Johnson syndrome.

29. Parkinsonism.

Answers

1. Answer: C

Suicide accounts for 1.5% of all deaths, with 80% of suicides occurring in low- and middle-income countries. Epidemiologically, completed suicide rates are highest in older males, while self-harm is highest in young people and women.

Suicide risk factors are often investigated in terms of predisposing and precipitating factors, at both population and at individual levels. Predisposing factors include neuropsychiatric disorders and family history of suicidal behaviour with strong association, with moderate association previous suicide attempt and adverse childhood experiences, and with a weak association socioeconomic deprivation. The strongest predisposing factors include psychiatric disorders including depression, bipolar disorder, schizophrenia spectrum disorders, substance use disorders, epilepsy, and traumatic brain injury, which increase the suicide risk threefold.

Precipitating factors include drug and alcohol misuse with the strongest association, then access to lethal means, life events, and new diagnosis of a terminal or chronic physical illness with a moderate association, and media effects with a weak association. While twin studies suggest the contribution of genetics to suicidal behaviour is 30–50%, associated gene mutations have not been identified.

There are five factors in the approach to a person at risk of suicide: (i) Assess for suicidal thoughts, irrespective of symptoms of a psychiatric disorder. Many tools for assessing suicide risk exist, but often have poor sensitivities and specificities. (ii) Consider predisposing and precipitating factors, including recent life events. (iii) Manage patients at risk of suicide with regular psychotherapy, and pharmacological therapy if symptoms of a psychiatric disorder. (iv) Counsel the suicidal person and their family to ensure a safe environment, including removal of means of suicide. (v) If the person is deemed at high risk of suicide, they should be referred to mental health services.

Fazel S, Runeson B. Suicide. New England Journal of Medicine. 2020;382(3):266–274.
https://www.nejm.org/doi/pdf/10.1056/NEJMra1902944

2. Answer: B

The mainstay of management of manic episodes of bipolar disease is lithium. Lithium provides the benefits of mood stabilisation, prevention of relapses, protection against suicide, reduction of the frequency and severity of relapses of bipolar disorder. Lithium is usually well-tolerated. However, due to lithium's narrow therapeutic index, careful monitoring of lithium level, renal function, thyroid function, serum calcium (including ionised calcium level), PTH level, weight, and ECG changes is important to ensure a patient has the maximum treatment benefit without unwanted side effects. Initially blood tests weekly, monthly, then quarterly may be required to ensure plasma lithium level is within the therapeutic range. Clinicians can refer to the 'Lithiumeter' which provides a practical guide of adjusting lithium dosage in clinical management of bipolar disease. Frequently patients need combinations of medications including antidepressants, mood stabilisers, and second-generation antipsychotics. Valproate can be added in combination with lithium treatment if necessary.

Careful planning prior to pregnancy is important to ensure no relapse of bipolar disorder during pregnancy by referring patients with bipolar disease to the psychiatry team and high-risk pregnancy clinics. Sodium valproate is known to cause congenital malformations and intellectual impairment in children who have been exposed to the medication in utero. Valproate should be avoided in women of child-bearing age for all non-seizure indications and for seizure indications, to consider alternatives. Carbamazepine is also known to increase risk of neural tube defects (e.g. spina bifida) in foetus although the risk is less than that with valproate. Carbamazepine exposure may also cause vitamin K deficiency in the foetus. Lithium has been associated with a small increased risk of foetal cardiac defects. For women with severe bipolar disorder lithium seems to be the safest option amongst different mood stabilisers. Pregnant women should have folic acid supplementation and have high resolution ultrasound to monitor whether a foetal abnormality is present. If mood stabilisers are to be withdrawn, the dose needs to be tapered slowly to avoid relapse of bipolar disorder, peripartum psychosis, suicide, and infanticide.

Malhi G, Outhred T, Morris G, Boyce P, Bryant R, Fitzgerald P et al. Royal Australian and New Zealand College of Psychiatrists clinical practice guidelines for mood disorders: bipolar disorder summary. Medical Journal of Australia. 2018;208(5):219–225.
https://onlinelibrary.wiley.com/doi/10.5694/mja17.00658

3. Answer: C

Clozapine is an atypical antipsychotic of the dibenzodiazepine class and is used for treatment resistant schizophrenia in patients who are unresponsive to, or intolerant of other antipsychotics.

Neutropaenia, agranulocytosis, and myocarditis are the severe adverse effects of clozapine. It is mandatory that all patients on clozapine be registered on to the national database CPMS and attend blood monitoring of WBC and neutrophil count regularly whilst receiving clozapine. Attendance at clozapine clinics is also a requirement for patients receiving this drug. Other side effects include hypotension, sedation, weight gain, exacerbation of diabetes, tachycardia, and neuroleptic malignant syndrome.

For initiation and titration, there is strict protocol (Table 14.1). In most patients, antipsychotic efficacy can be expected between 200–450mg per day. The total daily dose may be divided unevenly after initial titration, with the larger portion at bedtime. The maximum permissible dose of clozapine is 900mg per day. After the maximum therapeutic benefit has been achieved, the minimum effective dose should be used to maintain clinical remission and reduce occurrence of adverse effects.

Table 14.1   Initiation of clozapine

Day	Daily dose (mg)	Day	Daily dose (mg)
1	12.5	8	125
2	25	9	150
3	25	10	150
4	50	11	175
5	50	12	175
6	75	13	175
7	100	14	200

1. Titration above 200 mg per day: increase daily dose in increments of 25–50mg
2. Day 1 Lying and standing BP, temperature, and pulse to be attended 15 minutes prior to the first dose, 15 minutes after dose and then hourly for six hours
3. Day 7 FBE, Troponins, ECG
4. Day 14 FBE, Troponins, ECG

Other ongoing monitoring includes:
- Fasting lipid studies and glucose – 6-monthly
- Troponins – 12-monthly
- Clozapine level – 6 monthly or as ordered depending on individual need or compliance monitoring
- ECG – at 3 months, then 12-monthly
- Echocardiogram – at 6 months, then 12-monthly.

Patients may miss doses of clozapine for other reasons such as in this case. However, taking a full dose of clozapine after a 72-hour interruption poses a great risk of potentially life-threatening seizures. Retitration and monitoring is required and dependent on the period of time since the last dose was taken.

Period of interruption (time since last dose was due)	Dosage and monitoring requirements
< 48 hours	No change to dosage or monitoring
Between 48 hours and 72 hours	Start on 12.5 mg and titrate up No additional monitoring requirements
Between 72 hours and 28 days	Start on 12.5 mg and titrate up For monthly patients – weekly monitoring for 6 weeks. If no abnormalities, resume monthly monitoring For weekly patients – weekly monitoring for 6 weeks and as long as needed to reach 18 weeks (whichever is greatest)
> 28 days	Follow new patient initiation protocol

Warnez S, Alessi-Severini S. Clozapine: a review of clinical practice guidelines and prescribing trends. BMC Psychiatry. 2014;14(1).
https://bmcpsychiatry.biomedcentral.com/articles/10.1186/1471-244X-14-102

4. Answer: A

Conversion disorder (CD), also known as functional neurological symptom disorder as defined in the Diagnostic and Statistical Manual of Mental Disorders (DSM-V), involves the following:

1. One or more symptoms of altered voluntary motor or sensory function.
2. Clinical findings showing incompatibility between the symptom/s and recognised neurological or medical conditions.
3. These symptoms or deficits are not better explained by another medical or mental health disorder.
4. The symptom/s cause clinically significant distress or impairment in social, occupational, or other important areas of functioning that warrants medical attention.

The precise prevalence of CD is not known, although true CD is thought to be rare. It has associations with rural setting, lower socioeconomic status, and military veterans.

Individuals with CD will typically present to tertiary health services with debilitating symptoms, whereby diagnosis and treatment can be difficult, protracted, and costly. CD is also difficult to differentiate from chronic pain disorders such as chronic regional pain syndrome as there are no specific diagnostic tests and the reliability of clinical judgement is unclear. This is especially difficult given the overlap and correlation between chronic fatigue and chronic pain, which have been reported in children with diagnosed CD at rates of 56% and 34% respectively.

An adequate assessment of CD requires detailed history taking and a thorough neurological examination, as well as laboratory and neuroimaging tests. It is important to keep in mind that a history of depression, anxiety and panic attacks are common in patients with CD. There are many tests that seek to distinguish between functional and organic cause of symptoms. Hoover's sign is the most commonly used, it is present if the patient does not push down with their normal leg when the examiner is lifting the weak, contralateral leg.

Neuroimaging tests may include CT and MRI, although in some cases CT angiogram or MR angiogram may also be indicated. EEG may also be helpful to determine if episodes that are suspicious for seizures are true seizures. It is important to consider that some neurological diseases, such as amyotrophic lateral sclerosis, may also be unremarkable on investigation, thus a neurology follow-up is advised to keep monitoring symptoms.

The most successful and evidence-based treatment of CD is multidisciplinary inpatient treatment, conducted by a team including rehabilitation specialists and psychologists. There is also some support for cognitive behavioural therapy and hypnosis.

 Tsui P, Deptula A, Yuan DY. Conversion Disorder, Functional Neurological Symptom Disorder, and Chronic Pain: Comorbidity, Assessment, and Treatment. Current Pain and Headache Reports. 2017;21(6):29. https://link.springer.com/article/10.1007%2Fs11916-017-0627 7

5. Answer: A

Depression in older adults is an under-recognised and under-treated condition, with well under half of patients with a diagnosis of depression receiving adequate treatment. Cohort studies have shown a high mortality rate (around 20%) and high rates of ongoing depression (around 1/3) after a 2-year follow-up. Indications and considerations for treatment are largely the same as for younger adults, with most treatment modalities showing very similar response rates in younger adults as in older adults. Psychotherapy is effective first-line treatment, with a number needed to treat (NNT) of around 3. However, depression resistant to first-line treatments is common in older adults, and additional treatment is often required. Class switching of antidepressant, combining pharmacological with non-pharmacological treatment, augmentation therapy with antipsychotics or lithium, or even ECT in severe cases, are all potentially successful second-line therapies. Prescribing antidepressants for older patients needs to take into consideration comorbidities, drug interactions, polypharmacy and side effects, however specific evidence to support decision making in these areas is lacking. In general, SSRIs are preferred as first line therapy, considering potential CYP450 interactions, and tricyclic antidepressants or monoamine oxidase inhibitors are usually avoided as first line therapy.

 Kok RM, Reynolds CF. Management of depression in older adults. JAMA; 317(20): 2114–22. https://jamanetwork.com/journals/jama/article-abstract/2627976

6. Answer: C

This gentleman has mild depression without other red flags. The first-line treatment for mild depression is psychotherapy and symptom monitoring. A mild depression is defined as few, if any, symptoms more than those required to make the diagnosis are present, the intensity of the symptoms is distressing but manageable. The depressive symptoms have minor impact on social or occupational function.

A mnemonic, SIG-E-CAPS has been developed to screen for patients with major depression:

Sleep disorder (either increased or decreased sleep)
Interest deficit (anhedonia)
Guilt (worthlessness, hopelessness, regret)
Energy deficit
Concentration deficit
Appetite disorder (either decreased or increase)
Psychomotor retardation or agitation
Suicidality.

Patients who have four of the symptoms plus depressed mood or anhedonia for at least two weeks fulfil the diagnostic criteria of major depression. In patients with mild depression, the first-line treatment is psychotherapy and symptom monitoring without pharmacotherapy. In patients with moderate to severe depression, psychotherapy, pharmacotherapy, or both are the first-line treatment. SSRIs, serotonin-norepinephrine-reuptake inhibitors (SNRIs), and mirtazapine are the first-line medications for moderate to severe depression.

Depressive symptoms are also observed in other medical conditions, such as anaemia, hypothyroidism, chronic medical diseases, diabetes, Parkinson's disease, dementia, HIV infection, B_{12} and folate deficiency, and substance use, etc. Treatment of the underlying conditions is important to improve the mental health and quality of life of the patients. Involvement of alcohol and other drugs treatment services may be required in some cases.

Assessing suicidal ideation or behaviour, previous suicide attempts, and thoughts of harming others should be routine for all patients with depression to ensure safety of patients, health care workers, patients' friends, and family, and the public.

Park L, Zarate C. Depression in the Primary Care Setting. New England Journal of Medicine. 2019;380(6):559–568.
https://www.nejm.org/doi/full/10.1056/NEJMcp1712493

7. Answer: A

ECT has a long and chequered history emblematic of paternalistic and inhumane medical treatment, which has adversely affected the perceptions and assumptions that many within society have regarding its usefulness, including many medical doctors. Despite this, ECT is the most effective treatment for several severe psychiatric conditions, although due to its invasiveness and public perceptions, it is often reserved for situations in which pharmacotherapy has failed. The main indication for ECT is treatment-resistant major depression, for which there is a large body of randomised trial data supporting its use. However, multiple severe psychiatric conditions also respond well to ECT.

Catatonia is an uncommon cause of mutism and severe anorexia which can be life threatening. First line treatment of catatonia involves the use of benzodiazepines, but this often fails, and ECT is usually effective. It would seem that ECT is effective even if the cause of catatonia is medical in origin, associated with schizophrenia, mania, or even autism. ECT is also effective for treatment resistant mania or schizophrenia with difficult to treat positive symptoms (i.e., psychotic symptoms).

The major adverse effect of ECT is impairment of cognitive function, in particular retrograde and anterograde amnesia. Multiple technical factors can be modified to decrease the risk to an individual. Given the severe nature of conditions treated with ECT, it is not surprising that recent studies often show an improvement in cognitive function after treatment with ECT compared with baseline. Importantly, with appropriate education, consent, patient-centred care and good anaesthesia, patients show high levels of satisfaction with ECT as a treatment for severe psychiatric illnesses.

Weiner R, Reti I. Key updates in the clinical application of electroconvulsive therapy. International Review of Psychiatry. 2017;29(2):54–62.
https://www.tandfonline.com/doi/full/10.1080/09540261.2017.1309362

8. Answer: A

Self-harm is a strong predictor of suicide, with the risk being at its highest in the first 6 months after a harming episode, but it persists for many decades. Once a person has self-harmed, the likelihood that he or she will die by suicide increases 50–100 times, with one in 15 dying by suicide within 9 years of the index episode. In studies of risk factors for suicide, a history of self-harm or suicide attempts is the strongest factor, present in at least 40% of cases. Male sex, older age, and multiple episodes of self-harm have been identified as epidemiological associations with later suicide, but such risk factors are poor predictors for an individual's suicide risk. It is important to carefully enquire about each individual's current suicidality. This can inform likely suicide risk. If significant risk for suicide is identified, a clearly articulated plan should be formed with management that might include planned engagement with health professionals, environmental interventions to reduce risk (e.g., restricting access to lethal means, increased supervision, detention), psychotherapeutic or medication interventions, and facilitating access to community services. Other risk factors for suicide after self-harm include:

- Past psychiatric care
- Psychiatric disorder such as depression, anxiety disorder, and personality disorder
- Substance misuse (especially in young people)
- Social isolation
- Repeated self-harm
- Medically severe self-harm
- Strong suicidal intent
- Avoiding discovery at time of self-harm
- Hopelessness
- Poor physical health.

Psychiatric disorders are present in up to 90% of people who kill themselves, with increased risk in those suffering from depression, bipolar disorder, alcohol misuse, anorexia, and schizophrenia. Of patients with bipolar disorder, 10–15% die by suicide. Risk of suicide is increased in health-care professionals, including nurses, physicians, dentists, and pharmacists, and may relate in part to ready access to medicinal drugs.

Hawton K, van Heeringen K. Suicide. The Lancet. 2009;373(9672):1372–1381.
https://www.thelancet.com/journals/lancet/article/PIIS0140-6736(09)60372-X/fulltext

Skegg K. Self-harm. The Lancet. 2005;366(9495):1471–1483.
https://www.thelancet.com/journals/lancet/article/PIIS0140-6736(05)67600-3/fulltext

9. Answer: B

Both neuroleptic malignant syndrome (NMS) and serotonin syndrome (SS) are severe and potentially fatal adverse consequences of psychotropic medications. As both diagnoses manifest with hyperthermia, delirium, and autonomic instability, differentiating between the two can be challenging. In such situations, supportive therapy including cessation of psychotropic medication, cooling, hydration, electrolyte management, treatment of agitation and muscular rigidity are safe regardless of the specific diagnosis. However, medications that specifically target the underlying pathophysiology pose higher risk. In this case, the dopamine agonist bromocriptine used in NMS has serotonin agonist properties, can thus worsen symptoms of SS if there has been diagnostic misattribution.

Schönfeldt-Lecuona C, Kuhlwilm L, Cronemeyer M, Neu P, Connemann B, Gahr M et al. Treatment of the Neuroleptic Malignant Syndrome in International Therapy Guidelines: A Comparative Analysis. Pharmacopsychiatry. 2019;53(02): 51–59.
https://www.thiemeconnect.com/products/ejournals/abstract/10.1055/a-1046-1044

10. Answer: D

Schizophrenia is the most common psychotic disease. It has a global prevalence of less than 1% and is slightly more common in men. Symptom onset is usually between late adolescence and mid-30s. There are two categories of symptoms, positive and negative. Positive symptoms include delusions, hallucinations, disorganised speech, and catatonia. While negative symptoms include apathy, avolition (lack of motivation), alogia (poverty of speech), and affective flattening.

The diagnosis of schizophrenia is based on criteria established in the Diagnostic and Statistical Manual of Mental Disorders (DSM-V), it is as follows:

A. Two (or more) of the following, each present for a significant portion of time during a 1-month period (or less if successfully treated). At least one of these must be (1), (2), or (3):
  1. Delusions
  2. Hallucinations
  3. Disorganised speech

4. Catatonic behaviour

5. Negative symptoms.

B. For a significant portion of the time, level of functioning is impaired in one or more major areas, such as work, interpersonal relations, or self-care.

C. Continuous signs of the disturbance persist for at least 6 months, which must include at least 1 month of symptoms that meet Criterion A.

D. The symptoms must not be caused by another psychiatric disorder, such as schizoaffective disorder and depressive or bipolar disorder with psychotic features.

E. The disturbance is not attributable to the physiological effects of a substance or a medical condition.

F. If there is a history of autism spectrum disorder or a communication disorder of childhood onset, the additional diagnosis of schizophrenia is made only if prominent delusions or hallucinations, in addition to the other required symptoms of schizophrenia, are also present for at least 1 month (or less if successfully treated).

This patient fulfils the criteria for schizophrenia, as he has been experiencing paranoid delusions and disorganised speech for at least one month, as well as experiencing prodromal, or negative symptoms for at least 6 months. In addition, he has significant functional impairment.

Schizophreniform disorder is a psychiatric disorder on the schizophrenia spectrum; however, the total duration of symptoms is at least one month, but less than 6 months and thus does not meet the criteria for schizophrenia.

A brief psychotic disorder includes symptoms such as delusions, hallucinations, and disorganised speech that last for at least one day, but less than one month.

Schizoaffective disorder includes the presence of mood symptoms occurring concurrently with the psychotic episode. In schizoaffective disorder, there must be psychosis predominance, that is a period where the delusions are present for two weeks without prominent mood symptoms.

Depression with psychotic features has a mood predominance, and psychotic features will occur exclusively during periods of mood disturbance.

 Marder S, Cannon T. Schizophrenia. New England Journal of Medicine. 2019;381(18):1753–1761.
https://www.nejm.org/doi/full/10.1056/NEJMra1808803

11. Answer: B

Switching antidepressants is best done cautiously in most settings as synergistic serotonergic toxicity is a well-recognised adverse effect, which can be life threatening. However, in cases of severe mental illness, the risks of discontinuation effects or emergent severe mental illness are also important to consider. When switching from one short-acting SSRI to another, tapering the first and then starting the second at a low dose is a reasonable strategy, but for agents with a longer half-life, a washout period is often advisable. Fluoxetine and its active metabolite together have an unusually long half-life of 4–16 days, meaning that a washout period is usually required, however a taper is not usually needed. Fluoxetine is also a strong inhibitor of CYP2D6, for which many antidepressants are a substrate, further increasing the risk if there is an overlap of medications. If, for mental state reasons a cross-taper of medications is required, this is best done under the supervision of a psychiatrist.

 Keks N, Hope J, Keogh S. Switching and stopping antidepressants. Australian Prescriber [Internet]. 2016 [cited 9 May 2020];39(3):76–83.
Available from: https://www.nps.org.au/australian-prescriber/articles/switching-and-stopping-antidepressants

12. Answer: C

This patient has an established major mental illness and has not received appropriate treatment. The confidentiality of the doctor/patient therapeutic relationship can be breached if the patient is at imminent risk of harming others or self-harm due to mental illness. The doctor is acting in the public interest by taking reasonable steps to protect the potential victim from an unwell patient's actions.

According to the AMA guidance (https://ama.com.au/system/tdf/documents/Guidelines_for_Doctors_on_Disclosing_Medical_Records_to_Third_Parties_2010_0.pdf?file=1&type=node&id=36689. A doctor may disclose information from a patient's medical record without consent if the doctor reasonably believes the patient may cause imminent and serious harm to themselves, an identifiable individual or group of persons. In such circumstances, disclosure may be necessary to lessen or prevent a serious and imminent threat to an individual's life, health, safety, or welfare, or a serious threat to public health, public safety, or public welfare.

In a medical emergency where the patient cannot provide consent, a doctor may disclose information from a patient's medical record to the extent necessary to protect the patient's life or health.

There may be circumstances where the law requires a doctor to disclose a patient's medical record, regardless of whether or not the patient has consented. There are other situations where doctors may be required by statute to disclose information from a patient's medical record in cases of mandatory disease notification or mandatory notification of child abuse. In cases where there is a warrant, subpoena, or court order requiring the doctor to produce a patient's medical record, some doctors may wish to oppose disclosure of clinically sensitive or potentially harmful information. The records should still be supplied but under seal, asking that the court not release the records to the parties until it has heard argument against disclosure. Whether disclosure of information from a patient's medical record is permitted or required by law without patient consent, where appropriate the patient should be informed of that having occurred and this information should be documented in the medical record.

 Mental health legislation Australia and New Zealand | RANZCP [Internet]. Ranzcp.org. 2020 [cited 9 May 2020]. Available from: https://www.ranzcp.org/practice-education/guidelines-and-resources-for-practice/mental-health-legislation-australia-and-new-zealan

13. Answer: H

14. Answer: J

15. Answer: F

16. Answer: A

17. Answer: D

18. Answer: C

19. Answer: G

20. Answer: E
Descriptors of psychiatric symptomatology can be extremely useful in diagnosing and assessing severity of psychiatric problems. A delusion is a foundational concept encompassing fixed beliefs that are not endorsed by other members of their societal group and cannot be challenged by reasonable evidence to the contrary. This contrasts with obsessions, which are preoccupations which the individual can recognise as being not rational, and compulsions, which are repetitive actions that occur as a result of obsessions. Delusions often take on the theme of unseen forces such as magic, secrecy, microscopic agents, or spirituality, as this makes them easier to perpetuate as irrefutable contrary evidence is difficult to find.

Hallucinations refer to any sensory experience that cannot be validated by objective reality. In schizophrenia, the most common form of hallucination is auditory, sometimes in recognisable grammatical forms, sometimes in the form of a command, but sometimes also random, which can be interpreted as a code of some kind. They are usually experienced as being out of control of the individual. Given the overlap of hallucinations and delusional beliefs, it is not uncommon for the hallucination to assume delusional attribution, such that the individual might believe, for example, that a famous historical figure, religious figure or microelectronic device might be talking to them.

Ideas of reference are a common manifestation in psychotic illnesses. Examples include the misperception of a stranger's eye contact as directed personally at the self or hearing random words that others say and attributing them to the self. This phenomenon is often seen in schizophrenia and highlights the tendency for individuals in this situation to come to concrete conclusions based on insufficient data in this disease.

Thought broadcasting is where a patient experiences what is believed to be others reading, receiving, or knowing their thoughts.

Looseness of association, word salad, echolalia, and flight of ideas are terms used to delineate types of 'formal thought disorder,' which is where a patient's conversational content is used to infer disordered flow from one idea to another. Looseness of association is one of the more severe forms of formal thought disorder where a patient's conversational content moves between seemingly unconnected topics, but with grammatically correct content. More severe formal thought disorders are generally associated with more severe psychiatric illnesses such as schizophrenia and bipolar disorder; some milder degrees of formal thought disorder such as tangentiality and circumstantiality are more often seen in major depressive illnesses, cognitive impairment or schizotypal personality disorder.

Word salad is a very severe formal thought disorder where the vocalisations are not grammatically linked and little to no inference of meaning is possible. Often associated with severe psychosis, neologisms are often present in this type of conversational content.

A slightly less severe type of formal thought disorder is flight of ideas, where a patient's conversational content moves from one frame of reference to another with a tenuous but recognisable link between the ideas. In some cases, the associated ideas may be linked by phonetic rather than semantic relation, termed 'clang association'. Flight of ideas is typically associated with pressured speech and is often seen in mania, medical conditions, or substance induced psychosis.

Thought blocking is a type of poverty of content of speech and refers to the inability to articulate a thought process. This often occurs where the patient's 'mind goes blank' but can also occur in the setting of racing thoughts that travel too fast to articulate. Thought blocking is usually accompanied by significant anxiety, which can perpetuate the state. Poverty of speech syndromes are most closely associated with schizophrenia and major depression.

Echolalia is the repletion of the phrase or word spoken by the interviewer. Catatonia is an important presenting complaint which can be caused by or mimic a hypoactive delirium, often with an underlying severe mental illness. Associated symptoms include waxy flexibility, mutism, or severe thought blocking. Catatonia can be a presentation of schizophrenia, severe depression, or an underlying medical condition.

Another phenomenon worth mentioning in this context is that of dissociation. Dissociation can be defined as the splitting off of cognitive, somatic, emotional or behavioural experience from integrated awareness. Dissociation is observed as normal phenomena for example in dissociative anaesthesia, hypnosis, or even somnambulism. Dissociation may also exist as a coping mechanism to past or present traumatic events, although prolonged dissociation in this setting represents a maladaptive response. Derealisation is a relatively common form of dissociative disorder where the individual feels removed from the world or that the sensations of the environment are inaccessible. Derealisation and similar experiences are often seen in exhaustion or bereavement and can be a part of many psychiatric disorders. Psychiatric amnestic states or and dissociative identity disorder are rarer, but very dramatic forms of dissociation.

 Hoffman RE, Lehrer DS, McGlashan. Chapter 35: Alterations of speech, thought, perception and self-experience. In Tasman A et.al., Psychiatry. 2015. Wiley and Sons.
https://onlinelibrary.wiley.com/doi/abs/10.1002/9780470515167.ch35

21. Answer: E

22. Answer: D

23. Answer: A

Despite incomplete understanding of the neuropathogenesis of depression, there are several measures, both pharmacological and non-pharmacological, with significant positive effects on symptoms, and function for patients with depression. Initially, observations that monoamine depletion causes depression, and that monoamine augmentation can effectively treat depression, led to the monoamine hypothesis – that depression is essentially a state of lack of monoamine function within the brain. Multiple medications impacting the monoamine system have been found to be efficacious for the treatment of depression.

Firstly, monoamine oxidase inhibitors (phenelzine, moclobemide, tranylcypromine, etc.) were found to have potent antidepressant activity, although their widespread use has been limited by toxicity and potential for significant drug-drug interaction. Tricyclic antidepressants (TCAs; amitriptyline, doxepin, etc.) exert antidepressant effects through inhibition of serotonin and noradrenaline reuptake, but have several adverse off-target effects, leading to significant anticholinergic side-effects, and significant cardiac risk when taken in overdose. SSRIs (citalopram, fluoxetine, paroxetine, etc.) exert their effect through reuptake inhibition of serotonin over that of noradrenaline, but also have significantly fewer side effects than TCAs and are safer in overdose. Serotonin and noradrenaline reuptake inhibitors (SNRIs; venlafaxine, desvenlafaxine, duloxetine) inhibit reuptake of serotonin and noradrenaline like TCAs, but unlike TCAs, their off-target effects are less, with fewer anticholinergic side effects, and they are safer in overdose. Noradrenaline reuptake inhibitors (bupropion, reboxetine, and atomoxetine) have lower efficacy than other antidepressants but have some limited therapeutic uses. Mirtazapine acts by antagonising inhibitory autoreceptors; principally α-2 receptors, enhancing monoamine activity – however, it has multiple inhibitory effects at other monoamine receptors, accounting for some of its particular adverse effect profile.

The observation of disordered hypothalamic-pituitary-adrenal (HPA) axis hormones in depression has long been thought to be of significance in depression, although pharmacological agents targeting this system have not been efficacious. Neurotrophic effects not directly related to monoamine oxidase function have also been thought to be important in the development of depression, and this may be an important consideration in the HPA axis hypothesis; other factors potentially implicated in this process include brain-derived neurotrophic factor, glycogen synthase kinase 3, and glutamate/NMDA receptor. It is felt that these factors may contribute to neuronal loss in critical areas – a process, which is reversed by antidepressant therapy, including medications, exercise, and ECT.

Rang H, Ritter J, Flower R, Henderson G, Loke Y, MacEwan D et al. Rang and Dale's pharmacology. 9th ed. Edinburgh: Elsevier; 2019.
https://www.elsevier.com/books/rang-and-dales-pharmacology/ritter/978-0-7020-7448-6

24. Answer: G

Olanzapine and clozapine are the psychotropic medications associated with the highest amount of weight gain. Other agents implicated in causing some weight gain include chlorpromazine, sodium valproate, lithium, tricyclic antidepressants, and mirtazapine. Most antipsychotics cause some weight gain, with the possible exceptions of ziprasidone and aripiprazole. Most weight gain occurs early in the usage of medication, is most pronounced in psychotropic naïve patients, and should trigger a search for alternative agents if possible.

25. Answer: E

Lithium is by far the most common psychotropic medication implicated in diabetes insipidus (DI). In this setting, the pathophysiology is due to increased renal resistance to ADH leading to a nephrogenic DI. Up to 40% of patients treated with lithium long term develop irreversible polyuria: higher doses, longer duration and recurrent acute lithium toxicity are all associated with greater risk. In the setting of a patient with polydipsia and polyuria on lithium, high serum sodium is diagnostic of DI, low serum sodium is suggestive of primary polydipsia and normal serum sodium is equivocal – usually necessitating a therapeutic trial of cessation. Clozapine is a rare cause of DI.

26. Answer: B

Sexual dysfunction is a common side effect of psychotropic medications, with antidepressants being the most commonly implicated. Generally, the antidepressants with the highest serotonergic activity have the most effect on sexual function, manifest as low libido, delayed orgasm, and erectile dysfunction. Antipsychotics cause similar effects, although delayed orgasm is less commonly reported.

27. Answer: H

Prolongation of the QT interval, and occasionally sudden cardiac death or torsades des pointes, is associated with multiple psychotropic medications. Most commonly, antipsychotics are implicated, and ziprasidone is the most likely to cause QT prolongation. However, haloperidol (particularly intravenously) seems to be associated with the highest risk of malignant arrhythmia or sudden death. Citalopram is the antidepressant with the highest risk. Guidelines for managing antipsychotics and QT prolongation are unclear, although some authors recommend not using QT prolonging medications in patients with a baseline QTc already above 440 ms, and ceasing a QTc prolonging drug if QTc is above 500 ms, or if there is a change of >60 ms from baseline.

28. Answer: A

Carbamazepine is the drug most associated with Stevens–Johnson syndrome/toxic epidermal necrolysis (SJS/TEN) – a severe mucocutaneous reaction associated with high mortality and morbidity. Other psychotropic medications that less commonly cause SJS/TEN are lamotrigine and sodium valproate. While the absolute risk is small with carbamazepine at 1%, the severity of SJS/TENS warrants a high index of suspicion and counselling when initiating the medication. These same medications can also lead to drug reaction with eosinophilia and systemic symptoms (DRESS), both of which are examples of T-cell mediated hypersensitivity reactions (type IV hypersensitivity).

29. Answer: F

Given their dopamine blocking actions, all antipsychotic agents can precipitate drug induced Parkinsonism, with typical antipsychotic agents a more common cause. Of the drugs listed, haloperidol is the most likely. In contrast to Parkinson's disease, tremor is often less prominent, and more likely to be postural, bilateral, and symmetrical. Cessation of the causative agent usually resolves Parkinsonism in 4–6 weeks, but symptoms persist in around 7% – it is felt that, in these cases, the antidopaminergic drug probably unmasks an underlying Parkinson's disease.

Annamalai A. Medical Management of Psychotropic Side Effects. 1st ed. Springer International Publishing; 2017.
https://link.springer.com/book/10.1007%2F978-3-319-51026-2

15 Nephrology

Questions

Answers can be found in the Nephrology Answers section at the end of this chapter.

1. An 18-year-old Aboriginal and Torres Strait Islander (ATSI) man presents to the local community hospital with a 2-week history of headaches, a puffy face, and swollen ankles. He is hypertensive with a BP of 160/95 mmHg. Urine dipstick shows moderate haematuria. There are two skin sores on his right lower limb. Your provisional clinical diagnosis is acute post-streptococcal glomerulonephritis (APSGN).

Which one of the following is **NOT** correct at this point?
  A. Every single case of APSGN requires notification, contact identification, and contact tracing.
  B. He will make a full recovery without prednisolone treatment and is not at risk of developing CKD.
  C. Intramuscular benzathine penicillin should be given.
  D. Swabs should be taken from 2 different skin sores and sent for culture.

2. What is the mechanism of action of tolvaptan in the treatment of autosomal dominant polycystic kidney disease (ADPKD)?
  A. A vasopressin V_2-receptor agonist that induces vasopressin release.
  B. A vasopressin V_2-receptor antagonist that reduces the cAMP within tubular epithelial cells.
  C. An anti-metabolite to reduce the formation of new renal cysts.
  D. An antihypertensive via the renin-angiotensin-aldosterone pathway.

3. A 30-year-old man presents to the emergency department after tripping over his cat and fracturing his right neck of femur. He has a medical history of ESKD due to fibrillary glomerulonephritis on maintenance haemodialysis. His medications include irbesartan, darbepoetin, calcitriol, and calcium carbonate with meals. His blood test results are shown below. He underwent a right hip replacement.

Tests	Results	Normal values
Serum calcium	2.70 mmol/L	2.10 – 2.60
Serum phosphate	2.50 mmol/L	0.75 – 1.50
Serum albumin	40 g/L	34 – 48
PTH	1 pmol/L	0.8 – –5.5
ALP	257 U/L	30 – 110
Vitamin D	42 nmol/L	>50
Haemoglobin	90 g/L	135 – 175

Which one of the following recommendations reduces the risk of developing adynamic bone disease in this patient?
  A. Change calcium carbonate to a non-calcium-based phosphate binder.
  B. Commence a calcimimetic agent.
  C. Increase his calcitriol dose.
  D. Using a high calcium dialysate.

4. A 57-year-old woman with no significant medical history or regular medications presented to her GP with a two-week history of bilateral leg swelling, erythema, and minor discomfort (see picture below). She was afebrile. Her initial blood tests revealed a normal CRP and WBC count. Her liver function tests, and renal function were normal. She was diagnosed with bilateral leg cellulitis and treated with oral flucloxacillin. Two weeks later, her lower limb swelling was worse, and she noticed a decline in urine output.

How to Pass the FRACP Written Examination, First Edition. Jonathan Gleadle, Jordan Li, Danielle Wu, and Paul Kleinig.
© 2022 John Wiley & Sons Ltd. Published 2022 by John Wiley & Sons Ltd.

Her GP repeated her blood tests, which revealed a serum creatinine of 210 µmol/L [45-90] and CRP of 11 mg/L [0-8]. Urine analysis showed 1+protein, 5 RBC/hpf, 20 WBC/hpf and 1 WBC cast.

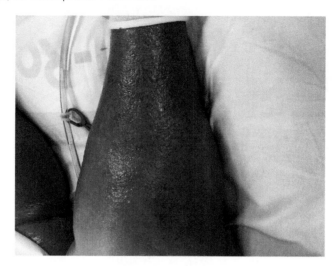

Apart from stopping flucloxacillin, the most appropriate next step is:
  A. Commence clindamycin and repeat renal function in 3 days.
  B. Commence prednisolone 60mg daily and repeat renal function in 3 days.
  C. Perform a kidney biopsy.
  D. Wait and repeat renal function test in 3 days.

5. Which one of the following has been identified in Indigenous Australians as the leading risk factor for AKI?
  A. Dehydration.
  B. Infection.
  C. Nonsteroidal anti-inflammatory drugs.
  D. Urinary tract obstruction.

6. Regarding antibody-mediated rejection in renal transplantation, which one of the following statements is correct?
  A. C4d is a sensitive maker in patients with antibody-mediated rejection.
  B. It can be caused by antibodies directed to HLA antigens.
  C. It is associated with activation of alternative complement pathway.
  D. It occurs only within 12 months after renal transplant.

7. A 32-year-old current smoker presents to the emergency department with dyspnoea, haemoptysis, and reduced urine output. His serum creatinine is 460 µmol/L [60-110] and his baseline creatinine 3 months ago was 86 µmol/L. Her anti-GBM and ANCA antibodies are pending. He undergoes an urgent renal biopsy which is shown below. There is a strong linear ribbon-like appearance on direct immunofluorescence.

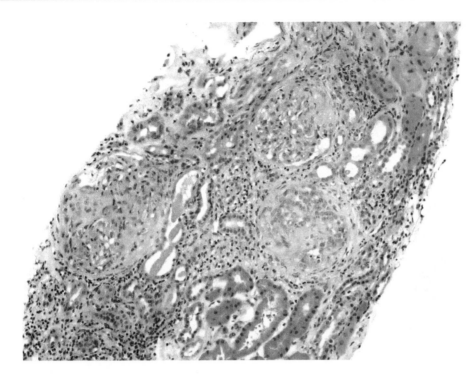

What is the most appropriate treatment?
   A. Cyclophosphamide and prednisolone.
   B. Plasma exchange, cyclophosphamide, and prednisolone.
   C. Plasma exchange, mycophenolate mofetil, and prednisolone.
   D. Rituximab and prednisolone.

8. C3 glomerulopathy is associated with abnormal activation or repression of which one of the following pathways?
   A. Alternative complement pathway.
   B. Classical complement pathway.
   C. Lectin pathway.
   D. STING (STimulator of INterferon Genes) pathway.

9. Which one of following medications is a risk factor for the development of calciphylaxis?
   A. Cinacalcet.
   B. Sevelamer.
   C. Vitamin K.
   D. Warfarin.

10. Which one of the following recommendations regarding chronic kidney disease–mineral and bone disorders (CKD-MBD) is correct?
   A. Biomarkers of bone turnover should be measured in patients with CKD-MBD.
   B. Bone mineral density (BMD) measurements can distinguish the type of renal osteodystrophy in CKD.
   C. Cinacalcet therapy is ineffective at ameliorating reduced BMD.
   D. In patients with CKD not on dialysis, calcitriol and vitamin D analogues should be routinely used to prevent progressive hyperparathyroidism.

11. A 75-year-old independent man with stage 5 CKD has been followed up in the renal clinic for 2 years. He has been educated about renal replacement options and wants haemodialysis if he needs. His recent blood tests show creatinine 460 µmol/L [60-110] with eGFR: 9 mL/min/1.73 m², urea 19 mmol/L [2.7-8], and haemoglobin of 101 g/L [135-175]. His medical history includes type 2 diabetes, hypertension, obesity (BMI 35 kg/m²), smoking, AAA repair, ischaemic heart disease and heart failure with preserved ejection fraction. His BP is 165/75 mmHg, SpO2 96% on room air. He feels a bit more fatigued than he used to and can only manage 400 metres of walking.

What is the most appropriate next step of management for his renal disease?
A. Initiate erythropoietin and review renal function in 2 months.
B. Initiate haemodialysis via a tunneled central catheter.
C. Start dialysis access planning.
D. Start renal transplant workup for the patient.

12. Which one of the following medications can cause hyperkalaemia in a patient with CKD by blocking sodium channels in the luminal membranes of principal cells?
A. Atenolol.
B. Digoxin.
C. Heparin.
D. Trimethoprim.

13. A 32-year-old man presents to the emergency department because his urine colour has changed to a 'dark tea colour', and this colour has persisted despite having drunk a large amount of water. He is taking a 'nature therapy pill' for his cold symptoms, including sore throat and cough which started yesterday. He has no significant medical history and no known allergies. On examination, he is afebrile, BP is 170/100mmHg, there is pharyngeal erythema without tonsillar exudates. Urine analysis is positive for blood and 3+ protein and RBC casts are seen on microscopy. Initial blood and urine test results are shown below:

Tests	Results	Normal values
WBC	8.2 x 10⁹/L	4 – 11
Platelet	452 x 10⁹/L	150 – 450
Creatinine	136 µmol/L	60 – 110
Urine albumin/creatinine ratio	352 mg/mmol	<2.5

In this patient, which one of the following is **NOT** a poor prognostic indicator?
A. He has renal impairment.
B. He has significant proteinuria.
C. He is hypertensive.
D. His urine microscopy has RBC casts.

14. Which one of the following is correct concerning the therapeutic use of lithium?
A. Haemodialysis should be considered for severe lithium toxicity.
B. Lithium is associated with hypocalcaemia.
C. Polyuria affects 20% of patients on long-term lithium.
D. Polyuria is caused by central diabetes insipidus.

15. A 21-year-old woman is diagnosed with lupus nephritis after presenting with fever, rash, and AKI. At diagnosis she has active urinary sediment with non-nephrotic range proteinuria, a creatinine of 427 µmol/L [45–90] and urea of 31 mmol/L [2.7–8.0]. A renal biopsy is performed and shows mesangial and subendothelial immune complex deposition with segmental endocapillary proliferation and >50% of glomeruli with crescents.

Which of the following is the most appropriate management strategy?
A. Mycophenolate mofetil and pulse intravenous methylprednisolone for three days followed by high dose oral prednisolone.
B. Oral high dose prednisolone 1mg/kg and oral cyclophosphamide.
C. Pulse intravenous methylprednisolone for three days, followed by high dose prednisolone.
D. Plasma exchange and pulse methylprednisolone for three days, followed by high dose prednisolone.

16. Patiromer is a new agent for treatment of hyperkalaemia. Which one of the following is correct?
A. It causes hypomagnesemia.
B. It selectively binds potassium in exchange for sodium and hydrogen.
C. The location where potassium binding occurs is in the upper gastrointestinal tract.
D. The median time of onset of effect is 2 hours.

17. Which one of the following serological markers can be used to prognosticate the course of primary membranous nephropathy?
A. Complement C3, C4.
B. M-type phospholipase A2 receptor (PLA2R) antibody.
C. Serum urokinase–type plasminogen activator receptor (suPAR).
D. Thrombospondin type 1 domain-containing 7A (THSD7A) antibody.

18. A 29-year-old man presents with muscle pain after strenuous exercise for 3 days trying to lose weight. At presentation, his creatine kinase (CK) is 42,000 U/L [0-250] and serum creatinine is 160 μmol/L [60-110]. He is not taking other medications or supplements. After 3 days of aggressive fluid resuscitation with 0.9% normal saline, his CK is 41,000 U/L and renal function is slightly improved. His urine output is 1.5L/24hr. He is haemodynamically stable.
The most appropriate next step is:
A. Change intravenous fluid to sodium bicarbonate alternating with 5% dextrose.
B. Check urine myoglobin level and discharge if negative.
C. Continue intravenous normal saline until CK trending down.
D. Encourage oral water intake to 3 litres a day and discharge home.

19. A 58-year-old Jehovah's Witness has anaemia due to his stage 4 CKD. He is having darbepoetin injections but suffers from needle phobia. His GP calls you to inquire about oral roxadustat.
Which one of the following is correct regarding the mechanism of roxadustat?
A. It is an erythropoietin receptor agonist.
B. It is a hepcidin agonist.
C. It is a hypoxia-inducible factor prolyl hydroxylase (PHD) inhibitor.
D. It increases red cell survival.

20. A 71-year-old man is admitted to hospital following an unwitnessed fall. His medical history includes osteoarthritis for which he takes ibuprofen as needed. His vital signs and mental status are normal. He is clinically euvolaemic and has a normal neurological examination. His TFTs, CXR and CT head are normal. His investigation results are shown below:

Tests	Results	Normal values
Serum sodium	124 mmol/L	135-145
Potassium	4.4 mmol/L	3.5-5.0
Creatinine	80 μmol/L	45-90 μmol/L
Serum osmolality	250 mOsm/kg	>275
Serum glucose level	5 mmol/L	3.2-5.5
Urine osmolality	140 mOsm/kg	<100
Urine sodium	38 mmol/L	<20

What is the mainstay of management of this patient?
A. Administration of intravenous hypertonic saline (3%) in the intensive care unit .
B. Fluid restriction 800 – 1200 ml over 24 hours.
C. Correction of sodium level to achieve a sodium level of 135 mmol/L over 24 hours.
D. Administration of normal saline (0.9%) to increase the sodium level to 130 mmol/L.

21. A 60-year-old man with ESKD due to membranoproliferative glomerulonephritis received a deceased donor kidney transplant four months ago. Post-transplantation, he had one episode of severe vascular rejection which was treated with a course of anti-thymoglobulin (ATG). His graft function has been stable with serum creatinine of 140 μmol/L [60–110]. His immunosuppressants include tacrolimus, mycophenolate, and prednisolone. His renal function has worsened over the past two weeks. His blood and urine BK virus PCR levels are remarkably high. His kidney biopsy result reveals significant tubulitis and interstitial lymphocyte infiltration and tubular epithelial cell nuclear positivity for BK virus.
Your first action would be to:
A. Intravenous cidofovir.
B. Intravenous immunoglobulin.
C. Reduce tacrolimus and mycophenolate doses.
D. Switch mycophenolate to leflunomide.

22. A 66-year-old man with stage 4 CKD due to biopsy proven diabetic nephropathy is receiving darbepoetin 40 mcg weekly. His other medical problems include smoking related COPD, ischaemic heart disease with exertional angina, CCF, hypertension, peripheral vascular disease, and type 2 diabetes. His most recent blood test shows a haemoglobin level of 140g/L [135-175] and normal iron studies. You contact him to ask him to hold darbepoetin as his haemoglobin is too high. He insists on continuing as he has been recently winning his golf games.

    You would advise him if he continues on darbepoetin, he is at higher risk of developing the following complications **EXCEPT**:
- **A.** Difficult control of hypertension.
- **B.** Stroke.
- **C.** Venous thromboembolism.
- **D.** Worsening diabetic control.

23. In a patient with stage 4 CKD which one of the following regarding the bone-kidney endocrine axis involving fibroblast growth factor 23 (FGF–23) is true?
- **A.** Elevated plasma FGF–23 level is seen with rising serum phosphate.
- **B.** FGF–23 inhibits urinary phosphate excretion.
- **C.** Elevated plasma FGF–23 level is associated with reduced risk of cardiovascular events in patients with CKD.
- **D.** FGF–23 is primarily synthesised by the kidney.

24. Which one of the following is **NOT** a key pathologic feature that is consistently and independently associated with renal outcome in a patient with IgA nephropathy?
- **A.** Mesangial hypercellularity.
- **B.** Podocyte foot process effacement.
- **C.** Segmental glomerulosclerosis.
- **D.** Tubular atrophy and interstitial fibrosis.

25. A 65-year-old man is reviewed in the clinic for his known stage 3B CKD with an eGFR of 31 ml/min/1.73m^2 due to presumptive diabetic nephropathy. His other medical issues include hypertension, type 2 diabetes, and Sjogren's syndrome. He is taking ramipril, thiazide, felodipine, and rosuvastatin. His most recent blood test shows potassium 5.1 mmol/L [3.2-5.2] and bicarbonate level of 16 mmol/L [22-32] which is similar to his previous two blood tests.

    What is the most appropriate next step regarding his metabolic acidosis?
- **A.** Increase the dose of insulin.
- **B.** Increase the dose of thiazide.
- **C.** Start oral sodium bicarbonate.
- **D.** Stop ACE inhibitor.

26. Which one of the following is correct for patients on peritoneal dialysis (PD)?
- **A.** In patients with PD related peritonitis, PD should be transferred to haemodialysis until infection is resolved.
- **B.** Peritoneal dialysis can lead to weight gain.
- **C.** The most common causative organism for PD related peritonitis is *S. aureus*.
- **D.** The peritoneal dialysate contains variable concentrations of potassium.

27. Which one of the following descriptions regarding podocyte structure and function is **INCORRECT**?
- **A.** Podocytes have unlimited ability to proliferate.
- **B.** Podocytes produce vascular endothelial growth factor.
- **C.** Podocytes synthesise and repair the glomerular basement membrane.
- **D.** Slit diaphragms between foot processes are permeable to water and solutes.

28. What is the most important risk factor for the development of post-transplant lymphoproliferative disorder (PTLD) in solid organ transplantation?
- **A.** EBV status mismatched transplant with donor positive and recipient negative for EBV immunity.
- **B.** Kidney transplantation as opposed to other solid organ transplants.
- **C.** The use of everolimus in maintenance immunosuppression regimen.
- **D.** The use of T-cell depleting induction therapy.

29. Which of one the following is **NOT** a risk factor for contrast-induced nephropathy (CIN)?
   A. Congestive heart failure.
   B. Metformin.
   C. Multiple myeloma.
   D. Sepsis.

30. Which one of the following conditions is most likely to cause nephrotic syndrome?
   A. Sarcoidosis.
   B. Sjögren's syndrome.
   C. Systemic amyloidosis.
   D. Systemic sclerosis.

31. Dapagliflozin exert its effect on which part of the renal tubule?
   A. Collecting duct.
   B. Proximal renal tubule.
   C. Thin ascending limb of Henle's loop.
   D. Thick ascending limb of Henle's loop.

32. A 65-year-old woman has stage 4 CKD due to membranous nephropathy with serum creatinine of 196 μmol/L [45-90]. She was diagnosed with a UTI 4 days ago and is taking trimethoprim 300 mg daily. Her GP contacts you because her renal function is deteriorating with creatinine 253 μmol/L and thinks she needs an urgent review. You explain that the increased serum creatinine is likely due to:
   A. Trimethoprim increases water loss leading to dehydration.
   B. Trimethoprim interferes with the serum creatinine assay in the lab.
   C. Trimethoprim reduces creatinine secretion in the proximal tubule.
   D. Trimethoprim reduces the glomerular filtration rate.

33. A 32-year-old man with ESKD secondary to IgA nephropathy received a living donor renal transplant 12 months ago. He has not been attending his renal appointments regularly. He reports no urinary symptoms, abdominal pain, fever, or difficulty with urination. His medications include tacrolimus, mycophenolate mofetil, and prednisolone 5mg daily. He is afebrile and normotensive. There is no graft tenderness. His creatinine has increased from a baseline level of 87 μmol/L to 164 μmol/L [60-110]. Tacrolimus trough level is 3 ng/mL [recommended range 7–8], BK viral PCR is negative in the blood, but the urine is positive with low viral count, CRP is normal, and urine culture is negative. An ultrasound of his transplant kidney did not reveal urinary tract obstruction.
   He is scheduled for a renal biopsy, what is the most likely finding in the biopsy?
   A. Allograft rejection.
   B. BK nephropathy.
   C. Calcineurin inhibitor toxicity.
   D. Recurrence of IgA nephropathy in the transplant kidney.

34. Which one of the following statements regarding malignancy post-renal transplant is correct?
   A. Breast cancer and prostate cancer incidence are increased post renal transplant.
   B. Incidences of colon cancer and lymphoma increases substantially post renal transplant.
   C. Melanomatous skin malignancy is the commonest cancer post renal transplant.
   D. Screening for malignancy with yearly CT chest and abdomen is recommended post renal transplant.

QUESTIONS (35–38) REFER TO THE FOLLOWING INFORMATION

Match the following immunosuppressants with their primary mechanism of action:
   A. Anti-thymocyte globulin (ATG).
   B. Basiliximab.
   C. Belatacept.
   D. Bortezomib.
   E. Everolimus.
   F. Mycophenolate.
   G. Tacrolimus.
   H. Tocilizumab.

35. Which one of the following immunosuppressants targets T cell signal 1 activation via the antigen presentation pathway?

36. Which is an IL-6 inhibitor that has been used as an immunomodulatory therapy for severe acute respiratory distress syndrome (ARDS) caused by COVID-19 infection?

37. Which one is an IL-2 receptor antagonist to limit activated T cell proliferation and has been used in induction therapy for kidney transplantation?

38. Which immunosuppressant inhibits lymphocyte cell cycle progression G1 to S phase and thus cell proliferation?

QUESTIONS (39–47) REFER TO THE FOLLOWING INFORMATION
For each of the scenarios, select the most likely renal disease:
- **A.** Acute interstitial nephritis.
- **B.** Alport's disease.
- **C.** Chinese herbal nephropathy.
- **D.** Collapsing focal segmental glomerulosclerosis (FSGS).
- **E.** Diabetic nephropathy.
- **F.** Goodpasture's disease.
- **G.** Idiopathic membranous nephropathy (MN).
- **H.** IgA nephropathy.
- **I.** Membranoproliferative glomerulonephritis (MPGN).
- **J.** Minimal change disease (MCD).
- **K.** Post infectious glomerulonephritis.
- **L.** Primary FSGS.
- **M.** Rapidly progressive glomerulonephritis.
- **N.** Thin basement membrane nephropathy.

39. Which glomerular disease is most likely to rapidly recur in a renal allograft?

40. An 18-year-old college student is struggling to keep up in class despite wearing a hearing aid. His vision is suboptimal and has difficult focusing. He is reviewed by a GP in the student wellbeing clinic. A urine dipstick finds haematuria and ++ proteinuria. His serum creatinine is 308 µmol/L [60-110]. His mother mentions that she also has haematuria.

41. A 32-year-old woman is discovered to have microscopic haematuria during a routine life insurance examination. She has no other medical history. Her father and sister also have persistent microscopic haematuria. There is no family history of deafness or known kidney disease requiring specific therapy. She is normotensive and the rest of her physical examination is unremarkable. Her urine shows 10 to 15 dysmorphic erythrocytes and one to two leukocytes per high-power field. A 24-h urine collection reveals 105 mg of protein. Her serum creatinine is 60 µmol/L [45-90] and the renal USS is normal.

42. A 45-year-old Māori man presents with new onset of peripheral oedema. He has been previously well except for removal of a ruptured spleen due to a motor bike accident. He is hypertensive. There is microscopic haematuria and a 24-hour urine protein of 3.5g. His serum creatinine is 196 µmol/L [60-110]. His histopathology is shown below. What is the most likely diagnosis?

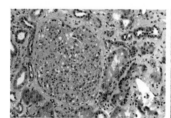
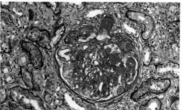

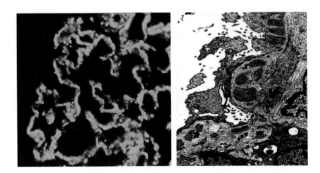

43. A 60-year-old Aboriginal man undergoes a kidney biopsy because of significant proteinuria of 7.6 g/day and rapid deterioration of renal function with serum creatinine of 200 μmol/L [60-110]. He was diagnosed with type 2 diabetes 3 years ago and maintains reasonably good blood glucose control. You are concerned that he may have other glomerular disease. Many of his glomeruli show the following features.

What is the most likely diagnosis?

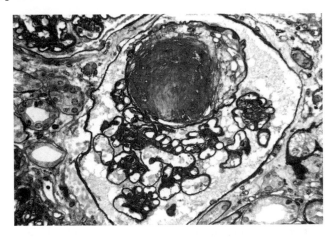

44. A 65-year-old woman presents with AKI and a serum creatinine of 650 μmol/L [45-90]. Urinalysis reveals 3+ protein and urine sediment with many casts as shown below. Renal biopsy is performed urgently. Light microscopy and result of immunofluorescence staining for IgG are provided below. Her autoimmune screen tests are all pending. On the basis of this information alone, you determine the patient has which glomerular disease?

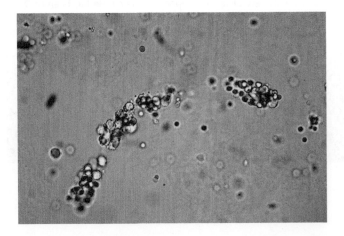

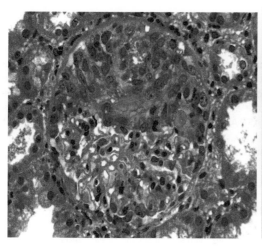
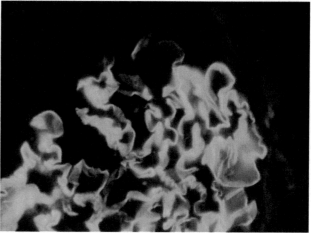

45. A 60-year-old man presents with a two-week history of bilateral leg swelling. He is found to have nephrotic syndrome with proteinuria 11 g/day, serum albumin 10 g/L [34-48], and serum creatinine 89 μmol/L [60-110]. He undergoes a kidney biopsy, and the result is pending. He noticed reduced urine output the next day. His haemoglobin is stable but renal function has deteriorated with creatinine 170 μmol/L. An urgent renal USS revealed no complications from kidney biopsy but bilateral leg and renal vein thrombosis. Based on the above clinical information, what is the most likely histopathology diagnosis from the kidney biopsy?

46. A 35-year-old man presents with a two-week history of bilateral leg swelling. He is found to have nephrotic syndrome with proteinuria 11 g/day, serum albumin 10 g/L [34-48] and serum creatinine 89 μmol/L [60-110]. He took a course of ibuprofen 3 weeks ago because of his painful right tennis elbow. He undergoes a kidney biopsy. All his glomeruli (total 26 in the sample) have the same appearance as shown below. The interstitial and blood vessels are reported as normal. Immunofluorescence staining is negative and electron microscopy result is pending. Which glomerulonephritis is most likely in this case?

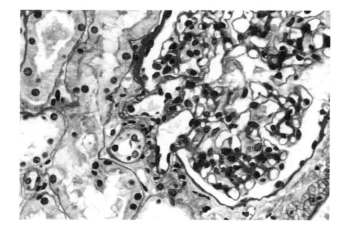

47. A 26-year-old man presents with a four-week history of bilateral leg swelling. He is known to have HIV infection 4 years ago but refuses treatment but is taking "Chinese herbal medicine". On examination, he is normotensive, BMI is 20 kg/m². There is bilateral pitting oedema. His initial investigation reveals nephrotic syndrome with proteinuria 11 g/day, serum albumin 10 g/L [34-48] and serum creatinine 89 μmol/L [60-110]. He is not anaemic. His CD4 cell count is 140/μL and HIV viral load is 120 000 copies/mL. Hepatitis B and C serology are negative. ANA, ds-DNA, ANCA are negative. Serum light chains levels are normal. Kidney USS reveals bilaterally enlarged but otherwise normal kidneys. The renal veins are patent. The kidney biopsy is most likely to show which glomerular disease?

Answers

1. Answer: B

Acute post-streptococcal glomerulonephritis (APSGN) is caused by immune-mediated glomerular injury due to the host's response to bacterial infection. Although the incidence of APSGN has declined in most parts of Australia and other developed countries, the Aboriginal community continues to have the highest documented global rate of APSGN. It is a disease associated with poverty and social disadvantage. It most commonly affects children but can occur at any age. In Aboriginal communities, outbreaks of APSGN are usually caused by specific strains of group A streptococci (GAS). APSGN is a major risk factor for the development of CKD in the Indigenous population, especially in adults.

A probable diagnosis of APSGN can be suspected if the patient has at least two of the following:
- Facial oedema and/or peripheral oedema
- Hypertension
- Haematuria on dipstick (2+ red blood cells).

APSGN can be confirmed in a probable case if the patient has the following:
- Haematuria on microscopy
- Evidence of recent streptococcal infection [positive Group A Streptococcal culture from skin or throat, or elevated anti-streptolysin O (ASO) titre or Anti-DNase B]
- Reduced C3 level.

In patients with a provisional diagnosis of APSGN, one must examine their skin for evidence of skin sores or scabies. If skin sores are present, swabs should be taken from two different skin sores. If indicated on history, a throat swab should be taken for identification of GAS. Blood should be collected to check renal function, ASOT, anti-DNase B titres, C3 and C4. All clinical cases of APSGN should be given intramuscular benzathine penicillin regardless of whether skin sores or pharyngitis are present at the time of presentation. All clinical cases of APSGN with severe hypertension should be considered for hospitalisation. All cases should be medically reviewed no later than 6-8 weeks after discharge or identification.

Every case of APSGN requires notification, contact identification, and contact tracing. Names of family, household, and close contacts of the suspected case including adults and children who have been staying in the household 2 weeks prior to the onset of APSGN should be collected. This is essential to assist with prompt contact tracing if the case is confirmed.

Subclinical cases usually have only one clinical symptom and may not have hypertension but on laboratory investigation are found to have haematuria, evidence of a streptococcal infection, and a reduced C3. Possible subclinical cases can be found when screening individuals who have been contacts of a case of APSGN. They are usually caused by specific strains of GAS, which can spread very quickly, thus resulting in many cases of APSGN particularly among children.

 Chaturvedi S, Boyd R, Krause V. Acute Post-Streptococcal Glomerulonephritis in the Northern Territory of Australia: A Review of Data from 2009 to 2016 and Comparison with the Literature. The American Journal of Tropical Medicine and Hygiene. 2018;99(6):1643–1648.
http://www.ajtmh.org/content/journals/10.4269/ajtmh.18-0093

2. Answer: B

Autosomal dominant polycystic kidney disease (ADPKD) is the fourth leading cause of ESKD in adults. Patients with ADPKD often experience symptoms of hypertension, abdominal fullness, haematuria, pain from the cysts, back pain, urinary tract infection, nephrosclerosis, liver cysts, pancreatic cysts, hernias, diverticulosis, mitral valve prolapse, cardiovascular complications, and intracranial aneurysms. Once progression of CKD begins, the mean decline in eGFR is approximately 4-6 ml/min/1.73 m^2 per year. 50% of patients with ADPKD develop ESKD by the age of 60.

In patients with genetic deficiency in genes encoding polycystin 1 (PKD1) and polycystin 2 (PKD2), tubular epithelial cells in the vasopressin-sensitive distal nephrons and collecting ducts show enhanced proliferation causing development of the cysts associated with an elevated level of cyclic adenosine monophosphate (cAMP) and destruction of the renal parenchyma. Tolvaptan is a vasopressin V2-receptor antagonist which decreases cAMP within cells.

The Tolvaptan Efficacy and Safety in Management of Autosomal Dominant Polycystic Kidney Disease and Its Outcomes, (TEMPO) trial, showed that in patients with an eGFR > 60 ml/min/1.73 m^2 , tolvaptan slowed the rate of kidney growth and reduced the decline in eGFR. However, more participants in the tolvaptan group in comparison to the placebo group discontinued the medication due to adverse events related to polyuria, polydipsia, nocturia, and urinary frequency. Reversible elevated liver enzyme levels after cessation of tolvaptan were also observed in the tolvaptan treatment group. The subsequent REPRISE (Replicating Evidence of Preserved Renal Function: an Investigation of Tolvaptan Safety and Efficacy in ADPKD) trial found tolvaptan led to a slower rate of decline in kidney function than placebo over a period of up to 12 months in patients with more advanced CKD from stage 2 to stage 4 (mean eGFR 41 ml/min/1.73 m^2).

Patients who are on tolvaptan treatment require routine liver enzyme test monitoring, initially monthly for a total duration of 18 months then every 3 months. Patients need to maintain adequate oral hydration due to its side effect of polyuria to avoid dehydration. It is unclear whether enhanced water intake might produce similar benefits.

Ingelfinger J. Tolvaptan and Autosomal Dominant Polycystic Kidney Disease. New England Journal of Medicine. 2017;377(20):1988–1989.
https://www.nejm.org/doi/10.1056/NEJMe1714276

3. Answer: A

Systemic disorders of bone and mineral metabolism due to CKD has been redefined as CKD-MBD by the Kidney Disease Improving Global Outcomes (KDIGO) group. These disorders include osteitis fibrosa cystica (OFC), osteomalacia, adynamic bone disease (ADB), and mixed lesions. In cases of unclear type of CKD-MBD, bone biopsy is the gold standard to determine the underlying aetiology and is used to guide treatment. However, a bone biopsy is invasive, not always readily available, and not often used.

ADB is the most prevalent type of CKD-MBD among patients with CKD, with a prevalence of 18% in those with CKD stage 3 to 5 CKD. ADB is a condition of low bone turnover in the absence of aluminium overload, whereas OFC is a condition of high bone turnover. Patients are typically asymptomatic at the time of diagnosis although some may have bone pain. They can present with fragility fractures, hypercalcaemia, and vascular calcification, the latter of which is associated with increased morbidity and mortality.

ABD is characterised by a reduced number of osteoclasts and osteoblasts without osteoid accumulation on bone histology. In contrast, OFC is a disorder characterised by increased bone turnover with a subsequent increase in bone formation and resorption. ABD is due to either the resistance of PTH on bone metabolism or the oversuppression of PTH release. The use of calcium-containing phosphate binders, calcimimetics, high dialysate calcium, active vitamin D analogues, and the presence of increased age and diabetes, have all been identified as risk factors for ABD. Currently, KDIGO recommends a target PTH levels at two to nine times the upper limit of normal.

Among dialysis patients, ADB is suggested by a persistently low intact serum PTH and hypercalcaemia. Among patients who are not on dialysis, the diagnosis of ADB is suggested by a PTH concentration that was initially high and progressively decreases to less than the upper limit of normal for the PTH assay in the setting of treatment with active vitamin D analogues. All patients with ABD have a normal or low bone-specific alkaline phosphatase (BSAP). However, routine testing of bone turnover markers such as BSAP and serum C-telopeptide crosslink, or bone imaging such as X-ray and dual-energy X-ray absorptiometry are not recommended since these tests do not reliably distinguish between the various types of renal bone diseases.

To allow the PTH to increase, ABD should be treated by using non-calcium-containing phosphate binders rather than calcium-containing phosphate binders, using a low calcium dialysate for patients on haemodialysis, and by reducing the dose or stopping calcitriol.

Sista S, Arum S. Management of adynamic bone disease in chronic kidney disease: A brief review. Journal of Clinical & Translational Endocrinology. 2016; 5:32–35.
https://www.ncbi.nlm.nih.gov/pmc/articles/PMC5644430/

4. Answer: D

Cellulitis presents as erythema, swelling and pain/discomfort. A lack of reliable microbiologic and laboratory gold standards combined with bedside diagnostic uncertainty makes it difficult to distinguish cellulitis from non-infectious causes of pseudocellulitis, which includes chronic venous stasis, lymphoedema, and lipodermatosclerosis. Bilateral lower leg cellulitis is very rare, so you should think of differential diagnosis or other non-infectious causes before starting antibiotics. This patient should not have been treated with flucloxacillin as it is a typical lipodermatosclerosis. The patient has no other symptoms to suggest infection; in particular, her CRP and WBC were normal.

Lipodermatosclerosis can be acute or chronic. Acute lipodermatosclerosis is often tender and bright red in colour and occurs with or without oedema as shown in the picture. Systemic symptoms and signs of infection are absent. Treatment includes compression stockings, weight reduction, ultrasound therapy, topical steroid ointment, and medications such as pentoxifylline. There is no role for antibiotics.

Acute interstitial nephritis (AIN) is an important cause of AKI resulting from immune-mediated tubulointerstitial injury. It can be caused by drugs, infection, and other causes. It is the cause of AKI in about 15% of patients hospitalised for AKI.

Drug hypersensitivity accounts for 75% of AIN. All drugs can cause interstitial nephritis, but the common ones are:
- Antibiotics: penicillin, cephalosporins, ciprofloxacin, rifampicin, sulphonamides, vancomycin, and acyclovir
- NSAIDs
- Diuretics: frusemide, thiazides

- Allopurinol
- Proton pump inhibitors (PPIs)
- Cocaine
- Carbamazepine.

Drug-induced AIN is characterised by slowly worsening renal function, usually 7 to 10 days after exposure. However, it can occur within 1 day of exposure if the patient has been exposed previously. It can also occur months after exposure, especially with PPIs.

This patient's clinical features are consistent with drug-induced AIN, especially the temporal relationship with the commencement of flucloxacillin and WBC casts on urine microscopy. Discontinuation of the offending drug is the mainstay of treatment. Most patients will recover and there is no need to perform kidney biopsy or give glucocorticoids immediately, and close follow-up is usually adequate. Kidney biopsy is only indicated in the setting of inconsistent clinical and investigation findings or if renal function does not improve immediately after ceasing the offending drug. The role of glucocorticoids remains controversial and they are generally reserved for patients who do not respond to discontinuation of the offending medication.

 Moledina D, Perazella M. Drug-Induced Acute Interstitial Nephritis. Clinical Journal of the American Society of Nephrology. 2017;12(12):2046–2049.
https://cjasn.asnjournals.org/content/12/12/2046

 [Internet]. Choosing Wisely: Don't routinely use antibiotics to treat bilateral swelling and redness of the lower leg unless there is clear evidence of infection. Aafp.org. 2019 [cited 18 August 2019]. Available from:
https://www.aafp.org/afp/recommendations/viewRecommendation.htm?recommendationId=287

5. Answer: B

A retrospective population-based study of AKI events in the Kimberley region of Western Australia identified the age distribution of AKI events in the Aboriginal and Torres Strait Islander residents was skewed to younger groups in comparison to national data on AKI. Infections were identified in 59% of patients (324 AKI events) with AKI, with pneumonia (12% of the events), skin, subcutaneous tissue (10%), and urinary tract infections (7.7%) the leading causes.

Streptococcal skin infections are associated with acute post-infectious glomerulonephritis and CKD. Risk factors for skin infections among Indigenous Australians in rural and remote areas include housing problems, overcrowding as environmental risk factors, and access to health care. Acute dialysis service and intensive care unit care are not available in some of the rural and remote areas in Australia.

In 2013 to 2014, there were 186,268 hospitalisations for acute dialysis of Indigenous Australians, a rate ten times higher than that for other Australians. As AKI is a risk factor for CKD, prevention of skin infections and AKI is important in the community health setting to minimise hospitalisations, development of CKD, reliance on hospital-based dialysis treatment, and to improve health outcomes of Indigenous Australians.

 Mohan J, Atkinson D, Rosman J, Griffiths E. Acute kidney injury in Indigenous Australians in the Kimberley: age distribution and associated diagnoses. Medical Journal of Australia. 2019;211(1):19–23.
https://www.mja.com.au/journal/2019/211/1/acute-kidney-injury-indigenous-australians-kimberley-age-distribution-and

 Cass A, Hughes J. Acute kidney injury in Indigenous Australians: an unrecognised priority for action. Medical Journal of Australia. 2019;211(1):14–15.
https://www.mja.com.au/journal/2019/211/1/acute-kidney-injury-indigenous-australians-unrecognised-priority-action

6. Answer: B

Pre-formed donor-specific anti-HLA antibodies, which were present before transplantation, donor-specific anti-HLA antibodies that form after transplantation and many non-HLA antibodies are found in patients with a diagnosis of antibody-mediated rejection (AMR). AMR is now recognised to be a disease process that can happen at any time post-transplantation with different severity. Activation of the classical complement cascade can lead to allograft damage, dysfunction, and loss.

Microvascular inflammation in the renal allograft is typically observed in patients with AMR. These changes include capillary dilatation, the presence of inflammatory cells, enlargement and vacuolization of the endothelial cells, and cytoplasmic swelling. Chronic vascular lesions are seen in the glomeruli, peritubular capillary basement membrane, and arterioles. Macrovascular lesions are also increasingly recognised, including mild or severe intimal arteritis, the presence of inflammatory cells in the intima, with or without transmural necrosis.

C4d, an endothelial membrane-associated complement split product, is a specific marker of AMR in renal allografts the stain is deposited in the capillaries. However, C4d is not a sensitive marker in patients with AMR since about 50% of patients with AMR have negative C4d staining.

Current treatment of AMR includes removal of circulating donor-specific anti-HLA antibodies and reduction of antibody production. Plasma exchange, IVIG, or both, and corticosteroids are mainstays of treatment options. However, more clinical trials are required to identify the best treatment regimen for AMR to improve long-term outcome.

7. Answer: B

Loupy A, Lefaucheur C. Antibody-Mediated Rejection of Solid-Organ Allografts. New England Journal of Medicine. 2018;379(12):1150–1160.
https://www.nejm.org/doi/full/10.1056/NEJMra1802677

Anti–glomerular basement membrane (anti-GBM) disease is a rare small vessel vasculitis affecting the capillaries in the lungs and the kidneys. It is an autoimmune disease in which pathogenic autoantibodies target autoantigens are expressed in the basement membrane of one or both of these organs. It has a bimodal age distribution, with peak incidences in the third decade and in the sixth and seventh decades. Infections such as Influenza A, upper and lower respiratory tract infections may trigger the disease in genetically susceptible patients. There is a strong HLA-gene association, with approximately 80% of patients inheriting an HLA-DR2 haplotype. Pulmonary haemorrhage is more commonly reported in patients with a smoking history or inhalation of hydrocarbon.

Although it is a rare disease, timely recognition, diagnosis, and initiation of treatment may significantly improve survival rate and reduce morbidity and mortality.

The majority (80 – 90%) of patients present with features of rapidly progressive glomerulonephritis (RPGN) with widespread crescent formation of uniform age and glomerular necrosis such as in this case. Around 50% of patients also present with alveolar haemorrhage. A small minority of patients may present with only pulmonary disease.

Urgent serologic testing for anti-GBM antibodies should be undertaken, particularly if there are any contraindications to renal biopsy. Urgent renal biopsy should be considered since serology test results may not be immediately available. Direct immunofluorescence for IgG on a renal biopsy showing a typical strong linear ribbon-like appearance is a typical finding of anti-GBM disease. Renal biopsy can also exclude other concomitant renal pathologies such as ANCA-associated vasculitis and membranous nephropathy. Lung biopsy results are rarely helpful in making the diagnosis of anti GBM disease.

The aim of treatment is to rapidly remove pathogenic autoantibodies and to inhibit further production of new autoantibodies by suppressing the immune system.

The latest Kidney Disease Improving Global Outcomes (KDIGO) guideline recommends the following treatment regimen for anti-GBM glomerulonephritis:

- Plasma exchange
- Oral cyclophosphamide
- Oral corticosteroids
- Prophylaxis treatments for oropharyngeal fungal infection, peptic ulcer disease, *Pneumocystis jiroveci* pneumonia, CMV infection and hepatitis B viral infection, osteoporosis whilst on long-term corticosteroids treatment.

IV methylprednisolone, cyclophosphamide, and plasma exchange are the first line treatment. Mycophenolate mofetil, cyclosporin, and rituximab currently have insufficient data to support them as first-line therapy but may be used in patients who have contraindications or intolerance to oral cyclophosphamide therapy.

Current recommendation for cytotoxic treatment is 3 months. Relapse of the disease is linked to ongoing use of pulmonary irritants such as cigarette smoke and hydrocarbons. The risk of relapse of anti-GBM disease is usually low.

Poor renal outcome is predicted by the severity of renal dysfunction, oligoanuria at presentation, and the proportion of glomeruli affected by crescents. Some patients may require dialysis or ventilatory support.

It is uncommon to have recurrence of anti-GBM disease post-renal transplantation if the patients have at least 6 months of sustained negative serological tests for anti-GBM antibodies prior to transplantation and good adherence to standard immunosuppressive medications. However, *de novo* anti-GBM disease post-renal transplantation for patients with Alport's syndrome is a well-recognised phenomenon.

McAdoo S, Pusey C. Anti-Glomerular Basement Membrane Disease. Clinical Journal of the American Society of Nephrology. 2017;12(7):1162–1172.
https://cjasn.asnjournals.org/content/12/7/1162

8. Answer: A

C3 glomerulopathy is a group of rare diseases with an incidence of one to two cases per million with an equal distribution between genders. C3 glomerulopathy can be divided into three subgroups: dense deposit disease (DDD), C3 glomerulonephritis, and the complement factor H-related 5 (CFHR5) glomerulopathy. Some cases of C3 glomerulopathy are associated with genetic mutations (abnormal genes for factors H and I and membrane cofactor protein) while others are associated with antibodies that either block inhibitory complement components (e.g., antibodies to factor H) or slow the activation of the alternative complement cascade or have antibodies that accelerate the alternative complement pathway (e.g., C3 nephritic factor).

These renal diseases are characterised by abnormal action of the alternative complement pathway with abnormal deposition of C3 in the glomeruli and variable progression to ESKD. In some cases, C3 glomerulopathy may develop after upper respiratory tract infection. Clinical presentations are heterogenous and may include micro- or macroscopic haematuria, microalbuminuria to nephrotic-range proteinuria, hypertension, and progressive renal failure. The diagnosis is based on history, family history, complementary studies, and renal biopsy. The key finding on biopsy is isolated C3 deposition in the glomeruli.

STING pathway is a signalling hub in innate immunity. It orchestrates the response to pathogenic, tumour, or self-DNA in the cytoplasm and autoimmune process. Currently there is no evidence that STING pathway plays a role in the pathogenesis of C3 glomerulopathy.

The lectin pathway is one of three pathways by which the complement system can be activated. Upon activation, it proceeds through the action of C4 and C2 to produce activated complement proteins further down the cascade. In contrast to the classical complement pathway, the lectin pathway does not recognises an antibody bound to its target. Subsequent activation of complement cascade leads to opsonisation, phagocytosis, and lysis of target microorganisms through the formation of the membrane-attack complex. It may induce several inflammatory effects, such as expression of adhesion molecules, chemotaxis and activation of leukocytes, release of reactive oxygen species, and secretion of cytokines and chemokines. The lectin pathway starts with mannose-binding lectin (MBL) or ficolin binding to certain sugars. Patients with MBL deficiency are prone to recurrent infections, including infections of the upper respiratory tract and other body systems.

Immunosuppressants (corticosteroids, cyclophosphamide, mycophenolate mofetil and rituximab) and the monoclonal antibody eculizumab have been used to treat C3 glomerulopathy with variable success. Some cases are also treated with plasma exchange. With eculizumab, there is an increased risk of meningococcal infection and it is crucial to ensure vaccinations is up to date. Vaccinations against *Streptococcus pneumoniae*, *Neisseria meningitides*, and *Haemophilus influenzae* are important to prevent infection in patients receiving immunosuppressants or anticomplement agents. (vaccinate at least 2 weeks before starting eculizumab; if vaccinating after this time, give prophylactic antibiotics for 2 weeks) and monitor for meningococcal infection during treatment.

Due to the rarity of this disease group, knowledge regarding its natural history is sparse and specific treatments for each subgroup remain to be determined. Current recommendations are drawn from observational studies and case series. Large, randomised trials are necessary to establish the ideal treatment regimen for each subgroup of C3 glomerulopathy.

Schena F, Esposito P, Rossini M. A Narrative Review on C3 Glomerulopathy: A Rare Renal Disease. International Journal of Molecular Sciences. 2020;21(2):525.
https://www.mdpi.com/1422-0067/21/2/525

Barbour T, Pickering M, Cook H. Recent insights into C3 glomerulopathy. Nephrology Dialysis Transplantation. 2013;28(7):1685–1693.
https://academic.oup.com/ndt/article/28/7/1685/1854991

9. Answer: D

Calciphylaxis, also known as calcific uremic arteriolopathy is a rare, life-threatening condition involving occlusion of microvasculature in the subcutaneous adipose tissue and dermis causing skin ischaemia and severe pain. It is sometimes accompanied by tactile hyperesthesia. It is an under-recognised skin condition, affecting mostly patients with ESKD who often have extraskeletal calcification.

The interval between the initiation of dialysis and the appearance of calciphylaxis ranges from 30 to 105 months. Patients treated with peritoneal dialysis have a higher incidence of calciphylaxis than patients treated with haemodialysis. Risk factors for calciphylaxis include ESKD, obesity, diabetes, female gender, dialysis-dependence for more than 2 years, repetitive skin trauma from subcutaneous injections, elevation in calcium or phosphate levels, primary/secondary hyperparathyroidism, over-suppressed PTH levels with adynamic bone disease, elevated alkaline phosphatase levels, Vitamin K deficiency, warfarin use, hepatobiliary disease, thrombophilia, SLE, hypoalbuminaemia, metastatic cancer, recurrent hypotension, rapid weight loss, exposure to ultraviolet light, exposure to aluminum, and elevated FGF-23 levels.

Warfarin, a Vitamin K antagonist which blocks MGP carboxylation, promotes vascular smooth muscle cell transdifferentiation and matrix mineralisation. Warfarin use increases the risk of calciphylaxis by 3- to 13-fold. Vitamin K deficiency from malabsorption and other causes may also play a role.

Once the diagnosis of calciphylaxis is made, patient survival is usually < 1 year. The presence of ulcerated skin lesions reduces the 6-month survival rate to 20%. Calciphylaxis has also been described in patients with CKD, AKI, in patients with prior renal transplant, and even rarely in patients with normal renal function.

Sepsis due to wound infection is the most common cause of death in patients with calciphylaxis. It is a debilitating condition that compromises quality of life. Patients report symptoms of pain, insomnia, nausea, anorexia, depression, and are often wheelchair-bound, bedridden, or require hospitalisations for symptom management.

Skin biopsy is the standard way to make the diagnosis of clinically suspected calciphylaxis. However, there is some risk of provoking new, non-healing ulcers and infection. Biopsy is contraindicated for acral, penile, or infected lesions.

It is important to seek advice from pain specialists in patients with intense pain from calciphylaxis. Operative debridement accompanied by negative-pressure wound therapy is recommended for patients with infected wound and large necrotic areas with drainage. In patients with peripheral lesions, hyperbaric oxygen therapy can be considered. Intake of Vitamin D and calcium should be eliminated. In patients with hyperparathyroidism, a calcimimetic agent or parathyroidectomy can be considered.

Intensified haemodialysis to increase the frequency or length of haemodialysis (more than the usual four hours per session, three times a week regimen) is recommended in haemodialysis patients with calciphylaxis to manage elevated calcium, phosphate, and parathyroid hormone levels. In ESKD patients on peritoneal dialysis, consider changing the patients from peritoneal dialysis to haemodialysis to accelerate wound healing. Consider stopping warfarin and changing to alternative anticoagulants if appropriate. If subcutaneous injections cannot be avoided, injection sites should be rotated to avoid repetitive trauma to the same area. Intravenous sodium thiosulfate has an increasingly favourable profile in management, but prospective randomised control trials are lacking. It has both cation-chelating and antioxidant properties. The chelation of calcium produces calcium thiosulfate, which may be more soluble than other calcium salts and, therefore, more readily cleared from the body. Sodium thiosulfate demonstrates beneficial effects in some patients, with partial to complete resolution of skin lesions

Nigwekar S, Thadhani R, Brandenburg V. Calciphylaxis. New England Journal of Medicine. 2018;378(18):1704–1714. https://www.nejm.org/doi/10.1056/NEJMra1505292

10. Answer: C

Current Kidney Disease Improving Global Outcomes (KDIGO) guidelines do not recommend routine measurement of bone turnover biomarkers in CKD patients. There is difficulty in interpretation of biomarkers of bone metabolism in CKD resulting from their use during the application of multiple simultaneous therapies, all of which can alter biomarkers of bone metabolism independent of other factors. Furthermore, the biomarkers cannot reliably determine the differing bony pathologies that may be present in CKD that include osteomalacia, adynamic bone disease, osteoporosis and renal osteodystrophy.

Dual-energy X-ray absorptiometry bone mineral density (DEXA BMD) scan can be considered in patients with CKD G3a–G5D with evidence of CKD-MBD and/or risk factors for osteoporosis if the results will impact treatment decisions. However, a low DEXA BMD result is unable to distinguish the type of renal osteodystrophy, which is defined by abnormal bone histology. Bone biopsy is the gold standard for the diagnosis and classification of renal osteodystrophy and this procedure can be considered if the results will impact on treatment decisions. Bone biopsy can be considered in patients with unexplained fractures, persistent bone pain, unexplained hypercalcaemia, unexplained hypophosphataemia, and possible aluminum toxicity to guide appropriate treatment.

Calcimimetics favorably alter serum calcium and PTH in hyperparathyroidism but do not significantly affect either bone turnover or BMD. Emerging evidence has suggested that calcium-based phosphate binders can worsen vascular calcification and restricting the dose of calcium-based phosphate binders is recommended in patients with CKD G3a-G5. Non-calcium-based phosphate binders are preferred but are considerably more expensive. Phosphate-lowering treatment includes low-phosphate diet, use of phosphate binders, and dialysis. It is not only limited to using phosphate-lowering medications.

Use of calcitriol and Vitamin D analogs should be reserved for patients with severe and progressive hyperparathyroidism in CKD G4–G5 and not routinely used in patients with CKD G3a–G5 not on dialysis due to significant risks of hypercalcaemia associated with use of the medication(s) compared to placebo in trials. Moderate PTH elevation may represent an appropriate adaptive response and does not require treatment.

Ketteler M, Block G, Evenepoel P, Fukagawa M, Herzog C, McCann L et al. Executive summary of the 2017 KDIGO Chronic Kidney Disease–Mineral and Bone Disorder (CKD-MBD) Guideline Update: what's changed and why it matters. Kidney International. 2017;92(1):26–36.
https://www.kidney-international.org/article/S0085-2538(17)30249-1/fulltext

11. Answer: C

Decisions about when to start dialysis remain complex and should be individualised to the patient. Options for renal replacement therapy (RRT) include haemodialysis, peritoneal dialysis, renal transplantation (usually after initiation of dialysis), and conservative or supportive care. Patient preference, frailty, medical comorbidities, place of residence, functional level, ability to provide self-care, family/carer's support, distance to the hospital, transport support, etc. are some of the factors to consider in determining the best treatment pathway for patients with ESKD.

Early referral of patients with CKD to nephrologists is important to identify and treat reversible cause(s) of CKD, optimise blood pressure, and symptom control, and to prepare for dialysis access if the patients are for dialysis in the future, and to identify patients who are potential transplant recipients. Increased morbidity, mortality, increased health care costs, and lower quality of life are associated with late referrals to nephrologists.

Absolute indications for dialysis in suitable candidates include symptoms related to uraemia such as uraemic pericarditis, encephalopathy, and bleeding diathesis. Common indications for dialysis include persistent fluid overload despite diuretics treatment; metabolic acidosis, hyperkalaemia, and hyperphosphataemia refractory to medical treatment; symptomatic uraemia such as nausea, vomiting, profound fatigue, and pruritus.

The Initiating Dialysis Early and Late (IDEAL) study found early dialysis initiation (i.e., at an eGFR > 10 mL/min/1.73m^2) was not associated with a morbidity and mortality benefit. In patients with stage 5 CKD who are asymptomatic, dialysis may be safely deferred until the eGFR is between 5–7 mL/min/1.73m^2 provided there is careful follow-up and adequate patient education to present to the hospital if they experience significant uraemic or fluid overload symptoms associated with ESKD.

Discussion about options for RRT with the patient and the patient's family is important to ensure success of the treatment, minimise complications, and improve quality of life.

If a patient chooses haemodialysis, it is important to refer for creation of an arteriovenous (AV) fistula/graft. Two to three months are usually required before an AV fistula can be used successfully. AV graft can be used soon after creation. Haemodialysis patients with a tunneled catheter have a two- to three fold increased risk of hospitalisations for infection and death compared with patients with an AV fistula or graft.

If patient opts for peritoneal dialysis (PD), patient will require Tenckhoff catheter placement, home visits by the dialysis staff, and training prior to the commencement of PD. Early discussion and consideration of the PD catheter referral is important to ensure a seamless commencement of PD.

Elderly patients with multiple comorbidities, nursing home resident status, frailty, lack of family/social support, and poor quality of life may be suitable candidates for conservative management in case of ESKD. Dialysis may not improve survival and may in fact increase morbidity, mortality, and worsen quality of life in these elderly patients.

Chen T, Lee V, Harris D. When to initiate dialysis for end-stage kidney disease: evidence and challenges. Medical Journal of Australia. 2018;209(6):275–279.
https://www.mja.com.au/journal/2018/209/6/when-initiate-dialysis-end-stage-kidney-disease-evidence-and-challenges

Brown M, Collett G, Josland E, Foote C, Li Q, Brennan F. CKD in Elderly Patients Managed without Dialysis: Survival, Symptoms, and Quality of Life. Clinical Journal of the American Society of Nephrology. 2015;10(2):260–268.
https://www.ncbi.nlm.nih.gov/pmc/articles/PMC4317735/

12. Answer: D

Potassium is the most abundant intracellular cation and is critical in many physiological functions. Serum potassium concentrations of 3.5–5.5 mmol/L are maintained by distinct renal and extrarenal mechanisms. Hyperkalaemia (potassium ≥ 6 mmol/L) can be a life-threatening condition. Common causes for hyperkalaemia include:

1. Excessive dietary intake in patients with CKD or AKI
2. Impaired elimination of potassium:
   - AKI or CKD leading to decreased renal excretion of potassium
   - Medications interfering with urinary potassium excretion (Table 15.1)
   - Primary or secondary hypoaldosteronism resulting in hyperkalaemia
   - Pseudohypoaldosteronism, a heterogeneous group of disorders characterised by hyperkalaemia, metabolic acidosis, and normal eGFR
   - Congenital adrenal hyperplasia
   - Distal tubular defect.

3. Redistribution of cellular potassium:
- Tissue injury
- Insulin deficiency
- Exercise
- Metabolic acidosis
- Hypertonic states.

Table 15.1 Commonly used medications that can cause hyperkalaemia and their mechanism.

Medication	Mechanism
ACE inhibitors, Angiotensin-II receptor antagonists	Reduces adrenal aldosterone biosynthesis through interrupting the renin-aldosterone axis Reduces effective glomerular filtration rate
Amiloride	Blocks sodium channels of luminal membrane of principal cells
Beta-blockers	Inhibits renin secretion Decreases cellular potassium uptake
Cyclosporin	Inhibits adrenal aldosterone biosynthesis Induces chloride channel shunt Increases potassium efflux from cells
Digoxin	Inhibits Na$^+$/K$^+$-ATPase
Heparin	Inhibits adrenal aldosterone biosynthesis Decreases number and affinity of angiotensin-II receptors
NSAIDs	Induces hyporeninemic hypoaldosteronism through inhibiting renal prostaglandin synthesis
Spironolactone	Mineralocorticoid receptor antagonist (competing with aldosterone) Inhibits adrenal aldosterone biosynthesis
Succinylcholine	Causes leakage of potassium out of cells through depolarisation of cell membranes
Tacrolimus	Inhibits adrenal aldosterone biosynthesis Induces chloride channel shunt Increases potassium efflux from cells
Trimethoprim	Blocks sodium channels in the luminal membrane of principal cells

 Palmer B, Clegg D. Diagnosis and treatment of hyperkalemia. Cleveland Clinic Journal of Medicine. 2017;84(12):934–942. https://www.mdedge.com/ccjm/article/152856/nephrology/diagnosis-and-treatment-hyperkalemia

13. Answer: D

This patient's clinical presentation is consistent with IgA nephropathy (IgAN). It can present with macroscopic haematuria immediately following upper respiratory tract infections, so called 'synpharyngitic nephritis' or 'synpharyngitic macroscopic haematuria'. This syndrome occurs in approximately 10–15% of IgAN and predominantly in patients under the age of 40. This is distinguished from post-streptococcal glomerulonephritis that occurs approximately 2 weeks after the pharyngitis or skin infection. Serum complement levels are normal in IgAN.

IgAN is the most common glomerulonephritis globally and is a leading cause of CKD and ESKD. A central finding in patients with IgAN is the presence of circulating and glomerular immune complexes comprised of galactose-deficient IgA1, an IgG autoantibody directed against the hinge region O-glycans, and C3.

The Oxford classification has been used in clinical-pathologic correlation in IgAN which includes mesangial hypercellularity (M), endocapillary hypercellularity (E), segmental glomerulosclerosis (S), tubular atrophy (T), MEST, and crescents (C).

Patients with IgAN who develop progressive disease typically have one or more of the following clinical or laboratory findings at the time of diagnosis, each of which is a marker for more severe disease and poor prognosis:
- Elevated serum creatinine
- Hypertension (>140/90 mmHg)
- Proteinuria above 1g/day.

Patients who have recurrent episodes of gross haematuria without proteinuria are at low risk for progressive kidney disease compared with patients who have persistent microscopic haematuria and proteinuria. This patient with IgAN has glomerular haematuria therefore, it is not surprising to see RBC casts and the presence of RBC casts is not a poor prognostic factor. However, persistent microscopic haematuria (especially with proteinuria) at presentation may be associated with progressive disease over time. The findings from renal biopsy (MEST-C score) can provide prognosis and identify patients who require treatment.

Rodrigues J, Haas M, Reich H. IgA Nephropathy. Clinical Journal of the American Society of Nephrology. 2017; 12(4):677–686.
https://cjasn.asnjournals.org/content/12/4/677

14. Answer: A

Lithium remains a key medication in the management of bipolar affective disorder (BPAD). It is indicated for treatment of acute mania, prevention of manic or depressive episodes in BPAD as well as schizoaffective disorder. The onset of action of lithium for severe mania may be delayed for 6 to 10 days. When initiating lithium treatment, consider adding a benzodiazepine or antipsychotic to control acute symptoms.

Lithium's exact mode of action is unknown, but it can inhibit dopamine release, enhance serotonin release, and decrease formation of intracellular second messengers.

Lithium has a narrow therapeutic index. The therapeutic range during acute mania is 0.5 to 1.2 mmol/L and the therapeutic range for prophylaxis is 0.4 to 1 mmol/L. Symptoms of lithium toxicity are commonly observed when the lithium level is > 1.5 mmol/L (> 1.2 mmol/L in the elderly). Sometimes symptoms of toxicity are noted at lower lithium concentrations in patients with organic neurological damage.

Polyuria and polydipsia are among the most common adverse effects associated with lithium usage (around 70% in long-term patients). Lithium interferes with the collecting tubules' ability to generate cyclic adenosine monophosphate (cAMP) in response to antidiuretic hormone (ADH) stimulation. As a result, kidneys do not respond to ADH and excessive diluted urine is lost (nephrogenic diabetes insipidus). This effect is initially reversible after cessation of lithium. However, chronic lithium use causes structural and irreversible changes.

Possible risk factors for polyuria/polydipsia associated with lithium use include duration of treatment, higher serum lithium levels, previous episodes of lithium intoxication, and the ingestion of antipsychotics. The optimal treatment for polyuria is prevention: keeping lithium levels at the lower end of therapeutic range, avoiding toxicity, and using once-daily lithium dosing before chronic structural damage occurs. In some cases, patients may still progress to ESKD. Amiloride can be a helpful remedy for lithium-induced polyuria.

Other common adverse effects of lithium include metallic taste, diarrhoea, muscle weakness, epigastric discomfort, weight gain, vertigo, leukocytosis, hypothyroidism (usually asymptomatic), hypercalcaemia, hyperparathyroidism, and benign T wave changes on ECG. In patients with severe lithium toxicity, increased muscle tone, hyperreflexia, myoclonic jerks, coarse tremor, dysarthria, disorientation, psychosis, seizures, and coma may be present. Infrequent side effects of lithium include memory impairment, arrythmias, hyperthyroidism, sexual dysfunction, and reduced libido.

Baseline ECG, weight, renal function, serum calcium (including ionised calcium), PTH, TFTs should be obtained and then repeat again every 3 to 6 months with lithium level (at least annually) to ensure no side effects/toxicity from lithium treatment. It is important to monitor serum lithium levels more frequently during acute illness, especially in patients with dehydration, CKD (use a lower therapeutic lithium level), AKI, gastroenteritis, concomitant diuretics/NSAIDs use, changes in weight, manic or depressive phases, and pregnancy.

Gitlin M. Lithium side effects and toxicity: prevalence and management strategies. International Journal of Bipolar Disorders. 2016;4(1).
https://journalbipolardisorders.springeropen.com/articles/10.1186/s40345-016-0068-y

15. Answer: A

Renal involvement in SLE is very common, with the most common presentation being proteinuria and renal impairment. Renal biopsy is important to determine the type and severity of lupus nephritis. Pathological classification uses the International Society of Nephrology/Renal Pathology Society (ISN/RPS) criteria. Classes III (mesangial and subendothelial immune complexes/segmental endocapillary proliferation in <50% glomeruli) and IV (mesangial and subendothelial immune complexes/segmental or global endocapillary proliferation in ≥ 50% of glomeruli) lupus nephritis typically warrant immunosuppressive treatment.

Current accepted treatment regimens are based on severity of disease, and typically involve high dose steroids and an additional immunosuppressive agent. The Kidney Disease: Improving Global Outcomes (KDIGO) clinical practice guidelines, American College of Rheumatology (ACR), and the joint European League Against Rheumatism and European Renal Association–European Dialysis and Transplant Association (EULAR/ERA–EDTA) guidelines recommend steroids combined with either cyclophosphamide or mycophenolate for induction therapy.

The decision between pulse IV methylprednisolone and high dose oral steroids hinges on whether the patient has severe active disease or not. The patient in this scenario has crescentic glomerulonephritis with AKI, therefore requires pulse IV methylprednisolone.

The decision between cyclophosphamide or mycophenolate is often guided by patient factors. A large international randomised controlled trial comparing IV cyclophosphamide to mycophenolate in patients with Class III to V lupus nephritis found no significant difference in urine protein/creatinine ratios or serum creatinine between groups. In women of childbearing age, mycophenolate is usually preferred due to the negative effect of cyclophosphamide on fertility but both agents carry risk of foetal malformation. Plasma exchange is not a recognised treatment for class IV lupus nephritis.

Almaani S, Meara A, Rovin B. Update on Lupus Nephritis. Clinical Journal of the American Society of Nephrology. 2016;12(5):825–835.
https://cjasn.asnjournals.org/content/12/5/825

Rovin B, Caster D, Cattran D, Gibson K, Hogan J, Moeller M et al. Management and treatment of glomerular diseases (part 2): conclusions from a Kidney Disease: Improving Global Outcomes (KDIGO) Controversies Conference. Kidney International. 2019;95(2):281–295.
https://iris.unito.it/retrieve/handle/2318/1689922/473486/KDIGOKI.pdf

16. Answer: A

Hyperkalaemia is a common, sometimes fatal electrolyte disturbance, often seen in patients with heart failure, AKI, or CKD. Acute treatment with insulin and dextrose causing intracellular translocation of potassium can be effective in the short-term, but they simply buy time until definitive potassium removal by dialysis or binding agents such as Resonium.

Patiromer is a non-absorbed, sodium-free potassium binding polymer that exchanges calcium for potassium in the GI tract, thereby increasing faecal potassium excretion and reducing serum potassium levels. Patiromer was approved in the USA and Europe in 2015 for the treatment of hyperkalaemia in adults. In clinical trials, patiromer reduced serum potassium levels and the risk of recurrent hyperkalaemia in patients with CKD and/or diabetic nephropathy with or without CCF, allowing the majority of patients to continue receiving renin-angiotensin-aldosterone system (RAAS) inhibitors. GI disorders and hypomagnesaemia were the most common adverse events; patiromer can cause hypomagnesaemia as it can bind magnesium or divalent cations. These were generally of mild or moderate severity. Therefore, oral patiromer is a valuable treatment option for the long-term management of hyperkalaemia.

Sodium zirconium cyclosilicate (ZS-9), a novel, non-absorbed, potassium-selective cation exchanger, has demonstrated activity in acutely lowering and maintaining normal potassium levels. It was approved for medical use in the Europe and the USA in 2018.

The main characteristics of Patiromer and Sodium zirconium cyclosilicate are summarised as below:

	Patiromer	Sodium zirconium cyclosilicate
Mechanism of action	Non-specific cation binding in exchange for calcium	Selective potassium binding in exchange for sodium and hydrogen
Location of action	Distal colon	Upper and lower GI tract
Onset of effect	7 hours	2.2 hours
Drug-drug interaction	Yes, must be taken 3 hours before or after other oral drugs	No
Main side effects	Hypomagnesaemia and GI side effects	Peripheral oedema and GI side effects

Rosano G, Spoletini I, Agewall S. Pharmacology of new treatments for hyperkalaemia: patiromer and sodium zirconium cyclosilicate. European Heart Journal Supplements. 2019;21(Supplement_A): A28–A33.
https://academic.oup.com/eurheartjsupp/article/21/Supplement_A/A28/5364191

17. Answer: B

Membranous nephropathy (MN) is the most common cause of nephrotic syndrome in non-diabetic patients over 40 years of age. MN has heterogenous presentation and clinical course. Initial features can include proteinuria (either with nephrotic-range or sub-nephrotic range proteinuria), microscopic haematuria, normal or impaired renal function, hypertension, nephrotic syndrome, hyperlipidaemia, and thromboembolic complications.

MN is divided into primary/idiopathic MN (around 70–80% of the patients) and secondary MN depending on the underlying cause or diagnosis. Secondary causes of MN include, but are not limited to, lupus nephritis, hepatitis B, hepatitis C, malignancy (lung, colon, stomach, and kidney) and medications (NSAIDs, gold, and penicillamine).

A renal biopsy is important to diagnose MN. Light microscopy may show late changes such as homogeneous thickening of capillary walls. Silver staining may show immune complex deposition in basement membrane giving rise to a characteristic 'spike and hole' appearance. Granular staining for IgG by immunofluorescence is noted in the subepithelial location. Electron microscopy shows electron-dense deposits in glomerular basement membrane in the subepithelial regions. Spike formation is indicative of new basement membrane material being laid between immune deposits.

Secondary MN is treated by addressing the underlying cause, whereas immunosuppressants are used to treat primary MN, including prednisolone, calcineurin inhibitors (CNIs), and rituximab can be appropriate therapies.

Complement C3 and C4 levels are usually normal in primary MN and low in other glomerulopathies. suPAR levels have been reported in focal segmental glomerulosclerosis (FSGS) and other primary glomerular diseases although its role remains controversial.

Anti-PLA2R antibody is present in 70–80% of primary cases. Patients with positive PLA2R antibody titres at the time of diagnosis have a lower rate of complete remission. Decreasing antibody titres suggest immunological remission which is generally followed by remission of proteinuria. Anti-PLA2R antibodies usually become undetectable prior to complete remission of proteinuria.

THSD7A (a 250kDa glycoprotein expressed by podocytes) antibodies have been found in 3–5% of patients with primary MN who were anti-PLA2R negative.

Keri K, Blumenthal S, Kulkarni V, Beck L, Chongkrairatanakul T. Primary membranous nephropathy: comprehensive review and historical perspective. Postgraduate Medical Journal. 2019;95(1119):23–31. https://pmj.bmj.com/content/95/1119/23

18. Answer: C

Rhabdomyolysis is characterised by the leakage of muscle-cell contents, including electrolytes, myoglobin, and other sarcoplasmic proteins (e.g. CK, aldolase, LDH, and AST) into the circulation. Exogenous agents that can be toxic to muscles, especially alcohol, illicit drugs, and statins are common non-traumatic causes. Recurrent episodes of rhabdomyolysis may be a sign of an underlying defect in muscle metabolism.

AKI is a potential complication of severe rhabdomyolysis, regardless of the cause, and the prognosis is substantially worse if renal failure develops. AKI related to rhabdomyolysis typically requires both myoglobinuria and volume depletion or some other nephrotoxic events. Studies show that AKI is rare unless the CK is >5000 U/L on admission. Many patients who have acute rise in CK occasionally as high as 12000 U/L following vigorous exercise do not always develop AKI.

Patient should be treated with aggressive hydration until the CK has decreased by at least 50%. Usually CK peaks at 24 to 36 hours after the event provided ongoing muscle damage has stopped and usually falls by the 3rd day. Myoglobin has a very short half-life and detection on day 3 suggests ongoing injury. Intravenous fluid treatment is to flush out the myoglobin, and to do so you need a sodium diuresis not just a water diuresis. Water diuresis only increases flow in the collecting duct. A sodium diuresis increases flow throughout the whole nephron where tubular toxicity occurs.

The clinical benefits of alkalinisation as compared with simple volume repletion are not firmly established. The disadvantage of alkalinisation is the reduction in ionised calcium, which can exacerbate the symptoms of the initial hypocalcaemic phase of rhabdomyolysis. The use of diuretics and other types of fluid replacement remains controversial. Mannitol may have theoretical benefits as an osmotic diuretic, but there is no clear evidence for clinical benefit in treating rhabdomyolysis.

Bosch X, Poch E, Grau J. Rhabdomyolysis and Acute Kidney Injury. New England Journal of Medicine. 2009;361(1):62–72. https://www.nejm.org/doi/full/10.1056/NEJMra0801327

19. Answer: C

Roxadustat is an orally bioavailable, reversible hypoxia-inducible factor (HIF) prolyl hydroxylase inhibitor. HIFs are transcription factors that regulate expression of genes in response to hypoxia, including genes required for erythropoiesis, and iron metabolism. In normoxia, a family of prolyl hydroxylases (PHDs) hydroxylate the HIF-α subunit, resulting in its rapid proteasomal degradation. In hypoxia, PHD activity is lessened causing HIF-α to accumulate, dimerise with HIF-β, and translocate into the nucleus activating transcriptional programs. This results in enhanced erythropoiesis. By inhibiting HIF-PHDs and mimicking the response to a cellular reduction in oxygen levels, roxadustat increases HIF activity, and promotes erythropoiesis. The short half-life of roxadustat, along with an intermittent dosing regimen, gives rise to transient bursts of HIF activity, which seem sufficient to stimulate effective erythropoiesis.

In clinical trials, roxadustat was superior to placebo in increasing haemoglobin levels in CKD patients with anaemia who were not undergoing dialysis and was non-inferior to erythropoietin in increasing haemoglobin levels in CKD patients with anaemia who were undergoing haemodialysis.

Roxadustat decreases levels of hepcidin, a regulator which allows access to existing iron stores as well as increased absorption of oral iron, thus avoiding the use of high doses of intravenous iron which has been associated with a pro-inflammatory state and increased mortality. Serum iron levels are usually stable during the roxadustat treatment and correspond with the effect of roxadustat on hepcidin and subsequent increase of ferroportin, allowing increased access to enteral iron and macrophage iron stores.

Roxadustat also decreases levels of total cholesterol, LDL, and triglycerides. These findings may be related to HIF dependent effects on acetyl coenzyme A and 3-hydroxy-3-methylglutaryl coenzyme A (HMGCoA) reductase.

Kaplan J. Roxadustat and Anemia of Chronic Kidney Disease. New England Journal of Medicine. 2019;381(11):1070–1072. https://www.nejm.org/doi/full/10.1056/NEJMe1908978

20. Answer: B

Hyponatraemia is one of the most common electrolyte abnormalities. The first step to determine the causes of hyponatraemia is to assess extracellular fluid volume status. Diagnosis of syndrome of inappropriate ADH secretion (SIADH) should be suspected in patients who are euvolaemic. Other common causes of hyponatraemia, such as hypothyroidism, cortisol deficiency, infection, intra-cranial pathology, diuretics, hyperglycaemia, pseudohyponatraemia due to hyperlipidaemia and hyperproteinaemia need to be excluded prior to the diagnosis of SIADH is made. A low serum sodium level, low serum osmolality, an increased urine sodium level, and increased urine osmolality confirm the diagnosis of SIADH.

In asymptomatic patients, fluid restriction of 800–1200 ml over 24 hours is the mainstay of management. This could be subsequently titrated to 500 ml below the daily urine output volume to improve serum sodium level.

Patients with severe symptomatic hyponatraemia (serum sodium level of <120 mmol/L) with seizures and altered mental status must be monitored frequently and corrected promptly because it can lead to cerebral oedema, irreversible neurologic damage, brainstem herniation, and death. Cerebral demyelination can occur if the sodium level is corrected too rapidly. It is recommended that increasing the serum sodium level should not exceed a rate of 10 mmol/L over 24 hours or 18 mmol/L over 48 hours. Treatment of patients with severe symptomatic hyponatraemia includes the use of intravenous hypertonic 3% saline infused at a rate of 0.5 to 2 mL per kg per hour until symptoms resolve.

At this time, vaptans, nonpeptide vasopressin receptor antagonists, have no established role in the treatment of hyponatraemia because of the potential for overcorrection of sodium and fluctuations in sodium levels.

Tee K, Dang J. The suspect – SIADH. Aust Fam Physician. 2017 Sep;46(9):677–680. PubMed PMID: 28892600 https://www.racgp.org.au/afp/2017/september/the-suspect-siadh/

21. Answer: C

The cause of rapid deterioration of graft function in this case is BK nephropathy (BKVN). BKVN is an important cause of premature graft failure. About 10%–30% of kidney recipients have BK viraemia, nephropathy occurs in 2%–5%. BKVN is most common early after transplant when immunosuppression is at its highest level. Patients are often asymptomatic, and the diagnostic standard is kidney biopsy. Risk factors include greater mismatching, extremes of age, men, diabetes, ureteric stents, lymphocyte-depleting induction, and aggressive immunosuppressive treatment during acute rejection, especially the usage of monoclonal antibody such as anti-thymocyte globulin (ATG).

The management of BKVN is challenging because no one therapeutic strategy is consistently effective. The reduction of overall immunosuppression is the cornerstone of treatment in BKVN. It is recommended to reduce the calcineurin inhibitor (CNI) by 25%–50% first. Alternatively, simultaneous dose reduction of both the antimetabolite and CNI can be considered. Another option is conversion from a CNI to sirolimus or everolimus. The patient's level of immunologic risk, the viral load, and the degree of kidney impairment all need to be considered.

Cidofovir can competitively inhibit viral DNA synthesis. The effect of cidofovir on BKVN has been reported in small case series with some benefit but its usage has been associated with substantial nephrotoxicity. Leflunomide is a pyrimidine synthesis inhibitor used in the treatment of rheumatoid arthritis. It is known to have both immunosuppressive and antiviral properties. Report of successful use of leflunomide for BKVN has been published as single centre experience. There is no randomised controlled trial data. Ciprofloxacin has been used in the treatment of BKVN. Quinolones may have anti-BK virus properties by inhibiting DNA topoisomerase activity and SV40 large T antigen helicase. An observational study reported that use of IVIG is safe and effective in treating BK viraemia and BKVN and preventing graft loss in patients who had inadequate response to immunosuppression reduction and leflunomide therapy.

Sawinski D, Trofe-Clark J. BK Virus Nephropathy. Clinical Journal of the American Society of Nephrology. 2018;13(12):1893–1896.
https://cjasn.asnjournals.org/content/13/12/1893

22. Answer: D

Erythropoietin (EPO) is a hormone that is produced by the kidney to stimulate RBC production in the bone marrow. EPO levels are inappropriately low in patients with CKD. Erythropoiesis stimulating agents (ESAs) boost the production of RBCs and increase haemoglobin levels. ESAs use can avoid blood transfusion and reduce fatigue in patients with anaemia associated with CKD. ESAs are listed on the Pharmaceutical Benefits Scheme (PBS) in Australia for treatment of anaemia secondary to intrinsic renal disease if fulfilling the following clinical criteria:

- Patient must require transfusion,
- Patient must have a haemoglobin level of less than 100 g/L,
- Patient must have intrinsic renal disease, as assessed by a nephrologist.

ESAs should be used with caution in patients with pre-existing hypertension, ischaemic cardiovascular disease, malignancy, epilepsy, history of seizures, or medical conditions associated with a predisposition to seizure activity such as CNS infections and brain metastases.

Most guidelines recommends a haemoglobin target between 100–115 g/L for patients on ESAs for treatment of anaemia secondary to intrinsic renal diseases. The US Food and Drug Administration (FDA) advises that using ESAs to target a haemoglobin level of greater than 110 g/L increases the risk of serious adverse cardiovascular events, including increased risks of death, myocardial infarction, stroke, difficult control of hypertension, VTE, and thrombosis of vascular access. It has no impact on diabetic control.

ESA treatment may have an impact on cancer progression. The FDA does not recommend the use of ESAs in patients with myelosuppressive chemotherapy when the anticipated outcome is cure. ESA treatment in CKD patients with cancer is complicated.

In patients with non-dialysis CKD or ESKD and active cancer, decisions to initiate ESAs or continue in patient already on ESAs when cancer is discovered must balance risks and benefits. Incremental risks of ESAs in CKD/ESKD patients with cancer primarily relate to a probable increase in the risk of thrombosis, probable increase in mortality risk, and a possible but unlikely risk of increased tumour progression.

Erythropoiesis stimulating agent [Internet]. Blood.gov.au. 2019 [cited 14 December 2019]. Available from: https://www.blood.gov.au/system/files/documents/companion-5-pbm-guidelines_0.pdf

Grandaliano G, Teutonico A, Allegretti A, Losappio R, Mancini A, Gesualdo L et al. The role of hyperparathyroidism, erythropoietin therapy, and CMV infection in the failure of arteriovenous fistula in hemodialysis. Kidney International. 2003;64(2):715–719.
https://www.kidney-international.org/article/S0085-2538(15)49381-0/fulltext

23. Answer: A

FGF–23 is a 251-amino acid protein synthesised and secreted by bone cells, mainly osteoblast. It plays an important role in the regulation of phosphate and 1,25-dihydroxy vitamin D metabolism. FGF–23 acts in the kidney to induce urinary phosphate excretion and suppress 1,25-dihydroxy vitamin D synthesis in the presence of FGF receptor 1 (FGFR1) and its co-receptor Klotho. Elevated plasma FGF–23 level is the earliest detectable abnormality in mineral metabolism in CKD as a physiological compensation to stabilise serum phosphate levels as the number of intact nephrons declines.

FGF–23 is increased in patients with advanced CKD by 100- to 1000-fold to compensate for persistent phosphate retention. This increase is due to decreased renal clearance but also to increased synthesis. FGF–23 is associated with vascular dysfunction, atherosclerosis, left ventricular hypertrophy, increased cardiovascular events, and increased mortality in patients with CKD.

Lu X, Hu M. Klotho/FGF23 Axis in Chronic Kidney Disease and Cardiovascular Disease. Kidney Diseases. 2016;3(1):15–23.
https://www.karger.com/Article/FullText/452880

24. Answer: B

IgA nephropathy (IgAN) is a leading cause of CKD and ESKD. A few key pathologic features are consistently independently associated with renal outcome in patients with IgAN, including mesangial hypercellularity (M), endocapillary hypercellularity (E), segmental glomerulosclerosis (S), tubular atrophy and interstitial fibrosis (T), and crescents (C), known collectively as the Oxford classification MEST-C scores. The clinical relevance and applicability of this score has been validated across multiple populations. The score overall consistently adds value to prognostication and treatment response.

Rodrigues J, Haas M, Reich H. IgA Nephropathy. Clinical Journal of the American Society of Nephrology. 2017;12(4):677–686.
https://cjasn.asnjournals.org/content/12/4/677

25. Answer: C

Maintenance of normal acid-base homeostasis is one of the most important kidney functions. The capacity of the kidneys to excrete the daily acid load as ammonium and titratable acid is impaired in CKD, resulting in acid retention and metabolic acidosis. The prevalence of metabolic acidosis increases with declining GFR. Metabolic acidosis is associated with CKD progression, bone demineralisation, skeletal muscle catabolism, and mortality.

Guidelines recommend treating metabolic acidosis in CKD with alkali therapy for serum bicarbonate level < 22 mmol/L. Given the persistent bicarbonate levels and mild hyperkalaemia in this patient, treatment of metabolic acidosis with sodium bicarbonate is appropriate. Although lisinopril may be contributing to the mild hyperkalaemia and low bicarbonate concentrations, treatment of metabolic acidosis with alkali therapy may reduce serum potassium concentration and permit continued use of the ACE inhibitor. Diuretics should not be used solely for the purpose of increasing serum bicarbonate levels. Insulin dose should be adjusted according to blood glucose level not bicarbonate levels.

Navaneethan S, Shao J, Buysse J, Bushinsky D. Effects of Treatment of Metabolic Acidosis in CKD. Clinical Journal of the American Society of Nephrology. 2019;14(7):1011–1020.
https://cjasn.asnjournals.org/content/14/7/1011

26. Answer: B

The peritoneal dialysate contains variable concentrations of glucose which often leads to weight gain because of the glucose load. Furthermore, patients with diabetes will often require enhanced diabetic treatment. Peritonitis continues to be a major cause of morbidity and mortality in peritoneal dialysis (PD) patients. *S. epidermidis* is the most frequently identified cause of PD-associated peritonitis. The most appropriate step in management of PD-related peritonitis is to give intraperitoneal antibiotics, which are administered during peritoneal dialysis exchanges. Routine transfer patient with PD-related peritonitis to hemodialysis is incorrect unless the peritonitis is refractory to treatment or caused by fungal infection or severe underlying surgical conditions. The peritoneal dialysate contains NO potassium, therefore hyperkalaemia is an uncommon finding in a patient with adequate PD.

Hansson J, Watnick S. Update on Peritoneal Dialysis: Core Curriculum 2016. American Journal of Kidney Diseases. 2016;67(1):151–164.
https://www.ajkd.org/article/S0272-6386(15)01064-1/fulltext

27. Answer: A

The podocyte is a highly differentiated epithelial cell sitting on the outside of the glomerular capillary loop. It connects to the underlying glomerular basement membrane (GBM) of the capillary loop by major cellular extensions from the cell body. Extensions terminate as foot processes on the GBM that interdigitate with those from adjacent podocytes. Podocyte foot processes are anchored to the GBM by $\alpha3\beta1$ integrins and α- and β-dystroglycans. Between foot processes, the filtration slit is bridged by a 40-nm wide zipper-like slit diaphragm. Slit diaphragm is highly permeable to water and small solutes.

The main functions of the podocyte include:

- Structural support of the capillary loop
- Major component of glomerular filtration barrier
- Synthesis and repair of the GBM
- Production of growth factors
  - Vascular endothelial growth factor (VEGF) traverses the GBM against the flow of glomerular filtration
  - Acts on VEGF receptors on glomerular endothelial cells

○ Effect is to maintain a healthy fenestrated endothelium
○ Platelet-derived growth factors (PDGFs) critical for the development and migration of mesangial cells into the mesangium
• Immunologic function
○ Podocytes may be a component of the innate immune system
○ Possibly have a surveillance role for pathogens or abnormal proteins in Bowman space.

28. Answer: A

Post-transplant lymphoproliferative disorder (PTLD) is a severe complication of solid organ transplants with an overall incidence of about 2%. The incidence of PTLD according to type of transplanted organ has been reported as follows: hematopoietic stem cell (0.5–1%), kidney (1%), pancreas (2.1%), heart (2.3%), lung (2.5%), liver (4.3%), heart–lung (10–20%), and bowel (10–20%) .

In about 85–90% of cases, PTLD is EBV–related. The most important risk factor is an EBV status mismatch, e.g., recipient seronegative/donor seropositive at the time of transplant, leading to a 10–75 times greater incidence of PTLD compared to seropositive recipients. Anti-thymocyte globulin and alemtuzumab have uncertain effects on PTLD risk. mTOR inhibitors such as everolimus has been associated with higher rather than lower risk for PTLD.

Clinical manifestation of PTLD is variable from asymptomatic to pleiotropic symptoms affecting any or multiple sites. PTLD has a high incidence of extranodal involvement, including the GI tract (20%–30% of patients), the solid allograft (10%–15% of patients), and the central nervous system (5%–20% of patients). The diagnosis of PTLD is made by histopathologic tissue examination. The treatment options for PTLD include a reduction in immunosuppression, often with a combination of chemotherapy and rituximab; surgical excision and radiotherapy are reserved for localised disease.

29. Answer: B

Contrast-induced nephropathy (CIN) is characterised by a decrease in kidney function that occurs within days after the intravascular administration of iodinated contrast material. It is the third most common cause of hospital-acquired AKI. The incidence is low (0.6–2.3%) in the general population but in high-risk groups especially in patients with advanced CKD the incidence may be up to 20%. Recent studies have suggested that the risk of AKI due to contrast material is overestimated.

Identification of patients at high risk for the development of CIN is of major importance. Non-modifiable and modifiable risk factors are summarised in Table 15.2 below.

Table 15.2   Risk factors for CIN.

Non-modifiable risk factors	Modifiable risk factors
Old age	Hypotension
Chronic kidney disease	Anaemia
Diabetes mellitus	Dehydration
Congestive heart failure	Low serum albumin
Cardiogenic shock	ACE inhibitors/ARBs
Renal transplant	Diuretics
Multiple myeloma	NSAIDs
Sepsis	Nephrotoxic antibiotics
	Volume of contrast volume

Metformin is not a nephrotoxic medication therefore it is not a risk factor of developing CIN. The rationale for stopping metformin before and after contrast exposure is that the worsening of renal function may increase the blood concentration of metformin which can rarely lead to lactic acidosis.

Mehran R, Nikolsky E. Contrast-induced nephropathy: Definition, epidemiology, and patients at risk. Kidney International. 2006;69: S11–S15.
https://www.kidney-international.org/article/S0085-2538(15)51387-2/fulltext

Mehran R, Dangas G, Weisbord S. Contrast-Associated Acute Kidney Injury. New England Journal of Medicine. 2019;380(22):2146–2155.
https://www.nejm.org/doi/full/10.1056/NEJMra1805256

30. Answer: C

Nephrotic syndrome can be classified as primary, being a disease specific to the kidneys, or secondary, being a renal manifestation of a systemic general illness. Secondary causes include the following, in order of approximate frequency:

- Diabetes mellitus
- Lupus nephritis
- Hepatitis B, hepatitis C, HIV
- Amyloidosis and paraproteinemias.

Renal manifestations in sarcoidosis include abnormal calcium metabolism, nephrolithiasis and nephrocalcinosis, and acute interstitial nephritis with or without granuloma formation. Sjögren's syndrome may affect renal function either as epithelial disease causing tubulointerstitial nephritis, or rarely as an immune complex–mediated glomerulopathy. Renal manifestations occur frequently in scleroderma. Commonest manifestation is a reduction in renal function due to chronic disease but most clinically important is the scleroderma renal crisis (SRC). This life-threatening complication occurs in up to 15% of the cases of diffuse cutaneous systemic sclerosis. Typically, patients present with accelerated hypertension and progressive renal impairment.

 Kodner C. Diagnosis and Management of Nephrotic Syndrome in Adults. Am Fam Physician. 2016 Mar 15;93(6):479–485.
https://www.aafp.org/afp/2016/0315/p479.html

31. Answer: B

The kidneys play a major role in the regulation of glucose in humans. All filtered glucose undergoes reabsorption in the kidney tubules and therefore, no glucose is present in the urine. The sodium-glucose co-transporter 2 (SGLT2) which is found primarily in the S1 segment of the proximal renal tubule, is essential for this process, accounting for 90% of the glucose reabsorption in the kidney, while SGLT1 located in the S2/S3 segment of proximal tubule reabsorb the remaining 10%. SGLT2s are also located in pancreatic a-cells and in the cerebellum, while SGLT1s are more widely distributed to intestine, heart, lungs, and skeletal muscles.

Selective inhibition of SGLT2 induces glycosuria in a dose-dependent manner and have beneficial effects on glucose regulation in individuals with type 2 diabetes. SGLT2 inhibitors are a class of glucose lowering agent whose mechanism of action involves blockade of SGLT2 co-transporters on the luminal surface of the proximal renal tubule. The resultant increase in glycosuria and natriuresis contributes to a broad range of metabolic benefits including reduction in glycosylated haemoglobin, body weight, blood pressure, and albuminuria.

Recent systemic review has concluded that SGLT2 inhibitors are associated with significantly lower major adverse cardiovascular events, heart failure hospitalisations, and all-cause mortality. The evidence is strongest in reducing heart failure hospitalisations. SGLT2 inhibitors are also associated with significantly lower adverse renal events and slow the progression of diabetic nephropathy, with these effects apparent even in the population with eGFR <60 mL/min/1.73 m^2.

 Zelniker T, Wiviott S, Raz I, Im K, Goodrich E, Bonaca M et al. SGLT2 inhibitors for primary and secondary prevention of cardiovascular and renal outcomes in type 2 diabetes: a systematic review and meta-analysis of cardiovascular outcome trials. The Lancet. 2019;393(10166):31–39.
https://www.thelancet.com/journals/lancet/article/PIIS0140-6736(18)32590-X/fulltext

32. Answer: C

Active tubular secretion in the proximal tubule is important in the elimination of many medications including trimethoprim. This energy-dependent process may be blocked by metabolic inhibitors. When drug concentration is high, secretory transport can reach an upper limit (transport maximum); each substance has a characteristic transport maximum. Creatinine is secreted actively by the proximal tubule and trimethoprim can competitively inhibit this process leading to an elevation in serum creatinine without reducing the glomerular filtration rate.

 Delanaye P, Mariat C, Cavalier E, Maillard N, Krzesinski J, White C. Trimethoprim, Creatinine and Creatinine-Based Equations. Nephron Clinical Practice. 2011;119(3):187–194.
https://www.karger.com/Article/FullText/328911

33. Answer: A

The low tacrolimus level at 3 ng/mL and failure to keep his renal appointments suggest possible poor adherence to medications and renal allograft rejection may be the cause of AKI post-transplant in this case. Twelve-hour trough levels are used to monitor tacrolimus levels. The recommended tacrolimus level is 8 to 10 ng/mL for the first few months post-transplant. After the first year, the tacrolimus target level is reduced to 5 to 7 ng/mL, and to a lower target level of 3 to 5 ng/mL in the presence of significant infection, malignancy, or BK viraemia.

A serum BK viral count > 10,000 copies/ml is associated with an increased risk of BK nephropathy. BK nephropathy is also unlikely due to an undetectable BK viral count in the blood. The positive urine BK virus is not correlated to BK nephropathy.

The recurrence of IgA nephropathy in the transplant kidney usually occurs after 10-year post-transplant.

The use of tacrolimus in prevention of allograft rejection is associated with AKI and chronic nephrotoxicity. Cyclosporin also shows similar adverse effect likely due to a drug class effect. Acute calcineurin inhibitor (CNI) nephrotoxicity is usually reversible after reduction of tacrolimus or cyclosporin dose. Chronic CNI nephrotoxicity can affect glomeruli, arterioles, and the tubulo-interstitium and can cause chronic progressive renal failure that is not reversible. CNI can also cause tubular dysfunction which may manifest as hyperkalaemia, hypomagnesaemia, hypophosphataemia, metabolic acidosis, and hyperuricaemia/gout. CNI very rarely causes thrombotic microangiopathy (TMA) leading to acute renal allograft loss. The low tacrolimus level in this case is unlikely to cause CNI toxicity.

Voora S, Adey D. Management of Kidney Transplant Recipients by General Nephrologists: Core Curriculum 2019. American Journal of Kidney Diseases. 2019;73(6):866–879. https://www.ajkd.org/article/S0272–6386(19)30161-1/fulltext

34. Answer: B

Malignancy is one of the most common causes of death in kidney transplant recipients. Non-melanotic skin cancer is the most common malignancy post-renal transplant. All renal transplant patients should wear sunscreen and have regular skin checks (at least yearly) with a dermatologist or a GP. Conversion from a calcineurin inhibitor to an mTOR inhibitor, which has better efficacy in control of epithelial cell–derived skin malignancy, should be considered in patients with recurrent skin cancers.

In renal transplant recipients, the incidence of cancer is generally increased two- to three fold compared with the general population. This increased cancer risk is not spread evenly over all types of cancers; while some cancer incidences are not increased such as breast, prostate, brain, and ovarian cancer, others are increased substantially such as lung, colon, liver, lymphoma (PTLD), melanoma and non-melanoma skin cancer. Immunosuppression is considered the most important risk factor for increased cancer risk in renal transplant patients, as it decreases the immunologic control of oncogenic viral infection and cancer immunosurveillance.

No guidelines currently exist in Australia or New Zealand for general malignancy screening post-renal transplant. Cancer screening should be tailored to patients based on their comorbidities, risk factors, overall prognosis, and preferences towards cancer screening.

Voora S, Adey D. Management of Kidney Transplant Recipients by General Nephrologists: Core Curriculum 2019. American Journal of Kidney Diseases. 2019;73(6):866–879. https://www.ajkd.org/article/S0272–6386(19)30161-1/abstract

Au E, Wong G, Chapman J. Cancer in kidney transplant recipients. Nature Reviews Nephrology. 2018;14(8):508–520. https://www.nature.com/articles/s41581-018-0022-6

35. Answer: G

36. Answer: H

37. Answer: B

38. Answer: E

Immunosuppressants which target T cell activation can be divided into three groups, dependent on which signal they target:

- Signal 1- activation via antigen presentation (T cell CD3- and APC MHC).
- Signal 2- co-stimulation, for optimal T cell activation (Signal 1-activated T cell CD28 and APC CD80/86).
- Signal 3- cytokine activation, for T cell proliferation (Signal 2-activated T cell and Cytokine, predominantly IL-2).

  Agents which target signal 1 (T cell CD3- and APC MHC)

- **Anti-T cell receptor agents** include **muromonab-CD3**, a murine (100% mouse-derived) monoclonal antibody which inhibits the CD3 subunit of T cells preventing initial T cell activation leading to rapid depletion of functional T cells. It has significant side effects and is no longer in clinical use.
- **Calcineurin inhibitors** including **cyclosporin** (via cyclophilin binding) and **tacrolimus** (via FKBP12 binding) inhibit calcineurin from dephosphorylating nuclear factor of activated T cells (NFAT), inhibiting T cell activation.
  <u>Agents which target signal 2</u> (activated T cell CD28 and APC CD80/86)
- **Anti-CD28/CTLA-Ig agents** (**Abatacept, Belatacept**) are human IgG heavy chains linked to cytotoxic T lymphocyte associated protein 4 (CTLA4), mimicking its action to competitively bind to CD80/86 and downregulate the T cell response.
- **Anti-CD40mAb agents (Bleselumab/ASKP1240)** competitively inhibit the interaction between activated T cell CD154 (also known as CD40L) and APC (antigen-presenting cell) CD40, which would otherwise lead to upregulation of CD80/86 on APCs and increased T cell co-stimulation.
- Anti-CD154 agents are no longer in development as early human studies showed increased thrombotic events, because CD154 is also present on platelets.
  <u>Agents which target signal 3</u> (activated T cell cytokine receptors and cytokines)
- **Anti-CD25/IL-2 receptor antagonists (Basiliximab, Daclizumab)** are humanised monoclonal antibodies to the a-subunit of IL-2 receptors (CD25), which competitively bind to the IL-2 receptors of activated T cells to limit activated T cell proliferation.

Other immunosuppressants include:
- **Anti-thymocyte globulin (ATG)**: Antibodies to human lymphocyte antigens created via immunising rabbits with human thymocytes, which induces lymphocyte depletion via complement dependent lysis and T cell activation-induced apoptosis.
- **Nonspecific cytokine inhibition (corticosteroids)**: corticosteroids bind to intracellular glucocorticoid receptors inhibiting cytokine transcription factors leading to numerous effects including depletion of T cells (via IL-2 inhibition, Th1 differentiation inhibition, and induction of apoptosis) eosinophil apoptosis (directly or via IL-5 inhibition) macrophage dysfunction (via inhibition of IL-1 and TNF-a).
- **Antimetabolites**
  - **Azathioprine (prodrug of 6-mercaptopurne):** purine analogues which interfere with de novo purine synthesis and thus DNA and RNA synthesis, and have other immunomodulatory effects including S-G2 cell cycle arrest.
  - **Mycophenolate:** inhibitor of inosine 5 monophosphate dehydrogenase involved in guanine nucleotide synthesis, critical for de novo purine synthesis, and thus DNA synthesis.
  - **Leflunomide:** inhibits dihydro-orate dehydrogenase inhibiting de novo pyrimidine synthesis and thus DNA synthesis and cell cycling from S to G2.
- **mTOR inhibitors (Sirolimus, Everolimus):** mammalian target of rapamycin (mTOR) inhibitors inhibit lymphocyte cell cycle progression G1 to S phase and thus cell proliferation, and has anti-proliferative, anti-viral, anti-inflammatory, and anti-tumor effects via receptors in other cells.
- **Anti-CD20 agents (Rituximab, Ocrelizumab, Ofatumumab, Veltuzumab):** Monoclonal antibodies which competitively inhibit CD20, a transmembrane protein present on pre-B and mature B lymphocytes (not present on stem cells, normal plasma cells, or other cell lines) inhibiting B cell regulation, activation for cell cycling, and B cell differentiation.
- **Anti-BAFF/Blys (Belimumab, Atacicept):** Belimumab (a-BAFFmAb) and Atacicept (TACI-Ig) inhibit the binding of cytokine B-cell activating factor (BAFF, also known as BlyS) to its B cell receptors (BAFF-R), and also in the case of atacicept transmembrane activator and CAML interactor (TACI) and cytokine-proliferation-inducing ligands to its B cell receptors, preventing the increase in NH-kB which would otherwise promote B cell differentiation and inhibit apoptosis.
- **Anti-plasma cell (Bortezomib)**: Proteasome inhibitor of plasma cells disrupting the regulation of plasma cells.
- **Anti-C5 complement (Eculizumab)** humanised monoclonal antibody to C5 inhibiting its cleavage to C5a and C5b, inhibiting the neutrophilic chemoattractant and membrane-attack complex properties respectively, leading to blockage of proinflammatory, prothrombotic, and lytic complement functions.
- **TNF-α antagonists** (monoclonal antibodies: **infliximab, adalimumab, golimumab, certolizumab**, and TNFR fusion protein bound to IgG: **etanercept**): Inhibit action of TNF-α, which binds to its receptors (TNF receptors 1 and 2: TNFR1 and TNFR2) to stimulate apoptotic pathways and NFκb signalling with diverse inflammatory actions including Th1 T cell proliferation.
- **IL-1 inhibitors (Anakinra, Rilonacept Canakinumab)**: Inhibits IL-1 and its numerous inflammatory effects including autoimmune conditions especially rheumatoid arthritis and Still's disease, mitigating injury in ischemic events including post myocardial infarction.
- **IL-6 inhibitor (Tocilizumab)**: Inhibition of IL-6 and thus inhibition of CD8 T cell differentiation, B cell differentiation, and activation of hepatic acute phase response.

- **IL-17 inhibitors (Secukinumab)** Inhibits IL-17 decreasing inflammatory cell migration and APC acidity to decrease adaptive immune response.
- **Intravenous Ig (IVIG):** Ig extract pooled from thousands of plasma donors which is anti-inflammatory at high doses (1–2g/kg) via numerous mechanisms including directly via binding to natural antibodies, immunomodulatory proteins and pathogens, and indirectly via Fc receptor induced anti-inflammatory pathways.
- **Anti-CD52 (Campath 1H, Alemtuzumab):** Humanised monoclonal antibodies that bind to CD52, present on B and T cells, which depletes both lymphoid cell lines.

 Wiseman A. Immunosuppressive Medications. Clinical Journal of the American Society of Nephrology. 2015;11(2):332–343. https://cjasn.asnjournals.org/content/early/2015/07/12/CJN.08570814/tab-article-info?versioned=true

 Halloran P. Immunosuppressive Drugs for Kidney Transplantation. New England Journal of Medicine. 2004;351(26): 2715–2729. https://www.nejm.org/doi/full/10.1056/NEJMra033540

 Zhang W, Egashira N, Masuda S. Recent Topics on The Mechanisms of Immunosuppressive Therapy-Related Neurotoxicities. International Journal of Molecular Sciences. 2019;20(13):3210. https://www.mdpi.com/1422-0067/20/13/3210

39. Answer: L

Primary focal segmental glomerulosclerosis (FSGS) may recur rapidly in the renal allograft. The rapidity of recurrence in some cases strongly suggests the presence in primary FSGS of a circulating factor in plasma, with resulting in toxicity to the glomerular capillary wall, glomerular basement membrane (GBM), and podocytes. The reported recurrence rate is 30–50% and is associated with poor renal allograft survival. There are two clinical presentations of FSGS after transplantation: an early recurrence, the most frequent, which is characterised by massive proteinuria within hours to days after implantation of the new kidney and a late recurrence which develops insidiously several months or years after transplantation. The management of patients with recurrent FSGS is difficult and not well established. The administration of high-dose ACE-inhibitors, angiotensin-receptor blockers and statins is recommended to exploit their antiproteinuric and antilipaemic effects. Increased doses of steroids and calcineurin inhibitors may protect from FSGS recurrence but may increase the risk of over-immunosuppression. The most commonly used therapeutic approach is the use of plasma exchange or immunoadsorption with protein A. In the absence of contraindication, a course of rituximab may be attempted if there is no response to plasmapheresis. In spite of the risk of recurrence, patients with FSGS should not be excluded from transplantation. In the case of living donation, the possibility of recurrence and its consequences should be clearly exposed to and discussed with the donor and the recipient and pre-emptive plasma exchange should be planned.

 Cravedi P, Kopp J, Remuzzi G. Recent Progress in the Pathophysiology and Treatment of FSGS Recurrence. American Journal of Transplantation. 2013;13(2):266–274. https://onlinelibrary.wiley.com/doi/abs/10.1111/ajt.12045

40. Answer: B

Alport's syndrome is an inherited disease characterised by progressive renal failure, hearing loss, and ocular abnormalities. Mutations in the COL4A5 (X-linked), or COL4A3 and COL4A4 (autosomal recessive) genes result in absence of the collagen IV α3α4α5 network from the basement membranes of the cornea, lens capsule, and retina and are associated with corneal opacities, anterior lenticonus. Results of pedigree analyses and Sanger sequencing suggested relative frequencies for the X-linked, autosomal recessive, and autosomal dominant forms of approximately 80%, 15%, and 5%, respectively. The demonstration of lenticonus is diagnostic of Alport's syndrome. Anterior lenticonus is present in 50% of men, but not women, with X-linked disease, where it is associated with early-onset renal failure and perimacular retinopathy. Patients have progressive difficulty in focusing because of their abnormal lens shape.

Female members of Alport families who have heterozygous mutations in COL4A5 and have hematuria have been considered to be carriers but recent reports demonstrate they have a significant lifetime risk of ESKD.

The diagnosis is confirmed if there is a lamellated GBM on kidney biopsy or a pathogenic mutation in the COL4A5 gene or two pathogenic COL4A3 or COL4A4 mutations. Genetic testing is at least 90% sensitive for X-linked disease.

Savige J, Gregory M, Gross O, Kashtan C, Ding J, Flinter F. Expert Guidelines for the Management of Alport Syndrome and Thin Basement Membrane Nephropathy. Journal of the American Society of Nephrology. 2013;24(3):364–375.
https://jasn.asnjournals.org/content/24/3/364

41. Answer: N

This patient has many of the clinical features that are strongly suggestive of thin basement membrane nephropathy (TBMN) such as persistent microscopic haematuria, no proteinuria, normal renal function and BP, absence of deafness, and possible autosomal dominant inheritance of haematuria.

TBMN is the most common cause of persistent haematuria in adults which affects at least 1% of the population, is a nonprogressive disorder associated with family history. Kidney biopsy reveals no other abnormalities except uniformly thinned glomerular basement membranes (GBM), as determined by electron microscopy.

It still is a major clinical challenge to differentiate between TBMN characterised by nonprogressive kidney disease and Alport's syndrome. The typical histopathologic feature of TBMN, i.e. uniform thinning of the GBM, could be found also at the early stages of Alport's syndrome. About 85% of Alport syndrome has X-linked inheritance with mutations in *COL4A5*, and most of the others have autosomal recessive disease with homozygous or compound heterozygous mutations in both copies (in trans) of *COL4A3* or *COL4A4*. Autosomal dominant inheritance is very rare and results from heterozygous *COL4A3* or *COL4A4* variants. On the other hand, TBMN is usually caused by heterozygous *COL4A3* or *COL4A4* mutations and can represent the carrier state of autosomal recessive Alport's syndrome.

In principle, DNA-based diagnosis of TBMN is possible. At present, the clinical diagnosis still is made mainly on the basis of persistent haematuria with minimal proteinuria and normal renal function, combined with electron microscopy examination of biopsy showing thinned GBM; the use of immunologic examination of the type IV collagen α3 to α5 chains is not being used extensively.

Savige J, Rana K, Tonna S, Buzza M, Dagher H, Wang Y. Thin basement membrane nephropathy. Kidney International. 2003;64(4):1169–1178.
https://www.kidney-international.org/article/S0085-2538(15)49452-9/fulltext

42. Answer: I

The renal biopsy shows the characteristic histologic features of type I membranoproliferative glomerulonephritis (MPGN). There is global and diffuse thickening of capillary walls. The capillary wall thickening is caused by mesangial interposition into the subendothelial zone of the capillary loops which leads to 'double contour' or 'train track formation'. There is also mesangial proliferation, hypercellularity and endocapillary proliferation. There is lobular accentuation, meaning that the segments or lobules are discernible because of cleft-like spaces between adjacent lobules. Immunofluorescence staining shows coarse granular pattern along the glomerular capillaries. Electron microscopy shows a segment of a glomerular capillary with large, discrete, electron-dense deposits in the subendothelial space. MPGN is often associated with hepatitis C infection.

Masani N, Jhaveri K, Fishbane S. Update on Membranoproliferative GN. Clinical Journal of the American Society of Nephrology. 2014;9(3):600–608.
https://cjasn.asnjournals.org/content/9/3/600

43. Answer: E

Clinically this patient is likely to have diabetic nephropathy. There are no standardised criteria for kidney biopsy in patients with a clinical diagnosis of diabetic nephropathy. Therefore, currently the decision to perform one is made by physicians. Up to 25% of all renal biopsies are done in patients with diabetes.

Rapid onset of proteinuria (regardless of the progression from microalbuminuria to macroalbuminuria), absence of retinopathy, presence of haematuria, active urinary sediment, rapid decrease of renal function, and suspicion of other nephropathies secondary to systemic disease, are some of the indications for renal biopsy in patient with suspected diabetic nephropathy.

This biopsy shows typical nodular intercapillary glomerulosclerosis (Kimmelstiel–Wilson nodules). It consists of nodular lesions containing areas of marked mesangial expansion forming large round fibrillar mesangial zones with palisading of mesangial nuclei around the periphery of the nodule and compression of the associated glomerular capillaries.

This patient has relatively short history of DM but has severe histopathological diabetic nephropathy and renal impairment. It is likely that the patient has a longer history of undiagnosed type 2 diabtes.

Alicic R, Rooney M, Tuttle K. Diabetic Kidney Disease. Clinical Journal of the American Society of Nephrology. 2017;12(12):2032–2045.
https://cjasn.asnjournals.org/content/12/12/2032

44. Answer: F

Goodpasture's syndrome refers to an anti-glomerular basement membrane (anti-GBM) disease that involves both the lungs and kidneys, often presenting as pulmonary haemorrhage and rapidly progressive glomerulonephritis (RPGN) with renal failure. This patient presents with AKI, active urine sediment with RBC casts. Renal biopsy shows crescent formation which is the histopathologic hallmark of anti-GBM disease. The average proportion of affected glomeruli is approximately 75%. The proportion of crescents observed in the biopsy sample correlates strongly with the degree of renal impairment at presentation. These crescents will typically be of uniform age, in contrast to other causes of RPGN, such as ANCA-associated vasculitis, where a mixture of cellular, fibrocellular, and fibrous crescents may be seen. Direct immunofluorescence for IgG on frozen kidney tissue has high sensitivity for detecting deposited antibodies, and is the gold standard for diagnosis of anti-GBM disease, typically showing a strong linear ribbon-like appearance as seen in this case.

McAdoo S, Pusey C. Anti-Glomerular Basement Membrane Disease. Clinical Journal of the American Society of Nephrology. 2017;12(7):1162–1172.
https://cjasn.asnjournals.org/content/12/7/1162

45. Answer: G

This patient has nephrotic syndrome and most common cause for nephrotic syndrome in adults is idiopathic membranous nephropathy.

Patients with the nephrotic syndrome are at increased risk for venous thrombosis, particularly deep vein and renal vein thrombosis (DVT and RVT). Pulmonary embolisation (mostly asymptomatic) is relatively common. Arterial thromboses (e.g. limb and cerebral) also occur with higher frequency than in the general population. In patients with nephrotic syndrome, the absolute risks of VTE (rate of 1.02% per year) and arterial thromboembolism (ATE) (rate of 1.48% per year) are each eight times higher than the estimated age- and sex-weighted annual incidences in the general population. Risks of both VTE and ATE are particularly high within the first 6 months of nephrotic syndrome. The annual incidence for thromboembolism in membranous nephropathy (MN) is 1.4%. The risk of thrombosis seems to be related to the severity and duration of the nephrotic state and is particularly increased with serum albumin concentrations less than 20 g/L. Furthermore, among the causes of nephrotic syndrome, the risk is highest with idiopathic MN, followed by membranoproliferative glomerulonephritis, and minimal change disease. The cause of the hypercoagulable state in patients with nephrotic syndrome is not well understood. A variety of haemostatic abnormalities have been described, including decreased levels of antithrombin and plasminogen (due to urinary losses), increased platelet activation, hyperfibrinogenaemia, inhibition of plasminogen activation, and the presence of high molecular weight fibrinogen in the circulation.

Lin R, McDonald G, Jolly T, Batten A, Chacko B. A Systematic Review of Prophylactic Anticoagulation in Nephrotic Syndrome. Kidney International Reports. 2020;5(4):435–447.
https://www.sciencedirect.com/science/article/pii/S2468024919315700

46. Answer: J

This patient has nephrotic syndrome. His kidney biopsy shows no abnormalities on light microscopy and immunofluorescent examination. The electron microscopy is pending but is likely to show foot process effacement. Overall, the clinical picture is consistent with minimal change disease (MCD). Most cases of MCD are idiopathic and not clearly associated with an underlying disease or event. With secondary MCD, the onset of nephrotic syndrome occurs concurrently or following an extraglomerular or glomerular disease process. MCD can be associated with the following:

- Medications
- Malignancy
- Infections
- Allergy.

NSAIDs and selective COX-2 inhibitors are the most common cause of secondary MCD.

Vivarelli M, Massella L, Ruggiero B, Emma F. Minimal Change Disease. Clinical Journal of the American Society of Nephrology. 2017;12(2):332–345.
https://cjasn.asnjournals.org/content/12/2/332

47. Answer: D

Collapsing glomerulopathy is a morphologic variant of FSGS characterised by segmental and global collapse of the glomerular capillaries, marked hypertrophy and hyperplasia of podocytes, and severe tubulointerstitial disease. It is most commonly seen in association with HIV, but also with other diseases such as TB, CMV, hepatitis B, and hepatitis C. Other causes include drugs such as bisphosphonates, opioids, and interferons; autoimmune diseases like SLE, adult Still's disease, and mixed connective tissue disease; and haematologic diseases including multiple myeloma, and acute leukaemia.

Although this patient is taking Chinese herbal medicine, his clinical features are not consistent with Chinese herbal nephropathy (CHN) which usually has mild low-molecular-weight proteinuria, hypertension, severe anaemia, and development of uroepithelial atypia. Renal histology in CHN shows unusual extensive, virtually hypocellular cortical interstitial fibrosis associated with tubular atrophy and global sclerosis of glomeruli decreasing from the outer to the inner cortex. Urothelial malignancy of the upper urinary tract develops subsequently in almost half of the patients. It is caused by aristolochic acid.

Chandra P, Kopp J. Viruses and collapsing glomerulopathy: a brief critical review. Clinical Kidney Journal. 2013;6(1):1-5.
https://academic.oup.com/ckj/article/6/1/1/470210

16 Neurology

Questions

Answers can be found in the Neurology Answers section at the end of this chapter.

1. A 45-year-old man presents to the emergency department with a left-sided facial droop with absent blink. His symptoms started 5 hours ago at work. He had flu-like symptoms 2 weeks ago and a left retro-auricular headache for the last 2 days. You diagnose him with Bell's palsy.

What is the most appropriate next step?
- **A.** Arrange CT scan of head.
- **B.** Commence oral prednisolone.
- **C.** Obtain nasopharyngeal swab for viral PCR.
- **D.** Order electromyography (EMG) and nerve conduction test.

2. A 60-year-old woman has presented with episodes of dizziness for last 24 hours. Symptoms occur on rolling over or getting out of bed with abrupt spinning sensation and imbalance, settling in minutes. She reports nausea but no vomiting or headache. There is no history of dysarthria, diplopia, dysphagia, weakness, or numbness. She denies any recent ear problems or respiratory tract illness. Her only past medical history is recurrent episodes of vertigo. On examination, she is afebrile, BP 130/70 mmHg, no postural hypotension, normal ear examination and neurological examination.

What should be the next step?
- **A.** CT Head and CT angiography.
- **B.** Dix–Hallpike manoeuvre.
- **C.** Hearing test with audiogram.
- **D.** Prochlorperazine.

3. Which of the following cannabinoids has shown efficacy in the treatment of some juvenile epilepsy syndromes?
- **A.** Δ9-tetrahydrocannabinol.
- **B.** Cannabinol.
- **C.** Cannabidiol.
- **D.** Tetrahydrocannabinolic acid.

4. A 50-year-old man presents to the emergency department with left hand clumsiness, which started suddenly whilst using a hand saw with his right hand at home. He has no significant past medical history and takes no regular medications. Systems review reveals mild neck pain which started at the time of the clumsiness.

On examination, his neck is mildly tender laterally on the right, but moves normally. Tone, power, reflexes, and sensation to light touch are normal in all four limbs, as is finger-nose, heel-shin, and rapid alternating movement tests. His gait is normal. Two-point discrimination is abnormal in the left hand, and proprioception is less accurate in the left hand compared to the right. Cranial nerve examination reveals right-sided ptosis, and anisocoria is present, with the left pupil measuring 4 mm and the right measuring 2 mm – these abnormalities have not been noticed previously. There is no anhidrosis, and cranial nerve function is otherwise normal. Plain CT brain reveals no acute abnormality.

Which of the following tests is most important?
- **A.** CT angiography of the head and neck.
- **B.** CT of the cervical spine.
- **C.** MRI of the cervical spine.
- **D.** MRI of the brain.

How to Pass the FRACP Written Examination, First Edition. Jonathan Gleadle, Jordan Li, Danielle Wu, and Paul Kleinig.
© 2022 John Wiley & Sons Ltd. Published 2022 by John Wiley & Sons Ltd.

5. A 32-year-old woman, G2P2, presents to the emergency department with a four-week history of worsening generalised headache, blurred vision (transiently worse when standing up from bending), lethargy, and dark urine. Her medical history include headache for 4 months, previous unprovoked left lower limb DVT and Budd-Chiari syndrome, she ceased warfarin 2 months ago. She is taking paracetamol and ibuprofen intermittently for headache. On examination, her BMI is 23 kg/m². Vital signs and temperature are normal. Fundoscopy shows papilloedema and blind spots are enlarged. She is mildly jaundiced. Neurological examination is normal. Abdominal ultrasound shows a spleen size of 15 cm. MRI of brain and MR venogram show evidence of sagittal and dominant transverse venous sinus thrombosis. Investigation results are shown below:

Tests	Test results	Normal values
Haemoglobin	100 g/L	115–155
White cell count	8 x 10⁹/L	4–11
Platelet	110 x 10⁹/L	150–450
Bilirubin	40 umol/L	2–24
LDH	1200 U/L	120–250
Reticulocyte	6%	0.2–3
Haptoglobin	0.02 g/L	0.3–2.0
Direct antiglobulin test	Negative	
Urine	Positive haemosiderin	
Creatinine	90 μmol/L	45–90
Urea	8 mmol/L	2.7–8.0
Serum beta-hCG	2 IU/L	< 5

What is the most appropriate next investigation?
  A. Bone marrow biopsy.
  B. Peripheral blood flow cytometry for GPI-linked proteins.
  C. Iron studies.
  D. JAK 2 mutation.

6. Which one of the following is ineffective in the induction treatment of chronic inflammatory demyelinating polyradiculoneuropathy (CIDP)?
  A. Intravenous immunoglobulin.
  B. Intravenous methylprednisolone.
  C. Oral methotrexate.
  D. Plasma exchange.

7. Which one of the biochemical compositions of cerebrospinal fluid (CSF) has the lowest concentration when compared with plasma in a healthy individual?
  A. Chloride.
  B. Lactic acid.
  C. Protein.
  D. Urea.

8. A 28-year-old woman with known epilepsy is seen in the clinic. She is 19 weeks pregnant. The visiting specialist has recently increased her lamotrigine dose despite the fact that she has been seizure-free for 3 years on the same dose.
  You would explain to her that the reason for increasing the dose is:
  A. A reduced drug absorption during pregnancy.
  B. An increase in the blood-brain barrier permeability during pregnancy.
  C. An increase in biotransformation during pregnancy.
  D. Pregnancy requires higher serum drug levels to prevent seizures.

9. A 36-year-old woman presents with a four-day history of progressive weakness of her lower limbs. Her medical history includes asthma, hypothyroidism, and type 1 diabetes which is under good control with HbA1c usually 6.5–7%. She had one episode of severe diarrhoea 10 days ago for which she required a short admission to an Acute Medical Unit. On examination, she is afebrile, BP is 110/60 mmHg, respiratory rate is 32/min and oxygen saturation on room air is 90%. She has symmetric weakness of bilateral proximal and distal extremity muscles. Sensation is intact. Tendon reflexes are absent, and the Babinski reflex is negative.

What is the most likely diagnosis?
- **A.** Diabetic radiculoplexus neuropathy.
- **B.** Guillain–Barré syndrome.
- **C.** Poliomyelitis.
- **D.** Necrotising autoimmune myositis.

10. Which one of the following headaches does **NOT** require neuroimaging?
- **A.** Recurrent headaches lasting 120 minutes located on the left side above the eye with conjunctival injection and eyelid oedema.
- **B.** A headache repeatedly triggered by coughing or physical activity.
- **C.** A new onset severe headache in a 28-year-old post-partum woman.
- **D.** Unilateral headache which has worsened following chiropractic intervention.

11. A 64-year-old woman presents with fever and speech disturbance over the past week. Her temperature is 37.9 °C. The patient is alert and oriented to time and place but unable to name objects properly. Dysarthria and occasional word substitution are noted. The patient is able to follow two- but not three-step commands. The MRI of brain is attached.

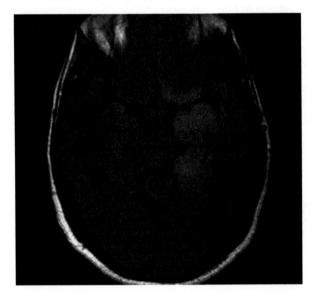

What is the most likely diagnosis?
- **A.** Cerebral toxoplasmosis.
- **B.** Herpes simplex encephalitis.
- **C.** Multiple sclerosis.
- **D.** Progressive multifocal leukoencephalopathy.

12. Regarding the treatment of intracranial parenchymal haemorrhage, which one of the following is correct?
- **A.** Craniectomy performed > 3 hours after the onset of haemorrhage has no survival benefit.
- **B.** Optimum blood pressure target for a patient with acute haemorrhagic stroke is <140/80 mmHg.
- **C.** Prophylactic anticonvulsant is indicated in all patients with haemorrhage stroke.
- **D.** Recombinant factor VIIa is effective and should be used routinely.

13. An 82-year-old woman with a 20-year history of Type 2 diabetes and a 10-year history of poorly controlled hypertension presents with right-sided incoordination and weakness progressing over hours. On examination she has mild pyramidal weakness in the right arm and leg, as well as marked ataxia in the same limbs. There is no sensory deficit, dysphasia, or visual field defect.
Which of the following vessels is most likely to be occluded?
- **A.** A left lenticulostriate artery.
- **B.** Left middle cerebral artery.
- **C.** Right anterior inferior cerebellar artery.
- **D.** Right posterior inferior cerebellar artery.

14. Endovascular thrombectomy of which of the following occluded arteries in patients with an acute ischaemic stroke has been shown to achieve significant improvement in functional outcome?
   A. Middle cerebral artery (M1 segment).
   B. Posterior cerebral arteries.
   C. Posterior inferior cerebellar artery.
   D. Vertebral arteries.

15. A 39-year-old male MCQ examination writer presents with worsening headache. Three months prior, he had been diagnosed with chronic migraine on the basis of frequent, hemicranial pain for the preceding 6 months with around 20 episodes per month, with debilitating episodes preceded by a visual aura (around four times a month). The pain is now bifrontal, near continuous and is not associated with aura. He takes no regular medications but uses ibuprofen daily for headache as well as naratriptan combined with two panadeine forte when the headache peaks (typically four times a week).
   Which of the following treatment strategies is the next most appropriate therapy?
   A. Amitriptyline 25mg daily.
   B. Avoidance of medications for acute therapy.
   C. Botulinum toxin therapy.
   D. Erenumab 70mg monthly.

16. Which variant of Guillain–Barré syndrome is most strongly associated with Anti-GQ1b antibodies?
   A. Miller–Fisher syndrome.
   B. Paraparetic variant.
   C. Pharyngeal–cervical–brachial (PCB) weakness variant.
   D. Pure motor variant.

17. You see a patient in the outpatient clinic for assessment for insertion of a gastrostomy tube. He tells you that he has a history of motor neuron disease (MND) and is having difficulty with swallowing. He initially presented to his GP with dysarthria six months ago, and on examination today you find significant dysarthria, slowed face jaw, and tongue movements disproportional to weakness, tongue wasting, and fasciculations with an exaggerated jaw jerk reflex. There is also mild asymmetrical upper limb weakness and hyperreflexia with wasting/fasciculations of the forearm muscles and thenar eminences.
   Which form of MND are these clinical findings most consistent with?
   A. Classic amyotrophic lateral sclerosis (bulbar onset variant).
   B. Classic amyotrophic lateral sclerosis with frontotemporal dementia.
   C. Isolated bulbar palsy.
   D. Primary lateral sclerosis (bulbar onset variant).

18. Which one of the following medications is **NOT** known to worsen myasthenia gravis symptoms?
   A. Azithromycin.
   B. Cephalexin.
   C. Ciprofloxacin.
   D. Gentamicin.

19. A 26-year-old woman is diagnosed with myasthenia gravis (MG) with muscle-specific tyrosine kinase antibodies. What is the feature of this condition when compared to MG with acetylcholine receptor antibodies?
   A. Axial weakness occurs in 50% of these patients.
   B. It is more commonly associated with bulbar dysfunction.
   C. Ptosis and double vision are more common and severe in these patients.
   D. Pyridostigmine is more effective in these patients.

20. A 29-year-old woman presents with visual impairment in her right eye and pain behind the eye with eye movement. Fundoscopy reveals optic neuritis in that eye. MRI of the head and CSF examination are normal.
   Which one of the following statements is true for this patient?
   A. Optic neuritis is a distinct clinical entity unrelated to multiple sclerosis.
   B. This patient's symptoms may progress to multiple sclerosis despite normal MRI head and CSF examination.
   C. Without treatment, this patient has a high likelihood of permanent unilateral visual loss.
   D. Treatment with high-dose methylprednisolone will preserve her vision.

21. A 75-year-old man from a nursing home presents to the emergency department with presyncopal symptoms, dizziness, and light-headedness on standing. His medical history includes Parkinson's disease, frequent falls, and previous left-sided neck of femur fracture. His medication chart from nursing home shows current medications of Levodopa with carbidopa 100 mg three times a day, perindopril 5 mg daily, and paracetamol 1000 mg qid. His sitting BP is 130/80 mmHg and standing BP is 90/50 mmHg.

What is the appropriate next stage of management?
- **A.** Start fludrocortisone.
- **B.** Start midodrine.
- **C.** Stop levodopa.
- **D.** Stop perindopril.

22. Which one of the following types of encephalitis is most commonly associated with small cell lung cancer?
- **A.** Acute disseminated encephalomyelitis (ADEM).
- **B.** Anti-N-methyl-D-aspartate (anti-NMDA) receptor encephalitis.
- **C.** Brainstem encephalitis.
- **D.** Limbic encephalitis.

23. Which of the following clinical features is more suggestive of Parkinson's disease than another neurodegenerative disease with Parkinsonism symptoms?
- **A.** Abnormal brain MRI.
- **B.** Postural hypotension.
- **C.** Resting tremor.
- **D.** Supranuclear ophthalmoplegia.

24. A 75-year-old man has a history of Parkinson's disease which was diagnosed 3 years ago. He has been on Levodopa/Carbidopa 250/25 mg three times a day for 2.5 years and has developed motor fluctuations and dyskinesia.

Which one of the following agents is efficacious in treating levodopa-induced dyskinesias?
- **A.** Amantadine.
- **B.** Bromocriptine.
- **C.** Entacapone.
- **D.** Rasagiline.

25. A 46-year-old woman presents to the emergency department with gradually worsening paraesthesia and tingling in both hands and feet for 8 weeks. She had been inhaling nitrous oxide from whipped-cream containers for several months. On examination there is slight weakness of finger extension and abduction bilaterally. She demonstrates mild weakness of leg flexors, as well as absent reflexes at the ankles, hyperreflexia at the knees and extensor plantar reflexes. Proprioception and vibration senses are impaired in both hands and feet. Romberg's sign is positive. Laboratory tests showed macrocytosis but no anaemia. Serum copper level is normal.

Which of the following investigations will help to establish the diagnosis of this patient's symptoms and signs?
- **A.** Fasting glucose and haemoglobin A1c (HbA1c).
- **B.** Serum B_{12} and serum methylmalonic acid.
- **C.** Serum folic acid level.
- **D.** Thyroid stimulating hormone (TSH).

26. A 69-year-old man with a history of poorly controlled hypertension, and heavy cigarette smoking presents to hospital with sudden onset of vertigo and unsteady gait. On examination he has right sided limb ataxia, uvula deviation to the left, severe dysphagia, dysphonia, and loss of pain sensation to the right face and left arm and leg. There is right-sided ptosis and miosis.

What is the most likely neuroanatomical site of the stroke?
- **A.** Right lateral medulla.
- **B.** Right medial medulla.
- **C.** Right lateral pons.
- **D.** Right medial pons.

27. Which one of the following primary brain tumours has the worst prognosis?
- **A.** Diffuse high-grade glioma.
- **B.** Ependymoma.

C. Glioblastoma.

D. Pilocytic astrocytoma.

28. A 64-year-old man presents with loss of feeling in the left little toe. On examination he has difficulty in standing on tiptoe on the left side and his left ankle jerk is absent. This is most likely due to:

A. Common peroneal nerve compression.

B. L5 radiculopathy.

C. Posterior tibial nerve compression.

D. S1 radiculopathy.

29. Which one of the treatment options has been shown to reduce risks of ischaemic stroke, myocardial infarction, or death from ischaemic vascular cause at 90 days if used within 12–24 hours post-ischaemic stroke in patients with minor stroke/high-risk TIA?

A. Aspirin + Clopidogrel.

B. Clopidogrel.

C. Direct oral anticoagulant.

D. Warfarin.

30. A 68-year-old woman is found to have a left-sided asymptomatic severe bifurcation carotid stenosis (80%) on ultrasound scan. Her medical history includes hypertension and hyperlipidaemia. She is not at high risk of surgical complications. Which one of following statements is correct regarding the primary composite endpoints of death, stroke, or myocardial infarction within 30 days after the procedure or ipsilateral stroke within 1 year comparing carotid-artery stenting and carotid endarterectomy?

A. Carotid artery stenting is not inferior to carotid endarterectomy.

B. Carotid artery stenting is inferior to carotid endarterectomy.

C. Carotid artery stenting is superior to carotid endarterectomy.

D. Surgical intervention should be avoided in asymptomatic severe carotid stenosis.

31. An 85-year-old man had a fall five days ago. His head hit the dinner table. He presents with progressive headache despite taking paracetamol. His wife reports that he has been vague over the last 2 days. He has hypertension and pulmonary fibrosis. His CT head is shown below.

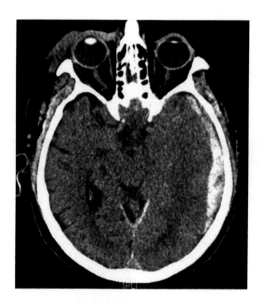

What is most likely cause of his condition?

A. Bleeding from artery of the circle of Willis.

B. Bleeding from branches of middle meningeal artery.

C. Hypertension.

D. Venous haemorrhage.

32. When assessing a patient for trigeminal neuralgia, which of the following is **NOT** consistent with trigeminal neuralgia?
   A. Pain at the angle of the mandible.
   B. Pain at the front of the ear.
   C. Pain of the lower jaw.
   D. Pain in the middle third of the scalp.

QUESTIONS (33–36) REFER TO THE FOLLOWING INFORMATION
Select the most appropriate anticonvulsant for the following questions.
   A. Carbamazepine.
   B. Ethosuximide.
   C. Gabapentin.
   D. Lamotrigine.
   E. Levetiracetam.
   F. Oxcarbazepine.
   G. Phenytoin.
   H. Topiramate.

33. Which antiepileptic drug has the non-linear pharmacokinetics when its plasma concentration is at steady state?

34. Which antiepileptic drug exert its effects via the calcium channel only?

35. Which antiepileptic drug is 100% renally excreted?

36. Which antiepileptic drug can be used in all types of seizure and also has level one evidence of benefit in migraine prophylaxis?

QUESTIONS (37–39) REFER TO THE FOLLOWING INFORMATION
For each of the following patients, select the mutated gene which is most likely to be responsible.
   A. *ATP1A1* gene.
   B. *APOE* gene.
   C. *KALIG-1* gene.
   D. *Retinoblastoma (RB)1* gene.
   E. *Neurofibromin 1* gene.
   F. *NOTCH3* gene.
   G. *Peripheral myelin protein-22 (PMP22) gene.*
   H. *PRPS1* gene.

37. An optic nerve glioma is seen on the head MRI in a 30-year-old man. The finding on examination is shown in the photo below.

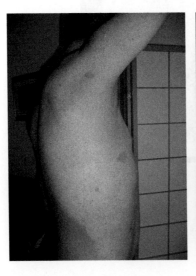
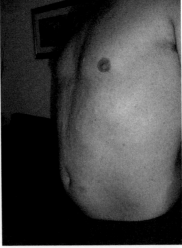

38. A 42-year-old woman is diagnosed with a TIA. Brain MRI shows severe microvascular ischaemic changes in the cerebral and brainstem white matter, there are multiple old lacunar infarcts in the periventricular white matter. There is strong family history of TIA. She is suspected to have cerebral autosomal dominant arteriopathy with subcortical infarcts and leukoencephalopathy (CADASIL).

39. The chief resident has recruited a patient with Charcot-Marie-Tooth (CMT) disease type 1 for RACP clinical exam.

QUESTIONS (40–48) **REFER TO THE FOLLOWING INFORMATION**
For each of the following clinical scenario and presentations, select the most likely site of lesion in the central nervous system.

- **A.** Brainstem.
- **B.** Broca's area.
- **C.** Cerebellum.
- **D.** Corpus callosum.
- **E.** Dorsal pons.
- **F.** Hippocampus.
- **G.** Interventricular foramen.
- **H.** Medial midbrain.
- **I.** Midbrain.
- **J.** Optic chiasm.
- **K.** Posterior parietal lobe.
- **L.** Substantia nigra.
- **M.** Subthalamic nucleus.
- **N.** Wernicke's area.

40. A 70-year-old man presents with tremor in his right hand which is most noticeable when he is watching television. It disappears when he is playing golf. His wife notices he is slowing down of his woodwork and his handwriting is difficult to read. He has no recent falls. On examination, there is a resting tremor in his right hand, and cogwheeling in the right wrist. There is decreased arm swing on the right. There is no ataxia and intact tandem gait. The power, reflexes, and sensation are grossly intact.

41. A 75-year-old woman develops sudden, uncontrollable movements of her arm where she throws it outwards and injures herself.

42. A 75-year-old man presents with sudden onset of right third cranial nerve palsy and a left hemiplegia involving the face, arm, and leg.

43. A 75-year-old man is seen in the clinic because of severe headache and vomiting. An MRI revealed the presence of brain tumour, complicated by a non-communicating hydrocephalus.

44. A 46-year-old woman has a traffic accident while driving a car to see her GP because of severe headache. She tells the police that she cannot see traffic on both sides of the midline, which is confirmed by her GP during the neurological exam.

45. A 73-year-old man suffers a stroke which produces a marked neglect of the opposite half body and visual space.

46. A 56-year-old woman is frustrated and depressed because she is unable to verbally express her thoughts in a meaningful way.

47. A 28-year-old man has been suffering from epilepsy for 10 years. Despite the extensive treatment with multiple anticonvulsants, the seizure activity has begun to spread to other region of the brain and opposite side of the brain. In order to reduce the spread of the seizures to other side, which structure would most likely be targeted by the neurosurgeon?

48. A neurological examination has revealed that the patient is unable to move his right eye to the right and the right side of his face is expressionless.

Answers

1. Answer: B

Bell's palsy is an acute, unilateral, peripheral, lower-motor-neuron facial nerve paralysis that gradually resolves over time in 80% to 90% of cases. It is the most common cause of unilateral facial paralysis, accounting for 70% of cases of acute unilateral facial paralysis.

The onset of Bell's palsy is typically sudden, and symptoms tend to peak in less than 48 hours. Early symptoms include the following:

- Weakness of the facial muscles
- Poor eyelid closure
- Aching of the ear or mastoid (60%)
- Alteration of taste (57%)
- Hyperacusis (30%)
- Decreased tearing
- Tingling or numbness of the cheek/mouth.

The diagnosis of Bell's palsy is made on the basis of a thorough history and physical examination. An otologic examination includes pneumatic otoscopy and tuning fork examination. An otologic cause should be considered if the history or physical examination demonstrates evidence of acute or chronic otitis media, including a tympanic membrane perforation, otorrhea, cholesteatoma, or granulation tissue, or if a history of ear surgery is noted. Concurrent rash or vesicles along the ear canal, pinna, and mouth should raise the suspicion for Ramsay Hunt syndrome (herpes zoster oticus). The external auditory canal should be inspected for vesicles, infection, or trauma. Testing for unilateral loss of taste (with coffee or sugar) may assist diagnostic certainty.

Guidelines do not recommend routine laboratory testing or diagnostic imaging in patients with new-onset Bell's palsy. Nerve conduction velocities and EMG may aid in assessing the outcome of a patient who has persistent and severe Bell's palsy. This testing is not part of the acute workup. This test should be performed 3 to 10 days after the onset of paralysis. EMG/nerve conduction studies do not show an abnormality for 3 weeks after a peripheral nerve injury.

Oral steroids should be prescribed within 72 hours of symptom onset for all patients with Bell's palsy. Oral antiviral therapy should not be given alone for patients with new-onset Bell's palsy. However, oral antiviral therapy may be offered in addition to oral steroids within 72 hours of symptom onset, especially if paralysis is severe.

Eviston T, Croxson G, Kennedy P, Hadlock T, Krishnan A. Bell's palsy: aetiology, clinical features, and multidisciplinary care. Journal of Neurology, Neurosurgery & Psychiatry. 2015;86(12):1356–1361.
https://jnnp.bmj.com/content/jnnp/86/12/1356.full.pdf

2. Answer: B

This presentation is typical of benign paroxysmal positional vertigo (BPPV), which can be diagnosed by the Dix–Hallpike manoeuvre.

BPPV is the most common vestibular cause of dizziness, caused by calcium debris deposition in the semicircular canals of the vestibular labyrinth, typically the posterior canal. In posterior canal BPPV the Dix–Hallpike manoeuvre produces a nystagmus which is characteristically upbeat and torsional, occurs after a latency period, duration usually < 1 minute, and is fatigable with repetition of manoeuvre. In contrast, central nystagmus is typically purely downbeat, horizontal, or vertical, has no latency period, persists > 1 minute, and is reproducible with similar nystagmus intensity. Repositioning manoeuvres including Epley manoeuvre is the best treatment for BPPV. Differentiating benign and serious causes is the most important part in assessing dizziness. Traditionally, this involved clarifying the 'type of dizziness', though there has been a recent focus on symptom timing and triggers, to decide the appropriate targeted bedside examinations then investigations:

1. Triggered episodic vestibular syndrome: Dix–Hallpike manoeuvre will differentiate between central paroxysmal positional vertigo causes (posterior fossa neoplasm, infarction, haemorrhage, demyelination) and BPPV (as described above.) Another common cause is orthostatic hypotension.
2. Spontaneous episodic vestibular syndrome: Atypical history and significant cardiovascular risk factors helps differentiate between concerning causes requiring further workup (TIA, arrythmia, MI, PE, hypoglycaemia) and benign causes (vestibular migraine, Meniere's disease, vasovagal episodes, panic attacks). The cardiovascular risk factors include IHD, hypertension, diabetes, previous TIA/CVA, PVD, smoker.
3. Triggered acute vestibular syndrome: History of trigger (head trauma, barotrauma, toxins, new medications i.e. gentamicin) will indicate the appropriate workup.
4. Spontaneous acute vestibular syndrome: Head Impulse Nystagmus and Test of Skew examination (HINTS) differentiates with greater sensitivity than CT or MRI posterior circulation stroke from benign causes (commonly vestibular neuritis or labyrinthitis), with at least one of: head impulse test with no corrective saccade, nystagmus predominantly vertical or torsional, and abnormal

test of skew with vertical correction on uncovering the eye. Less common causes include multiple sclerosis, cerebellar haemorrhage, thiamine deficiency, and autoimmune, infectious, and metabolic causes.

Newman-Toker D, Edlow J. TiTrATE. Neurologic Clinics. 2015; 33(3):577–599.
https://pubmed.ncbi.nlm.nih.gov/26231273/

3. Answer: C

Archaeological evidence of the use of cannabis for epilepsy arises from a period not long after the advent of written language, with Sumerian and Akkadian tablets outlining its use from around 1800 BC. Cannabis was in common use for epilepsy syndromes in the 19th century, with its use becoming less mainstream in the 20th century with the discovery of phenytoin and phenobarbital in the 1930s. The cannabis plant contains multiple active compounds and metabolites, with Δ9-tetrahydrocannabinol (THC), and cannabidiol (CBD), the most pharmacologically active. THC exerts most of its influence on the CB_1R receptor, expressed not only in brain tissue, but also in gut and heart tissue, and is responsible for the 'high' effects of cannabis, as well as the addictive properties. The pharmacological effects of cannabidiol are a little more elusive, although decreased activity of excitatory neurons appears to be key, perhaps by antagonising a G-coupled protein at synaptic excitatory neurons. Although the various parts of the endogenous cannabinoid system seem important in epilepsy, CBD seems to have the most potential as an antiepileptic medication.

There have been two successful randomised, placebo-controlled trials of cannabidiol in the treatment of severe childhood epilepsy syndromes. Dravet syndrome occurs in infancy. It is characterised by prolonged febrile and non-febrile seizures within the first year of life, progressing to multiple seizure types, associated with behavioural disturbance and developmental delay. Most cases are due to sodium channel nonsense mutations (SCN1A) gene. Cannabidiol reduced seizure frequency in comparison to placebo in this group but was associated with higher results of adverse effects (especially drowsiness and vomiting/diarrhoea). Lennox–Gastaut syndrome has onset slightly later in life (onset 3–5 years) but is also associated with significant developmental delay and treatment-refractory seizures. Cannabidiol was also effective in reducing seizure frequency for this diagnosis. Importantly, the response to placebo was fairly high in both trials, highlighting the necessity of randomised, placebo-controlled design in inferring efficacy from research in this area.

Friedman D, Devinsky O. Cannabinoids for the treatment of epilepsy. N Eng J Med. 2015; 373:1048–1058.
https://www.nejm.org/doi/full/10.1056/NEJMra1407304

4. Answer: A

The clinical signs suggest Horner's syndrome and evaluation depends on the clinical context. In the context of trauma, headache, or neck pain, acute onset of Horner's syndrome requires exclusion of vascular pathology (in particular carotid artery dissection) with CT angiography. In the case of subacute Horner's syndrome, CT angiography of the head, neck, and upper chest is recommended within several weeks in order to investigate for pathology along the sympathetic chain. Central causes of Horner's syndrome are due to pathology of the spinal cord, hypothalamus, or brainstem. When Horner's syndrome is combined with other brainstem neurological signs, MRI of the brain is warranted. Horner's syndrome may be due to pathology affecting central (hypothalamospinal), preganglionic, or postganglionic fibres. Anhidrosis is absent in postganglionic lesions but may be present central (face arm and trunk) and preganglionic (face only) lesions.

Carotid artery dissection can be associated with trauma, connective tissue disorders, or family history. Most cases of carotid artery dissection are idiopathic, although joint hypermobility is found on examination in around 50% (versus 5% of the general population). Median age is around the mid-forties, and diagnosis is more common in males. Overall, carotid artery dissection accounts for a small proportion of stroke; however, in young patients, it is estimated that around 20% of all strokes are caused by carotid artery dissection. Most strokes in carotid dissection are embolic rather than as a result of haemodynamic compromise of the carotid artery. The optimal management of extracranial carotid dissection has not been determined. Thrombolysis in acute stroke may be safely administered with the same inclusion and exclusion criteria as for ischaemic stroke not due to carotid dissection. Endovascular thrombectomy should be performed if other standard criteria are met, although stenting is often required and is complicated. Antithrombotic therapy is usually used in carotid artery dissection, but the optimal agents, duration, and investigations for guiding therapy have not been determined. Meta-analysis suggests that anticoagulation is not superior to an antiplatelet strategy for stroke prevention but carries higher bleeding risk.

Malem A. Unequal pupils and ptosis. BMJ. 2017; j643.
https://www.bmj.com/content/356/bmj.j643

5. Answer: B

This young female patient has a medical history of venous thromboembolism (VTE) in the left lower limb and previous Budd–Chiari syndrome (hepatic vein thrombosis) and now a sagittal sinus thrombosis. These atypical thrombotic sites warrant further investigation of the underlying cause of recurrent VTE. There is evidence of intravascular haemolysis, including a low Hb, an increased LDH level, an elevated reticulocyte count, a low haptoglobin, a negative direct antiglobulin test (DAT), and positive urine haemosiderin (haemoglobinuria). The findings of thrombocytopenia are likely related to mild splenomegaly as a consequence of portal hypertension given previous history of hepatic vein thrombosis.

The clinical picture and investigation results suggest a possible diagnosis of paroxysmal nocturnal haemoglobinuria (PNH). The next appropriate step of investigation is to collect peripheral blood for flow cytometry to identify reduced levels of glycosylphosphatidylinositol (GPI)-anchored proteins secondary to defective enzyme, phosphatidylinositol glycan A (PIGA) on the RBC membrane. Complement-medicated intravascular haemolysis is a consequence of deficiency of the complement inhibitory proteins decay accelerating factor (DAF, CD55) and membrane inhibitor of reactive lysis (MIRL, CD59). Eculizumab, a humanised monoclonal mouse antibody (IgG), is used to prevent activation of C5 and subsequent formation of the membrane attack complex in patients with PNH. Bone marrow biopsy is indicated if there is also clinical suspicion of aplastic anaemia or myelodysplastic syndrome that give rise to PNH. The clinical picture does not fit polycythemia ruba vera or haemochromatosis, so JAK 2 mutation and iron studies are not appropriate next step of investigation tests in this case. A small percentage of patients progress to have acute leukaemia from PNH.

Central venous sinus thrombosis (CVST) has varied clinical presentation, symptoms, and clinical courses. Acute, chronic intermittent, sudden-onset of thunder-clap headaches can occur with or without nausea. CVST causes around 1% of all strokes. CVST can cause increased intra-cranial hypertension due to venous thrombosis and sometimes also lead to cerebral oedema, infarction, haemorrhage, seizures, paresis, hemiplegia, and altered mental status. In patients with intracranial hypertension, imaging of the cerebral venous system is recommended to exclude CVST.

Risk factors for CVST include female gender, pregnancy, oestrogen-containing contraceptives, hormone replacement therapy, puerperium, malignancy, head trauma, infection, dehydration, autoimmune disease, thrombophilia, and systemic disease, such as sarcoidosis.

Accurate and timely diagnosis of CVST is important to avoid treatment delay. Treatment of CVST include body weight-adjusted subcutaneous low-molecular weight heparin, followed by oral anticoagulant treatment and cessation of oral estrogen-containing contraceptives or hormone replacement therapy. The optimal duration of long-term oral anticoagulation therapy after the first acute thrombotic event is unclear, but 6–12 months is reasonable. In patients with recurrent CVST and thrombophilia without reversible causes, consider life-long anticoagulation.

Careful monitoring is required to monitor intra-cranial pressure to avoid haemorrhagic and herniation complications. If cerebral oedema is severe, decompressive craniotomy appears lifesaving for many, with high rates of good recovery. Aggressive treatment of seizures is warranted. There is currently insufficient evidence to suggest the use of systemic or local thrombolysis, or thrombectomy.

MAGICapp – Making GRADE the Irresistible Choice – Medical Guidelines [Internet]. App.magicapp.org. 2020 [cited 19 March 2020]. Available from:
https://app.magicapp.org/#/guideline/4285

6. Answer: C

Chronic inflammatory demyelinating polyradiculoneuropathy (CIDP) must be treated to prevent accumulating disability. CIDP treatment can be divided into induction and maintenance treatment.

The goal of induction treatment is important to improve the patient's symptoms and to prevent secondary axonal degeneration.

1. IVIG contains antibodies that may neutralise immune factors mediating CIDP. Multiple clinical trials establish its efficacy. Patients usually require repeated treatments every few weeks or months to maintain remission or treat recurrences.
2. Corticosteroids can be the initial induction treatment. Several regimens are available and seem equally effective: oral prednisolone 60 mg/day, pulsed high-dose dexamethasone (usually starting with 40 mg for 4 days every 4 weeks), or intravenous methylprednisolone (starting with 1000 mg weekly or monthly). No specific corticosteroid treatment is proven to be most effective but pulsed oral and intravenous corticosteroid treatments possibly have fewer steroid-associated side effects. Studies have shown that 6 months of pulsed dexamethasone or 8 months of daily prednisone can achieve long-term remission in over 25% of patients.
3. Plasma exchange can remove antibodies and complement components that are responsible for immune-mediated damage of peripheral nerves. Two studies have confirmed benefit. It can be used as induction treatment and be considered in patients with CIDP not responding to IVIG.

When a patient does not improve after the first treatment regimen, the diagnosis should be reconsidered because misdiagnosis is common.

Randomised clinical trials have not shown that other immunosuppressive drugs are effective in the treatment of CIDP, including methotrexate, azathioprine, and ciclosporin. However, the use of immunomodulatory treatments (e.g. azathioprine, rituximab, and methotrexate) can have positive effects in individual patients, especially as add-on treatments or to reduce high doses of corticosteroids or IVIG. Chronic long-term treatment is often needed, but tailoring treatments to the lowest possible dose is important to reduce side-effects and associated costs. It is recommended to attempt dose reduction at least yearly.

Bunschoten C, Jacobs B, Van den Bergh P, Cornblath D, van Doorn P. Progress in diagnosis and treatment of chronic inflammatory demyelinating polyradiculoneuropathy. The Lancet Neurology [Internet]. 2019 [cited 20 June 2020]; 18(8):784–794.
https://www.thelancet.com/journals/laneur/article/PIIS1474-4422(19)30144-9/fulltext

7. Answer: C

Many diseases of central nervous system (CNS) can cause changes in the concentrations of individual components of cerebrospinal fluid (CSF). Testing the CSF plays an important role in the differential diagnostics and confirmation of a particular disease.

The total volume of CSF is approximately 150 ml and it is produced at a rate of 450 ml per day. CSF is produced in two ways: (i) Secretion (producing around 60% of the volume) occurs in the cells of the choroid plexus and ventricular ependyma, (ii) Ultrafiltration of blood plasma through choroidal capillaries. The resorption of liquor takes place in the arachnoid granulations. The composition of the CSF does not qualitatively differ much from the composition of blood plasma, but they differ quantitatively (see table below). This knowledge is essential for interpreting CSF results for diagnostic purpose. CSF has very low protein concentration because large protein molecules cannot cross the blood–brain barrier.

Component	CSF concentration	Plasma concentration	CSF concentration compared with plasma
Glucose	2.2–4.4 mmol/L	3.5–5.5 mmol/L	40% less
Protein	15–40 mg/dL	6300–8500 mg/dL	1% or less
Urea	3–6.5 mmol/L	3–6.0 mmol/L	Same
Lactic acid	1.2–2.0 mmol/L	0.2–2.0 mmol/L	Same
Sodium	140 mmol/L	145 mmol/L	Slightly lower
Potassium	2.8 mmol/L	4.5 mmol/L	40% less
Chloride	120 mmol/L	100 mmol/L	Higher than plasma level
Calcium	1.15 mmol/L	2.35 mmol/L	50% less
Bicarbonate	23 mmol/L	26 mmol/L	Similar
pH	7.3 mmol/L	7.4 mmol/L	Similar

RCPA – Cerebrospinal fluid examination [Internet]. Rcpa.edu.au. 2020 [cited 2 June 2020]. Available from: https://www.rcpa.edu.au/Manuals/RCPA-Manual/Pathology-Tests/C/Cerebrospinal-fluid-examination

8. Answer: C

Worsening control of epileptic seizures exposes the pregnant woman to risk of physical injury and psychological harm such as reduced social activities, impaired quality of life and loss of driver's licence. The increased mortality rate in pregnant women with epilepsy is mostly attributable to sudden unexplained death.

Studies have shown that, as pregnancy progresses, steady state plasma concentrations of antiepileptic drugs tend to fall unless the drug doses are increased. The main reasons are:

1. Increased renal clearance of unmetabolised drug because of the physiological increase in glomerular filtration rate during pregnancy, a phenomenon that is of greatest importance for antiepileptic drugs that undergo relatively little (e.g., levetiracetam) or no metabolism (e.g., gabapentin).
2. Increased biotransformation, because increased circulating levels of female steroidal sex hormones during pregnancy induce formation of the cytochrome P450 isoenzymes and glucuronosyl transferases that play the main roles in eliminating most antiepileptic drugs.
3. Dilutional effect from the increased maternal extracellular fluid, placental, and foetal volumes during pregnancy, an effect offset to an extent in late pregnancy when plasma albumin concentrations fall, so that there is an increased concentration of unbound drug relative to total drug in plasma.

The decrease in drug concentration tends to be small for drugs that are cleared by renal excretion and are larger for drugs cleared mainly through biotransformation. The greatest clearance increases among the currently commonly used antiepileptic drugs is lamotrigine, eliminated largely by N-glucuronidation. Doses of this drug may need to be doubled or tripled during pregnancy to maintain steady-state plasma drug concentrations at their pre-pregnancy values. The fall in plasma carbamazepine concentration tends to be relatively small and mainly due to increase in blood volume during pregnancy.

Seizure control tends to correlate with plasma antiepileptic drug concentrations. Dosages of antiepileptic drugs should therefore be adjusted in pregnancy due to falling plasma concentrations to avoid any deterioration in seizure control.

Epilepsy in Pregnancy (Green-top Guideline No.68) [Internet]. Royal College of Obstetricians & Gynaecologists. 2020 [cited 22 February 2020]. Available from: https://www.rcog.org.uk/en/guidelines-research-services/guidelines/gtg68/

9. Answer: B

Guillain–Barré syndrome (GBS) is a rapidly progressive and potentially life-threatening peripheral neuropathy that requires early diagnosis, monitoring, and treatment.

The pathogenesis is not completely understood, but GBS is believed to result from an abnormal immune response which causes damage to peripheral nerves. Up to 2/3 of patients report a preceding infection: *Campylobacter jejuni, Mycoplasma pneumoniae*, EBV, CMV, Hepatitis E virus, and Zika virus have all been temporally associated in case-control studies.

Diagnosis of GBS is based on clinical history and examination, supported by ancillary tests. CSF is mainly used to exclude alternate diagnoses. It may demonstrate 'albuminocytologic dissociation' (i.e., elevated protein but no pleocytosis); however normal protein and cell count are seen in 30–50% of cases, and a mild pleocytosis in a minority. Electrodiagnostic studies (EDS) commonly shows prolonged distal motor latencies, motor slowing, conduction block, prolonged F-waves temporal dispersion which can help support the diagnosis. EDS can also differentiate subtypes into acute inflammatory demyelinating polyradiculopathy (AIDP), acute motor axonal neuropathy (AMAN), and acute motor sensory axonal neuropathy (AMSAN.)

Features required for diagnosis:
- Progressive bilateral arm and leg weakness (initially legs may only be involved)
- Decreased or absent reflexes in affected arms and legs (may be temporary)

Features that strongly support the diagnosis:
- Progressive phase of disease lasts days to 4 weeks (typically < 2 weeks)
- Symmetry of symptoms and signs
- Milder sensory symptoms and signs
- Cranial nerve involvement, for example bilateral facial palsy
- Autonomic dysfunction, including labile blood pressure and fatal arrythmias
- Back or limb pain
- CSF with albumino-cytological dissociation
- Electrodiagnostic studies with features of motor or sensorimotor neuropathy.

Treatment is indicated if patients cannot walk more than 10 metres independently, or other concerning features. IVIG within 2 weeks and plasma exchange within 4 weeks of weakness onset has been shown to be efficacious. Prednisolone is ineffective.

ICU admission is recommended for patients with rapid progression of weakness, severe autonomic dysfunction, severe swallowing difficulties, or severe respiratory distress. Up to 20% of GBS patients develop respiratory failure and require mechanical ventilation. Mortality rates remain at 3–10% despite optimal medical care, mostly secondary to cardiovascular and respiratory complications and withdrawal of care in the severely affected elderly.

Leonhard S, Mandarakas M, Gondim F, Bateman K, Ferreira M, Cornblath D et al. Diagnosis and management of Guillain–Barré syndrome in ten steps. Nature Reviews Neurology. 2019;15(11):671–683. https://www.nature.com/articles/s41582-019-0250-9

10. Answer: A

Option A represents a cluster headache (trigeminal autonomic cephalgia): 15–180-minute episodes of unilateral peri-orbital or temporal headaches with ipsilateral conjunctival injection, lacrimation, nasal congestion, rhinorrhoea, eyelid oedema, sweating, flushing, ear fullness, miosis, or ptosis. At least five attacks are required for the diagnosis of cluster headache disorder, which is a primary headache disorder, and do not require neuroimaging.

Headaches are common, with headache disorders affecting up to half of the adult population globally. 90% of headaches are primary headaches: headaches not associated with any identifiable pathology, including tension-type headache, migraines, and cluster headaches. Secondary headaches represent the remaining 10% of headaches and are due to an underlying pathological cause (iatrogenic, infective, inflammatory, vascular, or structural) Most headaches can be diagnosed with a thorough history and targeted general and neurological examination, aiming to classify the type of headache, and screen for secondary headache. There are no diagnostic tests for primary headache. Most are benign and neuroimaging is usually not needed.

The red flags of a secondary headache, which head CT scan or MRI is required, are summarised in Table 16.1.

If any of the following headaches are suspected, urgent neuroimaging is indicated:

- Subarachnoid haemorrhage commonly presents with sudden onset of severe headache maximal in severity within the first minute, so called thunderclap headache. Investigation of choice is CT brain without contrast, then if normal, lumbar puncture.
- Reversible cerebral vasoconstriction syndrome.
- Space occupying lesion (Option B) can present with seizures, altered mental state, abnormal neurological signs, and symptoms of raised intracranial pressure, which can present as a headache worse in morning, coughing, or exertion. Investigation is ideally MRI brain with contrast or CT brain with contrast if MRI unavailable.
- Carotid or vertebral artery dissection (Option D) typically presents with unilateral headache, neck pain, Horner syndrome, or stroke symptoms, especially with the history of even minor neck trauma. Investigation is with CT/MRI brain and angiography.
- Cerebral venous sinus thrombosis (Option C) can present variably, commonly as a headache (thunderclap, acute, or gradual onset) in a young adult (mean age 39) with risk factors including pregnancy, postpartum, obesity, malignancy, and oral contraceptive pill use, typically with signs of raised intracranial pressure, focal neurological deficits, seizures, and altered mental state. CT/MRI brain and venography is investigation of choice.

Table 16.1   Red flag for a headache.

Headache associated with	New-onset headache in a patient who is
Head injury, especially with loss of consciousness	pregnant or post-partum
Focal neurological signs, papilloedema	taking contraceptive pills
Seizures but the person is not an epileptic	taking an anticoagulant
Progressive worsening	has taken amphetamine or cocaine
Abrupt onset with thunderclap character	young and obese
Worsening by coughing or physical activity	has a history of cancer
Fever and/or neck stiffness	HIV positive
Confusion	an organ transplant recipient and taking immunosuppressant
Vomiting	Onset after age of 50
Reduced GCS	
The person being woken from sleep	

Wronski M, Aagami AS. Investigation of patients presenting with headache. Medicine Today. 2015;16(11):41–46. https://endocrinologytoday.com.au/sites/default/files/cpd/MT2015-11-041-WRONSKI.pdf

11. Answer: B

Herpes simplex viruses (HSV-1 and HSV-2) produce a variety of infections involving mucocutaneous surfaces, the CNS, and occasionally visceral organs. HSV encephalitis is the most common identified cause of acute, sporadic viral encephalitis, and is usually localised to the temporal and frontal lobes in adults. Typically, it causes a flu-like illness with headache and fever followed by seizures, cognitive impairment, behavioural changes, and focal neurological signs, as in this case. However, its presentation is variable.

If HSV encephalitis is suspected, MRI brain and CSF analysis (if lumbar puncture is not contraindicated) should be performed urgently. The diagnosis of HSV encephalitis can be strongly suggested by the typical radiographic appearance that is oedema, haemorrhage, and necrosis in the inferomedial temporal lobe such as in this case. Brain involvement may be unilateral or bilateral. However, early in the clinical course of the disease, MRI results may be negative. A negative MRI does not rule out HSV encephalitis. Definitive diagnosis of HSV encephalitis is made by the detection of viral nucleic acid in the CSF by the PCR. This test has a sensitivity of 96–98% and specificity of 95–99% and has removed the need for brain biopsy. It remains positive for at least 5 to 7 days after starting antiviral therapy. Viral DNA may be undetectable in early disease, but, if so, a repeat examination by PCR on CSF three to seven days later can confirm the diagnosis.

Pending the confirmation of the diagnosis of HSV encephalitis, all adults with suspected encephalitis should be given acyclovir empirically, at a dose of 10 mg/kg, administered as intravenous infusions over one hour and repeated every eight hours for 14–21 days if renal function is normal. Higher doses are recommended for immunocompromised patients.

 Tyler KL. Acute Viral Encephalitis. N Engl J Med 2018; 379:557–566
https://www.nejm.org/doi/full/10.1056/NEJMra1708714

12. Answer: B

There is no effective targeted therapy for haemorrhagic stroke. Studies of recombinant FVIIa have yielded disappointing results. In an international, randomised, placebo-controlled trial of adults with intracerebral haemorrhage, 2325 participants received 1 g intravenous tranexamic acid bolus followed by an infusion of another 1 g intravenous tranexamic acid over 8 h, or matching placebo, within 8 h of symptom onset. It did not show any effect of tranexamic acid on the primary outcome of functional recovery at 90 days, there was a significant reduction in deaths within 7 days (but not at 90 days) and serious adverse events, and a modest attenuation (1 mL) of haematoma growth between the baseline and 24 h non-contrast CT.

The use of prophylactic anticonvulsant medication remains uncertain. In prospective and population-based studies, clinical seizures have not been associated with worse neurologic outcome or mortality. Indeed, two studies have reported worse outcomes in patients who did not have a documented seizure but who received antiepileptic drugs (primarily phenytoin).

No controlled studies have defined optimum BP levels for patients with acute haemorrhagic stroke, but greatly elevated BP is thought to lead to rebleeding and hematoma expansion. Stroke may result in loss of cerebral autoregulation of cerebral perfusion pressure. Intensive BP reduction (target BP <140 mmHg systolic) early in the treatment of patients with intracerebral haemorrhage appears to lessen the absolute growth of haematomas, particularly in patients who have received previous antithrombotic therapy, according to a combined analysis of the Intensive Blood Pressure Reduction in Acute Cerebral Haemorrhage Trials 1 and 2 (INTERACT).

For supratentorial intracerebral haemorrhage, early evacuation (<24 h after onset of haemorrhage) with open craniotomy may be lifesaving in deteriorating patients but is not clearly beneficial in deeply comatose or otherwise stable patients. In the first large clinical trial on surgical management of intracerebral haemorrhage, there was no overall benefit from early surgery compared with initial conservative treatment.

 Cordonnier C, Demchuk A, Ziai W, Anderson C. Intracerebral haemorrhage: current approaches to acute management. The Lancet. 2018;392(10154):1257–1268.
https://pubmed.ncbi.nlm.nih.gov/30319113/

13. Answer: A

Lacunar stroke syndromes occur as a result of occlusion of small perforating arteries in the deep structures of the brain. The pathophysiology of these strokes is through medial thickening and microatheroma formation, promulgated by hypertension and diabetes. Common presentations of lacunar infarcts are purely motor deficits, purely sensory deficits, ataxic hemiparesis syndrome, or mixed sensory and motor deficits without cortical signs.

Ataxic hemiparesis syndrome occurs due to involvement of both the corticospinal tract and either descending uncrossed cerebellar efferent fibres (corticopontocerebellar) or ascending efferent crossed fibres (superior cerebellar peduncle outflow). Commonest locations are thalamocapsular, paramedian pons, and centrum semiovale.

 Regenhardt R, Das A, Lo E, Caplan L. Advances in Understanding the Pathophysiology of Lacunar Stroke. JAMA Neurology. 2018;75(10):1273.
https://jamanetwork.com/journals/jamaneurology/article-abstract/2696969

14. Answer: A

Endovascular thrombectomy has emerged as a new standard of care in patients with acute large vessel occlusion (LVO) such as basilar, intracranial internal carotid artery (ICA), and proximal middle cerebral artery within 6 hours of stroke onset. Although not proven in a randomised controlled trial, most treatment guidelines support thrombectomy for acute basilar artery occlusion. Endovascular thrombectomy can reduce disability when started 6 to 24 hours from the time last seen well for patients with LVO who have a clinical deficit that is disproportionally severe compared with the volume of infarction on imaging studies and/or penumbral/core mismatch demonstrated with multimodal CT or MRI. The number needed to treat is around 3–4 for endovascular thrombectomy to prevent functional dependency at three months. Patients who present within 4.5 hours of the onset of ischaemic stroke signs or symptoms should still receive intravenous thrombolysis with recombinant tissue-type plasminogen activator where indicated.

Endovascular thrombectomy can be considered in patients with or without treatment with intravenous alteplase if they fulfil the following criteria:

- Large vessel occlusion when the procedure can be commenced within six hours of stroke onset.
- Ischaemic stroke caused by a large vessel occlusion in the ICA, proximal middle cerebral artery (M1 segment) if the procedure can be commenced between 6–24 hours after they were last known to be well if clinical and CT perfusion or MRI features indicate the presence of salvageable brain tissue.

Post-endovascular thrombectomy adverse events include perforation, dissection, subarachnoid haemorrhage, and intravenous contrast-related complications. As a result, endovascular thrombectomy should be performed in high-volume stroke centres that have experienced neurointerventionists, a multi-disciplinary stroke rehabilitation team, an ICU, and a neurosurgical team to streamline the process of clot retrieval and maximise the patient's outcome post-thrombolysis and post-thrombectomy. The earlier the reperfusion the more non-ischaemic brain tissue may be salvaged; 'time is brain'. Prior to the endovascular thrombectomy, it is essential to obtain a CT brain, CT brain angiogram and CT neck angiogram to determine the feasibility of access to the target artery occlusion. CT perfusion can assist determining the functional significance of the occluded vessel and help prognosticate.

MAGICapp - Making GRADE the Irresistible Choice – Medical Guidelines [Internet]. App.magicapp.org. 2020 [cited 9 March 2020]. Available from: https://app.magicapp.org/#/guideline/4473

Campbell B, De Silva D, Macleod M, Coutts S, Schwamm L, Davis S et al. Ischaemic stroke. Nature Reviews Disease Primers. 2019;5(1).
https://www.nature.com/articles/s41572-019-0118-8

15. Answer: B

Medication overuse headache is a common and debilitating headache disorder caused by the overuse of anti-migraine medications. Typically, the underlying pain problem is headache, however, use of analgesics for other pain problems can occasionally cause medication overuse headache. Diagnosis can be made on the basis of 15 headache episodes per month over a three month period, with medication use for acute therapy on at least 10 of 15 days, depending on the medication, or where headache classification does not fit another headache classification. Given the subjectivity of diagnostic criteria, prevalence studies vary, but may be as high as 7% in some countries.

Treatment of medication overuse headache revolves around cessation of intermittent use of medication for acute attacks, and this measure alone may be effective in around 50% of patients. Consequently, this is advised as the first step in managing medication overuse headache. However, the combination of withdrawal and initiation of prophylactic medication may be more effective than withdrawal of acute medications alone. Additionally, botulinum toxin, erenumab (a calcitonin-gene related peptide monoclonal antibody) and topiramate may prove to be effective with or without withdrawal of the offending medication.

Diener H, Dodick D, Evers S, Holle D, Jensen R, Lipton R et al. Pathophysiology, prevention, and treatment of medication overuse headache. The Lancet Neurology. 2019;18(9):891–902.
https://www.thelancet.com/pdfs/journals/laneur/PIIS1474-4422(19)30146-2.pdf

16. Answer: A

Guillain–Barré syndrome (GBS) is an acquired peripheral neuropathy, secondary to autoimmune inflammation of peripheral nerves and spinal roots. Up to two-thirds of patients with GBS describe an infection especially *Campylobacter jejuni* infection in the 6 weeks prior to symptom onset.

Classic sensorimotor GBS typically presents with distal paraesthesia, followed by motor weakness that ascends from the legs to the arms to the cranial muscles. GBS can also present as the following variants:

- Pure motor variant: Weakness without sensory symptoms or signs
- Bilateral facial palsy with paraesthesias: Weakness limited to cranial nerves
- Pharyngeal– cervical–brachial weakness: Upper limb weakness
- Paraparetic variant: Lower limb weakness
- Miller Fisher syndrome (MFS): Ophthalmoplegia, areflexia and ataxia which is associated with Anti-GQ1b antibodies.

GBS diagnostic criteria require progressive bilateral weakness of arms and legs (typically only legs at onset) and decreased or absent reflexes in affected limbs. Other suggestive features include progression of disease during the first days to four weeks, symmetry of limbs affected, sensory loss, cranial nerve involvement especially bilateral facial palsy, autonomic dysfunction, back or limb pain, and typical CSF and electrodiagnostic features.

MFS is observed in about 5% of all cases of GBS. Acute onset of external ophthalmoplegia is a cardinal feature. Ataxia tends to be out of proportion to the degree of sensory loss. Patients may also have mild limb weakness, ptosis, facial palsy, or bulbar palsy. Patients have reduced or absent sensory nerve action potentials and absent tibial H reflex. There is an overlap with Bickerstaff's brainstem encephalitis, which is characterised by encephalopathy and possibly hyper-reflexia in addition to MFS signs.

Anti-GQ1b antibodies are found in up to 90% of patients with MFS, but in as low as 5% of other GBS variants. Anti-GQ1b antibodies have a relatively high specificity and sensitivity for MFS. Dense concentrations of GQ1b ganglioside are found in the oculomotor, trochlear, and abducens nerves, which may explain the relationship between anti-GQ1b antibodies and ophthalmoplegia. Patients with acute oropharyngeal palsy carry anti-GQ1b/GT1a IgG antibodies. Recovery generally occurs within 1–3 months.

CSF findings in GBS are classically of 'albumin-cytological dissociation' with increased CSF protein but normal CSF cell count. However, protein levels are normal in up to 50% of patients in the first week of disease, and up to 30% in the second week. Additionally, a mild pleocytosis (up to 50 cells/µl) may sometimes be seen. Levels above 10 cells/µl should prompt consideration of other inflammatory, infectious, or neoplastic causes.

Electrophysiological examination reveals a sensorimotor polyradiculoneuropathy or polyneuropathy, with characteristic reduced conduction velocity, reduced sensory and motor evoked amplitudes, abnormal temporal dispersion, and in some cases partial motor conduction blocks. Classically there is "sural sparing" where the sural sensory nerve action potential is normal, but the median and ulnar sensory nerve action potentials are abnormal or absent. In the AMAN variant (acute motor axonal neuropathy) low or absent motor amplitudes without demyelinating features are seen.

Treatment is indicated if patients are unable to walk independently for more than 10 metres, rapidly progressive weakness, autonomic dysfunction, bulbar signs, or respiratory insufficiency. First line treatment is IVIG (0.4g/kg daily for 5 days) commenced within 2 weeks of onset or plasma exchange (200–250 ml plasma/kg in five sessions) commenced within 4 weeks of onset. There is no role for corticosteroids, and oral corticosteroids are associated with worse outcomes.

Leonhard S, Mandarakas M, Gondim F, Bateman K, Ferreira M, Cornblath D et al. Diagnosis and management of Guillain–Barré syndrome in ten steps. Nature Reviews Neurology. 2019;15(11):671–683.
https://www.nature.com/articles/s41582-019-0250-9

17. Answer: A

Motor neuron disease (MND) is a set of phenotypically distinct disease processes that can also be described as amyotrophic lateral sclerosis (ALS) and variants, such that the terms MND and ALS are often used interchangeably. Fundamentally, these diseases encompass degenerative pathology of upper and lower motor neurons, and there is increasing evidence of pathological degeneration of other parts of the central nervous system over time, which manifest mostly as cognitive and behavioural changes. MND is characterised by progressive motor deficits developing over weeks to months, and diagnosis is made by a consistent clinical picture with exclusion of other possible causes. As there is no gold standard imaging or pathological test for the diagnosis, this usually requires specialist neurological opinion, particularly in order to rule out other possible causes.

Clinical classification of MND is useful in prognostication and treatment decisions. Classical ALS presentations involve both upper and lower motor neuron signs in areas of symptom onset and can be divided into bulbar or spinal onset depending on the region first affected, and these two presentations account for around 70% of MND diagnoses. Similarly, primary lateral sclerosis can be bulbar or spinal onset, but involves only upper motor neurons. Bulbar only involvement without progression to limb involvement is possible with ALS and is classified as isolated bulbar palsy. Progressive spinal muscular atrophy is characterised by generalised lower motor neuron involvement. Frontotemporal dementia (FTD) is an important co-phenomenon with ALS and is seen early in diagnosis in ALS-FTD phenotype in around 13% of patients, with cognitive and behavioural impairment identified in up to 50% of patients over time. Rarer phenotypes include cachexia onset ALS, and respiratory onset motor neuron disease. There is ongoing debate about whether these phenotypes are pathologically distinct entities or not.

Prognosis with MND is variable and is related to phenotype. Young age at diagnosis, either lower or upper motor neuron dominant disease and long time to diagnosis are associated with longer survival; bulbar-onset ALS, comorbid FTD, neck flexor weakness and poor nutritional status are associated with short survival. Treatments associated with longer survival include riluzole, non-invasive ventilation, enteral feeding, and specialist multi-disciplinary care.

van Es M, Hardiman O, Chio A, Al-Chalabi A, Pasterkamp R, Veldink J et al. Amyotrophic lateral sclerosis. The Lancet. 2017;390(10107):2084–2098.
https://www.thelancet.com/journals/lancet/article/PIIS0140-6736(17)31287-4/fulltext

18. Answer: B

Myasthenia gravis (MG) is an autoimmune disorder of the postsynaptic neuromuscular junction characterised by fluctuating weakness involving variable combinations of ocular, bulbar, limb, and respiratory muscles. It is important to define disease subgroups since different subgroups have different treatment options and prognosis. Based on the age of onset, serum antibodies, affected muscle groups, and the presence of thymoma, MG can be divided into the following subgroups:

- early onset: < 50 years of age at onset, positive acetylcholine receptor antibody, thymus hyperplasia
- late onset: ≥ 50 years of age at onset, positive acetylcholine receptor antibody, thymus atrophy
- thymoma: positive acetylcholine receptor antibody, thymus lymphoepithelioma lipoprotein
- receptor-related peptide 4 (LRP4): LRP4 antibody is positive, normal thymus
- muscle specific kinase (MuSK): muscle specific kinase antibody is positive
- seronegative
- ocular

Treatment of MG include symptomatic therapy with an acetylcholinesterase inhibitor (pyridostigmine), chronic immunosuppressive therapies, rapid but transient immunomodulatory therapies (plasma exchange and IVIG), and thymectomy.

Chronic immunosuppressive therapies, such as prednisolone and azathioprine should be considered if patients do not achieve clinical remission with an acetylcholinesterase inhibitor, especially in non-ocular limited disease. If patients' symptoms are not controlled with the above regimen, mycophenolate mofetil (MMF) could be considered for mild or moderate symptoms and Rituximab for severe symptoms. In patients not responding to MMF and Rituximab, regular plasma exchange, methotrexate, cyclosporin, and tacrolimus can be used.

Clinicians and patients need to have awareness of medications with the potential to worsen symptoms of MG and should avoid the following medications, including fluoroquinolone, aminoglycoside, macrolide, ketolide antibiotics, magnesium sulfate, chloroquine, hydroxychloroquine, penicillamine, botulinum toxin, beta blockers, procainamide, quinidine, quinine, neuromuscular blocking agents, anti-PD-1 monoclonal antibodies. This is not a complete list of all medications that may exacerbate MG symptoms, and it is prudent to assume that any medication may exacerbate MG and to watch for worsening symptoms after a new medication is introduced.

Gilhus N. Myasthenia Gravis. New England Journal of Medicine. 2016;375(26):2570–2581
https://www.nejm.org/doi/full/10.1056/NEJMra1602678

19. Answer: B

Acetylcholine receptor antibodies are found in 80% of patients with myasthenia gravis (MG); muscle-specific tyrosine kinase antibodies are found in only 1 to 10%. Muscle-specific tyrosine kinase is a receptor tyrosine kinase at the postsynaptic membrane that plays an important role in the formation and maintenance of the neuromuscular junction by inducing acetylcholine receptor clustering and differentiation of nerve terminals. Disruption of this pathway by autoantibodies binding to muscle-specific tyrosine kinase leads to a neuromuscular transmission defect.

Both MG associated with acetylcholine receptor antibodies and MG associated with muscle-specific tyrosine kinase antibodies are characterised by fatigable weakness. However, patients with muscle-specific tyrosine kinase antibodies are more often female and have earlier disease onset (in the third decade of life) than patients with acetylcholine receptor antibodies. Ptosis and double vision are the most common manifestations with acetylcholine receptor antibodies but are less common and typically milder with muscle-specific tyrosine kinase antibodies. Muscle-specific tyrosine kinase antibodies are more commonly associated with bulbar dysfunction (in 67% of patients), axial weakness (in 92%), facial weakness (in 96%), and respiratory distress (in 60%), conditions that often lead to crisis and hospitalisation.

Pyridostigmine, an acetylcholine esterase inhibitor, may improve strength but should be used with caution during a myasthenic crisis, because its cholinergic effects cause increased salivation, which poses a risk of aspiration. Pyridostigmine is reportedly less effective in patients with muscle-specific tyrosine kinase antibodies than in patients with acetylcholine receptor antibodies.

Gilhus N, Verschuuren J. Myasthenia gravis: subgroup classification and therapeutic strategies. The Lancet Neurology. 2015;14(10):1023–1036.
https://pubmed.ncbi.nlm.nih.gov/26376969/

20. Answer: B

Optic neuritis is a demyelinating inflammation of the optic nerve that often occurs in association with multiple sclerosis (MS) and neuromyelitis optica (NMO). Typically, patients with optic neuritis are young, are often female (ratio of 3:1) and have subacute vision loss associated with pain on eye movement. A history of preceding viral illness may be present. The classical triad of inflammatory optic neuritis consists of loss of vision, periocular pain, and dyschromatopsia, and is unilateral in 70% of adults. The typical clinical course is that of retro-orbital pain usually exacerbated by eye movement, and loss of central vision. Visual loss varies from mild reduction to no perception of light and progresses over 7–10 days before reaching a nadir. A gradual recovery of visual acuity with time is characteristic of optic neuritis, although permanent residual deficits in colour vision and contrast and brightness sensitivity are common.

Investigations should be guided by the clinical presentation. The diagnosis of optic neuritis is usually made on clinical grounds. Early review is essential to ensure visual recovery has begun and the diagnosis reconsidered if it has not recovered.

Although more than half of all patients with MS have optic neuritis at some time, patients with optic neuritis who have completely normal MRI of brain and comprehensive CSF examination may not progress to MS. It has been reported that the risk of development of MS after an episode of isolated unilateral optic neuritis is 38% at 10 years and 50% at 15 years. Patients with MS may have recurrent attacks of optic neuritis. Whether optic neuritis is a distinct clinical entity or part of a continuum with MS is controversial.

Treatment with varying regimens of corticosteroids in patients with optic neuritis may result in hastened visual improvement, ameliorating the acute symptoms of pain caused by demyelinating inflammation of the nerve. Most patients begin to recover vision within 4 weeks even without treatment. Studies have demonstrated intravenous steroids do little to affect the ultimate visual acuity in patients with optic neuritis, but they do speed the rate of recovery and should be used in patients with either severe or bilateral vision loss.

NMO is characterised by often severe, bilateral optic neuritis and myelitis in a close temporal relationship. However, optic neuritis can occasionally precede the myelopathy. Eculizumab, a monoclonal antibody that targets C5, can be used to treat adults with neuromyelitis optica spectrum disorder (NMOSD) who are anti-aquaporin-4 (AQP4) antibody–positive.

Toosy A, Mason D, Miller D. Optic neuritis. The Lancet Neurology. 2014;13(1):83–99.
https://pubmed.ncbi.nlm.nih.gov/24331795/

21. Answer: D

Neurogenic orthostatic hypotension is very common (30–40%) in patients with Parkinson's disease. Orthostatic hypotension is defined as a drop in systolic BP by ≥ 20 mmHg or of diastolic BP by ≥10mmHg, within 3 minutes of standing or upon head-up tilt (minimum 60°) on a tilt table test. The accumulation of α-synuclein aggregates causes neurodegeneration and autonomic failure. Fall in BP causes presyncopal episodes, falls, and injuries. Treatment of orthostatic hypotension in patients with Parkinson's disease can improve cognition, balance, quality of life, and can reduce the risks of falls and injury.

The initial management strategy is to remove iatrogenic causes such as antihypertensive medications, review anti-Parkinson medications and to consider non-pharmacological interventions such as avoiding dehydration, alcohol, large meals, straining and standing up rapidly, eating smaller and more frequent meals, drinking water and increasing salt intake to increase plasma volume, wearing compression stockings to improve venous return and cardiac output, taking regular exercise in the horizontal position (e.g. swimming), and sleeping with the head of the bed raised. Failing these measures, pharmacological options can be considered based on the symptom severity and side effect profile. Levodopa reduces supine and standing BP but does not impair orthostatic adaptation and it is essential for patient with Parkinson's disease. Therefore, it is not the first choice of management here.

Fludrocortisone, a systemic corticosteroid which increases sensitivity to circulating catecholamines to increase plasma volume, is the first-line medication to be considered. The recommended dose is 0.1–0.2 mg/day and it can take up to 5 days to see the effect. The side effects include hypokalaemia and supine hypertension. Fludrocortisone is not recommended in patients with CKD and CCF.

In resistant cases, pyridostigmine, midodrine, ephedrine, and octreotide may be useful. Midodrine and ephedrine are not available in Australia but can be obtained via the Special Access Scheme (SAS).

Midodrine is a peripheral α-1 adrenoceptor agonist, exerts a pressor effect on both venous and arterial constriction to increase peripheral resistance. It is given in the morning, noon, and afternoon to avoid supine hypertension, a known adverse reaction of the medication, in the evening. Dosing should be at least 4 hours before the bedtime. The recommended dose is up to 10 mg three times a day. Other side effects of midodrine include bradycardia, supine hypertension, piloerection, itchiness, and urinary retention.

Wu C, Hohler A. Management of orthostatic hypotension in patients with Parkinson's disease. Practical Neurology. 2014;15(2):100–104.
https://pn.bmj.com/content/15/2/100.long

22. Answer: D

Encephalitis is the inflammation of the brain parenchyma due to infectious or autoimmune causes. It can lead to encephalopathy, seizures, focal neurological deficits, neurological disability, and death.

Paraneoplastic neurological syndromes (PNS) are neurological syndromes associated with cancer with no obvious metastatic, metabolic, infectious, or iatrogenic cause. Paraneoplastic limbic encephalitis (PLE) is a rare autoimmune neurological syndrome, most frequently associated with lung cancer (80% of these cases are small cell lung cancer), selectively affects limbic system structures, including the hippocampus, hypothalamus, and amygdala. The pathogenesis of this condition is likely an immune response directed against the central nervous proteins which are similar to tumour antigens. It leads to lymphocyte infiltration of perivascular and microglial cells followed by neuronal loss.

The presence of autoantibodies such as anti-Hu, anti-Ri, anti-Yo, anti-Ma/Ta, anti-amphiphysin, anti-Sox 1 and anti-CV-2 in serum and/or CSF are hallmarks of these syndromes. They are found in more than 80% of patients with PNS. PLE occurring in the setting of lung cancer is often associated with antibodies to the GABA-B receptor. Patients often present with cognitive impairment, personality change, short-term memory loss, and seizures. Anti-cancer treatment can improve neurological symptoms. Immunomodulators, such as steroids and IVIG, have been used to treat all types of PLE with variable results.

ADEM is typically a post-infectious or para-infectious condition. Of viral causes, Japanese encephalitis virus is the most commonly identified epidemic cause and HSV the most commonly identified sporadic cause.

Anti-NMDA receptor encephalitis is suggested by a prodromal influenza-like illness followed by subacute cognitive decline, behavioural changes, psychosis, movement disorders, seizures, and autonomic instability. The disease is more prevalent in women (female to male ratio 4:1) and about 37% of patients are younger than 18 years at presentation of the disease. About half of cases are associated with tumours, most commonly teratomas of the ovaries. Another established trigger is herpes viral encephalitis.

Brainstem encephalitis has distinct clinical characteristics and aetiologies when compared to encephalitis in general. Patients can have preserved consciousness and behaviour and thus might not strictly fulfil diagnostic criteria for encephalitis. However, focal neurological deficits such as ataxia, ocular dysfunction, bulbar dysfunction, and limb paresis suggest areas of inflammation in the midbrain, pons, and medulla. The majority of cases have non-infectious, inflammatory causes. Brain biopsy and histopathological diagnosis may play a role in the management of selected patients and can be useful in guiding treatment decisions. In immuno-competent patients, an empiric trial of steroids and/or other immunosuppressive agents may be warranted when CNS infection and neoplastic/paraneoplastic disorders are excluded.

Venkatesan A, Michael B, Probasco J, Geocadin R, Solomon T. Acute encephalitis in immunocompetent adults. The Lancet. 2019;393(101/2):702–716.
https://pubmed.ncbi.nlm.nih.gov/30782344/

23. Answer: C

Parkinson's disease is a neurodegenerative disorder characterised by the loss of dopaminergic neurons in the substantia nigra. The resultant dopamine deficiency leads to the characteristic Parkinsonian motor symptoms: bradykinesia, muscle rigidity, and resting tremor. Parkinson's disease also affects other neurotransmitters and regions of nervous system outside of the basal ganglia, leading to the non-motor symptoms of Parkinson's disease. Non-motor symptoms such as olfactory dysfunction, cognitive decline, and psychiatric symptoms can precede the motor symptoms of Parkinson's' disease by years.

Diagnosis of Parkinson's disease requires:

1. Bradykinesia: slowness in the initiation of voluntary movement, and progressive decrease in speed and amplitude of repetitive actions.
2. At least one of: muscle rigidity, 4–6 Hz resting tremor, and postural instability (not due to visual, vestibular, cerebellar, or proprioceptive pathology).
3. Three or more features including: unilateral onset, resting tremor, progression of disease, asymmetry with the side of unilateral onset worst, significant (70–100%) response to levodopa.

Diagnosis of Parkinson's disease also requires exclusion of clinical features which suggest an alternate cause including other degenerative diseases with Parkinsonism:

- Recurrent strokes with stepwise progression of Parkinsonian symptoms
- Recurrent head trauma
- Onset of symptoms consistent with onset of neuroleptics
- 1-methyl-4-phenyl-1,2,3,5-tetrahydropyridine (MPTP) exposure
- Negative response to high dose levodopa
- Prolonged remission

- Solely unilateral symptoms after 3 years
- Early significant autonomic involvement
- Early significant dementia with memory, language, and praxia disturbance
- Oculogyric crisis
- Supranuclear gaze palsy
- Babinski sign
- Cerebellar signs
- Hydrocephalus on CT/MRI.

Other neurodegenerative disorders usually do not have a resting tremor. Progressive supranuclear palsy (PSP) is a neurodegenerative disease characterised by supranuclear, initially vertical, gaze dysfunction accompanied by extrapyramidal symptoms and cognitive dysfunction. The diagnosis of PSP is purely clinical. The cranial nerve examination should include detailed analysis of ocular motility. The classic gaze palsy in PSP is supranuclear ophthalmoplegia. Supranuclear in this context refers to a lesion that is situated above the ocular motor nuclei, thus sparing the ocular motor nuclei, nerve fascicles, and neuromuscular junctional, and extraocular muscles.

Kalia L, Lang A. Parkinson's disease. The Lancet. 2015;386(9996):896–912.
https://www.thelancet.com/journals/lancet/article/PIIS0140-6736(14)61393-3/fulltext

24. Answer: A

Levodopa is considered the safest and most efficacious medication for treatment of Parkinson's disease and its early use following diagnosis should be considered. Amantadine has recently been studied in randomised trials and found to be efficacious in treatment of levodopa-induced dyskinesias. Amantadine increases dopamine release and blocks cholinergic receptors and acts as a N-methyl-D-aspartate (NMDA) antagonist in the glutamatergic pathway from subthalamic nucleus to globus pallidus. Entacapone is a catechol-o-methyl transferase (COMT) inhibitor and can increase the incidence of dyskinesias. Pergolide and bromocriptine are ergot-based dopamine agonists and are no longer in use due to the side effects of heart valve and pulmonary fibrosis.

Other approaches to reduce dyskinesia including minimising levodopa dose and supplementing with a dopamine agonist, and using smaller, more frequent doses of levodopa. In patients with severe medication-resistant motor fluctuations, subcutaneous apomorphine, deep-brain stimulation and a gel formulation of carbidopa/levodopa enteral suspension that can be infused directly into the small intestine using an externally worn medication pump can be considered to provide additional treatment options for patients with Parkinson's disease.

Okun M. Management of Parkinson Disease in 2017. JAMA. 2017;318(9):791.
https://jamanetwork.com/journals/jama/article-abstract/2650798

25. Answer: B

The patient's presenting symptoms raise the suspicion of subacute combined degeneration (SCD) of the spinal cord. In this case, it is related to nitrous oxide misuse causing vitamin B_{12} deficiency.

SCD is also related to other causes of vitamin B_{12} deficiency, such as a strict vegetarian diet without vitamin supplementation, post stomach surgery, after inhalation of nitrous oxide in dental procedures or inhalation of nitrous oxide as a recreational medication.

Vitamin B_{12} is usually found in animal products, such as fish, meat, poultry, eggs, milk, and milk products.

Although her blood test results showed macrocytosis, she does not have anaemia. Folic acid deficiency can cause macrocytosis, however, it does not cause the aforementioned neurological signs and symptoms. Neurological symptoms may occur in the absence of anaemia. SCD is characterised by demyelination of the dorsal and lateral spinal cord and is commonly associated with a B_{12}-related neuropathy. Other possible neurological manifestations of B_{12} deficiency include autonomic dysfunction, intellectual impairment, behavioural impairment, and impaired visual acuity.

Adding serum methylmalonic acid to a screen of serum B_{12} level improves the yield of identifying cellular B_{12} deficiency as a cause of neuropathy from 2% to 8% (elevated serum methylmalonic acid levels indicating cellular B_{12} deficiency.)

Copper deficiency can mimic B_{12} deficiency clinically with a myelopathy and sensory-predominant neuropathy. Copper deficiency should be considered when patients have a history of bariatric surgery or multiple nutritional deficiencies or if high zinc exposure (nutritional supplement or in some denture pastes).

Fasting glucose and HbA1c are used to rule out peripheral neuropathy secondary to diabetes. TSH is used to rule out thyroid disease.

Watson J, Dyck P. Peripheral Neuropathy: A Practical Approach to Diagnosis and Symptom Management. Mayo Clinic Proceedings. 2015;90(7):940–951.
https://www.mayoclinicproceedings.org/article/S0025-6196(15)00378-X/fulltext

26. Answer: A

Infarctions of the medulla most commonly occur as a result of occlusion of the intracranial vertebral artery, and occasionally the posterior inferior cerebellar artery. The most common clinical presentation of this form of stroke is lateral medullary syndrome, which presents with symptoms and signs such as those mentioned in the question. If the infarction occurs in conjunction with medial medulla infarction, contralateral hemiparesis, and tongue weakness can also occur. Ipsilateral facial sensory deficit occurs due to the trigeminal nucleus' location in the medulla, despite the trigeminal nerve exiting the brainstem at the level of the pons. Palatal and pharyngeal weakness occur as a result of infarction of the nucleus ambiguous. Other possible deficits in lateral medullary syndrome include skew deviation and ipsilateral lateropulsion (due to vestibular nucleus infarction), hiccups, and failure of automatic breathing.

Schulz U, Fischer U. Posterior circulation cerebrovascular syndromes: diagnosis and management. Journal of Neurology, Neurosurgery & Psychiatry. 2016;88(1):45–53.
https://jnnp.bmj.com/content/88/1/45.full

27. Answer: C

Primary central nervous system (CNS) tumours are a heterogeneous group of tumours arising from cells within the CNS and can be benign or malignant. Malignant primary brain tumours remain among the most difficult cancers to treat, with a 5-year overall survival no greater than 35%. The most common malignant primary brain tumours in adults are gliomas.

Glioblastoma, also known as glioblastoma multiforme (GBM) is the most lethal of the primary brain tumours in adults. Most patients do not survive beyond a year, and only 5% survive beyond 5 years. It can present as:

- Severe, refractory headache
- Progressive neurologic deficit, usually motor deficit
- Symptoms of increased intracranial pressure, including headaches, nausea and vomiting, and cognitive impairment
- Seizures.

MRI is the imaging modality of choice. GBMs do not have clearly defined margins; they tend to invade locally and spread along white matter pathways, creating the appearance of multiple GBMs or multicentric gliomas on imaging studies.

The treatment may include maximal safe surgical resection, radiotherapy, and concomitant and adjuvant chemotherapy with temozolomide. The addition of radiotherapy to surgery increases survival. The responsiveness of GBM to radiotherapy varies. Radiosensitisers, such as newer chemotherapeutic agents, targeted molecular agents, and antiangiogenic agents may increase the therapeutic effect of radiotherapy. In elderly patients with multiple comorbidities, less aggressive therapy is preferred by using radiation or temozolomide alone.

Lapointe S. Primary brain tumours in adults. Lancet. 2018; 392:432–446.
https://www.thelancet.com/journals/lancet/article/PIIS0140-6736(18)30990-5/fulltext

28. Answer: D

S1 innervates skin over the little toe and S1 radiculopathy is associated with loss of ankle jerk. Other findings of S1 radiculopathy can be decreased plantar and toe flexion.

L5 radiculopathy is associated with decreased foot dorsiflexion and toe extension with normal ankle jerk.

Common peroneal nerve compression leads to foot drop with weakness on foot dorsiflexion and eversion. It can be seen with prolonged immobilisation such as following general anaesthesia or from a plaster cast. Reflexes are preserved.

Posterior tibial nerve compression leads to sensory symptoms, such as aching or burning over the sole of the foot, with a positive Tinel's sign over the nerve posterior to the medial malleolus and sensory loss over the sole of the foot.

Berry J, Elia C, Saini H, Miulli D. A Review of Lumbar Radiculopathy, Diagnosis, and Treatment. Cureus. 2019.
https://www.ncbi.nlm.nih.gov/pmc/articles/PMC6858271/

29. Answer: A

In patients with high-risk TIA (ABCD2 score ≥4) or minor stroke (NIHSS ≤3), it is beneficial to treat these with a 300–600 mg clopidogrel load plus aspirin 100 mg on day 1 soon after the onset of symptoms and signs of ischaemic stroke, then dual anti-platelet therapy with clopidogrel 75 mg daily plus aspirin 100 mg daily for 21 days before returning to a single antiplatelet agent for ongoing secondary prevention of ischaemic stroke. In the Platelet-Oriented Inhibition in New TIA and minor ischemic stroke (POINT) trial which treated for 90 days there was no additional benefit from dual antiplatelet therapy beyond 21–30 days but a higher bleeding risk.

Anticoagulation in patients with an embolic stroke of undetermined source (ESUS) is not superior to antiplatelet therapies.

Prolonged cardiac monitoring with implantable loop recorder to identify paroxysmal atrial fibrillation or atrial flutter can be considered in patients with an ESUS since the pick-up rate is 10 times more than the intermittent and short-term cardiac monitoring. Anticoagulation needs to be considered in patients with atrial fibrillation/flutter to prevent ischaemic strokes.

Patent foramen ovale closure is considered in young patients (<60–65 years of age) with proven stroke and high risks features on echocardiogram such as inter-arterial septal aneurysm and moderate-large right-to-left shunting with agitated saline contrast.

Carotid endarterectomy can be considered in appropriate patients with ipsilateral carotid stenosis ≥ 50% within 2 weeks post-stroke.

Identification and management of the underlying cardiovascular risk factors such as hyperlipidaemia, obesity, diabetes, hypertension, thrombophilia in addition to the aforementioned conditions is important to minimise the risks of future TIAs or strokes.

Muller C, Roizman M, Wong A. Secondary prevention of ischaemic stroke. Internal Medicine Journal. 2019;49(10): 1221–1228.
https://onlinelibrary.wiley.com/doi/10.1111/imj.14454

30. Answer: A

In asymptomatic patients with carotid artery stenosis of greater than 60% of the diameter of the artery, the risk of stroke or death was lower when immediate carotid endarterectomy was performed than when surgery was deferred. A large randomised-controlled study found that in patients younger than 79 years of age with severe asymptomatic carotid stenosis, carotid artery stenting is not inferior to carotid endarterectomy with regard to the rate of the primary composite end point at 1 year. Analysis after five years of follow-up showed no significant difference between the carotid artery stenting and carotid endarterectomy treatment groups in the rates of non–procedure-related stroke, all stroke, and survival.

Rosenfield K, Matsumura J, Chaturvedi S, Riles T, Ansel G, Metzger D et al. Randomised Trial of Stent versus Surgery for Asymptomatic Carotid Stenosis. New England Journal of Medicine. 2016;374(11):1011–1020.
https://www.nejm.org/doi/full/10.1056/NEJMoa1515706

31. Answer: D

This patient's CT head shows a left subdural haematoma (SDH). SDH occurs not only in patients with severe head injury but also in patients with 'insignificant' head injuries or spontaneously, particularly in elderly patients and those receiving anticoagulants. SDH is characteristically caused by venous haemorrhage, most from veins that join the cerebrum to venous sinuses within dura. Generalised cerebral atrophy and increased venous fragility associated with ageing are the major predisposing factors. With ageing, the mass of the brain decreases leading to an increase in the space between the brain and the skull from 6% to 11% of the total intracranial space. This cause stretching of the bridging veins and the greater movement of the brain within the cranium makes these veins vulnerable to trauma. The mortality following SDH can be as high as 32%, and recurrence rates can reach 33%.

SDH can be classified as acute, subacute, or chronic. Generally, acute SDH is less than 72 hours old and is hyperdense compared with the brain on CT. The subacute phase begins 3–7 days after acute injury. Chronic SDH develops over the course of weeks and are hypodense compared with the brain. However, SDH may be mixed in nature.

The gradual expansion of chronic SDH may be due to: (i) recurrent bleeding from the haematoma capsule, (ii) the atrophied brain and lack of tamponading effect, (iii) normal or only slightly increased intracranial pressure.

The most important step in the diagnosis of SDH is a high index of suspicion. Treatment of SDH is by surgical evacuation, although small haematomas may resolve spontaneously. Reaccumulation of the haematoma is the most common postoperative problem. Around 11% of patients develop seizures after surgery.

Teale E, Iliffe S, Young J. Subdural haematoma in the elderly. BMJ. 2014;348(mar11 11): g1682–g1682.
https://www.bmj.com/content/348/bmj.g1682

32. Answer: A

Trigeminal neuralgia is defined by orofacial pain restricted to the distribution of the trigeminal nerve. Aetiology of classical trigeminal neuralgia (~ 75%) is neurovascular compression of the trigeminal nerve root. Secondary trigeminal neuralgia (~ 15%) is caused by neurological disease such as multiple sclerosis, cerebellopontine tumour, and arteriovenous malformations. The remaining cases (~10%) are idiopathic.

Trigeminal neuralgia is a clinical diagnosis, which most importantly involves confirming the pain is limited to the ophthalmic (V1), maxillary (V2), and/or mandibular (V3) divisions of the trigeminal nerve. This means exclusion of regions which cervical nerves innervate, including the posterior third of scalp, the back of the ear, and angle of the mandible. It is of sudden onset, severe, lasts seconds (to maximum 2 minutes) and of shooting stabbing sharp or electric-like quality. It is unilateral, except when caused by multiple sclerosis when it can be bilateral. The pain is reproducible upon light stimulation of the dermatomes of the affected nerve, especially near the midline, including innocuous stimuli such as light touch or cold air, or manoeuvres such as eating, talking, and smiling.

Evaluation often involves MRI brain to exclude a secondary cause, as well as to evaluate the anatomy of the trigeminal nerve for suitability of surgery. First line therapy is typically carbamazepine or oxcarbazepine. Second line therapy includes alternate medical agents, or referral for surgery including microvascular decompression, rhizotomy, and gamma knife radiosurgery.

Cruccu G, Finnerup N, Jensen T, Scholz J, Sindou M, Svensson P et al. Trigeminal neuralgia. Neurology. 2016;87(2): 220–228.
https://n.neurology.org/content/87/2/220

33. Answer: G

34. Answer: B

35. Answer: C

36. Answer: H

There is no proven algorithm for selecting an antiepileptic drug (AED) for patients with epilepsy. There are many factors that should be considered including the type of epilepsy/seizure being treated (i.e. focal vs generalised, specific syndrome, or if a clear first-line treatment exists), patient factors that narrow possible treatment options (such as comorbidities, drug interaction, pregnancy), medication factors such as tolerability, and side effects. It is important that clinician is familiar with common AEDs.

Ethosuximide exerts its effect via low voltage-activated calcium channel only. It is only effective in absence seizures. Phenytoin has non-linear pharmacokinetics. Topiramate can be used in all types of seizures and it has been used in treating migraine.

Gabapentin has 100% renal excretion. Other AEDs cleared renally, including pregabalin, levetiracetam, eslicarbazepine, lacosamide, and topiramate. In patients with renal impairment, these AEDs should be avoided or require dose adjustments. For patients who undergo dialysis, ethosuximide, gabapentin, lacosamide, levetiracetam, pregabalin, and topiramate are highly dialysable. Dose supplementation after dialysis may be needed for these AEDs.

Thijs R, Surges R, O'Brien T, Sander J. Epilepsy in adults. The Lancet. 2019;393(10172):689–701.
https://www.thelancet.com/journals/lancet/article/PIIS0140-6736(18)32596-0/fulltext

37. Answer: E

This patient has neurofibromatosis type 1 (NF1), also known as von Recklinghausen's disease. It is a multisystem genetic disorder characterised by cutaneous findings including café-au-lait spots and axillary freckling, by skeletal dysplasia, and by the growth of both benign and malignant nervous system tumours, most notably benign neurofibromas. NF1 is an autosomal dominant genetic disorder with an incidence of approximately 1 in 3000 individuals. Approximately one-half of the cases are familial; the remainder are new mutations. The *NF1* gene is located on chromosome 17q11.2. Neurofibromin, the cytoplasmic protein product encoded by the *NF1* gene, acts as a tumour suppressor, and is widely expressed, with high concentrations in the nervous system. Neurofibromin reduces cell proliferation by accelerating the inactivation of a cellular proto-oncogene, p21 ras, which is important in promoting tumour formation. Neurofibromin controls mammalian target of rapamycin (mTOR) via a common biochemical pathway with tuberin, the TSC2 gene product. The major disease features involve the nervous system, the skin, and bone, and the resulting complications are numerous, unpredictable, and vary even within families. However, many patients will not have substantial problems other than cutaneous neurofibromas and mild cognitive impairment.

38. Answer: F

Autosomal dominant arteriopathy with subcortical infarcts and leukoencephalopathy (CADASIL) is caused by a mutation in the *NOTCH3* gene on chromosome 19q12. *NOTCH3* codes for a transmembrane receptor protein which is located on the surface of smooth muscle cells of small arteries, particularly cerebral small arteries. Accumulation of the pathologic NOTCH3 receptor protein in small- and medium-sized cerebral arteries leads to thickening and fibrosis of the vessel walls. This arteriopathy causes cerebral infarction.

Ischaemic stroke can occur at any time from childhood to late adulthood, but typically occurs during mid-adulthood. Patients with CADASIL often have more than one stroke in their lifetime. Recurrent strokes can cause changes in mood and personality and early dementia. CADASIL is not associated with the common vascular risk factors such as hypertension or diabetes.

39. Answer: G

Charcot-Marie-Tooth (CMT) type 1 is a disorder of peripheral myelination resulting from a mutation in the *peripheral myelin protein-22* (*PMP22*) gene. CMT disease is the most common inherited neuromuscular disorder. It is characterised by inherited motor and sensory neuropathies without known metabolic derangements. CMT disease was subdivided into two types, CMT 1 and CMT 2, on the basis of pathologic and physiologic criteria. It has been subdivided further on the basis of the genetic cause of the disease. With the advent of genetic testing, it is likely that all the diseases currently falling under the heading of CMT syndrome will eventually become distinguishable. CMT type 2 is an axonal disorder, not a demyelinating disorder. It has been associated with mutations in the *ATP1A1* gene. CMT X (X-linked CMT) and CMT 4 also are demyelinating neuropathies. CMT X has been associated with mutations in the *PRPS1* gene.

40. Answer: L

This patient has cardinal symptoms of Parkinson's disease including resting tremor, stiffness, and slowness (bradykinesia) and poverty of movement (hypokinesia). Neuronal loss in the substantia nigra, which causes striatal dopamine deficiency, and intracellular inclusions containing aggregates of α-synuclein are the neuropathological hallmarks of Parkinson's disease.

Kalia L, Lang A. Parkinson's disease. The Lancet. 2015;386(9996):896–912.
https://www.thelancet.com/journals/lancet/article/PIIS0140-6736(14)61393-3/fulltext

41. Answer: M

Hemiballismus is a rare hyperkinetic movement disorder characterised by an involuntary, violent, coarse, and wide-amplitude movements involving ipsilateral arm and leg. The acute development of hemiballismus is often caused by focal lesions in the contralateral subthalamic nucleus and basal ganglia structures. There are many aetiologies but vascular causes and non-ketotic hyperglycaemia being the most common. Prognosis is favourable for most patients with complete resolution. It is first important to treat underlying causes such hyperglycaemia, infections, or neoplastic lesions. When pharmacological treatment is necessary, antidopaminergic drugs such as haloperidol and chlorpromazine can be helpful. Other treatments include topiramate, intrathecal baclofen and botulinum injections.

Hawley J, Weiner W. Hemiballismus: Current concepts and review. Parkinsonism & Related Disorders. 2012;18(2):125–129.
http://www.ncbi.nlm.nih.gov/pubmed/21930415

42. Answer: I

The involvement of the right third cranial nerve and the right pyramidal tract would suggest the lesion is at the level of the third cranial nerve nucleus in the midbrain. A midbrain infarct is most commonly a consequence of hypertensive cerebral vascular disease and may arise from an embolus with a cardiac origin or proximal atherosclerotic lesion. It is also sometimes known as Weber's syndrome and due to occlusion of paramedian branches of the posterior cerebral artery or of basilar bifurcation perforating arteries. The involvement of the third nerve excludes a lesion in the internal capsule, the medulla, the cervical cord, and occipital lobe. Sometimes contralateral Parkinsonism may develop due to involvement of the basal ganglia projections. On rare occasions, hemiparesis with contralateral third cranial nerve palsy can result from a hemispheric space-occupying lesion, which compresses the contralateral third cranial nerve and the cerebral peduncle against the clinoid process.

43. Answer: G

Noncommunicating hydrocephalus occurs when CSF flow is obstructed within the ventricular system or in its outlets to the arachnoid space, resulting in impairment of the CSF from the ventricular to the subarachnoid space:

- Interventricular foramen obstruction may lead to dilation of one, or if large enough (e.g. in colloid cyst), both lateral ventricles.
- The aqueduct of Sylvius can be obstructed by genetic or acquired lesions (e.g. atresia, ependymitis, haemorrhage, or tumour) and lead to dilation of both lateral ventricles, as well as the third ventricle.
- Fourth ventricle obstruction leads to dilatation of the aqueduct, as well as the lateral and third ventricles (e.g. Chiari malformation).

44. Answer: J

The optic chiasm or chiasma is the midline structure where the nasal (medial) fibres of the optic nerves decussate to continue posteriorly as the optic tracts. It lies in the chiasmatic cistern and along with the pituitary stalk, is completely encircled by the circle of Willis. Lesions compressing the chiasm classically produce the visual field defect of bitemporal hemianopia, where there is loss of the temporal visual fields such as in this case.

45. Answer: K

In unilateral neglect, patients fail to report, respond, or orient to meaningful stimuli presented on the affected side. It is a heterogeneous condition; different individuals may present with different symptoms and may involve various modalities, including visual, auditory, somatosensory, or kinetic. In most cases, the right parietal cortex is injured, and the left side of the body and/or space is/are ignored. The incidence rate for unilateral neglect following a right-sided stroke can be up to 80%. Right-sided unilateral neglect resulting from left hemisphere damage can be up to 43% of stroke patients.

46. Answer: B

The motor speech area or Broca's area in the cortex governs speech. It is situated in the inferior aspect of the frontal lobe immediately rostral and slightly ventral to the precentral gyrus. Damage of this area causes impairment of the ability to express words in a meaningful way or to use the words correctly.

47. Answer: D

The corpus callosum is the largest of the commissural fibres, linking the cerebral cortex of the left and right cerebral hemispheres. These connections can also be divided into: (i) Homotopic connections: those that link similar regions on each side (e.g. visual fields of motor/sensory areas of the trunk) (ii) Heterotopic connections: those that link dissimilar areas. In order to stop the spread of seizures from one hemisphere to the other. Incision of the corpus callosum is the surgery of choice.

48. Answer: E

This patient has a combination of VI and VII cranial nerve palsy indicating that the lesion is located in the dorsal pons at the site where the VII cranial nerve curves around the motor nucleus of VI cranial nerve.

 Assir M, M Das J. How to Localize Neurologic Lesions by Physical Examination [Internet]. StatPearls. 2020 [cited 14 March 2021]. Available from: https://www.ncbi.nlm.nih.gov/books/NBK493159/

17 Palliative Medicine

Questions

Answers can be found in the Palliative Medicine Answers section at the end of this chapter.

1. You are caring for a 72-year-old man dying from a malignant bowel obstruction due to metastatic gastric cancer. His nausea and vomiting are well controlled currently with dexamethasone 4 mg twice daily and haloperidol 0.5 mg twice daily. He has intermittent abdominal pain which is treated successfully with intermittent doses of morphine as required, only needing around two doses per day. He continues to pass no flatus or bowel motions. He is bed-bound, and examination shows significant global muscle wasting, low jugular venous pulsation, dry lips, and oral mucosa without ulceration or candidiasis, mild peripheral pedal oedema, mildly distended abdomen, and absent bowel sounds. His main symptomatic complaint is extreme dry mouth and thirst.
   Which of the following interventions is most appropriate for his thirst?
   A. Change subcutaneous morphine to fentanyl.
   B. Encourage oral intake with rehydration solution.
   C. Intravenous normal saline.
   D. Topical treatment with artificial saliva, lip moisturiser, and ice chips.

2. Which of the following statements is most true regarding malignant bowel obstruction?
   A. Interventional management of bowel obstruction is associated with longer survival.
   B. Most are due to a single point of obstruction.
   C. Most require procedural intervention such as stenting, resection, or bypass surgery.
   D. Surgery is most likely to be valuable as a bridge to further disease modifying treatment.

3. An 85-year-old man has been receiving haemodialysis three times a week for 8 years. He decides to withdraw from dialysis as he is deteriorating functionally, requiring frequent hospitalisation for haemodynamic issues, sepsis, and electrolyte imbalance. He feels the burden of attending dialysis is now not worth the effort and discomfort attendant to the procedure. He is aware that this will likely lead to his death within days, and he is admitted to the renal ward for end-of-life care. He does not take any regular opioid or benzodiazepine medications.
   On day 4 after withdrawing from dialysis, he experiences acute pulmonary oedema. His respiratory rate is 45/min, and oxygen saturation is 72% on room air. He is anxious, intermittently drowsy, and uncomfortable, with a high JVP and global inspiratory crackles globally in both lungs.
   Which of the following measures (in addition to sitting upright, and oxygen via nasal cannulae) is most likely to relieve his breathlessness, without causing further distressing symptoms?
   A. Midazolam 25 mg over 24 hours via continuous subcutaneous infusion.
   B. Morphine 25 mg over 24 hours via continuous subcutaneous infusion.
   C. Small boluses of intravenous midazolam titrated until comfort is achieved.
   D. Small boluses of intravenous morphine titrated until comfort is achieved.

4. A 56-year-old man has advanced motor neurone disease (MND). While discussing the palliative care plan, you will advise:
   A. Baclofen is effective in relieving fasciculations.
   B. Benzodiazepine is contraindicated due to the concern of respiratory failure.
   C. Non-invasive ventilation relieves respiratory failure symptoms and prolongs survival.
   D. Pain is not a common symptom as there is no sensory nerve involvement in MND.

How to Pass the FRACP Written Examination, First Edition. Jonathan Gleadle, Jordan Li, Danielle Wu, and Paul Kleinig.
© 2022 John Wiley & Sons Ltd. Published 2022 by John Wiley & Sons Ltd.

5. A 58-year-old woman with metastatic adenocarcinoma of the lung has had increasing left-sided chest pain in the context of recent disease progression. She has been treated with gefitinib since diagnosis 12 months ago, but her most recent CT scan shows progression of a left-sided mass invading her chest wall, and new liver metastases. She reports that her pain is similar to the pain that she has had since diagnosis but is increasing slowly in intensity over the past four weeks. The pain is pleuritic, worse at night, and is gnawing in quality. There are no apparent relieving or precipitating factors, or associated symptoms. Her dose of morphine in slow release preparation has increased in this time from 40 mg per day up to 120 mg per day, and her 'as required' immediate release morphine dose has increased from 5 mg per dose to 15mg per dose. In the last 24 hours she has had a total of 160 mg of oral morphine. She feels that the pain has worsened and her response to the 'as required' medication is now worse than it was previously.

On examination her observations are normal, and she looks comfortable at rest. Her chest examination shows mildly decreased chest excursion on the left and decreased air entry at the left base. Her lateral chest wall on the left is exquisitely tender to palpation, her spine is not tender in the midline. She is referred for palliative radiotherapy.

Which of the following analgesic regimes is most appropriate?

A. Increase slow release morphine to 80mg twice daily, and immediate release morphine to 20 mg as needed.
B. Rotate to slow release hydromorphone 40 mg daily, and immediate release hydromorphone 4–6 mg as needed.
C. Rotate to oxycodone 30 mg twice daily, and immediate release oxycodone 5–10 mg as needed.
D. Rotate to fentanyl patch 12 mcg/hr, and immediate release oxycodone 2.5-5 mg as needed.

6. You review a 73-year-old man in emergency department who has metastatic non-small cell lung cancer and COPD, with metastases to brain and liver. He has presented due to decreased conscious state. He has been becoming drowsier over the past two weeks and having decreased oral intake. Over the past two months he has been deteriorating and losing weight and stopped chemotherapy four weeks ago due to progressive disease and poor performance status. His goals of care are focused on comfort in this time. He is having 30mg of slow release oxycodone for chest pain and breathlessness and has been requiring 2–3 5mg doses orally as breakthrough analgesia every day. On examination, he is cachectic, and looks comfortable with a respiratory rate of 10/min, pupils of 2mm and no metabolic flap, he is rousable to voice, and oxygen saturations are 82% on room air and 90% on 4L of oxygen via nasal cannulae. When asked, he has no pain currently. Blood tests show slow deterioration in LFTs with normal bilirubin, normal creatinine, but low albumin and high neutrophils.

Which of the following statements is **LEAST CORRECT** regarding medication administration in this setting?

A. A bolus dose of 200-400 mcg of IV naloxone is warranted.
B. Administration of 400 mcg of naloxone will give this patient more pain.
C. Administration of 400 mcg of naloxone will make this patient more alert.
D. Holding the patient's slow release opioid is warranted.

7. You review a 94-year-old woman with metastatic breast cancer and brain metastases from home with her daughter. She is normally able to transfer by herself but needs help for showering. Her daughter is struggling with her care, however. She now has a diagnosis of new right lower lobe pneumonia and is delirious and non-communicative. She has AKI and has received intravenous antibiotics and fluids over the past 24 hours and has not improved clinically. On arrival into the emergency department, her daughter reports that she wants to be marked for intensive care unit (ICU) in the event of clinical deterioration and cardiopulmonary resuscitation (CPR) in the event of cardiac arrest. You estimate based on her comorbidities and age that her probability of surviving to hospital discharge if admitted to ICU is very low, and even lower in the event of her requiring CPR, the likelihood of return to her current level of function is almost non-existent. Her daughter reports that her mother's greatest fear is dying in a nursing home and is able to give you an Advance Care Directive that stipulates these wishes both for CPR and her strong wishes not to die in a nursing home.

Which of the following strategies is most appropriate at this stage?

A. Defer further discussion about resuscitation plans until consultant review the next day.
B. Engage the daughter in a discussion about the patient's goals and wishes, and how CPR and ICU would be unlikely to meet her goals.
C. Record a resuscitation plan that outlines that the patient is for ICU admission and CPR.
D. Record a resuscitation plan that outlines that the patient is not for ICU admission and CPR as these are futile measures in meeting the patient's goals and wishes.

8. You review a patient who has breathlessness due to lymphangitis carcinomatosis resulting from metastatic breast cancer. She is otherwise symptomatically and functionally well. Four days ago, she started on dexamethasone 4mg twice daily for control of breathlessness. Her symptoms have subsequently not improved, and she has not noticed any untoward effects of the medication. She has noticed an increase in appetite, energy, and oral intake.

What is the next most appropriate step in management?
   A. Add 40 mg frusemide twice daily.
   B. Cease the dexamethasone.
   C. Decrease the dexamethasone to 4 mg once daily.
   D. Increase the dexamethasone dose to 8 mg twice daily.

9. A 79-year-old man is dying from metastatic colorectal cancer. Over the past 24 hours, he has become progressively more sedated and is now not responsive to voice. On examination, he has a barely perceptible radial pulse at a rate of 110 bpm, has Cheyne-Stokes respirations, and dry mucous membranes, and his chest is clear to auscultation. His family report crackly breathing that is intermittently present and they ask you about its significance, they are not significantly distressed by the problem.
   What is the most appropriate management of the noisy breathing in this circumstance?
   A. Atropine drops.
   B. Education for his family.
   C. Hyoscine butylbromide subcutaneously.
   D. Oropharyngeal suction.

10. A 42-year-old man is admitted to hospital with aspiration pneumonia. He is physically dependent, bed-bound, fed by gastrostomy, non-verbal, and unable to communicate after suffering a significant traumatic brain injury two years previously. He has been hospitalised three times in the last twelve months as a result of aspiration events and pneumonia. His wife (who is his legally appointed guardian) gives a history that he shows no meaningful quality of life, seems to be distressed by the physical care that he requires, and that his children, who are now 7 and 9 years old, do not want to see him anymore as he is too distressed in their presence. She also reports that he would 'hate to see himself in this state'. Collateral history from the man's parents and friends is similar to his wife's description. At the time, the family were hoping that he might show some late recovery of meaning-ful function, but this has not occurred. The family requests that gastrostomy tube feeding be ceased so that he is allowed to die.
   Which of the following statements best encapsulates the ethical considerations around withdrawing tube feeding?
   A. A decision such as this can only be made by a state appointed guardian as opposed to a family member who is also guardian.
   B. As the benefits of tube feeding are always greater than the adverse consequence when a person cannot feed themselves, there is a responsibility to continue feeding until death from another cause other than malnutrition.
   C. The doctors looking after the patient have a responsibility to advocate for continued tube feeding as it represents a basic human right and deny the requests of the patient's wife.
   D. The patient's legally appointed guardian can, in conjunction with the treating medical team, elect to withhold tube feeding if the benefits are outweighed by the adverse effects.

Answers

1. Answer: D

Management of thirst and dry mouth at the end-of-life should predominantly be managed by topical therapies. Unfortunately, the symptom of dry mouth and thirst has multiple drivers not only related to dehydration, and enteral or parenteral fluid risks significant complications. Increased fluid intake in this setting increases gastric secretions, pulmonary secretions, peripheral oedema, and ascites, and should not be first line therapy. Subcutaneous fluid administration has a tendency to pool in the subcutaneous space near the site of infusion in patients near the end-of-life. Intravenous fluid is associated with discomfort from intravenous access. Oral fluid is difficult to manage and particularly in bowel obstruction, is associated with increased vomiting. All of these strategies may be appropriate in individual circumstances, but local topical therapies should be first line.

 Nabati L, Abrahm JL. Caring for patients at the end of life. Chapter 51 in Abeloff's clinical oncology. Niederhuber JE, Armitage JO, Doroshow JH et.al. eds. 6th Ed. 2020. Elsevier.
https://www.sciencedirect.com/science/article/pii/B9780323476744000517

2. Answer: D

Malignant bowel obstruction is a complex entity most commonly involving interplay between mechanical obstruction, often at multiple levels, and ileus due to chemical mediators via serotonergic pathways which lead to increased secretions and decreased motility. Bowel obstruction is a common event in disseminated intra-abdominal malignancy, with ovarian cancer being the most common cause, but colon, stomach, pancreas, and bladder cancer all being relatively common; extra-abdominal malignancies with peritoneal disease such as breast cancer, mesothelioma, and melanoma cause bowel obstruction less often.

Most malignant bowel obstructions resolve with non-interventional measures and gut rest, and medications such as steroids and anti-emetics can be useful to achieve adequate symptom control. The use of anti-secretory agents such as proton-pump inhibitors, ranitidine, and octreotide are also useful in managing symptoms. Correction of electrolyte imbalances such as hypokalaemia or hypercalcaemia is important. However, most patients eventually develop another episode of bowel obstruction, after the initial event has resolved. In advancing malignancy, particularly without treatment modifying options, bowel obstruction is usually a harbinger of poor prognosis, and reassessment of goals of treatment becomes critical at this time, particularly prior to consideration of surgical intervention.

Procedural intervention in bowel obstruction is a complex issue, with individualised, multidisciplinary care essential. Good results from surgical intervention are most likely where resection and re-anastomosis are possible, rather than bypass or stoma formation. Inoperable gastric outlet obstruction can be managed with stenting, and colonic stenting for inoperable large bowel obstruction can give reasonable results. Surgical intervention is best reserved for patients in whom reversal of enteral failure would make further anti-cancer treatment options viable.

 Ferguson H, Ferguson C, Speakman J, Ismail T. Management of intestinal obstruction in advanced malignancy. Annals of Medicine and Surgery. 2015;4(3):264–270.
https://www.ncbi.nlm.nih.gov/pmc/articles/PMC4539185/

3. Answer: D

A large number of patients die in hospital with acute and chronic illness. These patients have a high symptomatic burden and management of their symptoms is frequently suboptimal. Basic symptom management for the dying patient is a necessary skill for hospital clinicians, as specialist palliative care services may not be available, or as in this case, the time required to get palliative care specialist review may be longer than the patient's life-expectancy. Opioids have a high level of evidence for safety and efficacy in the management of dyspnoea at the end-of-life. The appropriate route of administration and dosage depends on the clinical setting. For the patient with chronic dyspnoea due to malignancy or organ failure, low-dose oral opioids are highly effective. For a patient who is dying in distress due to respiratory disease, speed of absorption is the critical factor. A continuous subcutaneous infusion of morphine will take hours to reach peak efficacy, which is inadequate in itself to manage acute distress – bolus doses are needed. In most circumstances, the subcutaneous route (with time to maximum concentration of around 20 minutes) is rapidly enough absorbed to be sufficient (for example with a patient with moderate dyspnoea due to new pulmonary embolus or infection). However, the practicalities of waiting 15 minutes to repeat a dose in a patient who is in respiratory distress may be inadvisable, and can be particularly distressing for the patient, family, and staff. In such settings, repeated intravenous administration of opioid is most likely to be efficacious, if feasible. In some settings, initiation of an emergency response call might be needed in order to provide intravenous opioid, as junior doctors may feel uncomfortable doing so.

In renal failure, accumulation of toxic metabolites of morphine can cause significant troubling neurotoxicity, and this is an important consideration if life expectancy is more than one day. Oxycodone and hydromorphone have active metabolites as well but seem better tolerated in renal failure. Fentanyl is metabolised and not renally cleared, but has the disadvantage of a very short half-life, and is potentially less efficacious for dyspnoea. Non-pharmacological measures are also effective for dyspnoea: oxygen if hypoxic, non-invasive ventilation if in type 2 respiratory failure, fans, cool air, relaxation techniques, walking aids, and upright positioning. The tolerability and suitability of such measures is situation specific. Other troubling symptoms in the dying patient include pain, dry mouth, nausea/vomiting, itch, constipation, and anxiety – which all have effective pharmacological treatments. Oral secretions and noisy breathing are not thought to be uncomfortable for patients, and treatment with anticholinergic medications in this setting is not usually indicated.

 Blinderman C, Billings J. Comfort Care for Patients Dying in the Hospital. New England Journal of Medicine. 2015;373(26):2549–2561.
https://www.nejm.org/doi/10.1056/NEJMra1411746

4. Answer: C

Motor neurone disease (MND) is a progressive neurodegenerative disease involving both upper and lower motor neurons. It is characterised by motor system failure due to the death of nerves responsible for all voluntary movements, leading to limb paralysis, weakness of the muscles of speech and swallowing, and ultimately respiratory failure. The aetiology is unknown, approximately 5–10% of patients have a family history, and for these patients an abnormal gene mutation can be found in up to 60%.

The prognosis for most patients is 2–3 years. The progression of the disease is very individual, but there is usually progressive loss of muscle power, which may affect the limbs, the bulbar area, the respiratory muscles, and the diaphragm. The most common cause of death is respiratory failure. Riluzole slows the progression in some patients, and edaravone (novel neuroprotective agent), has been shown to help certain patient groups. As there is no cure for MND, palliative care may be appropriate from the time of diagnosis, particularly as the prognosis is poor. Many patients may not be diagnosed for up to 12 months after their first symptoms and thus may have developed severe disability and may have a short prognosis.

Non-invasive ventilatory (NIV) support, which may relieve symptoms related to respiratory failure and prolong survival by up to 12 months and improve quality of life. Short acting benzodiazepine is used in relieving dyspnoea on exertion whilst long acting benzodiazepine can be used in dyspnoea at rest. Baclofen is usually used to relieve muscle spasm/spasticity. Carbamazepine and gabapentin are helpful in relieving fasciculations.

Although there is little evidence of sensory nerve involvement, pain is a common symptom, with studies showing a prevalence of up to 73%. The pain may be due to:
- Muscle stiffness and spasm in spasticity.
- Joint pains due to the altered muscle activity around the joint.
- Skin pressure pain due to immobility.

The development of dysphagia is a distressing and common symptom, affecting up to 87% of patients with MND. Cough and constipation are common. The placement of a percutaneous endoscopic gastrostomy (PEG) tube can be helpful in improving quality of life and there is evidence that it may increase survival. Emotional lability is common in MND patients, particularly those with bulbar disease, and one study showed a prevalence of 23%. There is increasing evidence that this symptom is related to frontal lobe damage and dysfunction. It can be particularly distressing to both patients and families.

 Oliver D. Palliative care in motor neurone disease: where are we now? Palliative Care: Research and Treatment. 2019; 12:117822421881391.
https://journals.sagepub.com/doi/10.1177/1178224218813914

5. Answer: C

Opioid rotation is an important tool in the management of cancer pain. Receptor dynamics, intracellular adaptations, and central nervous system adaptations all play important roles in the development of tolerance and hyperalgesia that develop with consistent opioid use. These consequences can easily result in reducing efficacy with increasing doses, or high levels of side effects in comparison to analgesia. Each opioid medication has differing interactions with the μ-receptor and differing intracellular consequences, resulting in incomplete cross-tolerance between opioids. These phenomena have rather useful clinical consequences, with rotation from one opioid to another often achieving an effective balance of analgesia and side effects. This occurs at dosages lower than expected by traditional dose-equivalence studies.

There is no compelling data to suggest that a particular opioid is a more effective choice to rotate to, however individual patient characteristics such as age, prior exposure, organ function, and interacting medications should influence drug choice. The pharmacokinetics of particular drugs also plays a role – whilst oxycodone, hydromorphone, and morphine have similar therapeutic half-lives, fentanyl is significantly shorter, and methadone significantly longer, resulting in significantly different analgesic profiles. Opioid rotation requires knowledge (or access to knowledge) of the relative dose-equivalence of the analgesic, but the final dosage needs to be reduced due to incomplete cross-tolerance (by 25–75%), to not dose to reduce risks significant toxicity. Average dose equivalence factors in comparison to oral morphine are 5–10 for oral methadone (i.e. methadone is 5–10 times more potent as an analgesic, mg for mg), 100 for transdermal fentanyl, 70 for transdermal buprenorphine, 5 for oral hydromorphone and 1.5 for oral oxycodone.

Mercadante S, Bruera E. Opioid switching in cancer pain: From the beginning to nowadays. Critical Reviews in Oncology/Hematology. 2016;99: 241–248.
https://www.sciencedirect.com/science/article/abs/pii/S1040842815301037?via%3Dihub

6. Answer: A

Management of potential respiratory depression due to opioid toxicity in cancer pain is more complicated than acute overdose or iatrogenic harm. In most cases of opioid overdose, rapid reversal of narcotisation is warranted, and this is reflected in international guidelines. However, in the setting of significant cancer pain, naloxone administration carries significant risk to the patient. In the setting of a patient in the last days of their life, such as is likely in this case, the risk of dying in significant pain almost always outweighs the risk of excess sedation in that timeframe. Diagnostic uncertainty also plays a part in this – in this clinical situation, his brain metastases, chronic lung disease, and progressive cancer all contribute to his multifactorial drowsiness, making the clinical indication for naloxone less obvious. Other common causes of drowsiness in advanced cancer include hypercalcaemia, benzodiazepines, and seizure. Earlier in the course of treatment of cancer pain, more aggressive treatment of narcotisation is warranted – but not at such high doses. In this situation, a large bolus of naloxone would probably wake the patient a little, at the expense of more pain.

In the setting of cancer pain and therapeutic opioid use, the most commonly used marker for opioid induced depression is a respiratory rate of 8 breaths/min. Naloxone should only be used in this setting if the patient cannot be roused by gentle stimuli. In this setting, 20–40 mcg naloxone aliquots can be administered at one minute intervals, until the respiratory rate is greater than 10 breaths/min, and the offending opioid held – low dose naloxone infusion could be considered, depending on the therapeutic half-life of the offending opioid, and the patient's goals of care. Larger bolus doses could be considered if the respiratory rate is less than 4 breaths/min. Ongoing assessment of pain state and as required analgesia is mandatory to prevent and manage rebound pain.

Howlett C, Gonzalez R, Yerram P, Faley B. Use of naloxone for reversal of life-threatening opioid toxicity in cancer-related pain. Journal of Oncology Pharmacy Practice. 2014;22(1):114–120.
https://journals.sagepub.com/doi/10.1177/1078155214551589

7. Answer: B

The advance planning of what to do in the event of clinical deterioration is a medical plan that is informed by the patients' wishes but is not beholden to them. Consequently, a medical practitioner is not under any obligation to offer treatment that they would deem to be futile. A rather obtuse but illustrative example of this concept is that you would not offer an appendectomy to treat pneumonia, similarly, you would not offer CPR to treat a dying patient. For this reason, it is not legally binding for an Advance Care Directive to demand a particular treatment, such as CPR. Having said this, it is certainly also acknowledged that consensus with a treatment plan is valuable, and time spent gaining this consensus is worthwhile, leading to improved outcomes. In situations where there is disagreement about resuscitation status, consensus can be achieved after one meeting in around 90% of patients, and this figure rises with subsequent meetings and discussions. There are many misconceptions about CPR and ICU interventions in the community and discussing the role and potential outcomes of these interventions is a valuable tool in discussion around the topic. Also important is developing a medical plan that best reflects the patient's goals of care, in light of what is possible with medical treatment.

In the event that a patient has a stable medical condition and is thus likely to benefit from CPR, simply gathering information about their preferences is sufficient. It is possible in this situation that an individual may not want CPR, but the likelihood is that they will, and either choice is appropriate. In the event that the patient has an advancing illness, and it is unclear whether CPR will meet their goals, a shared decision making model, where the patient and doctor engage meaningfully together in weighing up the risks and benefits of the intervention, is more appropriate. Where the patient is unlikely to benefit from CPR, the conversation should shift towards an informed consent framework, where recommendations against CPR are put to the patient in order to guide them in a difficult situation. This framework can be used in discussing any medical intervention, particularly where there is some uncertainty about benefits. These conversations typically take time, and often involve breaking bad news as part of the discussion. Patients and their family are most likely to perceive a benefit from these discussions if they feel that their concerns have been addressed, so patience, compassion, and active listening are also key skills in such an interaction.

 Jacobsen J, Tran K, Jackson V, Rubin E. Case 19–2020: A 74-Year-Old Man with Acute Respiratory Failure and Unclear Goals of Care. New England Journal of Medicine. 2020.
https://www.nejm.org/doi/10.1056/NEJMcpc2002419

8. Answer: B

Systemic corticosteroids are a useful adjunct for symptom management in palliative care, with evidence for short to medium term benefit of many different symptoms including poor energy, appetite, pain (particularly liver capsular pain and bony pain), breathlessness, and nausea. There are also potential uses in treating symptoms due to cerebral oedema, spinal cord compression, and bowel obstruction. Dexamethasone and betamethasone are the corticosteroids most studied in palliative care. Despite efficacy, long-term use of effective doses of corticosteroid is limited by multiple side effects, and loss of efficacy over time. In the short term, fluid retention, hyperglycaemia, dyspepsia, insomnia, and elevated mood (including psychosis on occasion) are the most common adverse effects. However medium term effects can be even more debilitating in patients with poor functional reserve – mood disorder and oropharyngeal candidiasis are common and debilitating enough, but more troubling is proximal myopathy, which may occur in up to 50% of patients with metastatic cancer treated with corticosteroid for over one month, resulting in functional loss that is usually not regained. Consequently, guidelines for using corticosteroid to treat symptoms due to metastatic cancer involve starting at a high enough dose to treat symptoms (8 mg per day for most indications, but 16 mg for cerebral oedema and cord compression); frequent re-evaluation for efficacy and side-effects; cessation if ineffective; and weaning rapidly to a minimum effective dose. Some guidelines recommend prophylactic nystatin and gastroprotectants.

 Moertel C, Schutt A, Reitemeier R, Hahn R. Corticosteroid therapy of preterminal gastrointestinal cancer. Cancer. 1974;33(6):1607–1609.
https://acsjournals.onlinelibrary.wiley.com/doi/abs/10.1002/1097-0142%28197406%2933%3A6%3C1607%3A%3AAID-CNCR2820330620%3E3.0.CO%3B2-V

9. Answer: B

Noisy breathing in the last days of life is an extremely common phenomenon caused by pooling of oropharyngeal secretions in the hypopharynx. The predominant mechanism for this in normal dying is decreased swallowing rather than hypersalivation or increasing lower respiratory secretions. There is no evidence that such a phenomenon causes any significant discomfort to the dying individual, although the phenomenon can be confronting for staff and family members. No single pharmacological measure has been shown to decrease noisy breathing in this setting once it has been established, and no method for predicting which patients it will occur. However, management strategies that theoretically might decrease noisy breathing, such as anticholinergic medications or suction, have potential side effects of their own, that can cause discomfort. As a consequence, a comprehensive communication strategy educating patients' families about the phenomenon, preferably ahead of time, is currently recommended.

This recommendation does not necessarily hold true for hypersalivation due to neurological disorders or complete upper gastrointestinal obstruction, where antisecretory medications may be appropriate. Similarly, copious lower respiratory secretions due to pulmonary oedema caused by central nervous system pathology, cardiac failure, or disseminated thoracic malignancy can cause significant cough and breathlessness, and these symptoms often need pharmacological management.

 Star A, Boland J. Updates in palliative care – recent advancements in the pharmacological management of symptoms. Clinical Medicine. 2018;18(1):11–16.
https://www.rcpjournals.org/content/clinmedicine/18/1/11

10. Answer: D

Withholding tube feeding is a complex and controversial issue in the event of permanent vegetative state. Within some particular frames of reference, the benefits of nutrition in terms of wound healing and prolonged life might always seem to outweigh any potential detrimental effects of care. Nutrition and hydration, in particular, despite often being delivered by artificial means, have particular controversies around withdrawal in many societies. However, a more nuanced ethical discussion around these issues points to the continued treatment despite no hope of meaningful recovery as futile and amounting to therapeutic obstinacy. In particular, where the care required to continue life sustaining treatment revolves around continued discomfort and loss of dignity for the individual involved, the costs of this treatment could easily be seen to outweigh any potential benefits. Additionally, where continued existence presents detrimental effects to a person's values and beliefs – for example, leaving a positive legacy for their family – the continuance of this state can easily be seen to be harmful. From a legal standpoint, in Australia at least, the natural provision of food and fluids is seen as a basic legal right, but not nutrition and hydration by artificial means. As a consequence, life sustaining artificial treatments including tube feeding can legally be withdrawn with appropriate discussion and assessment, if the decision is felt to represent an appropriate balance of harms and benefits, and the decision would be consistent with the patient's premorbid values and wishes. In the event of uncertainty, legal advice or second opinions may be prudent, but is not a necessity.

2011. Parenteral Nutrition Pocketbook. Chatswood, N.S.W.: Agency for Clinical Innovation, p.63.
https://www.aci.health.nsw.gov.au/__data/assets/pdf_file/0010/159805/aci_parenteral_nutrition_pb.pdf–

18 Pharmacology, Toxicology and Addiction Medicine

Questions

Answers can be found in the Pharmacology, Toxicology, and Addiction Medicine Answers section at the end of this chapter.

1. A drug is noted in pharmacological studies to achieve lower peak blood levels in healthy younger people compared to healthy older people. Which of the following pharmacokinetic phenomena associated with ageing is most likely to explain this finding?
  A. Decreased absorption.
  B. Decreased first pass metabolism.
  C. Decreased phase I metabolism.
  D. Decreased renal clearance.

2. Ampicillin elimination in a patient with stage 3b CKD is affected by which of the following mechanisms?
  A. Increased tubular reabsorption.
  B. Reduced glomerular filtration.
  C. Reduced glomerular filtration and reduced renal tubular secretion.
  D. Reduced renal tubular secretion.

3. In elderly patients, medicines with anticholinergic properties may be prescribed in which one of the following conditions:
  A. Alzheimer's disease.
  B. Benign prostatic hypertrophy (BPH).
  C. Bowel obstruction.
  D. Sinus bradycardia.

4. Azithromycin is used in the treatment of severe community acquired pneumonia. Which one of the following statements is correct?
  A. Azithromycin is a strong CYP3A4 inhibitor and cause significant drug-drug interactions.
  B. Azithromycin is bactericidal.
  C. Azithromycin binds to the 30S ribosomal subunit to inhibit RNA synthesis.
  D. Azithromycin is safe in pregnancy.

5. Biosimilar Rituximab has recently been introduced on the hospital medicines formulary whilst one of your patients is part way through his treatment schedule with R-CHOP for non-Hodgkins lymphoma.
  Which of the following statements is correct with respect to the consideration of biosimilar medicine use in this situation?
  A. A biosimilar medicine can be prescribed for all therapeutic indications for which the originator (or reference) biologic medicine is licensed.
  B. A biosimilar medicine is a generic version of an originator (or reference) biologic medicine and is considered to be bioequivalent.
  C. The use of a biosimilar medicine requires clinical input and monitoring due to a potentially different immunologic profile.
  D. The use of a biosimilar medicine should only be considered in a patient who is treatment naïve.

How to Pass the FRACP Written Examination, First Edition. Jonathan Gleadle, Jordan Li, Danielle Wu, and Paul Kleinig.
© 2022 John Wiley & Sons Ltd. Published 2022 by John Wiley & Sons Ltd.

6. Which one of the following regarding mechanism of action of bisphosphonates is correct?
   A. Bisphosphonates are the active fragments of human parathyroid hormone, promoting bone formation.
   B. Bisphosphonates reduce bone resorption by inhibiting osteoclasts and may have effect on osteoblasts.
   C. Bisphosphonates bind receptor activator of nuclear factor-kappa B ligand (RANKL) preventing activation of the RANK receptor, resulting in decreased formation and activity of osteoclasts.
   D. Bisphosphonates increase bone formation by osteoblasts.

7. Drug A is administered by continuous intravenous infusion at a rate of 1 mg/minute, and has a clearance of 120 mL/hr. What is the best approximation of its steady state concentration assuming a one compartment model?
   A. 0.5 mg/mL.
   B. 2 mg/mL.
   C. Unable to calculate – half-life needed to calculate.
   D. Unable to calculate – volume of distribution needed to calculate.

8. Clopidogrel has been observed to produce an inadequate response on platelet aggregation in some patients, when compared with ticagrelor and prasugrel.
   Which of the following situations could account for this observation?
   A. Co-administration of CYP3A4 inducers.
   B. Co-administration of CYP2D6 inhibitors.
   C. Loss of function mutations in CYP2C19.
   D. Mutations of $P2Y_{12}$ receptor gene.

9. An 85-year-old woman is seen in the geriatric assessment clinic accompanied by her family. Her family report a 12-month history of progressive memory loss and personality changes. She has become forgetful and can no longer manage to pay her bills and handle her finances. She has hypertension and often forgets to take her antihypertensive medication, telmisartan. Clinical examination reveals ideomotor apraxia and her mini-mental state examination (MMSE) is 23/30. Her CT head shows small vessel ischaemia but no other intracranial pathology.
   The available drugs approved by TGA to treat her condition target which one of the following neurotransmitters?
   A. Acetylcholine.
   B. Dopamine.
   C. Melatonin.
   D. Serotonin.

10. Which of one the following types of study for an investigational new drug 'Memory 100' involves each subject receiving a sequence of all the different treatments?
   A. Crossover clinical study.
   B. Parallel clinical study.
   C. Sequential clinical study.
   D. Triple-blind clinical study.

11. A 39-year-old woman has suffered from Addison's disease for 10 years. She is currently taking hydrocortisone plus fludrocortisone.
   Which one of the following additional treatments is most likely to induce an Addisonian crisis?
   A. Carbamazepine.
   B. Ketoconazole.
   C. Thyroxine.
   D. Spironolactone.

12. Which one of the following drugs does **NOT** exert its effects by competitive enzyme inhibition?
   A. Acyclovir.
   B. Allopurinol.
   C. Alpha methyldopa.
   D. Amlodipine.

13. You are prescribing intravenous ganciclovir for a patient with a severe CMV infection post allogeneic haemopoietic stem cell transplant. He is known to have stage 4 CKD and has morbid obesity. You are checking his renal function to adjust the dose. Which of the following should you use to obtain his eGFR?
   A. eGFR calculated by CKD-EPI formula.
   B. eGFR calculated by Cockcroft-Gault formula.
   C. eGFR calculated by MDRD formula.
   D. GFR measured by DTPA radionuclide scan.

14. A 53-year-old man consumed a bottle of liquid from his garage after an argument with his partner. He was found by his neighbour and brought in by ambulance. He has a Glasgow Coma Score of 6. BP is 95/70 mmHg, respiratory rate is 30/min with Kussmaul respirations, SpO_2 98% on room air. Initial ABG shows a pH of 7.07 with a pCO2 of 24 mmHg, pO2 of 100 mmHg, and bicarbonate of 8 mmol/L. His initial biochemistry results are shown below. His urine is sent for drug screen and microscope examination which is shown below. His ECG demonstrated sinus tachycardia but no QT prolongation.

Tests	Test results	Normal values
Sodium	140 mmol/L	135–145
Potassium	3.9 mmol/L	3.5–5.2
Chloride	93 mmol/L	95–110
Creatinine	130 μmol/L	60–110
Glucose	6.7 mmol/L	3.2– 5.5
Lactate	3.1 mmol/L	0.5–2.0

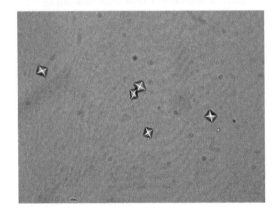

What is the most likely substance that he had consumed?
   A. Acetone based paint thinner.
   B. Ethylene glycol.
   C. Gasoline.
   D. Organophosphate insecticide.

15. Which of the following is **NOT** an implication of high first-pass metabolism?
   A. Enzyme inducers are associated with higher intrinsic clearance and reduced drug bioavailability.
   B. High extraction ratio of medication is related to decreased bioavailability.
   C. Non-oral routes of medication administration increase drug bioavailability significantly.
   D. Portal hypertension resulting in increased first-pass metabolism.

16. A 49-year-old woman is admitted to hospital with severe sepsis due to cellulitis and is discharged from the intensive care unit on day 7 still on intravenous flucloxacillin. She complains of shortness of breath, and CT pulmonary angiogram confirms four bilateral segmental PE despite prophylactic heparin 5000 units twice daily subcutaneously. Blood tests reveal the following (normal range in brackets):

Test	On admission	Now
Haemoglobin (115-155 g/L)	122 g/L	95 g/L
White blood cell count (4–11 x 10⁹/L)	22.7 x 10⁹/L	11.1 x 10⁹/L
Platelet count (150–450 x 10⁹/L)	487 x 10⁹/L	59 x 10⁹/L
Creatinine (45–90 umol/L)	249 umol/L	122 umol/L
INR	1.5	1.1
D–dimer (<0.50 mg/L)	2.1	3.0
Fibrinogen (1.5–4.0 g/L)	6.1 g/L	4.0 g/L

Which of one the following strategy is most appropriate for management of her pulmonary embolism?
   A. Bivalirudin infusion.
   B. Inferior vena cava filter now and anticoagulation once platelet count >100 x 10⁹/L.
   C. Therapeutic enoxaparin.
   D. Unfractionated heparin infusion.

17. Which diuretic inhibits the apical distal convoluted tubule epithelium sodium-chloride cotransporter and decreases peripheral vascular resistance?
   A. Amiloride.
   B. Acetazolamide.
   C. Eplerenone.
   D. Indapamide.

18. An 80-year-old man has had unstable angina, congestive heart failure, and type 2 diabetes. To which of the following medications is he most likely to develop tolerance?
   A. Carvedilol.
   B. Empagliflozin.
   C. Isosorbide mononitrate.
   D. Telmisartan.

19. A 62-year-old man is admitted with severe sepsis secondary to an infected diabetic ulcer in his right foot. The wound swap grew vancomycin-resistant *E. faecalis*, *Pseudomonas aeruginosa* and *MRSA*. His other medications include metformin, perindopril, bisoprolol, atorvastatin, aspirin, fluoxetine, and thyroxine. He has no known allergies.
   Which of the following antibiotics would be contraindicated in this patient?
   A. Ciprofloxacin.
   B. Daptomycin.
   C. Linezolid.
   D. Piperacillin/Tazobactam.

20. What is the best method to measure medication bioavailability?
   A. Time above minimum inhibitory concentration (MIC).
   B. Maximum/peak serum concentration (C max).
   C. Time to reach steady state (Tss).
   D. Area under the plasma concentration-time curve (AUC).

21. An 87-year-old nursing home man presents to the emergency department with confusion, hallucination, agitation, dry mouth, and urinary retention. He has a medical history of dementia, benign prostate hypertrophy, urge incontinence, coronary artery disease, stage 4 CKD, and hyperlipidaemia. On review of his medication list from the nursing home, which of the following medications has the most anticholinergic activity?
- **A.** Benztropine.
- **B.** Lorazepam.
- **C.** Oxybutynin.
- **D.** Zolpidem.

22. Which of the following conceptualisations is most appropriate for managing opioid use disorder?
- **A.** A chronic illness paradigm.
- **B.** A chronic pain paradigm.
- **C.** A criminal justice issue.
- **D.** A psychiatric problem.

23. Which of the following medications is most likely to result in significant toxicity if administered with a potent inhibitor of P-glycoprotein (P-gp) such as ketoconazole?
- **A.** Carvedilol.
- **B.** Digoxin.
- **C.** Fentanyl.
- **D.** Gentamicin.

24. Which one of the individual response variations is predominantly due to pharmacodynamic differences?
- **A.** Bioavailability.
- **B.** Enzyme activity.
- **C.** Liver function.
- **D.** Patient.

25. The efficacy of which of the following drugs is **LEAST LIKELY** to be influenced by inter-individual variability in the CYP2D6 gene?
- **A.** Codeine.
- **B.** Tacrolimus.
- **C.** Tamoxifen.
- **D.** Tramadol.

26. A 38-year-old woman is admitted to the hospital because of severe sepsis with a background of type 2 diabetes and morbid obesity with BMI 41 kg/m^2. While prescribing antibiotics you should consider:
- **A.** Alpha 1-acid glycoprotein (AAG) concentration is decreased in obese patients.
- **B.** The half-life of lipid soluble drugs is increased in obese patients.
- **C.** There should be a reduction in the dose of cephazolin.
- **D.** There is no need to increase dosage of prophylactic enoxaparin.

27. Which of the following agonists of the μ-opioid receptor (MOR) has the greatest effect on reuptake of serotonin?
- **A.** Cebranopadol.
- **B.** Fentanyl.
- **C.** Tapentadol.
- **D.** Tramadol.

28. An 85-year-old man is admitted to the Acute Medical Unit following a mechanical fall. He stated that he stood up quickly to answer the doorbell for a pizza delivery and ended up on the floor. He did not lose consciousness. He did not injure himself. His wife reports that he has had three falls in the past six months. This time he struggled to get himself off the floor, so an ambulance was called. His medical history includes type 2 diabetes, CKD, hypertension, ischaemic heart disease, and CCF. His current medications include metformin, linagliptin, aspirin, lipidil, ramipril, metoprolol, furosemide, isosorbide mononitrate, amlodipine, prazosin, sertraline, and esomeprazole.

Clinical examination reveals no evidence of CCF. His BP is 110/60 mmHg seated which falls to 100/50 mmHg within 3 minutes of standing, with mild light headedness. His initial investigation results and ECG are shown below:

Tests	Results	Normal values
Sodium	135 mmol/L	135–145
Potassium	4.5 mmol/L	3.5–5.2
Creatinine	139 µmol/L	60–100
Albumin	21 g/L	38–48
Glucose	3.8 mmol/L	3.2–5.5
ALP	238 U/L	30–110
GGT	159 U/L	0–60
ALT	179 U/L	0–55
AST	213 U/L	0–45
Hb	109 g/L	135–175
WBC	9.3×10^9/L	4.0–11.0
Platelet	320×10^9/L	150–450
MCV	85 fL	80–95
CRP	5 mg/L	0–8
Troponin	49 ng/L	<29
HbA1C	5.9%	

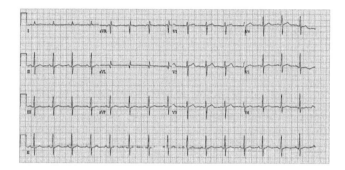

What do you need to do before discharging him to a private rehabilitation hospital?
- **A.** Commence bisphosphonate to prevent fall related hip fracture.
- **B.** Commence erythropoietin injection to treat anaemia which is a risk factor for falls.
- **C.** No further investigation or change of management plan as it is a mechanical fall.
- **D.** Review his medications despite good control of his diabetes, hypertension, and heart failure.

29. Which one of the following regarding pramipexole is correct?
- **A.** Diltiazem increases the renal excretion of pramipexole.
- **B.** Metoclopramide diminishes the effect of pramipexole.
- **C.** Pramipexole cannot be stopped without tapering.
- **D.** Pramipexole is an ergot-derived dopamine agonist.

30. Which one of the following drugs is **NOT** a prodrug?
- **A.** Enalapril.
- **B.** Famciclovir.
- **C.** Paracetamol.
- **D.** Prednisone.

31. You prescribe a small dose of risperidone for an inpatient diagnosed with delirium on the background of moderate dementia. Risperidone's therapeutic actions are primarily by which of the following mechanisms?

    A. Blocking dopaminergic transmission via D1 receptors and serotonin receptors 5HT1A in the mesolimbic system.

    B. Blocking dopaminergic transmission via D2 receptors and serotonin receptors 5HT2A in the mesolimbic system.

    C. Enhancing dopaminergic transmission via D2 receptors and anticholinergic effects in the mesocortical system.

    D. Enhancing dopaminergic transmission in the mesolimbic system, prefrontal cortex.

32. A 70-year-old man with smoking-related COPD and hyperlipidaemia is taking rosuvastatin. Which one of the following drugs for treatment of his infective exacerbation of COPD complicated by rapid atrial fibrillation produces the most significant drug interaction with rosuvastatin?

    A. Clarithromycin.

    B. Digoxin.

    C. Prednisolone.

    D. Rivaroxaban.

33. A 75-year-old man presents to the emergency department with acute onset right leg weakness beginning one hour ago. He reports no speech or vision difficulties. He takes no regular medications and has not been to see a doctor in over 20 years. A code stroke has been called. On examination, his BP is 190/100 mmHg. HR is 80 bpm and regular, he has severe right leg weakness predominantly affecting flexor groups with an extensor plantar response. The remaining peripheral neurological exam and cranial nerve examination are unremarkable. CT head and CT angiogram show a perfusion deficit in the left anterior cerebral artery territory with the remaining vasculature being normal.

    What is the most appropriate drug that the patient should receive next?

    A. Intravenous alteplase.

    B. Intravenous labetalol.

    C. Loading dose of aspirin and clopidogrel.

    D. Oral dabigatran.

34. A 58-year-old man is brought into Acute Assessment Unit by his wife. She reports her husband became suddenly confused whilst they were in the shopping mall this afternoon, asking questions like 'What are we doing here?' or 'How did we get here?'. She took him home and again he began asking 'How did we get here?' Given his ongoing symptoms, his wife brings him to hospital. She reports that he remembers her and the shopping mall. He has had no recent head trauma, loss of consciousness or seizure like activity. There are no infective symptoms, and his only past medical history is that of migraines. He has not had any alcohol in the last few days and has never used recreational drugs. These symptoms been ongoing for 2 hours now. On examination, he is not confused and is oriented to person, place, and time. However, he does not recall being in the shopping mall. His vital signs are normal, and he has no focal neurological signs on cranial nerve or peripheral neurological examination. He is able to perform serial 7s, spell 'world' backwards, and his mental state examination is normal. There are no electrolyte disturbances or abnormal liver function on blood test. His full blood examination is unremarkable.

    What is your evidence-based treatment to prevent this condition recurring?

    A. Commence aspirin.

    B. Commence lamotrigine.

    C. Commence perindopril.

    D. No pharmacotherapy.

35. Which one of the following statements regarding vancomycin is correct?

    A. A higher vancomycin dosage is required for the treatment of meningitis due to poor central nervous system penetration.

    B. A post-dialysis vancomycin level should be used to monitor vancomycin level in haemodialysis patients.

    C. Vancomycin level is not affected by haemodialysis.

    D. Red man syndrome is associated with a high serum vancomycin level.

36. Azithromycin has a very large volume of distribution when given orally. This indicates:

    A. Azithromycin has low lipid solubility.

    B. Azithromycin is eliminated by zero-order kinetics.

    C. Azithromycin is extensive bound to plasma protein.

    D. Azithromycin is extensively sequestered in tissues.

37. A 64-year-old man with a mechanical aortic valve is anti-coagulated with warfarin long term. Addition of which of the following medications is most likely to result in significant over-anticoagulation?

    A. Carbamazepine.
    B. Erythromycin.
    C. Flucloxacillin.
    D. Fluconazole.

38. Which one of the following β-blockers is a selective β1-adrenoreceptor blocker with nitric-oxide potentiating vasodilatory effects?

    A. Atenolol.
    B. Bisoprolol.
    C. Carvedilol.
    D. Nebivolol.

39. A 64-year-old woman is admitted with sepsis due to cellulitis and is initially treated with flucloxacillin, and her condition stabilises. On day two of her hospital stay, blood cultures become positive for MRSA and her antibiotic therapy is changed to vancomycin. During her first infusion of vancomycin she experiences neck flushing, back pain, widespread itch of a confluent macular erythematous eruption on the upper torso and neck. Her BP has dropped to 90/60 mmHg, and she is tachycardic at 115 bpm; there is no wheeze, stridor, or angioedema.

  Which of the following mechanisms best describes the most likely underlying pathology for her deterioration?

    A. Direct stimulation of mast cells leading to histamine release.
    B. Endotoxaemia due to rapid bacterial killing by vancomycin.
    C. Type I, IgE mediated hypersensitivity reaction leading to anaphylaxis.
    D. Type IV, T-cell mediated hypersensitivity reaction.

40. Which one of the following statements regarding cocaine use and overdose is correct?

    A. Benzodiazepines is the first-line treatment for cardiovascular toxicity due to cocaine use.
    B. Cocaine has a much longer pharmacokinetic and pharmacodynamic duration than methamphetamine.
    C. Hypothermia is a marker for severe cocaine toxicity and is associated with rhabdomyolysis.
    D. Intranasal use cocaine can cause chest pain and acute myocardial infarction within 10 minutes.

Answers

1. Answer: B

Normal ageing is associated with changes to pharmacokinetic profiles, the most clinically relevant of which are a consequence of decreased liver mass and blood flow. This change associated with normal ageing results in a decrease in first pass metabolism; the metabolism that occurs prior to the drug reaching the systemic circulation, and phase I metabolism; the early enzymatic reactions that alter drugs. Decreased first pass metabolism results in higher peak concentrations of orally administered drugs that are first pass metabolised in younger healthy individuals, such as many opioids, amitriptyline, and verapamil. Additionally, this same phenomenon can result in decreased plasma concentrations of prodrugs such as perindopril, codeine, and simvastatin, which require conversion into active compounds. In contrast, decreased phase I metabolism results in decreased clearance of many metabolised medications such as warfarin, phenytoin, but not increases in peak concentrations. Peak concentrations can also be influenced by absorption, which appears to be largely unaffected by healthy ageing for most drugs, except for medications that are actively transported, such as vitamin B_{12}. Distribution changes due to body composition and protein binding could also theoretically change peak concentrations, but this is felt to be unlikely due to the small magnitude of the changes involved. Decreased renal clearance is observed in older adults, but the extent to which this is a function of normal ageing as opposed to pathophysiology is unclear, this change would not alter peak concentration of a drug.

 Reeve E, Wiese MD, Mangoni AA: Alterations in drug disposition in older adults. Expert Opin Drug Metab Toxicol 2015; 11(5):1–18.
https://www.ncbi.nlm.nih.gov/pubmed/25600059

2. Answer: C

The half-life of ampicillin is short, from 0.7 to 1.5 hours in adults with normal kidney function because of a low volume of distribution and significant renal tubular secretion. Dosage adjustment of ampicillin in patients with renal impairment should include both glomerular and tubular function. Unfortunately, no practical ways to adjust medication dosage on the basis of tubular secretion have been developed clinically, which may lead to dosing difficulties in patients who mainly have their kidney tubular secretion function affected and mild reduction of glomerular filtration of ampicillin.

Ampicillin dosage needs to be adjusted in patients with renal impairment since the high parenteral doses and/or prolonged treatment may result in electrolyte disturbance due to sodium content and neurotoxicity (due to accumulation of the penicillin, such as seizures, coma). Risk of neutropenia may be increased in patients with renal impairment if ampicillin dosage is not adjusted according to the renal function.

The usual dosage of ampicillin is 0.25 to 2 g every 6 hours, dosage adjustment is based on eGFR (ml/min/1.73 m²). Suggested ampicillin dosing interval for patients with renal impairment: 0.25 to 2 g every 6 hourly for patients with eGFR > 50, 0.25 to 2 g every 6 to 12 hours in patients with eGFR between 10 to 50, and when eGFR is <10, 0.25 to 2 g every 12 to 24 hours.

 Eyler R, Shvets K. Clinical Pharmacology of Antibiotics. Clinical Journal of the American Society of Nephrology. 2019;14(7):1080–1090.
https://cjasn.asnjournals.org/content/14/7/1080

3. Answer: D

Many medications used in the elderly patients have intrinsic anticholinergic properties and they achieve the intended therapeutic effect through inhibition of acetylcholine-mediated responses by competitively binding any of the five muscarinic receptors (M1–M5) within specific organ systems. Other medicines have unintended anticholinergic effects that are not the primary therapeutic activity (Table 18.1).

Common anticholinergic side–effects include dry mouth, drowsiness, blurred vision, urinary retention, constipation, and tachycardia. At very high doses, anticholinergic delirium may occur.

Anticholinergics have complex gastrointestinal actions. Gastrointestinal motility and gastric secretions are reduced. Anticholinergic premedication does not provide protection against aspiration of gastric contents and chemical or bacterial pneumonitis. In the eye, anticholinergic drugs can precipitate narrow-angle glaucoma. Elderly men with prostatic hypertrophy are at risk for severe urinary retention after taking anticholinergics. Furthermore, confusion, agitation, and delirium are CNS side effects of anticholinergics, in particular antiparkinsonian drugs, phenothiazines, tricyclic antidepressants, antihistamines, and antispasmodics. Elderly patients may be more susceptible to anticholinergic effects such as confusion or delirium, which may increase their risk of falls or hospitalisation. Concurrently taking cholinesterase inhibitors and anticholinergic medications may reduce or nullify the effectiveness of both medications. In order to achieve maximum therapeutic effects, these drugs generally should not be used in combination with each other. The cumulative, sedative effect of taking one or more medicines with anticholinergic properties is known as the anticholinergic 'load' or 'burden'. This is commonly seen in patients with polypharmacy.

Anticholinergics should be avoided if possible, in people who have dementia. Higher cumulative anticholinergic use is associated with dementia risk. This increased risk is consistent across the various types of anticholinergic drugs.

Table 18.1   Medicines with anticholinergic properties.

Medicines with intended anticholinergic therapeutic effect	
Antispasmodics	Oxybutynin
Antidiarrheals	Loperamide
Bronchodilators	Ipratropium, theophylline, tiotropium
Antiparkinsonian	Biperiden, amantadine, benztropine
Atropine	

Medicines with unintended anticholinergic therapeutic effect	
Antipsychotics	Olanzapine, periciazine, chlorpromazine, haloperidol, quetiapine
Anxiolytics	Diazepam, alprazolam
Anticonvulsants	Carbamazepine
Antidepressant	Amitriptyline, bupropion, fluvoxamine, paroxetine, venlafaxine, dothiepin, doxepin
Antihistamines	Brompheniramine, cetirizine, chlorphenamine, diphenhydramine, hydroxyzine, pheniramine, promethazine
Analgesics	Codeine, fentanyl, morphine
Eye drops	Atropine, homatropine

Mintzer J, Burns A. Anticholinergic side-effects of drugs in elderly people. Journal of the Royal Society of Medicine. 2000;93(9):457–462.
https://www.ncbi.nlm.nih.gov/pmc/articles/PMC1298101/

4. Answer: D

Azithromycin is a broad-spectrum macrolide antibiotic with the main mechanism of action to bind to 50S ribosomal subunit to inhibit bacterial protein synthesis (bacteriostatic). Azithromycin also inhibits bacterial quorum-sensing, reduces biofilm and mucus production, and has immunomodulatory effects.

Azithromycin has a long half-life (70 hours and 50 hours for oral and IV doing respectively), permitting daily or single dose treatment. Azithromycin has a large volume of distribution (30 L/kg) due to excellent tissue penetration: azithromycin concentrations can reach up to 100-fold greater in tissues than plasma, and at least 200-fold greater in phagocytes than plasma. This leads to high tissue concentration of azithromycin at sites of inflammation. Azithromycin is minimally metabolised with no active metabolites and is largely eliminated unchanged in faeces via biliary excretion. Unique among the macrolides, azithromycin does not induce CYP3A4 leading to few drug–drug interactions. Notably, azithromycin does have a minor interaction with warfarin (increasing the anticoagulant effect) and rarely can cause QT prolongation (mainly in patients with pre-existing prolonged QT). Otherwise azithromycin is generally well tolerated and can be used in pregnancy.

Parnham M, Haber V, Giamarellos-Bourboulis E, Perletti G, Verleden G, Vos R. Azithromycin: Mechanisms of action and their relevance for clinical applications. Pharmacology & Therapeutics. 2014;143(2):225–245. https://www.sciencedirect.com/science/article/abs/pii/S0163725814000552?via%3Dihub

5. Answer: C

A biosimilar is a biological medication that emulates a bio-originator, or innovative biologic. The biosimilar should demonstrate no clinically meaningful differences in terms of safety and effectiveness from the innovator product. Each biologic/biosimilar is unique and cannot be considered as bioequivalent. A biosimilar is not a generic version of the innovator biological therapy. Generics are small-molecule copies of small-molecule innovators which have exact physio-chemical replicas of the originator drug. Biosimilars are biologics, which are large and complex molecules. Although biosimilar development and construction strive to utilises the same constituents in the same way as their bio-originators, it is usually not possible to make a biosimilar that exactly reproduces that development and construction of the bio-originator. Differences may occur due to the cell lines used to clone the biosimilar and differences in growth and purification processes. The regulatory approval pathway for biosimilar is higher than small molecule generics. The biosimilar must meet a predefined equivalence margin for difference in response rate, which is usually ±15%. The followings are key points when using a biosimilar:

1. A biologic and its biosimilar are not interchangeable.
2. The selection of a biologic / biosimilar as first-line therapy in treatment-naïve patients should be subject to evidence of safety, efficacy, and cost-effectiveness.
3. Patients should be fully informed when receiving treatment with a biologic/biosimilar.
4. Due to the potentially different immunological profiles of biological medicines, the decision to switch a patient who has already received therapy with a specific biologic/biosimilar to another requires appropriate clinical input and monitoring.
5. A patient who experiences adverse effects from one biologic/biosimilar may exhibit a different immunological response to an alternative biologic/biosimilar, potentially resulting in a varied adverse effect profile.
6. One of the key concerns when switching patients from bio-originator to biosimilar is the potential generation of anti-drug antibodies, which may make not only the biosimilar, but also the bio-originator ineffective.
7. Immunogenicity can also result in some serious adverse events, including infusion reactions and anaphylaxis.

McKinnon R.A. et al. Biosimilarity and interchangeability: principles and evidence: a systematic review. BioDrugs. 2018; 32: 27–52.
[Internet]. Www1.health.gov.au. 2020 [cited 22 February 2020]. Available from: https://www1.health.gov.au/internet/main/publishing.nsf/content/biosimilar-awareness-initiative/$File/Biosimilar-medicines-the-basics-for-healthcare-professionals-Brochure.pdf

6. Answer: B

Bisphosphonates inhibit bone resorption by inhibiting osteoclasts, decreasing osteoclast activity by reducing osteoclast progenitor development and recruitment as well as promoting osteoclast apoptosis. Bisphosphonates are structurally like pyrophosphate; a structure that gives the drugs a high affinity for bone and they likely remain in bone for many years.

Bisphosphonates are indicated for the treatment of osteoporosis, hypercalcaemia secondary to malignancy, prevention of skeletal-related events in patients with malignancies involving bone, and Paget's disease of bone. They have poor and variable intestinal absorption. As a result, they are never given at mealtimes nor with dairy products. Known side effects of bisphosphonate therapy include hypocalcaemia, oesophagitis, oesophageal erosions and ulcers, renal impairment, rarely atypical low-energy femoral fractures during long-term bisphosphonate treatment, and osteonecrosis of the jaw. Consider full dental assessment and complete any dental procedures before starting treatment to minimise risks of osteonecrosis of the jaw.

Optimal duration of treatment with bisphosphonates is uncertain and careful consideration should be taken before deciding whether the patient would benefit from a 'drug holiday' after a long-term treatment (Five years for on alendronate and risedronate, and three years for patients treated with yearly IV zoledronic acid) based on the risks for subsequent fractures and benefits of ongoing treatment.

Denosumab is a human monoclonal antibody that binds receptor activator of nuclear factor-kappa B ligand (RANKL) preventing activation of the RANK receptor. This results in decreased formation and activity of osteoclasts, therefore reducing bone resorption. Unlike bisphosphonates, denosumab's effects on bone do not persist after stopping treatment. Bone turnover markers increase, and bone mineral density rapidly decreases. Some reports found multiple vertebrae fractures occurring soon after denosumab cessation. Considering starting an alternate treatment such as bisphosphate may be an option. However, more studies are required to make recommendations to manage patients with osteoporosis after stopping denosumab.

Teriparatide is the active fragment of human parathyroid hormone. Teriparatide is a potent anabolic agent that activates osteoblasts and stimulates bone formation. It is recommended as a daily subcutaneous injection for up to 18 months due to risk of osteosarcoma.

Cremers S, Drake M, Ebetino F, Bilezikian J, Russell R. Pharmacology of bisphosphonates. British Journal of Clinical Pharmacology. 2019;85(6):1052–1062.
https://www.ncbi.nlm.nih.gov/pmc/articles/PMC6533426/pdf/BCP-85-1052.pdf

7. Answer: A

Therapeutic drug monitoring involves the approximation of known pharmacokinetic properties of individual medications, interacting with individual variability in order to reach a target effect, or in cases where the target effect might be less clinically obvious – a target concentration. The concepts of volume of distribution and clearance are mathematical calculations based on observed data of measured drug concentration and dosage given, rather than measured directly. Volume of distribution refers to the theoretical volume in which a drug would have to be distributed for the entire volume to have a consistent concentration. Clearance represents the theoretical volume of plasma that is cleared of a drug or metabolite in a particular amount of time, by all appreciable routes of drug elimination combined. One of the uses of these concepts is that, in a one-compartment model, a target steady state concentration can be calculated. As such, the steady state concentration equals the infusion rate divided by the clearance. Similarly, if the steady state concentration and the infusion rate (or removal rate) are measured and known, the clearance can be calculated, e.g. the principle of creatinine clearance.

Rang H, Ritter J, Flower R, Henderson G, Loke Y, MacEwan D et al. Rang and Dale's pharmacology. 9th ed. Edinburgh: Elsevier; 2019
https://www.elsevierhealth.com.au/rang-dales-pharmacology-9780702074486.html

8. Answer: C

Clopidogrel is a prodrug which is converted to its active metabolite by CYP450 enzymes, of which CYP2C19 is a significant contributor. The active compound then irreversibly binds the adenosine diphosphate $P2Y_{12}$ receptor on platelets to decrease platelet aggregation. Loss of function mutations in CYP2C19 therefore have a significant effect on the clinical efficacy of clopidogrel. Ticagrelor and prasugrel are also $P2Y_{12}$ inhibitors – ticagrelor is an active compound with an active metabolite, and prasugrel is an inactive compound requiring activation by CYP3A4 and CYP2B6. In clinical trials, ticagrelor and prasugrel have shown increased efficacy compared to clopidogrel for higher risk acute coronary syndromes, at the expense of higher bleeding rates. For patients without loss of function mutations in CYP2C19, however, clopidogrel remains efficacious, with lower rates of bleeding. Furthermore, therapeutic strategies based on genetic testing have shown promise in treatment of acute ST elevation myocardial infarction undergoing percutaneous coronary intervention and stenting.

Claassens D, Vos G, Bergmeijer T, Hermanides R, van 't Hof A, van der Harst P et al. A Genotype-Guided Strategy for Oral P2Y12 Inhibitors in Primary PCI. New England Journal of Medicine. 2019;381(17):1621–1631.
https://www.nejm.org/doi/full/10.1056/NEJMoa1907096

9. Answer: A

This patient's clinical presentation is typical of Alzheimer's disease (AD), which is the most common cause of dementia worldwide, with the prevalence continuing to grow because of the ageing population. AD is a neurodegenerative disease process is characterised classically by two hallmark pathologies: β-amyloid plaque deposition and neurofibrillary tangles of hyperphosphorylated tau. The diagnosis is clinical.

There are two classes of pharmacologic therapy available for patients with AD. The cholinesterase inhibitors such as donepezil, rivastigmine, and galantamine are recommended therapy for patients with mild and moderate AD dementia, as well as Parkinson's disease dementia. These drugs target the neurotransmitter, acetylcholine. Memantine, which has activity as both a non-competitive N-methyl-D-aspartate receptor antagonist and a dopamine agonist, is approved for use in patients with severe AD.

Melatonin is a hormone that regulates the sleep–wake cycle. It is primarily released by the pineal gland. It is used for the short-term treatment of insomnia and there is evidence that it is helpful in the treatment of AD.

Scheltens P, Blennow K, Breteler M, de Strooper B, Frisoni G, Salloway S et al. Alzheimer's disease. The Lancet. 2016;388(10043):505–517.
https://pubmed.ncbi.nlm.nih.gov/26921134/

10. Answer: A

A crossover clinical study or trial is a longitudinal study in which participants receive a sequence of different treatments (or exposures). While crossover studies can be observational studies, many important crossover studies are controlled experiments. Randomised, controlled, crossover experiments are especially important in obtaining high quality evidence for the effects of interventions. In a randomised clinical trial or study, the participants are randomly assigned to different arms of the study and receive different treatments. When the randomised clinical trial has a repeated measures design, the same measures are collected multiple times for each participant. A crossover clinical trial has a repeated measures design in which each participant is randomly assigned to a sequence of treatments, including at least two treatments (of which one 'treatment' may be a standard treatment or a placebo).

A crossover study has two advantages over a non-crossover longitudinal study. First, the influence of confounding covariates is reduced because each crossover participant serves as their own control. In a non-crossover study, even when randomised, different treatment groups may be unbalanced in some covariates. In a controlled, randomised crossover design, such imbalances are unlikely (unless covariates were to change systematically during the study). Second, optimal crossover designs are statistically efficient and so require fewer participants than do non-crossover designs. Other types of study are listed below:

- Single blind clinical study: the participant, but not the observer, does not know which of the possible treatments he is receiving.
- Double blind clinical study: neither the participant nor the observer knows which treatment is being given to the participant.
- Triple-blind clinical study: the participant, the observer-researcher and the researcher who analyses the data do not know which treatment is being received.
- Open clinical study is a clinical study without a control group, as opposed to a controlled clinical study.
- Explanatory clinical study is to acquire scientific knowledge and biological explanations about efficacy. It is usually done in the earliest phases of the development of a drug, with restricted inclusion criteria, in order to obtain a homogenous sample of participants, representative only of specific sub-groups of population, of a limited size.
- Parallel clinical study: in this type of study, each group of participants receives a single treatment simultaneously.
- Sequential clinical study: the observations are assessed as they are produced, and the total number of participants is not predetermined but depends on the accumulated results.

 CLINICAL TRIAL: A REVIEW [Internet]. Globalresearchonline.net. 2020 [cited 10 July 2020]. Available from: http://globalresearchonline.net/volume1issue2/Article%20019.pdf

11. Answer: A

The CYP3A4 enzyme is particularly susceptible to enzyme inducers (Table 18.2) and marked reductions in the plasma concentrations of CYP3A4 substrates may occur. Hydrocortisone is metabolised via CYP3A4. Commencing a strong inducer such as carbamazepine could precipitate Addison crisis. Ketoconazole as an inhibitor of CYP3A4 (Table 18.3) will increase the cortisol concentration, not decrease it.

Starting thyroxine in a patient with Addison disease having already received hydrocortisone should not precipitate a crisis, however, it may induce Addisonian crisis if not adequately replaced with hydrocortisone. Spironolactone is likely to block the effects of fludrocortisone but not the hydrocortisone and is less likely to cause a crisis.

Table 18.2 Common CYP3A4 Inducers

Carbamazepine	Phenytoin
Dexamethasone	Rifabutin
Griseofulvin	Rifampin
Nevirapine	St. John's wort

Table 18.3 Common CYP3A4 Inhibitors

Amiodarone	Imatinib
Amprenavir	Indinavir
Aprepitant	Isoniazid
Atazanavir	Itraconazole
Chloramphenicol	Ketoconazole
Clarithromycin	Lapatinib
Conivaptan	Miconazole
Cyclosporine	Nefazodone
Darunavir	Nelfinavir
Dasatinib	Posaconazole
Delavirdine	Ritonavir
Diltiazem	Quinupristin
Erythromycin	Saquinavir
Fluconazole	Tamoxifen
Fluoxetine	Telithromycin
Fluvoxamine	Troleandomycin
Fosamprenavir	Verapamil
Grapefruit juice	Voriconazole

 Drug Metabolism – The Importance of Cytochrome P450 3A4 [Internet]. Medsafe.govt.nz. 2019 [cited 22 August 2019]. Available from: https://www.medsafe.govt.nz/profs/puarticles/march2014drugmetabolismcytochromep4503a4.htm

12. Answer: D

The mechanism of action of many drugs in clinical practice involve enzyme inhibition. Inhibition of enzymes may be either reversible or irreversible depending on the specific effect of the inhibitor being used. The irreversible inhibitor destroys a functional group on the enzyme necessary for catalytic activity. Reversible enzyme inhibitors can be further classified as competitive, non-competitive, and uncompetitive. The difference between competitive and non-competitive inhibition is summarised below:

Competitive Inhibition	Non-competitive Inhibition
The molecule (inhibitor), other than the substrate, binds to the enzyme's active site.	The molecule (inhibitor) binds to a site other than the active site (an allosteric site).
The molecule (inhibitor) is structurally and chemically similar to the substrate.	The binding of the inhibitor to the allosteric site causes a conformational change to the enzyme's active site.
The molecule (inhibitor) blocks the active site and thus prevents substrate binding.	As a result of this change, the active site and substrate no longer share specificity, meaning the substrate cannot bind.
The molecule (inhibitor)'s effects can be reduced by increasing substrate concentration.	As the inhibitor is not in direct competition with the substrate, increasing substrate levels cannot mitigate the inhibitor's effect.
Km increases in the presence of inhibitor.	Km is unchanged in the presence of inhibitor.
Vmax is unchanged.	Vmax is decreased.

The following table summarises the common drugs that exert their effects by competitive enzyme inhibition. Amlodipine is a calcium channel blocker not an enzyme inhibitor.

Drugs	Enzyme inhibited
6-mercaptopurine	Adenylosuccinate synthetase
5-fluorouracil	Thymidylate synthetase
Acyclovir	DNA polymerase
Allopurinol	Xanthine oxidase
Alpha methyldopa	Dopa decarboxylase
Celecoxib	Cyclo-oxygenase-2
Methotrexate	Dihydrofolate reductase
Perindopril	Angiotensin converting enzyme
Rosuvastatin	HMG CoA reductase

Singh V, Sharma P, Alam M. Metabolism of Drugs with Inhibition of Enzymes. Journal of Drug Metabolism & Toxicology. 2018;09(01).
https://www.semanticscholar.org/paper/Metabolism-of-Drugs-with-Inhibition-of-Enzymes-Singh-Sharma/6f90c47e8731ac41 2deeee804aab6a07d958e989

13. Answer: B

Cockcroft-Gault formula is the only formula validated for drug dosing. The Modification of Diet in Renal Disease (MDRD) and Chronic Kidney Disease-Epidemiology Collaboration (CKD-EPI) formula are both used to screen and monitor patients with CKD but have never been validated for drug dosing. 99ᵐTc-DTPA radionuclide scan can obtain an accurate GFR but is invasive, expensive, and unnecessary. Furthermore, GFR determined by plasma clearance of 99ᵐTc-DTPA is inaccurate in patients with severe renal insufficiency (GFR<20ml/min).

Hudson J, Nolin T. Pragmatic Use of Kidney Function Estimates for Drug Dosing: The Tide Is Turning. Advances in Chronic Kidney Disease. 2018;25(1):14–20.–
https://www.ackdjournal.org/article/S1548-5595(17)30180-5/fulltext

14. Answer: B

This patient has classic features of ethylene glycol poisoning including high anion gap severe metabolic acidosis, typical oxalate crystals in the urine and renal impairment likely due to tubular blockage by the oxalate crystals. Ethylene glycol poisoning should be suspected in an intoxicated patient with the above clinical features. Early diagnosis and treatment will limit metabolic toxicity and decrease morbidity and mortality (between 2 to 22%).

Anion gap = $(Na^+ + K^+) - (HCO_3^- + CL^-)$. The reference range for the anion gap is 16 ± 4 mmol/L. The common causes of high anion gap metabolic acidosis are 'GOLD MARK'

- Glycols (ethylene glycol, propylene glycol)
- Oxoproline (pyroglutamic acid, the toxic metabolite of excessive acetaminophen or paracetamol)

- L-Lactate (standard lactic acid seen in lactic acidosis)
- D-Lactate (exogenous lactic acid produced by gut bacteria)
- Methanol (this is inclusive of alcohols in general)
- Aspirin (salicylic acid)
- Renal Failure (uremic acidosis)
- Ketones (diabetic, alcoholic and starvation ketosis).

Methanol and ethylene glycol are widely available in household and commercial products (automotive anti-freeze and de-icing solutions, solvents, cleaners, windshield wiper fluid, fuels, and other industrial products). Ethylene glycol is oxidised by alcohol dehydrogenase and then further metabolised to oxalic acid and other products. Oxalate crystals are eliminated in the urine.

Delays in treating toxic alcohol poisonings lead to worse outcomes. Therefore, therapy should commence as soon as there is a strong suspicion of toxic alcohol poisoning or when metabolic acidosis of unknown cause is present. There are three main treatments:

- Gastric lavage, induced emesis, or use of activated charcoal to remove alcohol from gastrointestinal tract needs to be initiated within 30 to 60 min after ingestion because gastrointestinal absorption of methanol or ethylene glycol is rapid.
- Administration of intravenous ethanol to keep serum ethanol concentration of >100 mg/dL (22 mmol/L) to provides competitive inhibition of the enzyme. This will delay or prevent generation of toxic metabolites. Fomepizole needs to be initiated while sufficient alcohol remains unmetabolised. Measurement of blood alcohol concentrations and/or serum osmolality can be helpful.
- Fomepizole is a strong inhibitor of alcohol dehydrogenase. It has an affinity for alcohol dehydrogenase 8000 times that of ethanol. Fomepizole is effective at low concentrations, has minimal side effects, and does not require monitoring in an ICU.
- Haemodialysis is helpful in removing unmetabolised alcohol and possibly toxic metabolites and delivering base to patient to ameliorate metabolic acidosis.

Kraut J, Mullins M. Toxic Alcohols. New England Journal of Medicine. 2018;378(3): 270–280.
https://www.nejm.org/doi/10.1056/NEJMra1615295

15. Answer: D

Medications taken orally must go through the intestine and liver to reach general circulation. First-pass metabolism may occur in the liver or in the intestine dependinging on enzyme activity, plasma protein and blood cell binding, and gastrointestinal motility, etc.

Portal hypertension can shunt portal venous blood into systemic circulation resulting in decreased first-pass metabolism and increases bioavailability of drugs in systemic circulation.

Administration of medications via an alternate route such as intravenous, intramuscular, sublingual, or transdermal avoids first-pass metabolism to optimise drug efficacy in systemic circulation. Drugs with high first-pass metabolism, such as morphine, diazepam, midazolam, ethanol, and glyceryl trinitrate (GTN), typically require a considerably higher oral dose than parenteral dose.

Extraction ratio (ER) is the fraction of drug that is removed from the blood or plasma as it crosses the eliminating organ such as liver or kidneys. Medications with higher ER have reduced bioavailability in general circulation.

Enzyme inducers increase the metabolic activities of enzymes and are associated with higher medication clearance and reduced drug bioavailability in general circulation.

Pond S, Tozer T. First-Pass Elimination. Clinical Pharmacokinetics. 1984;9(1):1–25.
https://link.springer.com/article/10.2165/00003088-198409010-00001–

16. Answer: A

This patient has a high pre-test probability for heparin-induced thrombocytopaenia (HIT), which is an immune-mediated prothrombotic state that occurs more commonly with unfractionated heparin than with low-molecular weight heparins. Guidelines recommend using the 4T score for grading pre-test probability and no laboratory testing if pre-test probability is low, as false positive results are common. If the 4T score indicates intermediate or high pre-test probability, cessation of heparin and substitution with a non-heparinoid anticoagulant is warranted. In this case of HIT with thrombosis, treatment for HIT is indicated whilst waiting laboratory testing. Treatment with heparin or low-molecular weight heparin in this instance risks worsening the prothrombotic state. Guidelines recommend cessation of the heparin whilst awaiting confirmatory testing and commencement of a non-heparinoid anticoagulation such as with bivalirudin (a direct thrombin inhibitor), fondaparinux (a synthetic mimic of one of the binding sites of heparin) or a direct oral anticoagulant such as rivaroxaban. Routine insertion of inferior vena cava filter is not recommended as the primary state is prothrombotic. Vitamin K antagonists are also not recommended as they can also worsen thrombosis in this setting. Platelet infusions are not recommended unless the patient is at high risk of bleeding or is actively bleeding.

 Cuker A, Arepally G, Chong B, Cines D, Greinacher A, Gruel Y et al. American Society of Hematology 2018 guidelines for management of venous thromboembolism: heparin-induced thrombocytopenia. Blood Advances. 2018;2(22):3360–3392. https://pubmed.ncbi.nlm.nih.gov/30482768/–

17. Answer: D

Similar to thiazide diuretics, indapamide inhibits the apical distal convoluted tubule epithelium sodium-chloride cotransporter where up to 10% of the filtered load of sodium is reabsorbed. In addition to its diuretic effects, total peripheral resistance is significantly decreased and it may also exert its antihypertensive effect by reducing vascular reactivity to various pressor stimuli by inhibiting the net inward flow of calcium and resultant phasic contractions in vascular smooth muscle. Its potency is 5 mmHg systolic greater than that of thiazide diuretics. It is a useful adjunctive antihypertensive medication in younger patients. Indapamide can cause hyponatraemia, confusion, and fall in elderly, especially in underweight elderly women. Furthermore, indapamide is superior in improving microalbuminuria in diabetics, reducing left ventricular mass index, inhibiting platelet aggregation, and reducing oxidative stress relative to thiazide diuretics. Indapamide has comparatively high lipid solubility; it is also bound to blood proteins and little is eliminated in the urine.

 Roush G, Sica D. Diuretics for Hypertension: A Review and Update. American Journal of Hypertension. 2016; 29(10):1130–1137. https://pubmed.ncbi.nlm.nih.gov/27048970/

18. Answer: C

Patients can rapidly develop tolerance to nitrates. Acute high-dose intravenous nitrates can cause loss of potency due to tachyphylaxis. Development of nitrate tolerance and clinical rebound should be considered with long-term nitrate use. Nitrate tolerance may develop within 1 to 2 days, resulting in decreased angina control. It is induced by nitrate regimens that produce continuous therapeutic levels. A nitrate free period may reduce development of nitrate tolerance. Unfortunately, breakthrough angina, or clinical rebound, can occur during the nitrate-free intervals used in some dosing strategies.

Isosorbide is a nitrate vasodilator available in various oral forms. Isosorbide dinitrate (ISDN) is an intermediate-acting nitrate approved for prevention of angina pectoris. It is also used in conjunction with hydralazine in treating CCF. Isosorbide mononitrate (ISMN) is the active metabolite of ISDN and is primarily used in the management of chronic stable angina. It is not FDA-approved for treating heart failure. It has higher bioavailability and a longer half-life (4–6 hours) than ISDN. The immediate-release form is typically given in two doses daily 7 hours apart to minimise tolerance, whereas the sustained-release form (Imdur®) can be given once daily.

Nitrate tolerance is a complex phenomenon, which involves neurohormonal counter-regulation, collectively classified as pseudotolerance, as well as intrinsic vascular processes, defined as vascular tolerance. Glyceryl trinitrate (GTN)-induced desensitisation of vasodilator responses to nitric oxide (NO) donors and endothelium-derived NO is termed cross-tolerance. A typical phenomenon associated with vascular tolerance is the worsening of anginal symptoms compared with pre-treatment state after cessation of nitrate therapy, which is known as the withdrawal or rebound effect.

 Münzel T, Daiber A, Mülsch A. Explaining the Phenomenon of Nitrate Tolerance. Circulation Research. 2005;97(7):618–628. https://www.ahajournals.org/doi/10.1161/01.RES.0000184694.03262.6d

19. Answer: C

Linezolid is used to treat patients with vancomycin-resistant *E. faecalis* infection. Other pathogens that linezolid has demonstrated activity against include penicillin-resistant *S. pneumoniae,* vancomycin-sensitive *E. faecalis*, methicillin-susceptible *S. epidermidis* and methicillin-resistant *S. epidermidis*, methicillin-susceptible *S. aureus* (MSSA), MRSA, *Corynebacterium sp*, *Moraxella catarrhalis*, legionella species, *Listeria monocytogenes*, *Pasteurella multocida*, and *Bacteroides fragilis*.

However, linezolid may increase serotonin as a result of monoamine oxidase-A (MAO-A) inhibition; thus, its use is contraindicated in patients taking fluoxetine. If linezolid must be administered, discontinue fluoxetine or any serotonergic drug immediately and monitor for CNS toxicity. Serotonergic therapy may be resumed 24 hours after the last linezolid dose.

Hashemian S, Farhadi T, Ganjparvar M. Linezolid: a review of its properties, function, and use in critical care. Drug Design, Development and Therapy. 2018; Volume 12:1759–1767.
https://www.dovepress.com/linezolid-a-review-of-its-properties-function-and-use-in-critical-care-peer-reviewed-article-DDDT

20. Answer: D

Medication bioavailability is the fraction of the administered dose intravascularly or extra-vascularly that reaches the systemic circulation. Bioavailability of an oral drug is affected by absorption and the first-pass metabolism of the medications by a few potential sites such as the liver, gastrointestinal tract, vascular endothelium, and lungs. The most reliable measure of a drug's bio-availability is area under the plasma concentration-time curve (AUC). AUC is directly proportional to the total amount of unchanged drug that reaches systemic circulation.

 Price G, Patel D. Drug Bioavailability [Internet]. Ncbi.nlm.nih.gov. 2020 [cited 4 July 2020]. Available from: https://www.ncbi.nlm.nih.gov/books/NBK557852/

21. Answer: C

Oxybutynin was used in this patient to treat urge incontinence. Oxybutynin inhibits the muscarinic actions of acetylcholine and has antispasmodic effects on smooth muscle and is indicated for detrusor over activity. It has strong anticholinergic effect and can cause the following side effects, including confusion, hallucination, delirium, dry mouth, pupil dilatation, blurred vision, urinary retention, constipation, tachycardia, and arrhythmias.

Older patients are in general on more medications than younger patients due to comorbidities. A higher total number of medications is associated with increasing risks of drug-drug interactions, financial burden, medication non-adherence, adverse drug reactions, and worse outcomes. Doctors should avoid the following medications in older nursing home patients:

- First-generation antihistamines, antispasmodics, antidepressants (highly anticholinergic).
- Antiparkinsonian agents such as benztropine (not recommended for prevention of extrapyramidal symptoms with antipsychotics).
- Conventional or atypical antipsychotics (increased risk of stroke and death in patients with dementia).
- Skeletal muscle relaxants (most muscle relaxants are poorly tolerated by older adults).
- Benzodiazepine (increased risk of cognitive impairment, delirium, falls, fractures, and motor vehicle crashes in older adults).
- Nonbenzodiazepine and benzodiazepine hypnotics (adverse events similar to those of benzodiazepines in older adults).
- Proton pump inhibitors (risk of *Clostridium difficile* infection, bone loss, and fractures).
- Tricyclic antidepressants in patients with dementia, narrow-angle glaucoma, cardiac conduction abnormality, prostatism, or history of urinary retention.
- Antimuscarinic drugs in patients with overactive bladder with concurrent dementia or chronic cognitive impairment.

 Kim L, Koncilja K, Nielsen C. Medication management in older adults. Cleveland Clinic Journal of Medicine. 2018;85(2):129–135.
https://pubmed.ncbi.nlm.nih.gov/29425085/

22. Answer: A

Opioid use disorder is vastly underdiagnosed and undertreated, defined as a hazardous pattern of opioid use over a 12-month period, or a 11-month period if usage is near to continuous. The maladaptive dependence on opioid medication has multiple pathways, for example recreational drug use, chronic pain, and self-medication for psychiatric issues. Whilst individualised care is appropriate and will lead to the best possible outcomes, the best over-arching model to view the problem for an individual is through the lens of chronic illness. By focussing on minimising the functional impact of the disorder for the individual over time, concepts such as remission, adaptation, and harm-minimisation become key concepts.

Medical management of opioid use disorder consequently becomes about minimising harm and maximising function. Withdrawal should be managed by decreasing opioid doses, often with buprenorphine. Symptomatic control in this time should be maximised to ensure long-term adherence. Loperamide for diarrhoea; clonidine for tachycardia, anxiety, sweating, and ondansetron for nausea are all commonly needed. For long term maintenance of opioid dependence opioid substitution with methadone or buprenorphine have long-established efficacy, naltrexone is gaining in its therapeutic scope, and other slow release opioids can be used if first line treatments are ineffective. Maintenance medications for opioid use disorder are associated with significant decrease in overdoses, overdose deaths, criminal behaviour, and infection. Naltrexone maintenance can be given via daily oral dosing or monthly depot injection; but supervised withdrawal needs to take place before initiation. Reducing barriers to naloxone injection becomes an important part of reducing harm from opioid overdose.

Blanco C, Volkow N. Management of opioid use disorder in the USA: present status and future directions. The Lancet. 2019;393(10182):1760–1772.
https://pubmed.ncbi.nlm.nih.gov/30878228/

23. Answer: B

P-glycoproteins (P-gp) are efflux transporters present at many sites within the body, gut, liver, kidneys, brain, and placenta in particular. They have a role in protecting eukaryotic cells from harmful substances and can serve to eliminate a substance from the body as well as from protected sites such as the CNS. There are a large number of medications that are substrates, inhibitors, and inducers of P-gp, but reports of clinically evident interactions are mostly found for drugs that have a narrow therapeutic window and heavy reliance on P-gp in their distribution. P-gp inhibitors are thus most likely to result in toxicity for medications like digoxin, cyclosporine, dabigatran, and loperamide. Some of the most potent P-gp inhibitors are azole anti-fungals, fexofenadine, and quinidine, whereas multiple cardiac drugs such as amiodarone, calcium channel blockers, and beta-blockers are moderate inhibitors, and polypharmacy plays a large role in adverse events. Rifampicin is a strong inducer of P-gp.

Lund M, Petersen TS, Dalhoff KP. Clinical implications of P-glycoprotein modulation in drug-drug interactions. *Drugs.* 2017; 77:859–883
https://www.ncbi.nlm.nih.gov/pubmed/28382570

24. Answer: B

Individual response variation to drugs may be pharmacodynamic (different response of receptors despite same concentrations of the drug at the receptor site) or pharmacokinetic (different response due to different concentrations of the drug throughout the body). Pharmacokinetics refers to how the body processes an unchanged drug and is often described in terms of absorption, distribution, metabolism, and excretion.

Absorption is the process of a drug moving from its site of delivery into blood. Drug absorption is determined by the drug's physicochemical properties, formulation, and route of administration. Drug bioavailability is the proportion of the administered dose which reaches systemic circulation. This is influenced by the proportion of the drug absorbed from the gastrointestinal tract, and furthermore the proportion of the first dose of the drug which is extracted by the liver.

Distribution is quantified in terms of the volume of distribution: the theoretical volume of fluid required to contain and uniformly distribute the drug in the body, at the same concentration as it would be in the blood. Ageing affects an individual's pharmacokinetics as it is associated with decreased muscle mass and total body water, and increased body fat. Decreased muscle mass and total body water results in smaller volumes of distribution for hydrophilic drugs in the elderly and thus decreased half-life. Meanwhile increased body fat results in larger volumes of distributions for lipophilic drugs and thus increased half-life.

Metabolism is the chemical modification of the drug, which occurs predominantly in the liver, and is mainly dependent on liver blood flow and function. Ageing is associated with a decrease in liver blood flow, which can decrease total and free drug clearance, even in the absence of liver disease.

Excretion is the clearance of the drug from the body, which occurs predominantly in the kidneys and is thus largely dependent on renal function. The kidneys are generally considered the organs most affected by ageing, where each decade of life is associated with a 10% decrease in renal parenchyma, as well as decreases in renal plasma flow, decreased tubular function secondary to oxidative stress, and tubular atrophy secondary to telomere shortening, and decreased expression of the klotho anti-ageing gene.

Pharmacodynamics describes the relationship between the drug concentration at the site of action, and the resultant effect of the drug. Drug–drug interactions and enzyme activity commonly affect the pharmacodynamics of a drug. Comparative to pharmacokinetics, older age affects pharmacodynamic relationships to a lesser extent, including increased sensitivity to CNS drugs, i.e. benzodiazepines (necessitating drug dose decreases), and decreased sensitivity to furosemide (necessitating drug dose increases).

van den Berg J, Vereecke H, Proost J, et al. Pharmacokinetic and pharmacodynamic interactions in anaesthesia. A review of current knowledge and how it can be used to optimize anaesthetic drug administration. British Journal of Anaesthesia. 2017;118(1):44–57.
https://bjanaesthesia.org/article/S0007-0912(17)30114-9/fulltext

25. Answer: B

The genes that encode drug metabolising enzymes (DMEs) are subject to wide inter-individual variation due to copy number variations, insertions, deletions, and single-nucleotide polymorphisms. This variance accounts for the wide range of metabolism seen between individuals for particular drugs. Prodrugs that require metabolism to become active compounds will theoretically be less efficacious in individuals with low activity of the required enzyme. Individuals with lower metabolism of drugs that require metabolism to be inactivated will theoretically require lower doses and potentially encounter more toxicity than those with higher levels of DME activity, who may require higher doses to achieve the same effect.

Genetic variance coding for CYP450 enzymes is clinically relevant for a number of medications. CYP2C9 has an impact on warfarin metabolism, but not as much impact on INR as genetic variance in the target enzyme (Vitamin K epoxide reductase complex subunit 1). CYP2C19 variations have potential to impact of clopidogrel, many antidepressants and possibly tamoxifen. Tacrolimus and cyclosporine metabolism are influenced by variations in CYP3A4 and 5. CYP2D6 converts codeine, tamoxifen, and tramadol into active compounds, and significant reduction in efficacy can be observed in poor metabolisers. Significant CNS toxicity can be observed in ultra-rapid metabolisers of codeine and tramadol.

 Sim S, Kacevska M, Ingelman-Sundberg M. Pharmacogenomics of drug-metabolizing enzymes: a recent update on clinical implications and endogenous effects. The Pharmacogenomics Journal. 2012;13(1):1–11.
https://www.ncbi.nlm.nih.gov/pubmed/23089672

26. Answer: B

Overweight is defined as a BMI of 25 to 29.9 kg/m² and obesity as a BMI >30 kg/m². Appropriate drug dosing in the obese patient is challenging. Obesity causes physiologic alterations which can affect drug pharmacokinetics. In the obese patient, body composition is characteriseds by a relatively higher percentage of fat and lower percentage of water and lean tissue mass than the non-obese. In spite of increased cardiac output and total blood volume, the blood flow per gram of fat is less than in the non-obese patient. Histological hepatic changes and an increased glomerular filtration rate have also been reported in obese individuals.

There is no general change in drug absorption in obese patients. Usually, lipid soluble drugs have an increased volume of distribution in obese patients. An increased volume of distribution can also result in an increased half-life.

Albumin and total protein concentrations are usually unchanged. Alpha 1-acid glycoprotein (AAG) concentrations may be increased, but changes in acidic drug binding are not clinically significant. Phase I metabolism – oxidation, reduction, or hydrolysis is increased or unchanged in obesity. Phase II metabolism – glucuronidation and sulfonation can be enhanced and cause an increased clearance of drug. Conjugation of drugs can be increased or unchanged. Drugs eliminated primarily through glomerular filtration such as cephazolin will tend to have increased renal clearance.

 Barras M, Legg A. Drug dosing in obese adults. Australian Prescriber. 2017;40(5):189–193.
https://www.ncbi.nlm.nih.gov/pmc/articles/PMC5662437/

27. Answer: D

Management of pain is a complex and multi-modal therapeutic enterprise. Traditional opioids have strong pain-relieving qualities through agonism of the μ-opioid receptor (MOR). Unwanted effects of drowsiness, respiratory depression, constipation, nausea, tolerance, and hyperalgesia limit the use of opioid medications in the long term. Improving therapeutic targets for analgesic medications have in recent times focussed on mechanisms surrounding the transmission of painful stimuli, with indirect effects on pain. For example, descending inhibitory control of pain is commonly modulated by noradrenaline and serotonin, whereas descending stimulation of pain sensation is modulated by separate excitatory neurotransmitters such as glutamate, through activation of N-methyl-d-aspartic acid (NMDA) receptor. Many other neuronal targets have been implicated in this system, such as α_2-adrenoreceptors, voltage-gated sodium ion channels, transient receptor potential V1 (TRPV1), neurokinin 1, calcitonin gene-related peptide (CGRP), and the opioid-like receptor nociception/orphanin FQ peptide (NOP). Other non-neuronal targets in pain transmission include cytokines, prostaglandins, nuclear factor-κB, and activated glial cells.

Theoretically, affecting these non-opioid targets should have therapeutic potential in decreasing toxicity, dependence, and hyperalgesia. Tramadol is an MOR agonist, which has multiple actions on the regulation of painful stimuli, including through serotonin and noradrenaline reuptake inhibition. Serotonin syndrome is often seen in tramadol overdose and serotonin effects limit upward dose-titration of the drug. Tramadol may also have action at voltage-gated sodium channels, NMDA receptors, cytokines, α_2-adrenoreceptors, and activated glial cells. Tapentadol acts as a MOR agonist and noradrenaline reuptake inhibitor.

Cebranopadol is a MOR agonist and NOP antagonist. Multiple CGRP antagonising therapies are being developed for treatment of migraine. Capsaicin has analgesic properties through agonising TRPV1. Local anaesthetics have analgesic properties through prolonging inactivation of voltage-gated sodium channels. These advances in the understanding of analgesia and pain perception have provided significant options in treating pain, but multimodal therapies involving functional goals, multidisciplinary care and harm minimisation remain key strategies in treating pain.

Barakat A. Revisiting tramadol: a multi-modal agent for pain management. CNS drugs. 2019; 33:481–501. https://link.springer.com/article/10.1007/s40263-019-00623-5–

28. Answer: D

Falls occur frequently in elderly. Approximately 30% to 40% of people aged 65 years and older who live in the community experience falls. About half of all falls result in an injury, of which 10% are serious and injury rates increase with age. Falls are a major threat to older adults' quality of life, often causing a decline in self-care ability and participation in physical and social activities. Fear of falling, which develops in 20% to 39% of people who fall, can lead to further limitation of activity, independent of injury.

Key assessment post-fall is to identify and treat the underlying causes or risk factors of falls. This is critical to prevent future falls. Many falls result from interactions of multiple risk factors, and the risk of falling increases linearly with the number of risk factors (see Table 18.4). Therefore, it is a multifactorial falls risk assessment with multifactorial intervention.

Table 18.4   Risk factors for falls.

Patient factors	Environmental factors
Ageing related physiological changes	Medications especially polypharmacy
Cognitive impairment	Alcohol and drugs
Urine and faecal incontinence	Assistive mobility devices
Visual impairment	Footwear
Gait, strength, or balance deficits	Home environment hazards
Mental health issues	
Acute illness such as sepsis	
Chronic disease such as diabetes, hypertension	

A critical part of risk assessment is a medication review. Several classes of medications such as psychoactive medications, benzodiazepines, antihypertensives, NSAIDs, and diuretics increase fall risk. Ageing population and prolonged survival of patients with multimorbidity is an important public health challenge in developed countries. The rising prevalence of multimorbidity leads to the application of multiple disease-specific guidelines and targeting disease-specific goals. This consequently results in high treatment burden and polypharmacy which is defined as the chronic co-prescription of multiple drugs (usually >5). Polypharmacy has been associated with an increased risk of hospitalisation, functional decline, cognitive impairment, non-adherence, adverse drug reactions, and drug–drug interactions. One study had demonstrated the population using five or more drugs was significantly associated with 21% increased rate of falls over a 2-year period.

This patient has polypharmacy. Given his excellent control of hypertension and BGL there is room to reduce his antihypertensive medications. His oral hyperglycaemic may be reduced to avoid hypoglycaemic episodes in the future. ACCORD trial had demonstrated no evidence that targeting a normal systolic BP compared with targeting a systolic BP of less than 140 mmHg lowers the overall risk of major cardiovascular events in high risk adults with type 2 diabetes. Furthermore, it showed a higher risk of serious adverse events with more intensive BP control. Other studies indicated that a comprehensive, customised, therapeutic strategy targeting glycated haemoglobin levels below 6.0% increased the rate of death from any cause after a mean of 3.5 years, as compared with a strategy targeting levels of 7.0 to 7.9% in patients with a median glycated haemoglobin level of 8.1% and either previous cardiovascular events or multiple cardiovascular risk factors. This patient has no fracture therefore he should not be started on bisphosphonate. His anaemia is mild so will have had no contribution to fall and is not severe enough to qualify for erythropoietin supplement according to PBS criteria.

Overview | Falls in older people: assessing risk and prevention | Guidance | NICE [Internet]. Nice.org.uk. 2020 [cited 10 July 2020]. Available from: https://www.nice.org.uk/guidance/cg161

29. Answer: B

Pramipexole is a non-ergot derived D2 and D3 selective dopamine agonist. Consequently, centrally active dopamine antagonists (i.e. antipsychotics or metoclopramide) diminish the effect of pramipexole and should not be used with pramipexole.

Pramipexole is approved for Parkinson's disease and primary severe restless leg syndrome. Pramipexole is only indicated for restless leg syndrome if International Restless Legs Syndrome Rating Scale of greater or equal to 21 points and all four diagnostic criteria are met:

- urge to move the legs that is
- worse during rest or inactivity
- relieved by movement
- worse in the evenings.

Secondary causes for restless leg syndrome must also be excluded, including iron deficiency, pregnancy, or CKD and differential diagnoses such as muscle cramps, arthritis, neuropathy, or drug-induced akathisia must be excluded before treatment with pramipexole.

Pramipexole is renally cleared, so some other renally cleared drugs can reduce the clearance of either or both drugs. These drugs include drugs which:

- Inhibit the active renal tubular secretion of anionic and cationic drugs, i.e. probenecid
- Are cleared by active renal tubular secretion (competitive inhibitors), i.e. digoxin, diltiazem, ranitidine, trimethoprim, and verapamil

Consider dose reductions when co-administering these drugs with pramipexole, and observe for signs of dopamine overstimulation, such as dyskinesias, agitation, or hallucinations. Pramipexole can be stopped without tapering.

Garcia-Borreguero D, Patrick J, DuBrava S, Becker P, Lankford A, Chen C et al. Pregabalin Versus Pramipexole: Effects on Sleep Disturbance in Restless Legs Syndrome. Sleep. 2014;37(4):635–643.
https://www.ncbi.nlm.nih.gov/pmc/articles/PMC4044751/

30. Answer: C

Prodrugs are molecules with little or no intended pharmacological activity. Prodrugs must be converted to the pharmacologically active agent in vivo; by enzymatic or chemical reactions or by a combination of the two. Paracetamol is not a prodrug as it is converted to toxic metabolites. Prodrugs can exist naturally such as many phytochemicals/botanical constituents and endogenous substances, or they can result from synthetic or semisynthetic processes – produced intentionally as part of a rational drug design or unintentionally during drug development. The design and development of prodrugs is the most common and effective strategy to overcome pharmacokinetic and pharmacodynamic drawbacks of active drugs.

The benefits of prodrugs include:

- Achieve optimal solubility.
- Improve the selective targeting of drugs to specific organ sites, tissues, and enzymes.
- Offer protection from rapid metabolism and elimination.
- Reduce the toxic effects of an active drug on other parts of the body.
- Enhance patient compliance as it can reduce the unpleasant taste or odour of the active drug.

The following is the list of example prodrug and active metabolite which are commonly used in clinical practice:

Prodrug	Active metabolite (active parent drug)
Allopurinol	Oxypurinol
Azathioprine	Mercaptopurine
Cortisone	Hydrocortisone
Diazepam	Oxazepam
Enalapril	Enalaprilat
Famciclovir	Penciclovir
Levodopa	Dopamine
Omeprazole	Omeprazole sulphonamide
Prednisone	Prednisolone
Ramipril	Ramiprilat
Simvastatin	Beta hydroxyl acid derivative
Sulfasalazine	5-Amino salicylic acid
Valganciclovir	Ganciclovir

Najjar A, Najjar A, Karaman R. Newly Developed Prodrugs and Prodrugs in Development; an Insight of the Recent Years. Molecules. 2020;25(4): 884.
https://pubmed.ncbi.nlm.nih.gov/32079289/

31. Answer: B

All antipsychotics have some degree of antagonism of dopaminergic transmission via D2 receptors. First-generation antipsychotics such as haloperidol produce antipsychotic effects at 60% to 80% D2 occupancy. Second-generation antipsychotics (SGA) like risperidone exhibit their therapeutic effects partially through D2 blockade specifically in the mesolimbic pathway, but more from the blockade of serotonin receptors like 5HT2A. SGAs have weak binding to D2 receptors and can quickly dissociate from the receptor, potentially accounting for the lower likelihood of causing extrapyramidal symptoms. Moreover, SGAs have agonism at the 5HT1A receptor. The ability of antipsychotics to block D2 receptors in the prefrontal cortex and nucleus accumbens is important in improving certain psychiatric symptoms. Risperidone does not cause anticholinergic effects, which makes it a preferred agent for the elderly with dementia.

 Goodman L, Brunton L, Chabner B, Knollmann B. Goodman & Gilman's the pharmacological basis of therapeutics. New York: McGraw-Hill; 2011.
https://www.amazon.com.au/Goodman-Gilmans-Pharmacological-Therapeutics-Twelfth-ebook/dp/B004HHP8SG

32. Answer: A

Statins are commonly prescribed cholesterol-lowering drugs which inhibit the rate-limiting step in cholesterol biosynthesis by competitively inhibiting HMG-CoA reductase. Statins are known to have a high risk for interactions with other drugs. The drugs most likely to interact with statins include macrolides, especially erythromycin and clarithromycin. Other drugs to watch for include fibrates (especially gemfibrozil), protease inhibitors, amiodarone, azole antifungal agents, and calcium channel blockers (most notably verapamil and diltiazem).

The mechanism by which statins interact with various drugs differ. Simvastatin is a major substrate of CYP3A4 and a substrate of OATP1B1. Simvastatin is contraindicated when co-administered with strong CYP3A4 inhibitors. Unlike simvastatin, rosuvastatin does not depend on metabolism by CYP3A4 and CYP2C9 to a clinically significant extent. However, rosuvastatin is a substrate of the OATP1B1 and BCRP transporters. Clarithromycin is a strong CYP3A4 inhibitor and inhibits OATP1B1 activity. The interaction between clarithromycin and rosuvastatin likely comes from clarithromycin inhibiting the transporter OATP1B1. The prescribing information for rosuvastatin includes significant interactions with known OATP1B1 inhibitors (e.g., cyclosporine, ritonavir, and simeprevir).

 Wooten JM A Brief Drug Class Review: Considerations for Statin Use, Toxicity, and Drug Interactions. South Med J. 2018; 111:39–44.
https://www.ncbi.nlm.nih.gov/pubmed/29298368

33. Answer: B

This patient has acute ischaemic stroke of unclear cause in the left anterior cerebral artery territory and presents within three hours after the onset. He is a potential candidate for thrombolysis treatment, as his stroke is disabling and there are no absolute contraindications. As per the Clinical Guideline Stroke Management Procedures and Protocols, a BP over 185mmHg systolic or 110mmHg diastolic is a relative contra indication to thrombolysis. In patients who are eligible for thrombolysis but have a systolic blood pressure > 185mmHg or > 110 mmHg diastolic, 10–20mg of intravenous labetalol can be administered via slow injection over 1–2 minutes. This dose may be doubled after 5–10 minutes. If BP remains >185/110 mmHg despite aggressive treatment, management with alteplase is contraindicated. If the BP can be reduced to below 185 mmHg systolic and 110 mmHg diastolic, then this patient would be suitable for thrombolysis as long as this was completed within 4.5 hours. Aspirin and clopidogrel would be reasonable in the setting of milder stroke. Acute anticoagulation should not be administered in the setting of an acute stroke, excepting cardioembolism with fully resolved symptoms and/or minimal infarction proven on imaging.

 Powers W, Rabinstein A, Ackerson T, Adeoye O, Bambakidis N, Becker K et al. 2018 Guidelines for the Early Management of Patients With Acute Ischemic Stroke: A Guideline for Healthcare Professionals From the American Heart Association/American Stroke Association. Stroke [Internet]. 2018 [cited 10 July 2020];49(3). Available from: https://www.ahajournals.org/doi/full/10.1161/str.0000000000000158

 InformMe – Clinical Guidelines for Stroke Management [Internet]. Informme.org.au. 2020 [cited 10 July 2020]. Available from: https://informme.org.au/Guidelines/Clinical%20Guidelines%20for%20Stroke%20Management

34. Answer: D

This presentation is likely due to transient global amnesia (TGA) as his only symptom is the inability to form new memories (anterograde amnesia). This is often described incorrectly as confusion.

The following diagnostic criteria must be met for TGA diagnosis:

- Attack must be witnessed and information available from a capable observer who was present for most of the attack.
- Clear-cut anterograde amnesia during the attack.
- Cognitive impairment limited to amnesia, without clouding of consciousness or loss of personal identity.
- No accompanying focal neurological symptoms during the attack and no significant neurologic signs afterwards.
- Absence of epileptic features.
- Resolution of the attack within 24 hours.
- Patients with recent head injury or active epilepsy are excluded.

The only known risk factors for TGA are age > 50 and previous history of migraines, both of which apply to this patient. As symptoms always resolve within 24 hours, he needs to be monitored over this time with the caveat that if symptoms persist past this point, he should be investigated further. As patients cannot lay down new memories during the attack, they will never be able to recall the episode itself, however as soon as the attack ends, any retrograde amnesia that they may have experienced will usually start to resolve.

There is no treatment for TGA. Most patients with TGA do not experience repeat episodes. Patients with repeat episodes of TGA should document the circumstances triggering the event to prevent TGA by avoiding triggers. There is no drug can prevent TGA recurring. Lamotrigine is used to treat absence seizure which is not in this case.

 Arena J, Rabinstein A. Transient Global Amnesia. Mayo Clinic Proceedings. 2015;90(2):264–272. https://pubmed.ncbi.nlm.nih.gov/25659242/

35. Answer: A

Vancomycin is a glycopeptide antimicrobial with antibacterial action. Vancomycin acts by inhibiting cell wall synthesis of bacteria. Vancomycin is used for treatment of infections resistant to penicillin or in patients with severe adverse reaction to penicillin. Appropriate vancomycin use can avoid increased generation of vancomycin-resistant enterococci.

Vancomycin is indicated in multidrug resistant Gram-positive infections, such as MRSA, *Streptococcus pneumoniae*, *Streptococcus pyogenes*, *Streptococcus bovis*, *Streptococcus viridans*, *Streptococcus agalactiae*, *Enterococcus*, *diphtheroids*, *Listeria monocitogenes*, *Actinomyces*, species of *Clostridium* (oral vancomycin for recurrent/refractory or serious cases of *C. difficile* infection), and species of *Lactobacillus*.

Vancomycin is not metabolised and is 80–90% excreted in the kidneys. Vancomycin's elimination half-life is highly dependent on renal function. Vancomycin level is significantly dialysed, with a rate ranging from 30–46%. There is a rebound effect of 16 to 36% at the end of the dialysis session after the medication is redistributed. Serum vancomycin level monitoring is done before the haemodialysis session.

Vancomycin has poor penetration into the lung and CNS and is poorly absorbed from the gastrointestinal tract, so it has a high risk of subtherapeutic tissue concentration at lower doses. Vancomycin's antibacterial action is time and concentration dependent. Appropriate vancomycin dosage based on actual body weight is important to ensure trough vancomycin levels are within therapeutic ranges.

Vancomycin is often given to patients with severe infections and in patients with septic shock. Other risk factors predispose patients to develop vancomycin-associated nephrotoxicity include advanced age, sepsis, impaired baseline renal function, dehydration, concomitant administration of aminoglycosides or other nephrotoxins, loop diuretics, amphotericin B, piperacillin-tazobactam, acyclovir, and intravenous contrast media, etc.

Pharmacokinetic changes in drug absorption, volume of distribution, metabolism, and elimination are noted in patients who are critically unwell. Careful monitoring of the renal function and vancomycin levels is important to ensure patients receive therapeutic dose of antibiotics and avoid adverse effects.

For twice daily dosing in patients with non-serious infections (vancomycin dose: 15–20 mg/kg), trough concentration should be 10–15 mg/L. Some experts recommend a trough level of 15–20 mg/L with a higher vancomycin dose (25–30 mg/kg) for more severe infections such as endocarditis, bacteraemia, meningitis, pneumonia, and osteomyelitis.

Vancomycin-associated nephrotoxicity is defined as an increase in 0.5 mg/dL (44 μmol/L) in serum creatinine or 50% increase above baseline in two consecutive measurements after several days of vancomycin after ruling out other causes of AKI. Reduction in renal function is likely associated with acute tubular necrosis and acute interstitial nephritis in patients with vancomycin-associated nephrotoxicity.

The most common side effects associated with vancomycin administration is red man syndrome (associated with histamine release), which is not related to serum concentration. Patients have histamine release, developing paraesthesia, and redness around face and torso, especially with rapid intravenous vancomycin infusion (> 500 mg in less than 30 minutes). Suggested vancomycin infusion time is 1 to 2 hours. Vancomycin can cause hypersensitivity reactions. Vancomycin may also cause ototoxicity with prolonged use, especially if it is used in conjunction with aminoglycosides (synergistic effect).

Zamoner W, Prado I, Balbi A, Ponce D. Vancomycin dosing, monitoring and toxicity: Critical review of the clinical practice. Clinical and Experimental Pharmacology and Physiology. 2019;46(4):292–301.
https://onlinelibrary.wiley.com/doi/full/10.1111/1440-1681.13066

36. Answer: D

Volume of distribution (Vd) can be described as fluid volume that would be required to contain the amount of drug present in the body at the same concentration as in the plasma. The volume is an apparent volume not a physical space. Vd is calculated as the ratio of the dose present in the body and its plasma concentration, that is Vd=A (amount of drug in the body)/C plasma concentration, when the distribution of the drug between the tissues and the plasma is at equilibrium.

A drug that accumulates in tissues, will have low plasma concentration with regard to the administered dose, and consequently the calculated Vd will be high. Drugs with a very small Vd (<10 L) are mainly confined to the intravascular fluid because the molecule is too large to leave this compartment or the drug binds preferably to plasma proteins. Some drugs cannot enter cells because of their low lipid solubility. These drugs are distributed throughout the body water in the extracellular compartment and have a relatively small Vd (12–20 L). Drugs that accumulate in organs either by active transport or by specific binding to tissue molecules have a high Vd, which can exceed several times the anatomical body volume. Vd is useful in estimating the dose required to achieve a given plasma concentration as Dose = plasma concentration x Vd.

Azithromycin reversibly binds to the bacterial ribosome and inhibits protein synthesis. The bioavailability of azithromycin is approximately 37%. Concomitant administration of oral azithromycin with food significantly decreases drug bioavailability by 50%. The plasma concentration of azithromycin is low because of extensive and rapid distribution from plasma to tissues. Plasma protein binding is low. Therefore, the Vd for azithromycin is very large, 25 to 35 l/kg. Tissue concentrations exceed the minimum inhibitory concentration that would inhibit 90% of likely pathogens (MIC90) after a single 500 mg oral dose. Mean concentrations in tissue are 10- to 100-fold higher than those reached in serum and persist for several days. Azithromycin also accumulates in phagocytes, with levels up to 200 times greater than in serum but penetrates poorly into cerebrospinal fluid and peritoneal fluid.

Azithromycin is mainly eliminated unchanged in the faeces via biliary excretion and transintestinal secretion. Urinary excretion is small. The half-life of azithromycin is 2 to 4 days. The pharmacokinetics of azithromycin are not significantly altered in elderly subjects and in patients with mild to moderate renal or hepatic insufficiency. Unlike clarithromycin, azithromycin does not interact significantly with cytochrome P450 3A4.

McMullan B, Mostaghim M. Prescribing azithromycin. Australian Prescriber. 2015;38(3):87–89.
https://www.ncbi.nlm.nih.gov/pmc/articles/PMC4653965/

37. Answer: D

Warfarin consists of a racemic mixture of two isomers: R- and S- forms, both of which are metabolised by cytochrome P450 enzymes. Of the two, the S- isomer is a far more active anticoagulant and is predominantly metabolised by CYP2C9. The R-isomer is metabolised predominantly by CYP3A4, but also by CYP2C19. Fluconazole inhibits all three CYP enzymes involved in warfarin metabolism.

Variations in INR in the setting of medication co-administration can be attributed to the effects of the treated condition (for example sepsis) as well as the effects of the drug on gut flora, and warfarin metabolism. On a population level, inhibitors of CYP2C9 are far more likely to result in an increase in INR of 50% or more, compared to drugs inhibiting CYP3A4. Consequently, amiodarone and azole antibiotic medications show the greatest likelihood of over-anticoagulation, for example fluconazole, metronidazole, resulting in increase in INR of greater than 50% around 50% of the time. Co-administration of inhibitors of CYP3A4 and CYP2C19 are also likely to result in increases in INR, but less predictably, and to a lesser extent such as macrolide antibiotics, omeprazole, and fluoxetine. In contrast, medications that induce CYP enzymes are often observed to lower INR, most frequently observed with carbamazepine. In clinical practice, knowledge of CYP P450 enzymes is critically important in using warfarin, and more active monitoring of INR in patients newly administered medications known to affect warfarin metabolism is warranted. Some authors advocate pre-emptive reduction of warfarin dose when starting amiodarone, fluconazole or metronidazole.

Martin-Perez M, Gaist D, Abajo FJ et.al: Population impact of drug interactions with warfarin: a real-world data approach. Thromb. Haemost. 2018; 118(3):461–470.
https://www.ncbi.nlm.nih.gov/pubmed/29433149–

38. Answer: D

Beta-blockers are useful in the treatment of angina, myocardial infarction, cardiac failure, hypertension, and cardiac arrhythmias. Beta-blockers given long-term have been shown in multiple randomised controlled trials to reduce mortality in patients with heart failure with reduced ejection fraction and following acute myocardial infarction., Beta-blockers slow the clinical progression of heart failure, as evidenced by reductions in hospitalisation rates and mortality.

Non-selective beta-blockers, such as propranolol, sotalol, timolol, and carvedilol, induce competitive blockade of both β_1 and β_2 receptors. Metoprolol and atenolol possess relative selectivity for the β_1 receptor. Although β_1(cardiac)-selective agents have the theoretical advantage of producing less bronchoconstriction and less peripheral vasoconstriction, a clear clinical advantage of cardio-selective agents is unestablished. Bronchoconstriction may occur when β_1-selective agents are administered in therapeutic doses.

Various beta-blockers differ in their water and lipid solubility. The lipophilic agents (e.g. propranolol, metoprolol, bisoprolol, and carvedilol) are readily absorbed from the gastrointestinal tract, metabolised by the liver, have large volumes of distribution, and penetrate the central nervous system well. The hydrophilic agents (e.g. atenolol, sotalol) are less readily absorbed, not extensively metabolised, and have relatively longer plasma half-lives, resulting in their ability to be administered once per day. Hepatic impairment may prolong the plasma half-life of lipophilic agents whereas renal impairment may prolong the action of hydrophilic agents. Nebivolol is a β1-receptor blocker with nitric oxide potentiating vasodilatory effect.

Carvedilol has both α_1-adrenoreceptor blockade and non-selective beta-blockade actions and is devoid of intrinsic sympathomimetic activity. Contraindications to beta-blocker therapy in patients with heart failure include severe decompensation requiring inotropic therapy, marked bradycardia, sick sinus syndrome, and partial or complete atrioventricular block, unless a permanent pacemaker is in place.

 Dézsi C, Szentes V. The Real Role of β-Blockers in Daily Cardiovascular Therapy. American Journal of Cardiovascular Drugs. 2017;17(5): 361–373.
https://link.springer.com/article/10.1007/s40256-017-0221-8

39. Answer: A

Vancomycin can cause both anaphylactoid and anaphylactic reactions. In anaphylactoid reactions (vancomycin red person syndrome), vancomycin itself causes direct stimulation of mast cells leading to profound systemic histamine release and a characteristic upper torso rash with truncal pain and widespread itch. The histamine release can cause profound hypotension and tachycardia due to direct negatively inotropic and vasodilatory effects, however angioedema, stridor, hives, and wheeze usually do not occur. Both anaphylactic and anaphylactoid reactions can be treated with intravenous fluid and antihistamines, but where there is some doubt about whether the reaction may be anaphylactic – e.g. non-specific rash, haemodynamic instability, angioedema, wheeze, stridor – adrenaline should also be administered. Repeated infusion with vancomycin should be avoided if other appropriate antibiotics are available, but, if needed, infusion rates below 10 mg/min should be enough to prevent future anaphylactoid events.

 Bruniera FR, Ferreira FM, Saviolli LRM et.al. The use of vancomycin with its and adverse effects: a review. *Eur Rev Med Pharmacol*. 2015; 19: 694–700.
https://pubmed.ncbi.nlm.nih.gov/25753888/

40. Answer: A

Methamphetamine has longer pharmacokinetic and pharmacodynamic half-life than cocaine. It may be as much as 10 times longer than that of cocaine.

Cocaine cardiovascular toxicity includes chest pain, acute myocardial infarction (AMI), arrhythmia, severe or malignant hypertension, and cardiomyopathy. In individuals with cocaine-associated AMI, median times to the onset of chest pain vary with the route or form of cocaine use: 30 minutes for intravenous use, 90 minutes for crack, and 135 minutes for intranasal use.

Hyperthermia is a marker for severe toxicity, and it is associated with numerous complications, including AKI, rhabdomyolysis, metabolic acidosis, DIC, and liver failure. Dopamine plays a role in the regulation of core body temperature, so increased dopaminergic neurotransmission may contribute to psychostimulant-induced hyperthermia in cocaine users.

The goals of pharmacotherapy in cocaine toxicity are to reduce the CNS and cardiovascular effects of the drug. Benzodiazepines are the treatment of choice.

 Heard K, Palmer R, Zahniser N. Mechanisms of Acute Cocaine Toxicity. The Open Pharmacology Journal. 2008;2(1):70–78.
https://openpharmacologyjournal.com/VOLUME/2/PAGE/70/

19 Respiratory and Sleep Medicine

Questions

Answers can be found in the Respiratory and Sleep Medicine Answers section at the end of this chapter.

1. Which of the following can cause reductions of serum α1-antitrypsin levels in patients being tested for α1-antitrypsin deficiency?
 A. Liver damage.
 B. Oral contraceptive pill use.
 C. Pneumonia.
 D. Pregnancy.

2. A 54-year-old woman has been treated with amiodarone 200 mg twice a day for one year for atrial fibrillation. She complains of shortness of breath, non-productive cough, and pleuritic chest pain. On examination, she has bilateral crackles on inspiration and no clubbing. Her FBE and CRP are normal.
 CXR shows localised right upper lobe opacity. High-resolution CT of the chest shows a high-attenuation right upper lobe consolidation and ground glass opacity. Pulmonary function test reveals a restrictive pattern and a reduction in diffusion capacity (DLCO). Flexible bronchoscopy and bronchial alveolar lavage (BAL) fluid finds foam cells, lymphocytosis, and neutrophilia.
 Which one of the following pulmonary toxicities associated with amiodarone use is most likely in this patient?
 A. Bronchiolitis obliterans organising pneumonia (BOOP).
 B. Diffuse alveolar haemorrhage.
 C. Eosinophilic pneumonia.
 D. Interstitial pneumonitis.

3. You review a 45-year-old woman in the respiratory clinic for worsening asthma control. She has had eight severe exacerbations of asthma in the last year. She takes an inhaled corticosteroid, an inhaled long-acting beta agonist, and an inhaled long-acting muscarinic antagonist. She has no significant past medical history and has never smoked. Her examination shows obesity with BMI of 42 kg/m². She has mildly reduced air entry globally, but no wheeze, and no evidence of fluid overload. Her puffer technique is good. Sputum analysis shows normal eosinophils and neutrophils and there is no significant growth of micro-organisms. Pulmonary function testing shows normal spirometry with significant airway hyper-responsiveness after methacholine challenge.
 Which of the following treatment measures has the best evidence for improving her asthma control?
 A. Aggressive weight loss.
 B. Increased inhaled corticosteroid.
 C. Omalizumab.
 D. Theophylline.

4. Omalizumab is used as a second line treatment of eosinophilic/Th2 asthma. What is the mechanism of action of omalizumab?
 A. An antagonist to IL-5.
 B. An antagonist to IL-13.
 C. An antibody to the IL-4 alpha-receptor.
 D. Blocking the interaction of IgE with its receptor.

How to Pass the FRACP Written Examination, First Edition. Jonathan Gleadle, Jordan Li, Danielle Wu, and Paul Kleinig.
© 2022 John Wiley & Sons Ltd. Published 2022 by John Wiley & Sons Ltd.

5. Which one of the following treatments reduces the frequency of exacerbations in a patient with bronchiectasis?
   A. Inhaled antibiotics.
   B. Inhaled long-acting bronchodilators & corticosteroids.
   C. Inhaled recombinant human deoxyribonuclease.
   D. Oral macrolides.

6. A 65-year-old patient with a background of COPD is diagnosed to have left lower lobe community acquired pneumonia. Which one of these organisms might urinary antigen testing be employed to confirm it as the most likely causative agent?
   A. *Haemophilus influenzae type B*.
   B. *Klebsiella pneumoniae*.
   C. *Staphylococcus aureus*.
   D. *Streptococcus pneumoniae*.

7. Ivacaftor monotherapy in cystic fibrosis is effective in a subset of cystic fibrosis patients because?
   A. It enhances CFTR endoplasmic reticulum transport.
   B. It functions as a DNase which is defective only in a subgroup of patients.
   C. It is a small interfering RNA that targets specific causative mutations.
   D. It potentiates CFTR channel function which is defective in a subgroup of patients.

8. A 73-year-old woman has been on warfarin since a diagnosis of PE a year ago. She has exertional dyspnoea with exercise tolerance of 15 metres. Her BP is 140/90 mmHg, heart rate: 85 bpm, respiratory rate: 18 per minute, and SpO2: 91% on room air. Her serum creatinine is 200 μmol/L [70-100] and eGFR is 21 mL/min/1.73m^2.
   Which one of the following management plans is appropriate?
   A. Consider insertion of an inferior vena cava filter to prevent further PE.
   B. Perform a computed tomography pulmonary angiography (CTPA) to rule out chronic PE.
   C. Perform a D-dimer test to rule out chronic PE.
   D. Perform a V/Q scan and an echocardiogram to rule out chronic thromboembolic pulmonary hypertension (CTEPH).

9. Community-acquired pneumonia (CAP) is a common admitting diagnosis to the medical inpatient unit. Which one of the following statements regarding CAP is **INCORRECT?**
   A. Atypical bacterium including *Mycoplasma*, *Chlamydia*, and *Legionella* constitute 20% of CAP.
   B. CXR with infiltrative changes is required for definitive diagnosis of CAP but will miss at least 25% of CAP.
   C. Majority of CAP is due to aspiration of bacteria from the upper respiratory tract.
   D. Microbiology evaluations are recommended for all hospitalised patients with CAP.

10. Which of the following enzymes is responsible for degradation of fibrin into D-dimer and fragment E?
   A. Antithrombin.
   B. Factor XIIIa.
   C. Plasmin.
   D. Thrombin.

11. A 66-year-old man had severe smoking-related COPD with typical clinical features of emphysema. He died of ischaemic bowel after presenting with abdominal pain to the emergency department.
   During the autopsy, which one of the followings is the most likely histologic findings in his lung?
   A. Airway centred inflammation with fibrosis and poorly formed non-necrotising granulomas.
   B. Bronchial smooth muscle hypertrophy with proliferation of eosinophils.
   C. Dilation of distal air spaces of terminal bronchioles and destruction of alveolar walls.
   D. Hyperplasia of bronchial mucus-secreting submucosal glands.

12. A 23-year-old man develops shortness of breath and cough over four days, he is febrile at 38 °C, and requires 6L of oxygen via face mask to maintain oxygen saturations above 94%. He is a professional musician and has recently started smoking. There is no significant past medical history and no recent medication. He is treated with intravenous ceftriaxone and azithromycin but deteriorates, requiring invasive ventilation. A wide ranging screen for infective causes is negative. An axial section of his CT chest scan is shown below:

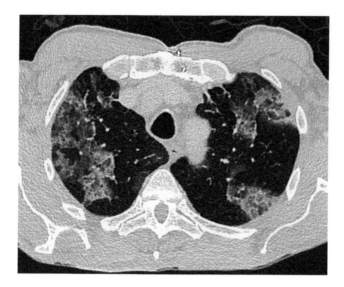

Transbronchial biopsy shows a marked increase in numbers of eosinophils infiltrating interstitial spaces, and very few within the alveoli.

What is the most likely diagnosis?
- **A.** Acute eosinophilic pneumonia (AEP).
- **B.** Allergic bronchopulmonary aspergillosis (ABPA).
- **C.** Eosinophilic granulomatosis with polyangiitis (EGPA).
- **D.** *Strongyloides stercoralis* infection.

13. With regards to Legionnaires' disease, which statement is **INCORRECT**?
- **A.** All *Legionella* species are Gram-positive bacteria.
- **B.** Legionnaire's disease is mainly transmitted via inhalation of infectious aerosols.
- **C.** Urinary antigen test is the first-line diagnostic test for Legionnaire's disease.
- **D.** Water is the major reservoir for *Legionella*.

14. A 65-year-old man with a history of aspergilloma and recurrent haemoptysis underwent bronchial artery embolisation one week ago. He presents to the emergency department with 600 ml of haemoptysis. His BP is 100/50 mmHg, HR is 98 bpm, respiratory rate is 24/min, temperature is 36.5 °C and SpO2 is 94% on room air. The haemoglobin is 92 g/L [135 – 175), the platelet count is 250 x 10⁹/L [150 – 450], INR is 1.0 [0.9 – 1.3], and APTT is 30 seconds [24 – 38).

What is the method of choice for treating massive and recurrent haemoptysis due to refractory aspergilloma?
- **A.** Bronchial artery embolisation.
- **B.** Bronchoscopy.
- **C.** Surgical treatment.
- **D.** Tranexamic acid.

15. Which one of the following is correct regarding patients with malignant mesothelioma?
- **A.** Malignant mesothelioma does not affect the peritoneum or pericardium.
- **B.** Malignant mesothelioma is insensitive to radiotherapy therefore it is not effective in temporarily relieving pain caused by disease.
- **C.** Talc pleurodesis is the preferred treatment over video-assisted thoracoscopic partial pleurectomy for pleural effusion caused by mesothelioma.
- **D.** The sensitivity of cytological examination of pleural fluid in suspected mesothelioma is over 50%.

16. Which one of the following causes of chronic sleepiness is characterised by early transition to rapid eye movement (REM) sleep after falling asleep, and REM sleep during daytime naps?
- **A.** Narcolepsy.
- **B.** Obstructive sleep apnoea.
- **C.** Sedative use.
- **D.** Shift work.

17. With regards to acute respiratory failure in COPD, which of the following clinical factors is an indicator for invasive ventilation, as opposed to non-invasive positive pressure ventilation (NPPV)?
- **A.** Persistent hypoxia despite supplemental oxygen therapy.
- **B.** Persistent inability to clear respiratory secretions.
- **C.** Respiratory acidosis.
- **D.** Severe dyspnoea with respiratory muscle fatigue.

18. CPAP treatment of moderate-severe OSA in patients with established cardiovascular disease is associated with which one of the following outcomes?
- **A.** Improved quality of life and mood.
- **B.** Reduced cardiovascular mortality.
- **C.** Reduced hospitalisation for heart failure.
- **D.** Reduced overall mortality.

19. A 52-year-old man has worked in an industry for 15 years. He presents with a 3-month history of cough and breathlessness. CXR shows diffuse interstitial shadowing. His sputum culture is positive for acid-fast bacilli. Which one of the following exposures is most likely to have predisposed this patient to tuberculosis?
- **A.** Beryllium.
- **B.** Cotton dust.
- **C.** Nanoparticle.
- **D.** Silica.

20. A 56-year-old man undergoes a sleep study because of daytime sleepiness. The apnoea-hypopnea index (AHI) is reported as 30/hour. Your appropriate response includes the following **EXCEPT**:
- **A.** His AHI indicates he should avoid evening alcohol and benzodiazepines.
- **B.** His driver's licence should be withheld until CPAP treatment result is assessed.
- **C.** He needs CPAP treatment.
- **D.** He qualifies for a disability pension from the government.

21. A 65-year-old ex-smoker with known COPD presents to the emergency department with shortness of breath and a cough with purulent sputum. He is suspected of having an infective exacerbation of COPD. On examination he is severely short of breath with an oxygen saturation of 86% on room air. An arterial blood gas is performed which shows the following:

pH	7.25
PaO_2	60 mmHg
$PaCO_2$	58 mmHg
HCO_3	30 mEq/L

In this patient, which of the following physiologic parameters is most likely to be facilitating the delivery of oxygen to tissues?
- **A.** Low body temperature.
- **B.** Low concentration of 2,3-diphosphoglycerate.
- **C.** Low PaO_2.
- **D.** Low pH.

22. A 65-year-old woman is seen in the high-risk pre-operative assessment clinic before right radical nephrectomy for renal cell carcinoma. She has severe kyphoscoliosis, and you arrange pulmonary function testing. Which one of the following abnormalities of the lung function test is most likely to be found?

    A. Decreased vital capacity (VC).

    B. Increased functional residual capacity (FRC).

    C. Increased maximal inspiratory pressure (MIP).

    D. Reduced forced expiratory volume-one second (FEV_1) to forced vital capacity (FVC) ratio.

23 A 64-year-old woman presents to the emergency department with dyspnoea. Her CXR shows bilateral moderate pleural effusions. She is afebrile, BP is 145/67 mmHg, HR is 89 bpm, RR is 20/min, and SpO_2 is 93% on room air. Her diagnostic pleural fluid results show protein 35.8 g/L (serum proteins 69 g/L), and LDH 820 U/L (serum LDH 563 U/L). The erythrocyte count is 2,500,000 cells/μL, and leukocytes count is 3,700 cells/μL with 55% neutrophils, 40% lymphocytes and 5% monocytes. The Gram stain and cultures are sterile.

    Which one of the following is the most likely cause of her pleural effusion?

    A. Liver cirrhosis.

    B. Left ventricular failure.

    C. Nephrotic syndrome.

    D. Malignant pleural effusion.

24. A 68-year-old man undergoes a CXR before his right hip replacement as a pre-operative assessment. He is a retired boilermaker and is an ex-smoker. He is asymptomatic, and his chest was clear on auscultation. His CXR is displayed below. You explain to him:

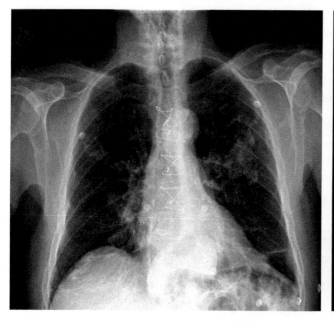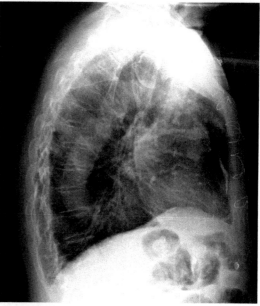

    A. This is a benign condition which does not need follow up.

    B. This is a malignant disorder with poor prognosis.

    C. This is a premalignant condition and requires annual CXR and follow up.

    D. This is a progressive disease; he will develop exertional dyspnoea within 12 months.

25. A 22-year-old man presents to hospital with chest pain and shortness of breath. His oxygen saturation is 90% on 6L/min of oxygen, he is tachycardic, and tachypnoeic, with distended neck veins and a systolic BP of 85 mmHg. His CXR is shown below. Which of the following is the best treatment?

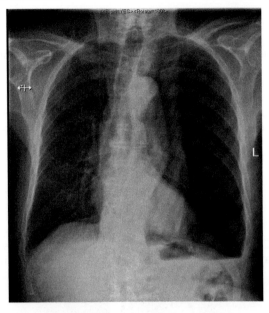

A. Intravenous inotropes and broad-spectrum antibiotics.
B. Needle aspiration.
C. Tube thoracostomy.
D. Video-assisted thoracoscopic surgery (VATS) pleurodesis.

26. A 66-year-old woman is referred by her GP because of a 12-month history of weight loss, fatigue, dry cough, and severe exertional dyspnoea. Her CXR and CT chest are displayed below. When you are performing a physical examination which one of the following signs would be **UNEXPECTED**?
  A. Bibasal fine end-inspiratory crackles.
  B. Digital clubbing.
  C. High pitched, holosystolic murmur at the left lower sternal border.
  D. Pulsus paradoxus.

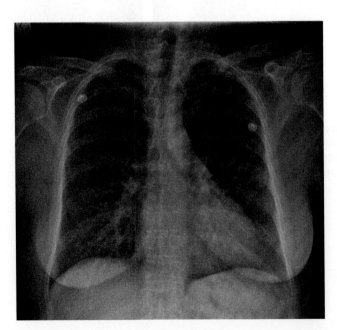

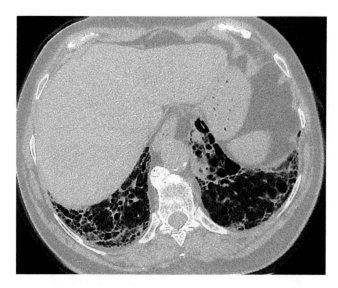

27. A 57-year-old truck driver is referred for assessment of 'difficult-to-control hypertension' despite being on three antihypertensive medications. He is a current smoker and has typical features of metabolic syndrome including recent weight gain with a BMI of 36 kg/m², glucose intolerance, OSA and hyperlipidaemia. On examination, his BP is 160/95 mmHg. He has acne, central obesity with adipose deposits on the dorsal upper thorax, and abdominal striae. His CXR is shown below. He undergoes an endobronchial ultrasound guided (EBUS) biopsy which reveals clusters of malignant cells.

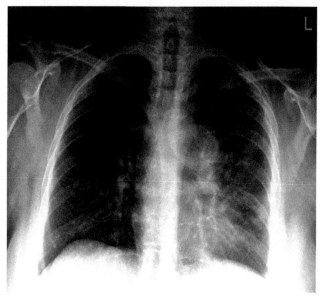

What type of lung cancer is he most likely to have?
  A. Carcinoid tumour of the lung.
  B. Adenocarcinoma of the lung.
  C. Small cell lung cancer.
  D. Squamous cell lung cancer.

28. A 22-year-old overseas nursing student is referred by the University Health Clinic with a three week history of general malaise, low grade fevers and night sweats. She has also developed right-sided chest pain in the last three days. She returned from Sri Lanka five weeks ago, following a holiday.

She has no significant medical history and takes no medications. Her initial investigation results and CXR are shown below. Thoracentesis yields yellow fluid. The initial microscopy and biochemistry results demonstrate RBC 500/µl; WBC 3600/µL with 15% neutrophils, 65% lymphocytes, 10% macrophages, 5% mesothelial and 5% eosinophils. Total protein 41g/L; LDH 265 U/L (serum LDH 120); pH 7.39; Gram stain shows no organisms and culture is pending.

Tests	Results	Normal values
Haemoglobin	123 g/L	120–170
White blood cells	8.8 x 10⁹/L	4.0–11.0
Platelet	177 x 10⁹/L	150–400
Creatinine	90 μmol/L	60–120
CRP	56 g/L	0–20
INR	1.2	1

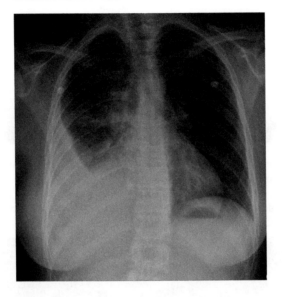

What is the most appropriate next step?
- **A.** Arrange a bronchoscopy and send lavage for culture.
- **B.** Give low-molecular-weight heparin and order a CT pulmonary angiogram (CTPA).
- **C.** Intravenous ceftriaxone and azithromycin, then repeat CXR four weeks later.
- **D.** Perform a pleural biopsy.

29. A 75-year-old man with no history of smoking and no significant past medical history presents with progressive dyspnoea and hypoxia over one year. An axial image from his CT chest is shown below.

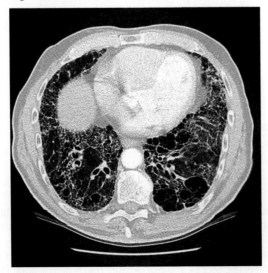

Which one of the following patterns of lung injury best describes the above changes?
- **A.** Cryptogenic organising pneumonia.
- **B.** Hypersensitivity pneumonitis.
- **C.** Non-specific interstitial pneumonia.
- **D.** Usual interstitial pneumonia.

30. A 30-year-old man is reviewed in the respiratory clinic for chronic breathlessness and wheeze which started six months ago, and initially was responsive to inhaled salbutamol. Symptoms have progressively worsened despite addition of inhaled corticosteroid, long-acting beta agonist, and long-acting muscarinic antagonist. He is a non-smoker, of normal body habitus and has a history of allergic rhinitis. He now lives in rural Victoria, where he has been working in the poultry industry; however, his childhood years were spent in Darwin, where he visits family every six months or so. On examination, his observations are normal except for a mildly elevated respiratory rate. His chest examination shows widespread polyphonic expiratory wheeze. His puffer technique is good, and his prescriptions are filled regularly. His pulmonary function tests show a severe ventilatory deficit with an obstructive pattern and significant reversibility post-bronchodilator, diffusing capacity of carbon monoxide was normal when corrected for volume. His FBE is as follows:

Tests	Results	Normal values
Haemoglobin	107 g/L	115–155
Mean Cell Volume	92 fL	80–98
White Blood Cell Count	11.5 x 10⁹/L	4–11
Neutrophils	3.2 x 10⁹/L	2.0–7.5
Lymphocytes	1.7 x 10⁹/L	1.5–4.0
Monocytes	0.9 x 10⁹/L	0.2–0.8
Eosinophils	5.7 x 10⁹/L	0–0.4

Which of the following measures is **LEAST** likely to be useful in ruling out diagnoses other than asthma?
- **A.** CT chest.
- **B.** IgE to aspergillus.
- **C.** IgG to bird antigens.
- **D.** Strongyloides serology.

QUESTIONS (31–35) **REFER TO THE FOLLOWING INFORMATION**
For each patient described below, select the most likely arterial blood gas findings while breathing room air.

	pH (7.35–7.45)	P_aO_2 (80–110mmHg)	P_aCO_2 (35–45mmHg)	Bicarbonate (23–33mmol/L)
A	7.50	55	33	25
B	7.45	100	24	17
C	7.49	60	24	23
D	7.40	100	40	25
E	7.33	54	55	38
F	7.25	54	65	26
G	7.26	99	16	7.1
H	7.15	96	33	11

31. A 36-year-old woman with type 1 diabetes presents with a two day history of general unwellness and abdominal pain. There is a history of poor compliance with treatment. On examination, she is afebrile, BP is 110/60 mmHg. Abdominal examination reveals mild tenderness. Urinalysis shows: +++ ketones, ++++ glucose.

32. A 63-year-old man has smoking-related COPD. He stopped smoking two years ago and is currently on domiciliary oxygen. He has previously been admitted to hospital with acute exacerbation of COPD and required non-invasive ventilation. He is currently well.

33. A 56-year-old woman suffering from depression and chronic back pain is admitted to the Acute Medical Unit after her son found her unresponsive, shallow, and slow breathing on the floor. An empty pack of oxycodone was found next to her. She was well two hours ago before her son left for his dental appointment.

34. You are seeing a 56-year-old man on the ward because of his chest pain and shortness of breath. He is a life-long non-smoker without other medical history. He was admitted four days ago after a motor bike accident and fractured his right tibia which required open reduction internal fixation three days ago. He is afebrile, cardiovascular and respiratory examination are unremarkable except a respiratory rate of 22/min. His WBC count is normal, CRP and troponin are mildly elevated.

35. A 56-year-old woman is brought into the emergency department after ingesting sixty 300 mg aspirin tablets. Her usual weight is 50 kg. She is semi-conscious but responding to painful stimuli. Her BP is 125/80 mmHg, HR is 100 bpm, and respiratory rate of 36 /min.

QUESTIONS (36–42) REFER TO THE FOLLOWING INFORMATION
Provide the most likely clinical diagnosis for each of the following clinical presentations and CXR findings:

    A. Acute pulmonary oedema.
    B. Aspiration pneumonia.
    C. Goodpasture's syndrome.
    D. Granulomatosis with polyangiitis.
    E. Metastatic lung cancer.
    F. Primary lung cancer.
    G. Pneumothorax.
    H. Pulmonary embolism.
    I. Pulmonary sarcoidosis.
    J. Pulmonary tuberculosis.

36. A 22-year-old man with acute onset of chest pain, dyspnoea, and hypoxia. His CXR is shown below.

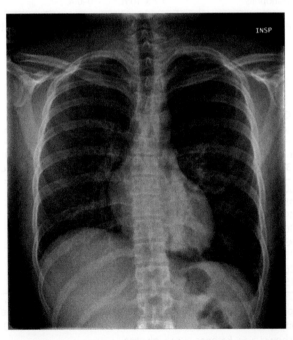

37. A 66-year-old man is admitted for investigation of weight loss of 10kg over the past 12 months, cough, and exertional dyspnoea for one month. His initial CXR is shown below.

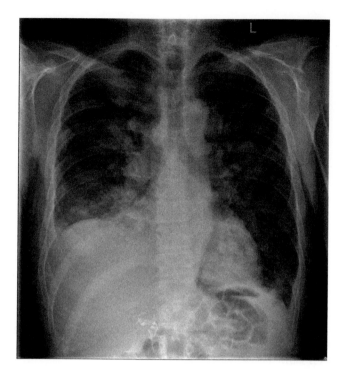

38. 64-year-old man with brainstem infarct in a rehabilitation ward develops fever, cough, and shortness of breath.

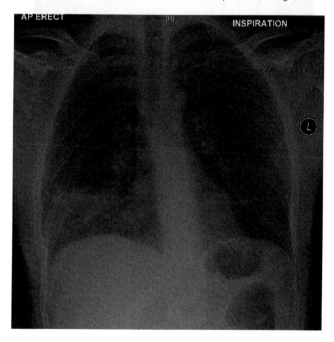

39. You are asked to review a 78-year-old woman with sudden onset of chest pain, severe dyspnoea, and requiring 6L of oxygen to keep oxygen saturation above 90% in an orthopaedic ward. She had a right hip replacement two weeks ago. Her CXR is shown below.

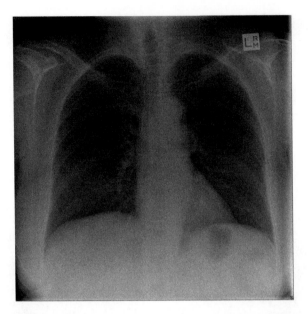

40. You are asked to review a 78-year-old man with sudden onset of chest pain, severe dyspnoea, and requiring 6L of oxygen to keep oxygen saturation above 90% in an orthopaedic ward. He had an open reduction and internal fixation following left intertrochanteric fracture. His CXR is shown below.

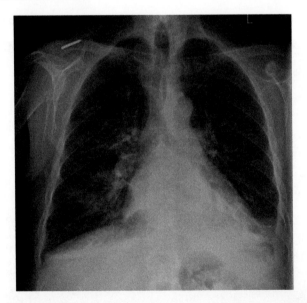

41. A 75-year-old man presents with small volume haemoptysis and low-grade fever. He has lost 4 kg of weight in the past three months. Blood test reveals AKI with serum creatinine 450 μmol/L [60–110]. There is no urine output for urine analysis. CXR is shown below.

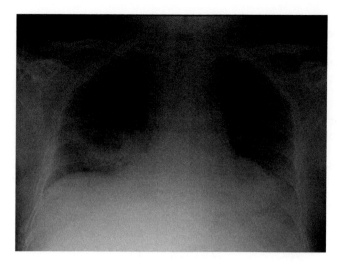

42. 75-year-old man has a CXR done before his elective hernia repair because he is a current heavy smoker. His pre-operative blood test shows serum creatinine of 210 μmol/L [60–110], hypercalcaemia but not anaemia.

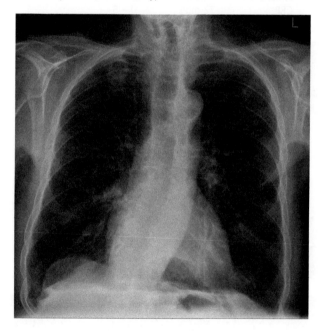

QUESTIONS (43–49) REFER TO THE FOLLOWING INFORMATION
Which of the following diagnoses best explains the constellation of clinical findings and radiological changes?

    A. Acute interstitial fibrosis (Hamman–Rich syndrome).

    B. Allergic bronchopulmonary aspergillosis.

   C. Alveolar proteinosis.

   D. Churg-Strauss syndrome [eosinophilic granulomatosis with polyangiitis (EGPA)].

   E. Cryptogenic organizing pneumonia (COP).

   F. Desquamative interstitial pneumonitis (DIP).

   G. Idiopathic pulmonary fibrosis (IPF).

   H. Löffler syndrome.

   I. Löfgren syndrome.

   J. Lymphangioleiomyomatosis.

   K. Granulomatosis with polyangiitis (GPA).

43. A 39-year-old woman presents with a four months history of lethargy and unproductive cough. She has had no fevers or weight loss. She also developed painful rashes/lesions on both lower limbs one week ago (see below). She is a farmer and a current smoker. On examination, she has low grade fever and SpO$_2$ is 95% on room air. The respiratory examination is unremarkable. Initial investigation results and CXR are showed below.

Tests	Results	Normal values
WBC	12.0 x 10^9/L	4 – 11
Neutrophil	10.5 x 10^9/L	1.8 – 7.5
Eosinophil	0.15 x 10^9/L	0.02 – 0.5
Lymphocyte	1.05 x 10^9/L	1.5 – 3.5
CRP	72 mg/L	0 – 8

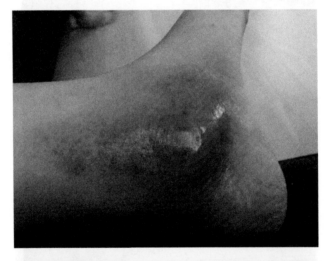

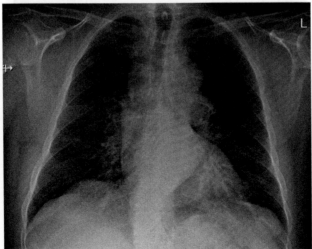

44. A 45-year-old woman who has had asthma for 20 years presents with progressive dyspnoea, wheezing and productive cough. She is taking a regular inhaled corticosteroid and both short- and long-acting β-agonists. On examination, she is afebrile but has mild tachypnoea and SaO$_2$ 93% on room air. Respiratory examination reveals moderate air movement, diffuse wheezes and ego-phony in the left upper lung zone without change in tactile fremitus. Initial investigation results are showed below. CXR shows patchy infiltrate in both upper lobes and prominent lung markings. Chest CT further reveals mucus plugging and central bronchiectasis.

Tests	Results	Normal values
WBC	8.5 x 10^9/L	4 – 11
Neutrophil	3.8 x 10^9/L	1.8 – 7.5
Eosinophil	0.1 x 10^9/L	0.02 – 0.5
Lymphocyte	0.85 x 10^9/L	1.5 – 3.5
CRP	52 mg/L	0 – 8

45. A 64-year-old woman is referred by her GP because of an eight week history of dyspnoea, dry cough, low grade fever, night sweats, weight loss, and lethargy. She had been treated with intravenous ceftriaxone and oral azithromycin followed by two weeks of amoxicillin/clavulanic acid for pneumonia with no obvious improvement. She was well before this illness and is a non-smoker. She is a high school teacher and has not travelled abroad in the past five years. On examination, her temperature is 38 °C; SpO$_2$ 96% on room air. There are scattered crepitations in the bilateral lung fields with occasionally expiratory wheeze. There is no clubbing. The rest of the physical examination is unremarkable. Her initial investigation results are shown below. Her high-resolution CT (HRCT) of chest demonstrates patchy consolidation with a predominantly subpleural and peribronchial distribution. There are small, ill-defined peribronchial and peribronchiolar nodules.

Tests	Results	Normal values
WBC	13 x 10^9/L	4 – 11
Neutrophil	9 x 10^9/L	1.8 – 7.5
Eosinophil	0.1 x 10^9/L	0.02 – 0.5
Lymphocyte	1.1 x 10^9/L	1.5 – 3.5 x 10^9/L
CRP	68 mg/L	0 – 8

46. A 64-year-old Caucasian man presents with a one year history of worsening dyspnoea on exertion and mild non-productive cough. He reports previous asbestos exposure when he worked in a shipyard but has never smoked. He has been treated with several inhaled beta-agonists, without any improvement. The physical examination is significant for dry inspiratory crackles and clubbing of his digits. A CXR shows a diffuse infiltrative process, without lymphadenopathy or effusions. The patient undergoes an open lung biopsy, which shows minimal inflammatory round cell infiltrate, widening of alveolar septa and fibrosis with fibro-blastic foci.

47. A 34-year-old man presents with a cough of abrupt onset, fever, and chest pain. He has no significant medical history. He is admitted to the ICU due to progressive respiratory failure requiring mechanical ventilation. The patient's CXR shows diffuse, patchy ground-glass opacities and intralobular septal thickening. Bronchoscopy with bronchoalveolar lavage (BAL) show copious amounts of grossly turbid exudates in the airways with material that tests positive with periodic acid–Schiff (PAS) reagent on pathological examination.

48. A 32-year-old woman is referred by the emergency department to the respiratory outpatient clinic because she has had three episodes of spontaneous pneumothorax. You note she has an appointment to see a nephrologist because of renal lesion which is likely an angiomyolipoma according to the renal ultrasound report. She is a non-smoker. She has exertional dyspnoea and a non-productive cough for the past three months. Her chest CT is shown below.

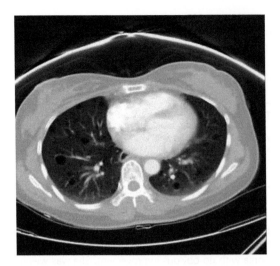

49. A 34-year-old man presents with complaints of fever for seven days, and a cough, breathlessness, tingling of hands and feet, and weakness of both hands and feet for four days. He has history of asthma and recurrent sinusitis. On examination, he is afebrile with SpO_2 93% on room air. He has a bilateral polyphonic wheeze and evidence of distal asymmetric sensory neuropathy with motor weakness. His initial investigation results are showed below. P-ANCA (ELISA) is positive. Pulmonary function test shows reversible airway obstruction. nerve conduction studies confirm mononeuritis multiplex.

Tests	Results	Normal values
WBC	10.2×10^9/L	4–11
Neutrophil	7.3×10^9/L	1.8–7.5
Eosinophil	2.3×10^9/L	0.02–0.5
Lymphocyte	0.1×10^9/L	1.5–3.5
CRP	62 mg/L	0–8

Answers

1. Answer: A

α1-antitrypsin deficiency (AATD) is the major genetic cause of COPD. Even a moderate deficiency of serum α1-antitrypsin may cause lung damage, especially in smokers. AATD occurs due to autosomal co-dominant inheritance of mutations in the *SERPINA1* gene on chromosome 14, causing quantitative and/or qualitative deficiency of the protease inhibitor α1-antitrypsin (AAT). Serum AAT of less than 1.1 g/L is suggestive of the AAT genotype with associated clinical risks. Serum AAT of less than 0.57 g/L suggests severe AATD, with a high risk of clinical consequences.

Medical conditions associated with AATD include COPD, difficult-to-treat asthma, early-onset lung disease, bronchiectasis, liver disease, panniculitis, and vasculitis. Testing for AATD is recommended in patients with these conditions and in patients who have a family history of AATD. In cases for which a suspicion of AATD exists, serum AAT concentrations and genotype or phenotype should be requested. However, most cases of AATD unfortunately remain undiagnosed due to clinicians' unfamiliarity with the disease or appropriate tests.

It is important to be aware of other causes of abnormal AATD levels. Acute phase response to infection or inflammation, pregnancy, and oral contraceptive pill use can result in increase in serum AAT levels. Liver damage and protein-losing enteropathies can reduce serum AAT concentrations. Measurement of CRP with AAT concentrations is important to rule out acute inflammation/infection, which may cause transient elevation of serum AAT level.

Appropriate smoking cessation advice should be given to patients with AATD to prevent further progression of lung damage.

 Franciosi A, Carroll T, McElvaney N. Pitfalls and caveats in α1-antitrypsin deficiency testing: a guide for clinicians. The Lancet Respiratory Medicine. 2019. https://www.thelancet.com/journals/lanres/article/PIIS2213-2600(19)30141-9/fulltext

2. Answer: D

Amiodarone is associated with multiple pulmonary side effects, which include interstitial pneumonitis, eosinophilic pneumonia, ARDS, diffuse alveolar haemorrhage (DAH), pulmonary nodules and masses, and rarely pleural effusions.

This clinical vignette is consistent with the diagnosis of interstitial pneumonitis, the most common pulmonary toxicity associated with amiodarone use. In addition to the symptoms above, patients may also report fever and weight loss. The onset of the symptoms of interstitial pneumonitis usually develops 6 to 12 months after initiation of amiodarone. However, symptoms of interstitial pneumonitis can happen within two months after initiation of amiodarone or several years after treatment.

HRCT of the chest and upper abdomen usually shows ground glass and reticular opacities and increased attenuation in the lungs, liver, and spleen in patients with interstitial pneumonitis associated with amiodarone use.

Flexible bronchoscopy with bronchial alveolar lavage (BAL) is useful to differentiate between the possible pulmonary adverse effects of amiodarone use. The presence of 'foam' cells (alveolar macrophages full of amiodarone-phospholipid complexes) is suggestive of pulmonary interstitial pneumonitis.

In addition to cessation of amiodarone, patients with moderate to severe symptoms of interstitial pneumonitis are usually treated with systemic glucocorticoids.

In patients with DAH, BAL fluids usually contain haemosiderin-laden macrophages and abundant eosinophils (typically >25%). Patients with bronchiolitis obliterans organising pneumonia (BOOP) may present with clinical symptoms that are similar to that described in this case vignette. BOOP is suspected if the patients are treated for chest infection without clinical improvement. To confirm the diagnosis, a lung biopsy via video-assisted thoracoscopic surgery (VATS) is necessary. BOOP is also a known less common pulmonary side effect associated with amiodarone use.

Amiodarone is indicated for treatment and prophylaxis of serious tachyarrhythmias refractory to other treatment, including VT, AF, and supraventricular tachycardia; it has a long half-life (25 to 100 days) and amiodarone toxicity is associated with duration of therapy and cumulative dose.

Other adverse effects of amiodarone include anorexia, taste disturbance, transient elevation of hepatic aminotransferases, thyroid dysfunction (hypo or hyperthyroidism, iodine-induced thyrotoxicosis, and destructive thyroiditis), photosensitivity, skin pigmentation (blue-grey), reversible benign corneal microdeposits, photophobia, neurotoxicity (tremor, ataxia, paraesthesia, peripheral neuropathy, limb weakness), moderate bradycardia, atrioventricular block, and arrythmias.

Prior to starting amiodarone, it is important to check baseline serum electrolytes, TFTs, LFTs, PFTs, CXR, and ECG. It is also important to correct electrolyte disturbances (hypokalaemia, hyperkalaemia, and hypomagnesaemia) and check QT interval

(< 500 milliseconds), prior to starting amiodarone to avoid arrythmias. If chronic amiodarone use is required, check TFTs, LFTs, and serum electrolytes every six months and monitor CXR and ECG yearly. Due to amiodarone's long half-life, the risk of thyroid dysfunction and liver damage persist for up to a year after cessation of amiodarone.

 Papiris S, Triantafillidou C, Kolilekas L, Markoulaki D, Manali E. Amiodarone. Drug Safety. 2010;33(7): 539–558. https://link.springer.com/article/10.2165%2F11532320-000000000-00000

3. Answer: A

Phenotypic characterisation of asthma has advanced significantly in recent years. The greatest advances in this area are in the mechanisms and treatment of Type 2 asthma – so called as it involves CD4+ Type 2 lymphocytes driving eosinophilic inflammation through interleukins (IL)4, 5, 13 and IgE. This asthma phenotype is characterised by inhaled corticosteroid responsiveness and can be classified further as allergic (accompanied by evidence of atopy), or eosinophilic. In both allergic and eosinophilic asthma sub-types, sputum eosinophilia is an expected finding. These phenotypes have been successfully targeted with monoclonal antibodies targeting IgE (omalizumab), IL-5 (mepolizumab) and IL-4 and IL-13 in combination (dupilumab). Additionally, dupilumab showed efficacy in a randomised trial which included poorly controlled asthmatics with normal eosinophil count (sputum eosinophilia was not reported), but subgroup analysis showed no significant benefit for these patients.

Non-Type 2 asthma is less well defined and therapeutic strategies are less well developed. Broadly speaking, non-Type 2 asthma occurs either as a result of excess neutrophilic inflammation or as a so-called paucicellular phenotype. There is also a group of patients with mixed findings, or in whom neutrophilic sputum reverts to eosinophilic sputum after treatment of infection. Non-Type 2 asthma is usually later in onset, with the neutrophilic phenotype associated with smoking and poor air quality, the hyper-sensitive phenotype often occurring in obese women resulting in frequent exacerbations and poor control. Targeting neutrophilic asthma with therapies aimed at implicated cytokines and mediators such as IL-1, tumour necrosis factor-α, IL-17, IL-6, C-X-C motif chemokine receptor 2 and interferon has not been successful. In such patients, treating infection is important, as is smoking cessation. Weight loss, including bariatric surgery, has shown benefit in treating patients with poorly-controlled asthma and obesity, low dose macrolide therapy may be beneficial in this patient population, and bronchial thermoplasty has been used with some success in some centres. Add on therapy with tiotropium as a mist inhaler form is efficacious in improving lung function and reducing exacerbations. three

 Sze E, Bhalla A, Nair P. Mechanisms and therapeutic strategies for non-T2 asthma. Allergy. 2019. https://onlinelibrary.wiley.com/doi/full/10.1111/all.13985

4. Answer: D

Asthma is a complex disease characteriseds by inflammation and airway abnormalities. Asthma can broadly be separated into two categories: eosinophilic (T-helper 2 [Th2]) and non-eosinophilic (non-Th2). Each category has a different underlying immunobiology. For patients with eosinophilic/Th2 asthma, the disease is typically exacerbated by inhaled 'triggers'. Triggers include allergens, pollutants, and infections that contact with the airway epithelium and induce an inflammatory cascade. This cascade includes multiple cytokines, or cellular messengers, that help coordinate an immune response to a given trigger. Cytokines, such as interleukins (ILs), interact with cells and immunoglobulins to activate eosinophils, mast cells, and leukotrienes, and stimulate mucus and histamine release. The end result for the patient is bronchoconstriction, chest congestion, cough, dyspnoea, and wheezing.

Recently developed monoclonal antibodies, also referred to as 'biologics', target different levels of the eosinophilic/Th2 asthmatic response. No biologic is recommended as a first-line treatment for asthma. They should be considered for patients with eosinophilic/Th2 asthma who do not achieve disease control using oral and inhaler therapies (i.e. those with moderate to severe asthma). No trial has directly compared any one of these drugs with another, so choices between the drugs are largely based on patient biomarkers, cost, and ease of administration. It is impossible to recommend one biologic over another as better therapy at this time.

Omalizumab has a high affinity for IgE and blocks its binding to mast cells, basophils, and other antigen presenting cells. It was the first monoclonal antibody approved for asthma. It is endorsed by the Global Initiative for Asthma (GINA) guidelines as step 5 treatment for moderate to severe asthma in patients with serum IgE levels of 30–700 IU/mL and positive skin testing to at least one perennial allergen. Outcomes studies show reductions in asthma exacerbation rates, emergency department visits, and inhaled corticosteroid dose, along with improvements in symptoms and quality of life.

Mepolizumab is an IL-5 antagonist administered subcutaneously every 4 weeks, and benralizumab is an IL-5 receptor antagonist administered 8-weekly after a 4-weekly run in period. Studies showing proven benefit in patients with moderate to severe asthma and serum eosinophil counts of 150–300 cells/mL, and efficacy is linearly related to baseline eosinophil count. As is the case with omalizumab, the GINA guidelines recommend IL-5 inhibitors as step 5 treatment.

Benralizumab is an IgG1 antibody directed against the IL-5 receptor-alpha (IL-5Ra). IL-5 is a major cytokine responsible for the growth, differentiation, recruitment, activation, and survival of eosinophils. Benralizumab blocks the effect of IL-5 on eosinophils and induces antibody-mediated cell cytotoxicity, causing eosinophil cell death. As a result, eosinophil numbers are reduced in the blood and airways following benralizumab treatment. Benralizumab is indicated for the treatment of severe eosinophilic asthma.

Omalizumab, Mepolizumab, and Benralizumab are the three currently approved monoclonal antibody treatments for severe asthma available on the PBS in Australia. Dupilumab is an IL-4 alpha-receptor antibody that blocks IL-4 and IL-13 and is administered subcutaneously every two weeks. Two recent trials found benefit in patients with asthma. Dupilumab is now approved by the FDA for use in asthmatics. The first trial found a reduction in exacerbation rates and improvements in asthma symptoms and FEV_1, and the second trial proved a reduction in oral corticosteroid use. However, benefits were related to serum eosinophils and were seen at higher counts.

 2019 GINA Main Report – Global Initiative for Asthma – GINA [Internet]. Global Initiative for Asthma – GINA. 2020 [cited 19 February 2020].
https://ginasthma.org/gina-reports/

 Drazen J, Harrington D. New Biologics for Asthma. New England Journal of Medicine. 2018;378(26): 2533–2534.
https://www.nejm.org/doi/full/10.1056/NEJMe1806037

5. Answer: D

Bronchiectasis is a chronic lung disease of heterogeneous aetiology, characterised by chronic cough, sputum production, and recurrent pulmonary exacerbations. It is defined radiologically by permanent abnormal bronchial dilatation. The prevalence of bronchiectasis continues to increase worldwide.

An exacerbation is defined as deterioration from baseline in three or more of the following symptoms for at least 48 hours, and which a clinician decides requires a change in treatment: cough, sputum volume and/or consistency, sputum purulence, breathlessness and/or exercise tolerance, fatigue and/or malaise, and haemoptysis.

Several multicentre trials of inhaled antibiotics do not demonstrate reduction in exacerbation frequency. However, these agents continue to be used in some patients with bronchiectasis. Macrolides exert immunomodulatory effects on innate and adaptive immune responses in a biphasic manner, initially by promoting host defence by stimulating immune and epithelial cells and later by reducing tissue injury by interactions with structural cells, leukocytes, and modulation of transcription factors to promote inflammation resolution. Three well-conducted clinical trials have demonstrated statistically significant reductions in exacerbations.

Effective airway clearance remains the cornerstone of bronchiectasis management. Nebulised saline and mannitol increase hydration of the airway surface, alter mucus rheology, and increase mucociliary clearance. They should be used in patients who have copious sputum production, difficulty expectorating sputum, poor quality of life, and frequent exacerbations despite standard airway clearance techniques. However, recombinant human deoxyribonuclease is contraindicated in bronchiectasis without cystic fibrosis. The large multicentre randomised double-blind, placebo-controlled trial of deoxyribonuclease in non-cystic fibrosis bronchiectasis found a deleterious effect on lung function and exacerbation frequency. The routine use of long-term inhaled corticosteroids and/or long-acting bronchodilators has not been demonstrated to reduce exacerbations and should be avoided unless concomitant COPD or asthma exists.

 McShane P, Tino G. Bronchiectasis. Chest. 2019;155(4): 825–833.
https://journal.chestnet.org/article/S0012-3692(18)32705-3/fulltext

6. Answer: D

Urinary antigen tests (UATs) can be performed to detect pneumococcal capsular antigen from *Streptococcus pneumoniae* infection and antigen from *Legionella pneumophilia*. UATs, along with blood and sputum cultures, can identify the pathogen of community-acquired pneumonia (CAP) in up to 75% of cases. This can lead to narrowing of antibiotic spectrum and consequently limitation of antimicrobial resistance.

UATs are generally considered the most sensitive test, reported as 54-92% in the literature. Hyponatraemia, diarrhoea, fever, and recent travel are strongly associated with a positive *Legionella* UAT, but no characteristics are strongly associated with positive pneumococcal UAT.

Sputum and blood cultures are considered more useful, as they can also identify antibiotic sensitivities. Sensitivities for sputum Gram staining, PCR, and culture are reported variably in the literature anywhere from 20–94%: higher sensitivities are reported among subset analysis of only good quality samples prior to antibiotic treatment. Blood cultures are generally reported as positive in up to 20% of pneumococcal pneumonias.

Viruses now predominate as the most frequent pathogens associated with pneumonia, with *Streptococcus pneumonia* third most common following rhinovirus and influenza. Pathogenesis is now thought to include dysbiosis of the lung microbiome causing aspiration of commensal bacteria into sterile alveoli. The trigger of this may be viral, in which case antibiotics may hinder normalisation of the lung microbiome. Supportive evidence comes from a recent study showing reduced clinical cure rate of 88% vs 91% with 7-day vs 1-day ceftriaxone courses. Furthermore, recent studies suggest up to 15% of patients with CAP can be safely treated without antibiotics when driven by procalcitonin levels.

 Wunderink R, Waterer G. Advances in the causes and management of community acquired pneumonia in adults. BMJ. 2017: j2471.
https://www.ncbi.nlm.nih.gov/pubmed/28694251

 Bellew S, Grijalva C, Williams D, et al. Pneumococcal and Legionella Urinary Antigen Tests in Community-acquired Pneumonia: Prospective Evaluation of Indications for Testing. Clinical Infectious Diseases. 2018;68(12): 2026–2033.
https://www.ncbi.nlm.nih.gov/pubmed/30265290

7. Answer: D

Cystic fibrosis (CF) is an autosomal recessive condition resulting from mutations in the gene coding for the cystic fibrosis transmembrane conductance regulator (CFTR). This protein is responsible for maintaining low viscosity of epithelial secretions by transporting chloride ions out of epithelial cells. There have been hundreds of mutations identified in the CFTR gene, the most common of which is the Phe508del, which results in decreased CFTR transport due to misfolding of the protein leading to retention in the endoplasmic reticulum. Around 50% of patients with CF are homozygotes for the Phe508del gene and another 40% are compound heterozygote with Phe508del and another CF causing gene. Around 10% of patients have a Gly551Asp mutation, which results in impaired gating of a normally inserted CFTR protein. In all, CF mutations are classified into seven groups, with therapies being directed at each of the dysfunctional processes.

Treatment of CF has advanced significantly in recent times, with average life expectancy well into middle age. Symptomatic treatment of the highly aberrant microenvironment caused by CFTR dysfunction has been the main reason for this advance, prior to the advent of directed therapies. Therapies that restore airway surface liquid and mucociliary clearance include inhaled hypertonic saline, mannitol, and recombinant DNase-1. Anti-inflammatories, in particular those directed at leukotriene and neutrophil interactions are currently being evaluated. Anti-bacterial therapy in both nebulised and systemic forms are critical in the treatment and prevention of infection in CF.

Therapies directed at the primary functional deficit of CFTR work at different classes of CFTR mutations. For example, patients with mutations leading to decreased function of CFTR channels, such as Gly551Asp and Arg117His, respond to ivacaftor, which potentiates CFTR function. However, as CFTR is not transported from the endoplasmic reticulum in patients who are Phe508del homozygotes, ivacaftor monotherapy is not efficacious in this patient group. However, in combination with lumacaftor, which partly rescues CFTR transport, ivacaftor has been shown to improve outcomes for this patient group.

 De Boeck K, Amaral M. Progress in therapies for cystic fibrosis. The Lancet Respiratory Medicine. 2016;4(8): 662–674.
https://www.thelancet.com/journals/lanres/article/PIIS2213-2600(16)00023-0/fulltext

8. Answer: D

The patient's prolonged dyspnoea following previous treated PE should raise the suspicion of chronic thromboembolic pulmonary hypertension (CTEPH). CTEPH represents group 4 pulmonary hypertension, characteriseds by organiseds thromboembolic material and pulmonary arteriopathy secondary to defective angiogenesis, impaired fibrinolysis, or endothelial dysfunction. The definition of CTEPH is pulmonary hypertension despite effective anticoagulation for three months, although diagnosis is usually delayed. The incidence of CTEPH after acute PE is around 3.4%. It is associated with right ventricular failure and untreated CTEPH portends poor prognosis with a five year survival rate of 30%.

In patients with ongoing dyspnoea after treatment of PE, it is important to perform a V/Q scan and a transthoracic echocardiogram (TTE) to assess for residual pulmonary obstruction and screen for pulmonary hypertension to rule out CTEPH. V/Q scan is the preferred imaging test for CTEPH screening, with sensitivity 90–100% and specificity 94–100%. Digital subtraction angiography is the gold standard for subsequent characterisations of vessel morphology, however CTPA is more widely used to assess operability.

The patient's poor renal function makes CTPA a second choice as it requires iodinated contrast and could potentially worsen her renal function.

A negative D-dimer result is useful in ruling out patients with non-high clinical probability of venous thromboembolic disease (VTE) in the acute setting. However, it would not be useful in a patient with high suspicion of a chronic PE as the D-dimer levels are likely to be positive. Elevated D-dimer levels are also noted in other medical conditions, such as inflammation, infection, malignancy, trauma, and pregnancy.

Inferior vena cava filter insertion may prevent PE in patients with acute VTE who have an absolute contraindication to anticoagulation, such as active bleeding. It is not recommended in patients treated with anticoagulants for acute VTE.

Pulmonary endarterectomy (PEA) is first line treatment and should be offered to all eligible patients. Three-year survival increases significantly from 70% to 90% with operation.

Around 40% of patients with CTEPH are unsuitable for PEA, for reasons including suspicion of inaccessible vascular obstruction, pulmonary artery pressure disproportionate to pathogenic pulmonary lesions, and significant medical comorbidities. These patients should be offered medical therapy and balloon pulmonary angioplasty (BPA).

- Medical therapy, including phosphodiesterase type 5 inhibitors, oral/inhaled prostanoids, and endothelin receptor antagonists, i.e. macitentan.
- BPA is associated with improved haemodynamic, symptom control, exercise capacity, and right ventricular function.

Tran H, Gibbs H, Merriman E, et al. New guidelines from the Thrombosis and Haemostasis Society of Australia and New Zealand for the diagnosis and management of venous thromboembolism. Medical Journal of Australia. 2019; 210(5): 227–235.
https://www.ncbi.nlm.nih.gov/pubmed/30739331

9. Answer: D

Community-acquired pneumonia (CAP) carries significant morbidity and mortality rates of up to 50% for patients requiring intensive care admission and up to 18% for general hospitalisation.

The most common pathogens are *Streptococcus pneumoniae* (35%) and *Haemophilus influenzae* (12%.) Viruses especially influenzas, rhinovirus, and coronavirus are detected next after *Haemophilus influenza*. However, viruses are often not recognised as a cause of pneumonia in the clinical practice. Atypical bacterium including *mycoplasma*, *chlamydia*, and *legionella* account for about 20% of pneumonias in a large worldwide cohort. Micro-aspiration of bacteria, which usually colonise the nasopharynx and oropharynx of healthy individuals, is the predominant cause of pneumonia. It is a descending process which progresses from the oropharynx to the trachea, to the terminal bronchioles and finally to the alveoli. Less than 5% of pneumonia is caused by haematologic spread from a bacteraemia.

Laboratory evaluation can assess inflammatory state, associated organ damage, and disease severity. NICE guidelines recommend measuring CRP, and not offering antibiotics if CRP < 20 mg/L with no convincing evidence of CAP. Procalcitonin (PCT) measurement can reduce antibiotic exposure and cost of treatment without increase in mortality or treatment failure, when used to discourage antibiotics with PCT < 0.1 and encourage antibiotics if PCT > 0.25.

Microbiology evaluations are recommended for higher risk patients when it will change empiric antibiotic treatment. Nonetheless, the pathogen is still not detected in up to 50% of cases. It is not recommended for every patient admitted with pneumonia. CXR is classically required for definitive diagnosis. However, CXR misses 25% of alveolar consolidation on CT.

Prina E, Ranzani O, Torres A. Community-acquired pneumonia. The Lancet. 2015;386(9998): 1097–1108.
https://www.thelancet.com/journals/lancet/article/PIIS0140-6736(15)60733-4/fulltext

10. Answer: C

The fibrin degradation product D-dimer is most commonly used in the diagnosis of venous thromboembolism (VTE) and disseminated intravascular coagulation (DIC). D-dimer can be used as a surrogate marker of fibrin-based thrombus formation, as any formation of fibrin clot activates plasminogen to plasmin, which breaks down fibrin into its constituent parts. Factor XIIIa is responsible for strengthening fibrin monomers by cross-linking them, thrombin converts fibrinogen to fibrin, and antithrombin antagonises this process.

D-dimer is a sensitive but non-specific test for diagnosis of VTE. D-dimer can also be utilised in risk stratification models to determine optimum duration of anticoagulation therapy after VTE. D-dimer can be used to identify medical patients at high risk for VTE after hospital discharge who might benefit from additional prophylactic anticoagulation.

DIC is characterised by excessive thrombin generation, leading to excessive fibrin production and breakdown, typically leading to very high levels of D-dimer, low fibrinogen, platelet consumption and coagulopathy with elevated prothrombin time. D-dimer has been shown to be of limited utility in predicting stroke in atrial fibrillation and is of limited value in excluding aortic dissection in patients already at low risk for the diagnosis.

 Weitz J, Fredenburgh J, Eikelboom J. A Test in Context: D-Dimer. Journal of the American College of Cardiology. 2017;70(19):2411–2420.
https://www.onlinejacc.org/content/70/19/2411/F4

11. Answer: C

COPD is a progressive inflammatory condition of the airways and lung parenchyma and represents a spectrum of phenotypes. Smoking is the key environmental risk factor; indoor pollution and biomass fuel smoke are significant contributors in developing nations. Genetics and epigenetics also play a large role in the development of COPD, with alpha-1-antitrypsin deficiency the most widely known.

Emphysema is one of the two main types of COPD. Emphysema is characterised by abnormal and permanent dilation of distal air spaces of terminal bronchioles, destruction of alveolar walls, and mild fibrosis. These pathological changes result in loss of respiratory surface area, reduced and altered perfusion, decrease of elastic recoil, and hyperexpansion.

Chronic bronchitis is another type of COPD. Early changes in chronic bronchitis show hypersecretion of mucus in large airways with hypertrophy of submucosal glands in tracheobronchial tree. Later an increase in goblet cells in small airways contributes to airway obstruction due to excessive mucous. Submucosal mucous glands occupy an increasing proportion of bronchial wall.

The clinical features for these two types of COPD are summarised below but note significant overlap does occur.

	Chronic bronchitis	Emphysema
Clinical feature	'Blue bloater' – cyanosis, obesity,	'Pink puffer' – cachexia, hyperinflated chest
Main symptoms	Productive cough	Dyspnoea
Chest signs	Expiratory wheeze, signs of Cor pulmonale	Hyperinflated, reduced breath sounds
CXR	Increased lung markings	Hyperinflation, decreased lung markings, bullae
PaO_2	Markedly reduced	Slightly reduced
$PaCO_2$	CO2 retention	Normal
Spirometry	Decreased FEV_1	Decreased FEV_1
Total lung capacity	Normal	Increased
DLCO	Normal	Decreased
Haematocrit	Tend to increase	Normal

Airway centred inflammation with fibrosis and poorly formed non-necrotising granulomas is a key finding in patients with hypersensitivity pneumonitis. Classic histologic findings in the airway of asthma especially severe asthma include mucous plugging, eosinophilic inflammation and airway oedema, epithelial desquamation and hyperplasia, goblet cell metaplasia, subbasement membrane thickening, subepithelial fibrosis, smooth muscle hypertrophy/hyperplasia and submucosal gland hypertrophy. Charcot–Leyden crystals, an eosinophilic protein crystal, can also be seen.

 Rabe K, Watz H. Chronic obstructive pulmonary disease. The Lancet. 2017;389(10082): 1931–1940.
https://www.thelancet.com/journals/lancet/article/PIIS0140-6736(17)31222-9/fulltext

12. Answer: A

Pulmonary diseases with an eosinophilic infiltrate as the predominant histologically finding (eosinophilic pneumonias) have a wide range of causes with differing clinical syndromes and pathological features. Acute eosinophilic pneumonia (AEP) presents with rapidly progressive respiratory failure with cough and fever. It is proposed to be an immune mediated response to an inhaled precipitant, with fine dust particles, change in smoking behaviour, and heavy exposure to second-hand smoke likely precipitating factors. Radiographically, AEP typically presents with peripheral ground glass infiltrates as seen clearly in the apical section of this CT, and interstitial opacity, seen underlying the ground glass opacity. Pathological diagnosis is best made by biopsy, as the alveolar infiltrate in AEP is usually mixed, whereas the interstitial findings are characteristically eosinophilic. Treatment with corticosteroids is usually very effective.

Other causes of eosinophilic pneumonia are usually more chronic and have differing histological features. Allergic bronchopulmonary aspergillosis (ABPA) usually presents with refractory asthma-like symptoms, elevated total IgE, elevated specific IgG or IgE to *Aspergillus fumigatus,* peripheral eosinophilia, central bronchiectasis, and peripheral infiltrates – although not all features are necessary to make the diagnosis. Pathological testing is not necessary to diagnose ABPA, and findings are variable, with bronchocentric granulomas, alveolar eosinophils, and mucoid impaction all possible. Eosinophilic granulomatosis with polyangiitis (EGPA, previously Churg-Strauss syndrome) usually presents more gradually, with a prodrome of asthma-like symptoms and rhinosinusitis, prior to an infiltrative phase with multiple organ involvement and then a vasculitic phase. Pulmonary infiltrates are common, and histology typically shows perivascular inflammation or frank vasculitis. *S. Stercoralis* lung infection can present either with chronic infection or an asthma-like illness in immunocompetent individuals, or as a manifestation of hyper-infection in immunocompromised individuals. Eosinophilic and *Paragonimus* species usually present with chronic illness and appropriate exposure history. Multiple drugs, including NSAIDs and antibiotics can precipitate eosinophilic pneumonia, as can the hyper-eosinophilic syndrome.

Cottin V. Eosinophilic Lung Diseases. Clinics in Chest Medicine,2016;37(3): 535–556.
https://doi.org/10.1016/j.ccm.2016.04.015

13. Answer: A

There are over 50 different species of *Legionella* bacteria. In Australia, the most common species that are known to cause human disease are *Legionella pneumophila* and *Legionella longbeachae*. *Legionella* are ubiquitous in the environment. They are often isolated from water and wet areas in the natural environment, such as creeks, hot springs, sea water, woodchips, mulch, and soil. Potting mix is often colonised with *L. longbeachae*.

The term given to the severe pneumonia and systemic infection caused by *Legionella* is Legionnaires' disease. Legionnaires' disease is an 'urgent' notifiable disease under the different jurisdictions Public Health Acts. Legionella can also cause a less severe, and self-limiting infective condition without respiratory symptoms called Pontiac Fever.

Legionella are Gram-negative bacteria with strict growth requirements. They do not grow in the normal culture media. *Legionella* are generally acquired through inhalation of contaminated aerosols of water or soils. Micro-aspiration of contaminated water may be an important mode of transmission in certain subgroups, such as intubated patients and those receiving nasogastric feeding. *Legionellosis* is not contagious, with no human-to-human transmission being recorded. The incubation period for Legionnaires' disease is 2–10 days, most commonly 5–6 days. *Legionella* can cause outbreaks from contaminated water sources such as in hospitals or hotels.

Legionella pneumonia is considered an atypical pneumonia, and may manifest several extra-pulmonary features, particularly gastrointestinal and neurological symptoms. Additionally, hyponatraemia, elevation in liver transaminases, and high creatine kinase are often seen in association with Legionnaires' disease.

The *Legionella* urinary antigen test is the most rapid and sensitive test currently available, but will only detect the most common serogroup, *L. pneumophila* serogroup 1. The antigen test may not become positive for up to 5 days into the illness and should be repeated if the specimen was taken early in the illness and Legionnaires' disease is still strongly suspected. Detection of *Legionella* DNA in clinical specimens using PCR techniques is now available in some reference laboratories. The sensitivities and specificities of such tests are variable.

Legionella are intracellular pathogens, and generally respond well to macrolide, tetracycline, and quinolone antibiotics.

Cunha B, Burillo A, Bouza E. Legionnaires' disease. The Lancet. 2016;387(10016): 376–385.
https://www.thelancet.com/journals/lancet/article/PIIS0140-6736(15)60078-2/fulltext

14. Answer: C

Haemoptysis is defined as the expectoration of blood from the lower respiratory tract. It is important to rule out bleeding from the upper respiratory tract (mouth, nose, and throat) and the upper gastrointestinal tract. Mild haemoptysis is usually self-limiting. The definitions of the amount of blood that has to be coughed up for the haemoptysis to count as massive vary between 100 and

1000 mL in 24 hours, but most are in the range between 300 to 600 mL in 24 hours. However, cardiorespiratory compromise is arguably more important than volume of haemoptysis. Common causes of massive haemoptysis include inflammatory disease, infection, and malignancies of the airways.

Careful history taking and clinical examination may provide some pointers to the severity of the bleeding and risk factors of the underlying diseases. The primary blood tests include FBE, coagulation studies, and inflammatory markers. The secondary laboratory tests (e.g. c-ANCA, p-ANCA, ANA, ds-DNA antibody, anti-GBM antibody etc.) are indicated if history suggests the possibility of immunological or vasculitic diseases. Initial imaging studies include CXR in two planes, contrast-enhanced CT, and CT angiography.

Initial management of massive haemoptysis includes application of oxygen, positioning of the patient with the bleeding side down and securing an airway (generally in an intensive care setting with a double lumen endotracheal tube), addressing issues with over-anticoagulation, and treating infection or inflammation. Bronchoscopy is useful to localise the bleeding source and to apply local treatment to stop bleeding.

Bronchial artery embolisation (BAE) is the first line of treatment for haemorrhage from the pulmonary periphery. It is used to treat massive and recurrent haemoptysis and pre-surgically to provide successful haemostasis. Surgery is indicated if BAE alone is not successful, or for traumatic or iatrogenic pulmonary/vascular injury, and refractory aspergilloma.

Small studies have shown that haemoptysis in patients with cystic fibrosis can be controlled by antifibrinolytic treatment with tranexamic acid. However, tranexamic acid on its own may not be sufficient to control massive and recurrent haemorrhage in patients with aspergilloma refractory to BAE treatment.

 Ittrich H, Bockhorn M, Klose H, Simon M. The Diagnosis and Treatment of Hemoptysis. Deutsches Aerzteblatt Online. 2017. https://www.ncbi.nlm.nih.gov/pmc/articles/PMC5478790/

15. Answer: C

Malignant mesothelioma is an aggressive tumour that originates in the serosa membranes that line the thoracic and abdominal cavities. Peritoneal malignant mesothelioma is relatively uncommon, although the incidence has been steadily rising. It can cause ascites, abdominal pain, and occasionally bowel obstruction. In addition to the pleura and the peritoneum, mesotheliomas can rarely occur on other serosa surfaces, such as the pericardium and the tunica vaginalis.

Malignant pleural mesothelioma (MPM) is nearly always associated with prior exposure to asbestos, which may have happened decades earlier. Patients can have fairly extensive tumour involvement by the time they develop symptoms. Common initial presenting symptoms include dyspnoea due to pleural effusion, and chest wall pain. As the disease progresses, patients may experience a 'cancer syndrome', such as lethargy, poor appetite, weight loss, cachexia, fevers, night sweats, thrombocytosis, elevated CRP, anaemia, and hypoalbuminaemia.

There are no validated or recommended screening tools for those patients in high risk categories of developing MPM.

Video-assisted thoracoscopic surgery (VATS) is not only the gold standard for securing biopsy tissue for the pathological diagnosis but it also allows effective drainage of pleural effusion and talc pleurodesis. Medical pleuroscopy can be similarly efficacious allowing biopsy and pleurodesis but can be performed under sedation. FDG-PET CT is a very sensitive modality to detect possible lymph node involvement and distant metastatic disease which will influence a management plan and should be performed where available.

Mesotheliomas can be divided into three histological subtypes – epithelioid, sarcomatoid, and biphasic (mixed epithelioid and sarcomatoid). Epithelioid mesothelioma is the most common subtype (60% of all mesotheliomas) and is associated with better prognosis. Sarcomatoid malignant mesotheliomas represent about 20% of mesotheliomas.

A panel of immunohistochemical markers should be used for pathologic diagnosis of malignant pleural mesothelioma. The immunohistochemical panels should contain positive (mesothelial) and negative (carcinoma-related) markers for malignant mesotheliomas with an epithelioid component and include at least one cytokeratin marker, at least two mesothelial markers and at least two carcinoma-related markers. Cytological yield by examining the pleural fluid in suspected mesothelioma is poor with a sensitivity of only 32%. It is recommended that all patients fit enough should undergo a biopsy to confirm diagnosis.

Validated and reproducible poor prognostic markers for malignant mesothelioma include sarcomatoid histological subtype, poor performance status, male gender, weight loss, chest pain, high standardised uptake value ratios on PET scan, expression of cyclooxygenase-2, expression of VEGF, hypermethylation of the P16^{INK4a} gene, and high serum mesothelin levels.

From diagnosis, the median survival of patients with malignant mesothelioma is 12 months. Currently, there is no curative treatment for malignant mesothelioma. In rare cases of localised tumours, surgical treatment such as extrapleural pneumonectomy can be performed in selected patients. Mesothelioma is sensitive to moderately high radiation doses and radiotherapy is advocated for palliation of symptomatic tumour masses arising from the pleural cavity or metastases in other locations. The administration of prophylactic radiotherapy following pleural interventions in patients with mesothelioma has no significant effect on changing the disease course and is not recommended. Systemic therapy, in the form of combination chemotherapy, pemetrexed and cisplatin (± bevacizumab), demonstrate improved progression free survival compared to single agent chemotherapy. Investigations regarding immunotherapy show promise but further research is required.

Thoracoscopic talc pleurodesis is effective and the first treatment option to control recurrent malignant pleural effusions in mesothelioma, but tunnelled indwelling pleural catheters can also provide symptomatic relief of dyspnoea related to effusions. Multimodality therapy (surgery, chemotherapy, and radiotherapy) may offer some benefit, but further research is required to define the magnitude of this benefit.

 Penman A, Keena V, Candwijk N. Guidelines for the diagnosis and treatment of malignant pleural mesothelioma. Rhodes: Asbestos Diseases Research Institute; 2013.
http://adri.org.au/wp-content/uploads/2018/08/Guidelines-for-the-diagnosis-and-treatment-of-malignant-pleural-mesothelioma.pdf

 Scherpereel A, Opitz I, Berghmans T, Psallidas I, Glatzer M, Rigau D et al. ERS/ESTS/EACTS/ESTRO guidelines for the management of malignant pleural mesothelioma. European Respiratory Journal. 2020;55(6): 1900953.
https://erj.ersjournals.com/content/erj/early/2020/02/20/13993003.00953-2019.full.pdf

16. Answer: A

Narcolepsy is a cause of daytime sleepiness, with a prevalence of around 1 in 2000, but often remains undiagnosed for a significant period of time after symptoms have started. Narcolepsy is a disorder of orexin signalling – in type 1 narcolepsy, where orexin is absent in cerebrospinal fluid, there is an absence of the neurons responsible for secreting orexin in the hypothalamus. Orexin is responsible for inducing wakefulness during daytime and suppressing REM sleep, patients with cataplexy often experience a number of clinical phenomena that are felt to be due to overactivity of the REM state – where vivid dreams occur, and skeletal muscle paralysis is typical. The origin of narcolepsy may be autoimmune – it may be that in susceptible individuals; an influenza or streptococcal infection may induce an autoimmune process leading to damage to orexin secreting neurons. These theories have been fuelled by the observation that anti-streptolysin titres are commonly elevated when symptoms occur, and disease clusters occurring after large outbreaks of influenza. Patients with HLA-DQB1*06:02 are around 200 times more likely to experience narcolepsy that those without, which further suggests an autoimmune cause for the disease. Other genes controlling immune function also influence risk, but not to the same extent. People with type 2 narcolepsy do not have cataplexy and have normal orexin-A levels.

Symptoms that help to distinguish narcolepsy from other disorders causing chronic sleepiness include sleep that is refreshing, sleep paralysis, hypnogogic or hypnopompic hallucinations, and episodes of cataplexy. Sleep paralysis is a phenomenon where a person is unable to move while falling asleep or waking from sleep. Hypnogogic hallucinations are vivid hallucinations where dream-like states blur with reality on falling asleep, hypnopompic hallucinations occur on waking. Cataplexy is a dramatic manifestation of narcolepsy, where the patient, typically in response to a stark emotional trigger, loses muscle tone whilst retaining consciousness – this is highly suggestive of type 1 narcolepsy. Diagnosis of narcolepsy is confirmed by sleep studies, where early REM transition and disrupted sleep cycle is typical, and multiple sleep latency testing the following day, shows a mean sleep latency of ≤8 minutes with 2 or more sleep onset REM periods (SOREMP). Treatment of narcolepsy is partly behavioural, encouraging one good afternoon nap and sufficient night-time sleep, but wake promoting agents or even psychostimulants are often required – cataplexy can be reduced with antidepressants.

 Scammell T. Narcolepsy. New England Journal of Medicine. 2015;373(27): 2654–2662.
https://www.nejm.org/doi/full/10.1056/NEJMra1500587

 Bassetti C, Adamantidis A, Burdakov D, Han F, Gay S, Kallweit U et al. Narcolepsy — clinical spectrum, aetiopathophysiology, diagnosis and treatment. Nature Reviews Neurology. 2019;15(9): 519–539.
https://www.nature.com/articles/s41582-019-0226-9

17. Answer: B

Indications for non-invasive positive pressure ventilation (NPPV) have grown since being shown to be effective for COPD exacerbations resulting in hypercapnic respiratory failure. Since this time, NPPV has become first choice for respiratory failure due to COPD exacerbation, with respiratory muscle fatigue, respiratory distress, and hypoxia despite supplemental oxygen therapy. NPPV has been shown to effectively reduce carbon dioxide levels, increase pH, and increase oxygenation. NPPV also results in reduced mortality and morbidity due to intubation, and ventilator associated pneumonia. Invasive ventilation can be used where NPPV has failed, but also where acute respiratory failure is accompanied by other factors that make NPPV unlikely to be effective including; impaired consciousness or psychomotor agitation, after respiratory arrest, persistent cardiac arrhythmia, haemodynamic instability despite intravenous fluids and vasoactive drugs, inability to clear chest secretions or massive aspiration/vomiting for airway protection.

 Singh D, Agusti A, Anzueto A, Barnes P, Bourbeau J, Celli B et al. Global Strategy for the Diagnosis, Management, and Prevention of Chronic Obstructive Lung Disease: the GOLD science committee report 2019. European Respiratory Journal. 2019;53(5): 1900164.
https://erj.ersjournals.com/content/53/5/1900164

18. Answer: A
The SAVE trial is the largest randomised trial in the management of OSA. Therapy with CPAP plus usual care, as compared with usual care alone, did not prevent cardiovascular events in patients with moderate-to-severe OSA and established cardiovascular disease. CPAP significantly reduced snoring and daytime sleepiness and improved health-related quality of life and mood.

OSA has been associated with multiple risk factors and medical conditions include:
- Obesity
- Congestive heart failure
- Higher androgen levels (male gender, use of androgen supplementation and polycystic ovarian disease, which increase the mass of the tongue)
- Atrial fibrillation
- CKD
- Metabolic syndrome
- Type 2 diabetes
- Treatment-refractory hypertension
- Pulmonary hypertension
- COPD
- Nocturnal dysrhythmias
- Stroke
- Hypothyroidism
- Acromegaly
- Alcohol
- Sedatives
- Opioids use.

Of these, obesity is the most commonly associated risk factor of OSA with the condition reported to be present in > 40% of patients with a BMI of >30 kg/m^2 and in 60% of patients with metabolic syndrome. However, it is important to note that OSA is also commonly seen in patients with normal weight.

Clinical symptoms or signs that should raise the suspicion for OSA include daytime somnolence, fatigue, unrefreshed sleep, poor concentration, poor memory, loud snoring, a large neck, crowded oropharynx, nocturia, dry mouth on awakening, and morning headaches, chocking or gasping in sleep.

OSA is associated with an increased risk of motor vehicle accident (three times that of the general population), arrhythmias (sinus bradycardia, atrioventricular block, and non-sustained VT), hypertension, stroke, coronary artery disease, heart failure, and even death.

In addition to medical history, sleep history, physical examination, and screening questionnaires to suggest a possible diagnosis of OSA, overnight polysomnography in a sleep laboratory is important to measure the frequency of obstructed breathing events. These include:
- Apnoeas – defined as near-complete (90%) cessations in airflow for more than 10 seconds in sleep, despite ventilatory effort, and
- Hypopnoeas – defined as reductions in airflow by more than 30% with concurrent reduction in oxyhaemoglobin saturation by at least 3% or arousals from sleep.

The number of apnoeas and hypopnoeas per hour of sleep is termed the apnoea–hypopnoea index (AHI). The AHI is used to categorise disease severity: persons with an AHI of 5 to 15, 16 to 30, or more than 30 events per hour are considered to have mild, moderate, or severe OSA, respectively.

To reduce the cost of in-lab sleep studies, home sleep apnoea tests have been developed and validated to measure the respiratory-event index (REI). This is calculated as the frequency of breathing events (all apnoeas and any hypopnoeas with oxyhemoglobin desaturation of ≥4%) for the entire recording time with exclusion of events scored because of arousal.

Treatment is recommended for patients with > 15 AHI or REI events and for patients with AHI or REI between 5 to 14 with symptoms suggestive of OSA on top of other coexisting medical conditions, such as ischemic heart disease, or a history of stroke.

Patients with mild OSA who decline or do not tolerate CPAP therapy may be candidates for positional therapy (avoiding a supine sleep position), an oral appliance to advance the mandible, or surgical correction of a collapsible pharynx. Furthermore, maxillomandibular advancement surgical procedures may be beneficial in patients with mild or moderate OSA. A newer treatment option is hypoglossal-nerve stimulation during sleep to move the tongue forward and open the airway. Lifestyle changes such as weight loss, cessation of alcohol, benzodiazepines, and opioids may also improve symptoms of OSA.

Veasey S, Rosen I. Obstructive Sleep Apnea in Adults. New England Journal of Medicine. 2019;380(15): 1442–1449.
https://www.nejm.org/doi/full/10.1056/NEJMc1906527

CPAP for Prevention of Cardiovascular Events in Obstructive Sleep Apnea R. Doug McEvoy et al. N Engl J Med 2016; 375: 919–931.
https://www.nejm.org/doi/full/10.1056/NEJMoa1606599

19. Answer: D

Occupational exposure to silica dust occurs in many industrial operations. Slate workers, stone masons, and miners are exposed to silica dust. Silicosis impairs macrophage function and predisposes to TB infection. In addition to silicosis, silica exposure is associated with COPD, malignancies, other mycobacterial, fungal, and bacterial lung infections. TB risk increases with severity of silicosis, and in acute and accelerated silicosis. Silica exposure increases TB risk even without silicosis. Additionally, active TB at baseline predicts radiological progression of silicosis. Smoking is another aggravating factor. Major morbidities and mortalities result when these epidemics of silicosis, TB, and smoking coexist.

Coal workers' pneumoconiosis is still a major concern in industrially developing countries. Coal dust causes emphysema with nodular fibrosis. Beryllium, which is used in the aerospace industry and in beryllium copper alloy machining, can cause granulomatous pneumoconiosis induced by a delayed hypersensitivity to beryllium, and is clinically indistinguishable from sarcoidosis. Exposure to cotton dust and endotoxins in these sectors is a major health issue with high rates of byssinosis—a progressive respiratory disease characterised by cough, shortness of breath, chest tightness, and airflow obstruction. Exposure to nanoparticles has emerged as a novel occupational exposure because there is a growing demand for engineered nanomaterials of very small dimensions and diverse chemistry. Inhaled nanoparticles contribute to cytotoxic reactions in the lungs. Non-specific pulmonary inflammation with fibrotic changes and foreign body granulomas have been observed among workers occupationally exposed to polyacrylate nanoparticles.

Cullinan P, Muñoz X, Suojalehto H, Agius R, Jindal S, Sigsgaard T et al. Occupational lung diseases: from old and novel exposures to effective preventive strategies. The Lancet Respiratory Medicine. 2017;5(5): 445–455.
https://www.thelancet.com/journals/lanres/article/PIIS2213-2600(16)30424-6/fulltext

20. Answer: D

OSA should be considered in all patients who report sleepiness. Other symptoms such as loud snoring, dry mouth on awakening, and morning headaches support pursuing evaluation for OSA. OSA is associated with increased cardiovascular morbidity and mortality. In addition, OSA is associated with an increased risk of diabetes, obesity, and hyperlipidaemia.

Obstructive apnoeas are defined as near-complete (>90%) cessations in airflow for more than 10 seconds in sleep, despite ventilatory effort, and hypopnoeas are defined as reductions in airflow by more than 30% with concurrent reductions in SaO_2 by at least 3% or arousals from sleep. Collectively, the number of apnoeas and hypopnoeas per hour of sleep is termed the apnoea–hypopnoea index (AHI), in which the presence of OSA is defined as an AHI of 5 or more events per hour. Patients with an AHI of 5 to 15, 16 to 30, and more than 30 events per hour are considered to have mild, moderate, and severe OSA, respectively. Currently, treatment is recommended for all patients with an AHI of 15 or more events per hour, as well as for persons with an AHI of 5 to 14 events per hour with symptoms of sleepiness, impaired cognition, mood disturbance, or insomnia or with coexisting conditions such as hypertension, ischemic heart disease, or a history of stroke. Lifestyle changes are effective in mitigating the symptoms of OSA. Weight loss is most important in patients with obesity. Both evening alcohol and benzodiazepines for insomnia treatment relax the pharyngeal muscles allowing the pharyngeal walls to collapse more easily. They should be avoided in patients with OSA.

Patients with untreated OSA have three times the risk of motor vehicle accidents as the general population. A person is not fit to hold an unconditional licence: if the person has established severe OSA on a diagnostic sleep study or if the person has had a motor vehicle crash caused by inattention or sleepiness; or if the person, in the opinion of the treating doctor, represents a significant driving risk as a result of a sleep disorder. A conditional licence may be considered by the driver licensing authority subject to periodic review, taking into account the nature of the driving task and information provided by the treating doctor as to whether the following criteria are met:

- The person is compliant with treatment.
- The response to treatment is satisfactory.

 Young T. Epidemiology of Obstructive Sleep Apnea: A Population Health Perspective. Am J Respir Crit Care Med Vol 165. pp 1217–1239, 2002
https://www.atsjournals.org/doi/full/10.1164/rccm.2109080

21. Answer: D

The haemoglobin oxygen dissociation curve (ODC) is a graphical representation of the relationship between oxygen saturation and oxygen partial pressure (PaO_2), which helps to understand the process of oxygen delivery to tissues.

The shape of ODC is such that at lower saturations of haemoglobin, oxygen will dissociate more readily and thus be more available for peripheral tissues to uptake. For partial pressures greater than 60mmHg, there is relatively little change in haemoglobin saturation. However, at partial pressures lower than 60mmHg there is a steep decline, often referred to as a 'slippery slope' as small reductions in PaO_2 can lead to a large reduction in haemoglobin saturation. Conversely this can be used to the clinician's advantage, whereby relatively small increases in the partial pressure of oxygen can be used to dramatically increase the patient's haemoglobin saturation.

Several physiologic factors can affect the oxygen dissociation curve by shifting it to the right, thereby decreasing the affinity oxygen has with haemoglobin and increasing peripheral oxygen delivery. These factors include:

- Higher partial pressure of CO_2 (PCO_2)
- Higher acidity (lower pH)
- Higher temperature
- Increased concentration of 2,3-diphosphoglycerate (2,3-DPG).

The effect of PCO_2 is known as the Bohr effect, and is mediated largely by the increased plasma acidity, however some studies have shown PCO_2 to independently affect the dissociation curve. These factors are present in hypoxic states, and thus offer a compensatory mechanism for low peripheral oxygenation.

2,3-DPG is an intermediate metabolite in the glycolytic pathway which binds to deoxyhaemoglobin. Higher concentrations of 2,3-DPG are seen, for example, in chronic hypoxia which shifts the curve to the right and facilitates the extraction of oxygen.

 Collins J-A, Rudenski A, Gibson J, Howard L, O'Driscoll R. Relating oxygen partial pressure, saturation, and content: the haemoglobin-oxygen dissociation curve. Breathe (Sheff). 2015;11(3): 194–201.
https://www.ncbi.nlm.nih.gov/pmc/articles/PMC4666443/

22. Answer: A

Kyphoscoliosis is associated with a restrictive pattern on pulmonary function testing. There is a decrease in vital capacity (VC) and total lung capacity (TLC) in proportion to the spinal deformity. FEV_1 and FVC are proportionately decreased. Hence the ratio of FEV_1: FVC remains normal or is increased.

Functional residual capacity (FRC) is decreased because of reduced compliance of the chest wall. Lung compliance eventually decreases due to progressive atelectasis and air trapping. This reduced compliance increases the work of breathing. In addition, chest wall compliance decreases with age, further increasing work of breathing and risk of respiratory muscle fatigue in elderly patients. Consequently, these patients tend to breathe with lower tidal volumes and increased respiratory rate. Although this breathing pattern decreases respiratory effort, dead space fraction may be increased, and alveolar hypoventilation may ensue with resultant hypercapnia. Hypoxaemia without hypercapnia is also seen in moderate-to-severe kyphoscoliosis, and ventilation–perfusion (V/Q) mismatch has been reported with severe kyphoscoliosis. Pulmonary hypertension develops in some patients as a result of persistent hypoxaemia.

Maximal inspiratory pressure (MIP) and maximal expiratory pressure (MEP) are decreased either because of muscle weakness or mechanical disadvantage from the rib cage distortion.

 Dempsey T, Scanlon P. Pulmonary Function Tests for the Generalist: A Brief Review. Mayo Clinic Proceedings. 2018;93(6): 763–771.
https://www.mayoclinicproceedings.org/article/S0025-6196(18)30282-9/fulltext

23. Answer: D

Light's criteria have been validated to help diagnose the nature of the pleural fluid and aetiology of the underlying lung condition(s). The criteria are sensitive but not specific. Pleural fluid is an exudate if one or more of the following conditions are met:

1. Pleural fluid protein to serum protein ratio > 0.5
2. Pleural fluid LDH to serum LDH ratio > 0.6
3. Pleural fluid LDH more than two-thirds of the upper limit of normal serum LDH.

Causes of pleural transudates:

Very common causes
- Left ventricular failure
- Liver cirrhosis

Less common causes
- Hypoalbuminaemia
- Peritoneal dialysis
- Hypothyroidism
- Nephrotic syndrome
- Mitral stenosis

Rare causes
- Constrictive pericarditis
- Urinothorax
- Meigs' syndrome

Causes of pleural exudates:

Common causes
- Parapneumonic effusion
- Malignancy
- TB

Less common causes
- Pulmonary embolism
- Rheumatoid arthritis and other autoimmune pleuritis
- Benign asbestos effusion
- Pancreatitis
- Post-myocardial infarction
- Post-coronary artery bypass graft

Rare causes
- Yellow nail syndrome (and other lymphatic disorders e.g., lymphangioleiomyomatosis)
- Fungal infections.

Some diseases typically cause exudative effusions, but in certain cases may be transudative: amyloidosis, chylothorax, constrictive pericarditis, malignancy, pulmonary embolism, sarcoidosis, and trapped lung. Additional pleural fluid studies such as cell count, differential, Gram stain, culture, cytology, triglycerides may be required depending on the possible causes of pleural effusion depending on the clinical context.

Feller-Kopman D, Light R. Pleural Disease. New England Journal of Medicine. 2018;378(8): 740–751.
https://www.nejm.org/doi/10.1056/NEJMra1403503

24. Answer: A

This boilermaker's CXR shows extensive pleural plaques. Exposure to asbestos can cause the following asbestos related diseases:
- Asbestosis (pulmonary fibrosis secondary to asbestos)
- Benign asbestos pleural effusion (BAPE)
- Diffuse pleural thickening
- Pleural plaques
- Rounded atelectasis (Blesovsky syndrome)
- Mesothelioma
- Non-small cell lung cancer.

Asbestos is a naturally occurring silicate mineral. There are two major forms of asbestos, the needle-shaped amphibole fibres, and the curly serpentine fibres (or white asbestos). All asbestos is thought to have toxicity, but amphibole fibres are more pathogenic as they can penetrate deeper into the lung and pleura and have a longer bio-persistence. Asbestos was mined and used commonly in Australia from the late 1800s to the mid to late 1900s, leaving a wide variety of potential occupational and environmental exposures. There is a significant delay between exposure and manifestation of disease in the order of decades.

Pleural plaques are the most common benign asbestos related disease. They do not cause any symptoms, as seen in this case. It almost exclusively involves the parietal pleura. These plaques usually occur 20 years later after the asbestos exposure. Pleural plaques are comprised of collagen fibers in an open basket-weave pattern and covered by a layer of mesothelial cells, and they may or may not be calcified. Pleural plaques may grow over time, but they are not a premalignant condition and there is no need for follow up.

Asbestosis is a diffuse parenchymal lung disease, or pulmonary fibrosis related to asbestos exposure. It has a strong dose dependent relation and appears as a usual interstitial pneumonia (UIP) pattern of fibrosis.

Mesothelioma and non-small cell lung cancer are both associated with asbestos exposure. It should be noted that the combination of smoking and asbestos exposure gives a several fold increase in risk (5–20 times relative risk) compared to each individual exposure.

Musk A, Klerk N, Nowak A. Asbestos exposure: challenges for Australian clinicians. Medical Journal of Australia 2016; 204(2): 48–49.
https://www.mja.com.au/system/files/issues/204_02/10.5694mja15.01072.pdf

Harris E, Musk A, de Klerk N, Reid A, Franklin P, Brims F. Diagnosis of asbestos-related lung diseases. Expert Review of Respiratory Medicine. 2019;13(3):241–249.
https://www.tandfonline.com/doi/abs/10.1080/17476348.2019.1568875

25. Answer: C

The patient has a tension pneumothorax with circulatory instability. CXR shows marked rightward deviation of the trachea, heart, and mediastinum. Clinically unstable patients, symptomatic or >2cm secondary pneumothorax patients, or patients with recurrent primary spontaneous pneumothorax (PSP), haemopneumothorax, or bilateral pneumothoraces, should undergo chest tube insertion which is more likely to be successful than needle aspiration. Given his instability, the most likely intervention to succeed and is more likely to resolve the patient's haemodynamic and respiratory compromise in a suitable timeframe is tube thoracostomy. Needle aspiration is suitable for smaller symptomatic pneumothoraces, and observation for asymptomatic pneumothoraces.

PSP occurs in people without clinical lung disease, due to the rupture of small subpleural blebs. The annual incidence of PSP is 22.7 per 100 000 with a sex ratio of 1:3.3 (women: men). It typically occurs in tall thin males between the ages of 10 and 30 years, with peak age in the early 20s and rarely in patients over the age of 40. Recurrences range from 25 to 50%, with most recurrences occurring within the first year. Factors that predispose patients to PSP include smoking, family history, Marfan syndrome, Birt–Hogg–Dubé syndrome, homocystinuria, and thoracic endometriosis. The risk of PSP is proportional to the amount of cigarette smoking, where cigarette induced respiratory bronchiolitis may be associated with PSP development and recurrence.

Wong A, Galiabovitch E, Bhagwat K. Management of primary spontaneous pneumothorax: a review. ANZ Journal of Surgery. 2018;89(4): 303–308.
https://onlinelibrary.wiley.com/doi/abs/10.1111/ans.14713

26. Answer: D

This patient's presentation is suggestive of idiopathic pulmonary fibrosis (IPF). The CXR will rarely be normal on presentation. The main abnormalities are peripheral reticular opacities predominantly at the lung bases as seen in this case. Honeycombing and lower lobe volume loss can also be seen on CXR in advanced cases.

HRCT findings are more sensitive and specific and are a mandatory component of the diagnostic pathway of IPF. The radiological appearance is that of a usual interstitial pneumonia (UIP) pattern of fibrosis. It is characteriseds by peripheral, subpleural reticular opacities in an apicobasal gradient (which refer to the fine network of lines from inter- and intralobular septal thickening), traction bronchiectasis (representing the radial tension of the fibrotic lung on the airways), and honeycombing (small 3–10 mm peripheral clustered cystic airspaces). Ground-glass opacities can be found but should be less extensive than reticular abnormalities. UIP fibrosis is not pathognomonic for IPF, and other causes of pulmonary fibrosis should be sought such as asbestosis or connective tissue disease.

IPF is a progressive lung disease with a poor prognosis, with a 4-year median survival. Antifibrotic agents (pirfenidone and nintedanib) have been shown to reduce decline in lung function, and potentially a mortality benefit.

Physical examination of most patients with IPF will reveal fine bibasilar inspiratory crackles (Velcro crackles). Digital clubbing is seen in 25–50% of patients with IPF. Pulmonary hypertension is a common complication in patients with IPF, estimated up to 40%

of patients with IPF who are evaluated or listed for lung transplantation have pulmonary hypertension. It is therefore no surprise to find signs of pulmonary hypertension on physical examination which include right ventricular heave, a loud P2 component of the second heart sound, a fixed split S2, a holosystolic tricuspid regurgitation murmur, elevated JVP, and peripheral oedema.

Pulsus paradoxus is an exaggerated fall in a patient's BP during inspiration by more than 10 mmHg. Pulsus paradoxus is caused by the alterations in the mechanical forces imposed on the chambers of the heart and pulmonary vasculature often due to pericardial disease, particularly cardiac tamponade, and constrictive pericarditis. However, pulsus paradoxus may be seen in non-pericardial cardiac diseases such as right ventricular myocardial infarction and restrictive cardiomyopathy. Non-cardiac disease states can occasionally lead to pulsus paradoxus such as severe asthma, tension pneumothorax, large bilateral pleural effusions, PE but not IPF.

 Lederer D, Martinez F. Idiopathic Pulmonary Fibrosis. New England Journal of Medicine. 2018;378(19): 1811–1823.
https://www.nejm.org/doi/10.1056/NEJMra1705751

27. Answer: C

Small cell lung cancer (SCLC) represents roughly 10–15% of all lung cancers and is the most aggressive. It is almost exclusively associated with a heavy smoking history. The location of this cancer is usually central, such as in this case, and patients often have bulky mediastinal lymphadenopathy. A large proportion of patients will present with metastatic disease.

SCLC originates from a neuroendocrine cell lineage and is associated with paraneoplastic syndromes. Commonly these are SIADH with secretion of antidiuretic hormone (ADH), or Cushing's syndrome with the secretion of adrenocorticotropic hormone (ACTH) such as in this patient. Symptoms include weight gain, fatigue, glucose intolerance, hypertension, moon face, buffalo hump, muscular weakness, acne, abdominal striae, depression, decreased libido, and fracture due to osteoporosis. Neurologic syndromes are also seen, such as Lambert-Eaton myasthenic syndrome, or limbic encephalitis.

Biopsy reveals small- to medium-sized, round, or oval cells with a high nuclear cytoplasmic ratio and necrosis. Nuclear features include finely dispersed chromatin with no distinct nucleoli, smudging, and a high mitotic rate.

SCLC can be staged using the AJCC TNM system, however clinical decisions are made on the basis of limited stage (LS-SCLC) or extensive stage disease (ES-SCLC). LS-SCLC can be encompassed into a radiation field, whereas extensive stage disease cannot. Surgery is rarely possible due to the extent of disease. Combined chemoradiotherapy with prophylactic cranial irradiation (PCI) is the treatment of choice for LS-SCLC. Palliative systemic therapy with chest radiotherapy +/– PCI is used in ES-SCLC. The role of immunotherapy In SCLC is still under investigation. Even though it is common to see remission early in treatment, relapse is very common and the prognosis for SCLC remains poor.

 Wang S, Zimmermann S, Parikh K, Mansfield A, Adjei A. Current Diagnosis and Management of Small-Cell Lung Cancer. Mayo Clinic Proceedings. 2019;94(8): 1599–1622.
https://www.mayoclinicproceedings.org/article/S0025-6196(19)30126-0/fulltext

28. Answer: D

This patient has a unilateral pleural effusion, and the underlying cause is likely to be TB as this patient is from TB endemic area with clinical symptoms consistent with TB.

A tuberculous pleural effusion is usually exudative by Light's criteria. Measurement of adenosine deaminase (ADA), interferon-γ or PCR for mycobacterial DNA can be used to establish the diagnosis of tuberculous pleuritis. An ADA level greater than 40 U/L has a sensitivity of more than 90% and a specificity of about 85% for the presence of TB.

A predominance of neutrophils in the pleural fluid (>50% of the cells) indicates that an acute process such as PE, parapneumonic effusion is affecting the pleura. A predominance of mononuclear cells indicates a chronic process while a preponderance of small lymphocytes can be related to tuberculous pleuritis, coronary artery bypass surgery, or cancer. In patients with tuberculous pleuritis the pleural fluid culture is only positive for *Mycobacterium* in <30% of cases. However, the combination of pleural biopsy for histopathologic examination and culture will be positive in about 65% of cases. The yield of bronchial lavage culture is low in the absence of a cough and the absence of pulmonary parenchymal abnormalities on the CXR. The CTPA would not be the most high-yield investigation in determining the underlying cause of the pleural effusion in this case.

 Vorster M, Allwood B, Diacon A, Koegelenberg C. Tuberculous pleural effusions: advances and controversies [Internet]. 2020 [cited 12 January 2020].
http://jtd.amegroups.com/article/view/4221/4848

29. Answer: D

Interstitial lung disease is a term used to capture a large spectrum of chronic lung diseases, most of which are rare, but which result in fibrosis of lung tissue. In many cases, an underlying cause can be found, such as concurrent autoimmune disease, drugs, chronic infection, allergens, and occupational exposure. However, many cases are idiopathic, in that they are not clearly caused by one of these causes and can be termed to broadly as idiopathic interstitial pneumonias (IIP). Imaging findings are important for diagnosis, but also for prognostication and prediction of response to treatment. For example, in a patient with an IIP presentation, a pattern of usual interstitial pneumonitis (UIP) is highly specific for a diagnosis of idiopathic pulmonary fibrosis (IPF), which has a poor prognosis, but may respond to anti-fibrotic medication. Currently, there are two treatments approved for IPF in Australia – Pirfenidone (Esbriet®) and Nintedanib (Ofev®). These drugs are not curative, only slow disease progression, and patients often discontinue use due to severe side effects. UIP is characterised by a subpleural basal predominance of findings, reticular abnormalities, honeycombing and absence of clearly inflammatory features such as alveolitis or consolidation; traction bronchiectasis is consistent with UIP but is not necessary for diagnosis; honeycombing is the main discriminatory feature.

Mikolasch, T., Garthwaite, H. and Porter, J. (2017). Update in diagnosis and management of interstitial lung disease. *Clinical Medicine*, 17(2), pp.146–153.
https://www.rcpjournals.org/content/clinmedicine/17/2/146

30. Answer: C

A patient who presents with significant eosinophilia and poor asthma control despite good puffer technique should be evaluated for other pulmonary diseases that can cause this clinical picture. Apart from Type 2 asthma (i.e. atopic or eosinophilic asthma) four main pathologies unify this combination of clinical issues: pulmonary strongyloidiasis, eosinophilic granulomatosis with polyangiitis (EGPA), allergic bronchopulmonary aspergillosis (ABPA), and chronic eosinophilic pneumonia.

Strongyloidiasis is suggested by gastrointestinal symptoms and urticarial lower trunk rash, and positive serology with peripheral blood eosinophilia confirm diagnosis. Respiratory symptoms typically occur during the pulmonary migration phase of filariform larvae. However, serology can remain positive for years after successful treatment. The typical case scenario for pulmonary strongyloides infection is eosinophilia associated with pulmonary symptoms which worsen after steroid treatment. Wheeze and obstructive deficit can occur in pulmonary strongyloidiasis; however, haemoptysis, breathlessness, cough, and pleural effusion are all possible manifestations.

EGPA is an eosinophilic vasculitis of medium-sized vessels that commonly presents in young to middle-aged adults with a history of asthma and allergic rhinitis with worsening respiratory symptoms. Eosinophil granulomas in infected tissue are the most characteristic finding, but other common manifestations include mononeuropathy, polyneuropathy, unfixed pulmonary infiltrates, renal disease, histological evidence of extravascular eosinophils, ANCAs are present in around 40% of cases. Vasculitis in this disease can cause severe gastrointestinal problems such as peritonitis, pancreatitis, or perforation. Heart and renal disease are poor prognostic signs.

ABPA usually occurs in patients with chronic lung disease (most commonly cystic fibrosis and asthma) who have decreased clearance of aspergillus species from lung tissue permitting germination of fungal spores. Both type I and type III hypersensitivity reactions occur in response to this which leads to further mast cell degranulation increased capillary permeability and immune-complex driven inflammation. Typically causing upper lobe mucous impaction and central bronchiectasis with or without cavitation and pulmonary infiltrates, which may eventually cause fibrosis. Diagnosis is suggested by high *Aspergillus sp*. IgE or IgG, high total IgE, and suggestive clinical and radiological features.

Eosinophilic pneumonia is discussed in detail elsewhere in this text, and can, rarely, present with wheeze and obstructive ventilatory deficit. Hypersensitivity pneumonitis, which in this case is suggested by the bird exposure, is usually a type III hypersensitivity reaction, and therefore eosinophilia is an unexpected finding. Additionally, restrictive deficits with reduced gas transfer are more typically associated with hypersensitivity pneumonitis.

Divakaran S, Dellaripa P, Kobzik L, Levy B, Loscalzo J. All That Wheezes. . . . New England Journal of Medicine. 2017;377(5): 477–484.
https://www.nejm.org/doi/full/10.1056/NEJMimc1613182

31. Answer: G

This patient's clinical presentation is suggestive of DKA. The underlying problem seems to be poor compliance, but other precipitants should be actively searched for especially infection given the history of abdominal pain. A suitable urine specimen should be sent for pregnancy test, microscopy, and culture.

A pH of 7.26 is an acidaemia so a net acidosis must be present. Both the PaCO$_2$ (16 mmHg) and the bicarbonate (7.1 mmol/L) are decreased significantly. This is consistent with the presence of a metabolic acidosis. The lactate level was not measured here so a contribution from lactic acidosis cannot be fully excluded.

32. Answer: E

It is likely that this patient has a chronic respiratory acidosis with low PaO2 hence he is on domiciliary oxygen. The elevated serum bicarbonate is due to renal compensation. Long term oxygen therapy (LTOT) reduces mortality in COPD. It may also have a beneficial impact on haemodynamics, haematological status, exercise capacity, lung mechanics and mental state. To qualify for LTOT (ideally at least 18 hours a day), the patient should have PaO2 consistently < 55 mmHg (SpO2 < 88%) when breathing air, at rest and awake.

33. Answer: F

The clinical presentation is consistent with narcotic overdose which suppresses the medullary respiratory centre leading to hypoventilation and CO2 retention. Renal compensation for respiratory acidosis takes hours to start and days to complete. In this case, there is not sufficient time for renal compensation to develop and increase plasma HCO3. Therefore, the ABG is likely to show an acute, uncompensated respiratory acidosis.

34. Answer: C

The number one differential diagnosis in this case is PE. ABG in patients with PE characteristically reveal hypoxemia, hypocapnia, and respiratory alkalosis; however, the predictive value of hypoxemia is quite low.

35. Answer: B

A patient with salicylate intoxication can have a primary respiratory alkalosis due to salicylate stimulating the respiratory centre causing hyperventilation. The other toxicity of salicylate overdose can be uncoupling of the oxidative phosphorylation leading to an accumulation of lactic acidosis and a resultant metabolic acidosis.

 Kaufman D. Interpretation of Arterial Blood Gases (ABGs) [Internet]. Thoracic.org. [cited 15 June 2020]. Available from: https://www.thoracic.org/professionals/clinical-resources/critical-care/clinical-education/abgs.php

36. Answer: G

This CXR shows lucency within the majority of the peripheral left lung field with a linear opacity at the interface between this and the more opaque lung tissue (visceral pleural white line. This combination is suggestive of a pneumothorax, in this case quite large, although without significant mass effect on surrounding structures.

37. Answer: E

This CXR demonstrates multiple large, well-circumscribed, round pulmonary metastases which is often termed cannonball metastases. The history of significant unintentional weight loss is consistent with malignancy. Metastases with such an appearance are classically secondary to renal cell carcinoma, choriocarcinoma or less commonly prostate cancer, synovial sarcoma, and endometrial carcinoma.

38. Answer: B

This CXR reveals confluent right lower zone opacity, with obscuration of the right heart border (silhouette sign) suggesting right middle lobe pneumonia. The right middle lobe is commonly involved in aspiration pneumonia for the patient who is ambulant or sitting, whereas the right lower lobe is more commonly involved in the recumbent patient.

39. Answer: H

The differential diagnosis for this patient's clinical presentation include PE, pulmonary oedema, ARDS, and hospital acquired pneumonia. However, his CXR is normal therefore the most likely clinical diagnosis is PE.

40. Answer: A

This posteroanterior (PA) CXR is showing many signs of acute pulmonary oedema. There is upper lobe diversion, which refers to engorgement of the upper zone vasculature, which should normally be smaller than the corresponding lower lobe vessels. This finding is more difficult to interpret on anteroposterior (AP) films, where the gravity dependent lower lobe filling is lost. The reticular opacity in the lower zones bilaterally is due to interstitial oedema, and the horizontal linear opacity across the mid-zone of the right lung is due to fluid in the horizontal fissure. The small linear opacities that reach the periphery in the lower zone on the right are Kerley B lines, which are fairly specific for interstitial oedema. There is a left-sided pleural effusion and possibly some left lingular opacity as the left heart border is obscured with decreasing opacity inferior to this. These findings may or may not be due to the heart failure, or may indeed be the precipitating factor for the decompensation (i.e. left lingular pneumonia). There is impression of batwing perihilar opacity.

41. Answer: D

CXR shows a cavitating mass in the right mid-zone. Cavitating lesions can be infective – abscess, septic emboli, TB, fungi; inflammatory – granulomatosis with polyangiitis; or neoplastic – squamous cell cancer, other metastatic cancer. The number, pattern, size, and distribution can be helpful in stratifying between these processes. In a patient with a history suggestive of primary bronchogenic carcinoma, a squamous cell primary is most likely, but other tumours can also cavitate. This patient has AKI, haemoptysis, and a pulmonary cavitating lesion which is suggestive of granulomatosis with polyangiitis.

42. Answer: F

CXR shows a right upper lobe lesion. Given his smoking history, weight loss and hypercalcaemia, this lesion is likely to be a primary lung cancer until proven otherwise.

 Gunderman R. Essential Radiology, 3rd Ed. Thieme Medical Publishers; 2013.
https://www.thieme.com/books-main/radiology/product/1600-essential-radiology

43. Answer: I

This patient's clinical presentation is suggestive of Löfgren syndrome which is an acute form of sarcoidosis. Löfgren syndrome presents with a triad of symptoms; erythema nodosum, bilateral hilar adenopathy and arthritis, typically of the ankles. Patients may also present with malaise and fevers. Löfgren syndrome has a favourable prognosis with complete resolution often occurring within six months.

Sarcoidosis is a multisystem disorder characterised by non-caseating granulomas of macrophages, epithelioid cells, mononuclear cells, and CD4+ and CD8+ T cells. Pulmonary sarcoidosis of the lungs and intra-thoracic lymph nodes is the most common manifestation in up to 90% of patients. Clinical features include cough, shortness of breath, chest tightness, or is asymptomatic. Pulmonary sarcoidosis is staged based on the radiology as described in the table below.

Stage	Radiography	Frequency at presentation	Frequency of spontaneous remission
I	Mediastinal and hilar adenopathy (often bilateral) without pulmonary involvement	40–50%	<80%
II	Mediastinal and hilar adenopathy (often bilateral) with pulmonary involvement	30–40%	33%
III	Pulmonary involvement, without adenopathy	15–20%	33%
IV	Pulmonary fibrosis with lung volume loss, without adenopathy	2–5%	–

Other symptoms are dependent on other system involvement:
- Cutaneous sarcoidosis (33%): papules/ plaques of various colours typically on extremities, head, and neck; subcutaneous nodules which are typically multiple and painless; erythema nodosum, and inflammation of tattoos and scars.
- Ocular sarcoidosis (10–25%): typically bilateral uveitis, which can be anterior uveitis (especially Caucasians, presenting with painful red eye with vision loss) or posterior uveitis and pan uveitis (especially of African ethnicity, presenting with painless visual loss and floaters) or less commonly conjunctivitis, conjunctiva nodules, scleritis, episcleritis, lacrimal gland involvement, orbital mass, and optic neuritis.
- Sarcoid arthropathy (5–15%): inflammatory arthritis, especially of large joints (ankle joint in > 90% of cases) and less commonly polyarthritis of small joints, or arthralgia.
- Hepatic sarcoidosis (5–20%): asymptomatic and non-specific symptoms, with abnormal liver function/imaging.
- Neurologic involvement (3–10%): commonly cranial nerves (II, VII, and VIII), meninges, and parenchyma.
- Renal sarcoidosis (3–20%): classically granulomatous interstitial nephritis, presenting as microscopic haematuria, aseptic pyuria, and proteinuria.

- Cardiac sarcoidosis (1–23%): granulomatous myocardial inflammation which can lead to cardiomyopathy and symptomatic and fatal arrhythmias, especially AV block (>50%).
- Gastrointestinal sarcoidosis (<1%): mucosal infiltration causing mucositis, ulcers, obstruction, and strictures most commonly presenting as epigastric pain.

Sarcoidosis diagnosis requires histopathologic evidence of noncaseating granuloma, suggestive clinical presentation, and exclusion of other causes of granulomas. Treatment is indicated for severe symptoms or severe organ involvement. Oral glucocorticoids are first line therapy, with immunosuppressants and biologics as second line agents.

 Ungprasert P, Ryu J, Matteson E. Clinical Manifestations, Diagnosis, and Treatment of Sarcoidosis. Mayo Clinic Proceedings: Innovations, Quality & Outcomes. 2019;3(3): 358–375.
https://www.ncbi.nlm.nih.gov/pmc/articles/pmid/31485575/

44. Answer: B

Allergic bronchopulmonary aspergillosis (ABPA) is caused by hypersensitivity reaction to the fungi *Aspergillus fumigatus* and primarily affects the central airways. Onset of disease occurs most often in the fourth and fifth decades, and virtually all patients have long-standing atopic asthma. The typical patient has a long history of intermittent wheezing, after which the illness evolves into a more chronic and more highly symptomatic disorder with fever, chills, and/or productive cough. The CXR may show a segmental infiltrate or segmental atelectasis, most commonly in the upper lobes. In the patient with typical symptoms, the branching, finger-like shadows from mucoid impaction of dilated central bronchi are pathognomonic of ABPA.

The disorder needs to be detected before bronchiectasis has developed because the occurrence of bronchiectasis is associated with poorer outcomes. Because many patients with ABPA may be minimally symptomatic or asymptomatic, a high index of suspicion for ABPA should be maintained while managing any patient with bronchial asthma, whatever the severity or the level of control. Complications that result from delay in treatment for ABPA are pulmonary fibrosis, bronchiectasis with chronic sputum production, and severe persistent asthma with loss of lung function.

 Patel A R, Patel A R, Singh S, et al. (April 27, 2019) Diagnosing Allergic Bronchopulmonary Aspergillosis: A Review. Cureus 11(4): e4550.
https://www.cureus.com/articles/19187-diagnosing-allergic-bronchopulmonary-aspergillosis-a-review

45. Answer: E

This patient's clinical presentations are suggestive of cryptogenic organising pneumonia (COP), previously called idiopathic bronchiolitis obliterans with organising pneumonia (BOOP). It is a consequence of alveolar epithelial injury due to an unknown insult and is characterized by the formation of organised buds of granulation tissue obstructing the alveolar lumen and bronchioles resulting in respiratory failure. COP is a pathologic diagnosis that can be idiopathic or be associated with other processes, such as connective tissue disease, drugs, and malignancy. The histopathological hallmark is an excessive proliferation of fibrous tissue within the alveolar sacs and alveolar ducts with extension into the bronchioles. Organised plugs of intraluminal granulation tissue are known as Masson bodies. The granulation tissue has a uniform appearance within the alveolar spaces with preservation of lung parenchymal architecture.

Patients typically present subacute (weeks in duration) with fever, malaise, cough, and dyspnoea. Patients frequently fail empiric antibiotics for presumed bacterial pneumonia.

The CXR findings in COP include patchy diffuse consolidations mostly involving bilateral lower zones. Other findings include migratory, irregular, linear, or nodular opacities and pleural effusions. HRCT of the lungs reveals bilateral patchy peripherally located consolidations or ground glass opacities. These are often asymmetric. Other less common findings include irregular nodular opacities and cavitary lesions. COP should be diagnosed only after exclusion of any other possible aetiology. Flexible bronchoscopy with bronchoalveolar lavage (BAL) is often performed to rule out infections, pulmonary haemorrhage, and malignancy. A targeted lung biopsy (either bronchoscopically, percutaneously or surgically) is often required to make a definitive diagnosis.

The vast majority of patients with COP are treated with oral prednisolone (1 mg/kg per day and weaning over 6 to 12 months) resulting in marked improvement in symptoms. Long-term outcomes when treated is excellent. Spontaneous remissions are seen in about 50% of mild cases.

 Cordier J. Cryptogenic organising pneumonia. European Respiratory Journal. 2006;28(2): 422–446.
https://erj.ersjournals.com/content/28/2/422

46. Answer: G

This patient's history and presentation is classical for idiopathic pulmonary fibrosis (IPF) – an insidious loss of pulmonary function and the absence of signs or symptoms of a systemic process. His biopsy specimen report describes usual interstitial pneumonitis (UIP), which is characteristic of IPF. Besides a CXR, HRCT of the chest and PFTs are useful non-invasive tests to evaluate patients. A diagnosis can be made with or without lung biopsy. The Fleischner Society suggest that lung biopsy is not necessary in patients who are deemed in a multidisciplinary setting to have UIP or 'probable-UIP' pattern fibrosis on CT. When lung biopsies are performed, they need to be correlated with the HRCT findings. Survival is usually two to three years after diagnosis. Although multiple medical therapies have been tried, currently, there are only two treatments approved for IPF – Pirfenidone (Esbriet®) and Nintedanib (Ofev®). These drugs are not curative, only slowing disease progression, and patients often discontinue use due to severe side effects. Lung transplantation is an option, and patients should be referred once the diffusing capacity for carbon monoxide (DLCO) has dropped below 40%. Patients with desquamative interstitial pneumonia (DIP) are usually younger; biopsy in these patients reveals a homogeneous pattern of involvement and characteristic pigmented alveolar macrophages. In patients with Hamman–Rich syndrome, cough, and dyspnoea rapidly progress to significant respiratory compromise. The onset of bronchiolitis obliterans organising pneumonia (BOOP) is more acute, and systemic symptoms such as fever and malaise are not uncommon.

Richeldi L, Collard H, Jones M. Idiopathic pulmonary fibrosis. The Lancet. 2017;389(10082): 1941–1952.
https://www.thelancet.com/journals/lancet/article/PIIS0140-6736(17)30866-8/fulltext

47. Answer: C

Clinical presentations of patients with pulmonary alveolar proteinosis (PAP) can vary considerably. The condition may progress, remain stable, or resolve spontaneously. Some patients are asymptomatic; others have severe respiratory failure. Most patients present with gradually progressive exertional dyspnoea and a cough that is usually unproductive. Diagnosis is made with bronchoalveolar lavage (BAL), which shows grossly turbid exudates in the airways and periodic acid–Schiff (PAS) positive material on pathological examination. Löffler syndrome is characterised by transient and migratory infiltrates on CXR and a predominance of eosinophils on BAL.

PAP is a rare pulmonary disease characterised by alveolar accumulation of surfactant. It may result from mutations in surfactant proteins or granulocyte macrophage–colony stimulating factor (GM-CSF) receptor genes, it may be secondary to toxic inhalation, haematological disorders or it may be autoimmune, with anti-GM-CSF antibodies blocking activation of alveolar macrophages. Autoimmune alveolar proteinosis is the most frequent form of PAP, representing 90% of cases. Although not specific, HRCT shows a characteristic 'crazy paving' pattern. In most cases, BAL findings establish the diagnosis. Whole lung lavage is the most effective therapy, especially for autoimmune disease. Novel therapies targeting alveolar macrophages (recombinant GM-CSF therapy) or anti-GM-CSF antibodies (rituximab and plasmapheresis) are being investigated.

Borie R, Danel C, Debray M, Taille C, Dombret M, Aubier M et al. Pulmonary alveolar proteinosis. European Respiratory Review. 2011;20(120): 98–107.
https://err.ersjournals.com/content/20/120/98

48. Answer: J

Lymphangioleiomyomatosis (LAM) is a multisystem disease of females, characterised by proliferation of abnormal smooth muscle-like LAM cells which cause pulmonary cysts formation, cystic structures in the axial lymphatics (e.g. lymphangioleiomyomas), and renal angiomyolipomas. LAM is caused by mutations of the *TSC1* or *TSC2* genes, which encode, respectively, hamartin and tuberin, two proteins with a major role in control of the mammalian target of rapamycin (mTOR) signalling pathway. LAM occurs sporadically or in association with (30% of cases) tuberous sclerosis complex, an autosomal dominant syndrome characterised by widespread hamartomatous lesions.

Clinically, LAM is characterised by progressive dyspnoea on exertion, recurrent pneumothoraces, abdominal and thoracic lymphadenopathy, and abdominal tumours, including angiomyolipomas and lymphangiomyomas. The pulmonary manifestations of LAM usually predominate. There are no proven therapies for LAM, but an improved understanding of the molecular pathogenesis of the disease has identified several promising molecular targets, such as mTOR. Sirolimus and everolimus, two mTOR inhibitors, are effective in stabilising lung function and reducing the size of lymphangioleiomyomas and angiomyolipomas.

Harari S, Torre O, Moss J. Lymphangioleiomyomatosis: what do we know and what are we looking for? European Respiratory Review. 2011;20(119): 034–44.
https://err.ersjournals.com/content/20/119/034

49. Answer: D

This patient has eosinophilic granulomatosis with polyangiitis (EGPA), previously known as Churg–Strauss syndrome. EGPA is a systemic necrotising vasculitis that affects small-to-medium-sized vessels and is associated with severe asthma and blood and tissue eosinophilia. The cause of EGPA is unknown but is likely due to autoimmune reaction to an environmental agent or drug. This supported by the presence of hypergammaglobulinemia, RF, ANCA, and high levels of IgE.

The American College of Rheumatology (ACR) established the following six criteria for the diagnosis of EGPA. The presence of four or more criteria yields a sensitivity of 85% and a specificity of 99.7%:

- Asthma
- Eosinophilia (>10% in peripheral blood)
- Paranasal sinusitis
- Pulmonary infiltrates
- Histological proof of vasculitis with extravascular eosinophils
- Mononeuritis multiplex or polyneuropathy.

ANCAs are present in approximately 40% of patients with EGPA. Most of these patients are perinuclear-ANCA (p-ANCA) positive (anti-myeloperoxidase antibodies). Other test results include eosinophilia, anaemia, elevated CRP, elevated serum IgE levels, hyper-gammaglobulinemia, and positive RF. On bronchoalveolar lavage (BAL), eosinophilia is evident in 33% of cases. The characteristic pathologic changes in EGPA, found especially in the lung and kidney, include small necrotising granulomas, as well as necrotising vasculitis involving small arteries and venules.

Glucocorticoids alone are usually adequate for the treatment of EGPA. Cytotoxic drugs are necessary in fewer than 20% of patients. Rituximab can be used in the treatment of steroid-resistant cases, as well as for prevention and treatment of relapse. The anti-IgE monoclonal antibody omalizumab has demonstrated a corticosteroid-sparing effect in refractory or relapsing EGPA.

Conron M. Rare diseases bullet 11: Churg–Strauss syndrome. Thorax. 2000;55(10): 870–877. https://pubmed.ncbi.nlm.nih.gov/10992542/

20 Rheumatology

Questions

Answers can be found in the Rheumatology Answers section at the end of this chapter.

1. A 45-year-old woman presents to the emergency department with left-sided hemiplegia. CT brain shows a right-sided lacunar infarct. Her medical history includes SLE, unprovoked pulmonary embolism, unprovoked right lower limb DVT, a transient ischaemic attack and three unexplained miscarriages before 10 weeks' gestation. She is on Warfarin with an INR of 2.5. Her APTT is prolonged and fails to correct on mixing with normal plasma.

   Which one of the following immunotherapies has been recommended as primary and secondary prophylaxis for patients with her condition?
   - **A.** Azathioprine.
   - **B.** Hydroxychloroquine.
   - **C.** Mycophenolate.
   - **D.** Prednisolone.

2. A 43-year-old woman presents with acute pain in the right eye, photophobia, and blurred vision. On further questioning, she reports lower back pain which started gradually around a decade ago with deep pain in the lower lumbar spine and alternating pain in the buttocks. The back pain sometimes wakes her up from sleep in the early hours of the morning. She also has morning stiffness in the lower back for around 45 minutes. There is some improvement of the back pain with exercise but no improvement with rest. She denies a history of trauma, fever, or recent infective episodes. Her temperature is 36.5 °C and vital signs are within normal limits. Physical examination reveals reduced range of movement of the lumbar spine, right eye conjunctival injection, and no nuchal rigidity. There is no pitting of her nails and no rash. There is tenderness on deep palpation in the right buttock area and on pelvic spring. X-ray of her pelvis demonstrated fusion of the sacroiliac joints bilaterally.

   What is the appropriate next investigation to confirm this woman's diagnosis?
   - **A.** Chlamydia and gonorrhea screen.
   - **B.** C-reactive protein (CRP).
   - **C.** HLA-B27.
   - **D.** No further investigation is required.

3. A 38-year-old woman with SLE has been receiving corticosteroid treatment for the past 4 years. Her maintenance prednisolone dose is 15mg/day. She complains of left groin pain and difficulty in walking for several weeks; the groin pain also has occurred at rest for the past few days. She reports no falls or trauma. On examination, she is afebrile; there is limited movement of the left hip.

   Which one of the following is the most likely diagnosis?
   - **A.** Avascular necrosis of the left femoral head.
   - **B.** Left trochanteric bursitis.
   - **C.** Osteoporotic fracture of the left neck of femur.
   - **D.** Severe left osteoarthritis.

4. Which one of the following statements about the role of antinuclear antibody (ANA) testing in the diagnosis and management of SLE is correct?
   - **A.** 95% of SLE patients are positive for ANA.
   - **B.** ANA titres can be used to monitor SLE.
   - **C.** ANA test has a specificity of 90% for SLE.
   - **D.** High level of ANA is predictive of renal involvement in SLE.

How to Pass the FRACP Written Examination, First Edition. Jonathan Gleadle, Jordan Li, Danielle Wu, and Paul Kleinig.
© 2022 John Wiley & Sons Ltd. Published 2022 by John Wiley & Sons Ltd.

5. Which one of the following is **INCORRECT** regarding bone turnover markers (BTMs) in the diagnosis and management of osteoporosis?

    A. BTMs can be used to diagnose osteoporosis.

    B. BTMs can be used to monitor therapeutic response to antiresorptive medications.

    C. BTMs can be used to assess compliance with antiresorptive therapy.

    D. BTMs can help to identify possible secondary osteoporosis.

6. A 52-year-old man presents with a painful and swollen left knee. He has no significant past medical history. Aspiration of the knee reveals calcium pyrophosphate crystals and 20,000/µL leukocytes with 95% neutrophils. The X-ray of his left knee is shown below.

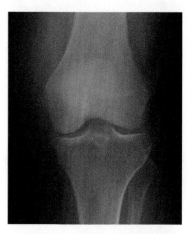

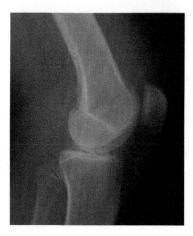

Which additional test should be performed?

    A. Parathyroid hormone.

    B. Serum anti-cyclic citrullinated peptide (anti-CCP) antibody.

    C. Serum electrophoresis and light chains.

    D. Serum telopeptides.

7. A 72-year-old man presents to the emergency department with a 2-day history of acute swelling and pain of his left knee. He had an ulcer on the left toe 2 weeks ago and was treated by his GP for infection. He is a kidney transplant recipient and is taking prednisolone 5mg daily and azathioprine 150 mg daily. He has chronic tophaceous gout (see below) but is not on allopurinol because of the concern of drug interaction. On examination, he is febrile, his left knee is irritable but vital signs are stable. His renal function is stable with serum creatinine 160 µmol/L [60-110]. There is neutrophilia. He undergoes an arthrocentesis.

The synovial fluid leukocyte count is 120,000/μL with 95% neutrophils. Polarised light microscopy examination reveals negatively birefringent monosodium urate crystals. Gram stain of the aspirated fluid is negative. Culture result is pending.

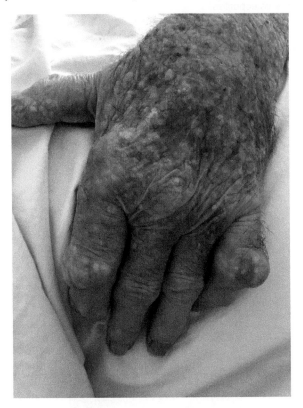

The most appropriate immediate treatment would be:
  A. Increase prednisolone dose to 50mg daily.
  B. Intra-articular corticosteroid injection.
  C. Intravenous ceftriaxone and vancomycin.
  D. Oral allopurinol 50mg daily and reduce azathioprine to 50mg daily.

8. A 40-year-old woman is referred to the outpatient department with gradually worsening proximal muscle weakness over three months. She has a periorbital blue–purple rash with oedema and an erythematous rash on the face, knees, elbows, neck, malleoli, anterior chest (in a V-sign), back, and shoulders and a violaceous eruption on the knuckles (see picture below). Her creatinine kinase (CK) level is markedly elevated.

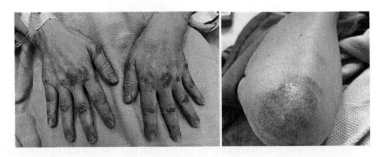

What laboratory test is most relevant to the likely diagnosis?
  A. Anti-3-hydroxy-3-methylglutaryl-coenzyme A reductase (anti-HMGCR) antibody.
  B. Anti-signal recognition particle (anti-SRP) antibody.

C. Anti-transcription intermediary factor 1γ (TIF1γ) antibody.

D. Anti-cytosolic 5'-nucleotidase 1A (anti-cNIA) antibody.

9. Regarding febuxostat and treatment of gout, which one of the following is correct?

A. Febuxostat can be used safely in patients taking azathioprine concurrently.

B. Febuxostat increases cardiovascular and all-cause mortality when compared to allopurinol.

C. Febuxostat is a purine inhibitor of xanthine oxidase.

D. Febuxostat is the first-line medication for gout in patients with stage 4 CKD.

10. You review a 56-year-old woman in the clinic who has a diagnosis of rheumatoid arthritis for the last 17 years, hypertension, stage 2 CKD and hyperlipidaemia. She denies productive cough, weight loss, dysuria, fever and rigors. Her regular medications include methotrexate 7.5 mg weekly, folic acid 10 mg weekly, perindopril 5 mg daily, atorvastatin 80 mg daily, and ibuprofen 200 mg as needed. On examination, her BP is 120/64 mmHg, HR is 80 bpm, respiratory rate is 12/min, SpO2 is 95% on room air and temperature is 36.5 °C. She has ulnar deviation, swan-neck deformity of fingers, Boutonnière deformity of the thumbs, rheumatoid nodules on her elbows as well as splenomegaly. There is no active tenosynovitis.

Tests	Results	Normal values
Haemoglobin	95 g/L	115–155
WBC count	2 x 10⁹/L	4–11
Platelet count	90 x 10⁹/L	150–450
Absolute neutrophil count	0.4 x 10⁹/L	1.8–7.5
CRP	12 mg/L	0–8
ESR	25 mm/hr	1–20
Rheumatoid factor (RF)	300 IU/ml	<14
Anti-cyclic citrullinated peptide antibody (anti-CCP)	40 u/ml	<20

What is the appropriate next step in management of her neutropenia?

A. Administration of granulocyte-colony stimulating factor (G-CSF).

B. Intravenous piperacillin+tazobactam.

C. Observation.

D. Splenectomy.

11. Which of the following classes of medications has the **LEAST** evidence for symptomatic benefit in patients with fibromyalgia?

A. 5-HT2A receptor antagonists.

B. Gabapentinoid anticonvulsants.

C. Non-steroidal antiinflammatory drugs.

D. Tricyclic antidepressants.

12. An 82-year-old man presents with sudden onset loss of vision in his left eye. Over the past three weeks he has experienced left retro-orbital headaches, fatigue, and low-grade temperatures. He also reports that he has been unable to finish meals due to pain when chewing. He has type 2 diabetes and is a current smoker. Fluorescein angiography shows signs consistent with anterior ischaemic optic neuropathy of the left eye. ECG shows atrial fibrillation. Carotid ultrasound shows 50–79% stenosis of the left internal carotid, just distal to the bifurcation. Biopsy of the left superficial temporal artery shows no evidence of vasculitis. Blood tests reveal normocytic anaemia, mild thrombocytosis, an elevated CRP of 94 mg/L [0–8.0 m], and ESR of 82 mm/hr [0–20].

Which of the following is the most appropriate management?

A. Anticoagulation.

B. Carotid endarterectomy.

C. Carotid stent.

D. High dose prednisolone.

13. A 55-year-old man has had progressive weakness of hands, forearms, and lower extremities for 10 years. He has recently noted an increased frequency of falls without dysphagia. He has atrophy and weakness in the quadriceps, forearm muscles, and finger flexors on examination. Deep tendon reflexes and sensory examination are normal. His CK level is 200 [0–250]. EMG shows active and chronic myopathic units. Muscle biopsy shows CD8+ cells invading healthy fibres, widespread expression of major

histocompatibility complex (MHC) class I antigen, autophagic vacuoles, ragged-red, ragged-blue fibres and congophilic amyloid deposits. Ultrastructure of the muscle biopsy reveals rimmed myeloid bodies and filamentous inclusion bodies.

What is the appropriate management of the patient?

A. Intravenous immunoglobulin (IVIG).

B. Methotrexate.

C. Physiotherapy, occupational therapy.

D. Prednisolone.

14. A 65-year-old man presents to the emergency department with bilateral knee pain and X-ray findings of loss of joint space, osteophytes, subchondral cyst, and subchondral sclerosis. Which one of the following treatment options has been shown to lead to less pain and functional disability at 1 year?

A. Intra-articular glucocorticoid injections.

B. Non-steroidal anti-inflammatory medications.

C. Opioids.

D. Physiotherapy.

15. The following right hip X-ray displays radiographic features of which of the following rheumatic disorders?

A. Osteoarthritis.

B. Osteoporosis.

C. Paget's disease.

D. Subcapital femoral neck fracture.

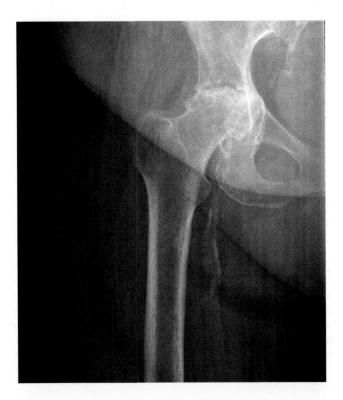

16. A 60-year-old man presents to the emergency department with shortness of breath, abdominal bloating, peripheral oedema, and generalised fatigue. On examination, his BP is 115/70 mmHg, HR is 105 bpm. There is bowing of the femur and tibia, warm and well-perfused extremities, an enlarged apical impulse, a third heart sound, a loud venous hum over the right-sided internal jugular vein, and ascites. Past medical history includes Paget's disease of bone, osteoarthritis, hearing impairment, and a giant cell tumour.

X-ray shows pelvis, bilateral femur, and bilateral tibia involvement consistent with Paget's disease. Additional bony involvement in the vertebrae and skull is noted on bone scan.

Tests	Results	Normal values
Haemoglobin	140 g/L	135–175
Creatinine	90 umol/L	60–110
Alkaline phosphatase (ALP)	250 U/L	30–110
Gamma-glutamyl transferase (GGT)	16 U/L	9–18
Bilirubin	18 µmol/L	2–24
Calcium	2.40 mmol/L	2.10–2.60
25-hydroxyvitamin Vitamin D	100 nmol/L	>75

Which one of the following treatment options is appropriate for his condition?
- **A.** Bisphosphonate.
- **B.** Calcitonin.
- **C.** Cinacalcet.
- **D.** Denosumab.

17. A 77-year-old man presents to the emergency department with a history of neck pain, shoulder, arm, hip, and pelvic girdle pain for 2 weeks. He notices the pain and stiffness particularly in the morning, lasting for > 1 hour. His investigation results are shown below:

Tests	Results	Normal values
ESR	70 mm/hour	Male (>50 years old): 1–15
Fasting glucose	5 mmol/L	3.2–5.5
HbA1c	6.7%	<6.5
Rheumatoid factor (RF)	2 IU/ml	<14
Antibodies to cyclic citrullinated peptides (anti-CCP)	Negative	

Which one of the following initial treatment options is appropriate for his condition?
- **A.** IV methylprednisolone 1 g daily for 3 days followed by oral prednisolone 1 mg/kg daily for 2 to 4 weeks with a tapering regimen.
- **B.** Oral prednisolone 1 mg/kg daily for 2 to 4 weeks with a tapering regimen.
- **C.** Oral prednisolone 15–20 mg daily for 1 to 2 months with a tapering regimen.
- **D.** Oral mycophenolate mofetil 1 g twice a day.

18. A 52-year-old woman has symptoms of dry eyes, dry mouth, lethargy, and joint pain. She also reports recurrent swelling of her parotid glands. Clinical examination finds splenomegaly. Her blood test results are shown below:

Tests	Results	Normal values
Haemoglobin	90 g/L	115–155
White blood cell count	10 x 10⁹/L	4–11
Platelet	80 x 10⁹/L	150–450
ESR	25 mm/hr	< 20
Creatinine	110 µmol/L	45–90
Rheumatoid factor (RF)	23 IU/ml	<14
Anti-nuclear antibody (ANA)	1:80 titre	Negative
Anti-SSA antibodies (Ro)	positive	Negative
C3	0.97 g/L	0.95–1.4
C4	0.02 g/L	0.16–0.32

Which one of the following malignancies is associated with the above condition?
- **A.** B-cell non-Hodgkin's Lymphoma.
- **B.** Breast cancer.
- **C.** Hairy cell leukaemia.
- **D.** Multiple myeloma.

19. A 19-year-old university student has had psoriasis for two years which affects 12% of her skin. She has no symptoms or signs to suggest psoriatic arthritis at this stage. She is studying music and majoring in piano. She consults you regarding the possibility that she may develop psoriatic arthritis in the future which may impact her career.

Which one of the following pieces of advice is appropriate?
 A. About 30% of psoriatic patients will develop psoriatic arthritis.
 B. Psoriatic arthritis only occurs after the onset of psoriasis.
 C. Serum markers can predict the occurrence of psoriatic arthritis.
 D. She has a high chance of developing severe psoriatic arthritis.

20. A 45-year-old woman has a history of systemic sclerosis. She reports pallor and cyanosis in her fingers when it is cold and when she has emotional stress. Her medications include pantoprazole, controlled release nifedipine 120 mg daily, and paracetamol. She reports the side effect of peripheral oedema with nifedipine treatment, which has been stopped today.

What alternative treatment is appropriate for controlling the symptoms in fingers?
 A. Captopril.
 B. Indomethacin.
 C. Pregabalin.
 D. Sildenafil.

21. A 25-year-old man presents to the emergency department with a swollen, red, warm right knee joint. He had a new sexual partner two months ago and had a history of dysuria and penile discharge around four weeks prior to presentation. He denies recent trauma. On examination his vital signs are within normal range and temperature is 36.8 °C. The right knee is tender, swollen, warm to touch and there is evidence of joint effusion. There is no associated rash.

Joint aspiration is performed. The synovial fluid is slightly turbid; WBC count is 25 000 x 10⁶/L with 50% polymorphonuclear leucocyte. There are no bacteria or crystals seen. Initial laboratory investigation results are shown below. The blood cultures and synovial fluid culture are pending.

Tests	Results	Normal values
White cell count (WCC)	11.5 x 10⁹/L	4–11
Absolute neutrophil count	8.1 x 10⁹/L	1.8–7.5
CRP	25 mg/L	0–8
ESR	30 mm/hr	1–10
INR	1	0.9–1.3
APTT	25 seconds	24–38

What is the most appropriate treatment for this patient at this stage?
 A. Colchicine.
 B. Intravenous flucloxacillin and ceftriaxone.
 C. Non-steroidal anti-inflammatory drug.
 D. Prednisolone.

22. Regarding the mechanism of action of rheumatoid arthritis therapy, select the option which correctly pairs the agent with its mechanism of action
 A. Tofacitinib: Janus kinase (JAK) inhibitor.
 B. Rituximab: anti-CD40 antibody.
 C. Abatacept: antibody to TNF.
 D. Etanercept: a T-cell costimulation blocker.

23. A 50-year-old man presents with a three-month history of painful and swelling of bilateral wrists and small joints of his hands. He is diagnosed to have rheumatoid arthritis. His hand X-ray is shown below.

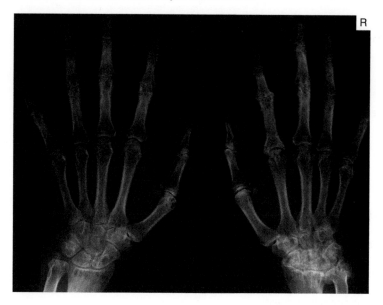

Which one of the following is associated with a good prognosis?
- **A.** Anti-citrullinated protein antibodies (ACPA) positivity.
- **B.** HLA_DRB1*04/04 genotype.
- **C.** The age of onset older than 30 years.
- **D.** The features of his hand X-ray.

24. A 45-year-old woman presents with oliguria, drowsiness, severe headaches and reduced visual acuity. Her medical history includes diffuse systemic sclerosis and hand disability. Current medications include pantoprazole and perindopril. Her BP is 200/100 mmHg, HR is 76 bpm, respiratory rate: 12/min, SpO2: 98% on room air and temperature is 37°C. Her baseline serum creatinine is 75 µmol/L [45–90]. Repeat blood tests today show a serum creatinine level of 250 µmol/L.
Which one of the following autoantibodies is most strongly associated with this clinical presentation?
- **A.** Anti-centromere autoantibody.
- **B.** Anti-RNA polymerase III autoantibody.
- **C.** Anti-Scl-70 autoantibody.
- **D.** A nucleolar pattern of ANAs.

25. A 24-year-old woman presented with a facial rash, fatigue, joint pain, and muscle aches.
Which one of the following statements is true regarding laboratory testing in SLE?
- **A.** An ANA titre of 1:2560 confirms a diagnosis of SLE.
- **B.** ANA and ENA testing should be repeated frequently to monitor disease activity.
- **C.** Detection of an anti-dsDNA antibody and an anti-Sm antibody confirms a diagnosis of SLE.
- **D.** Elevated complement levels are seen with increased disease activity.

26. A 60-year-old woman presents with a six-month history of weight loss, breathlessness, Raynaud's phenomenon, dysphagia, and skin contractures which are impairing her ability to hold a pen and write.
The detection of which of the following autoantibodies would cast doubt on a diagnosis of systemic sclerosis?
- **A.** Anti-centromere.
- **B.** Anti-DFS70.
- **C.** Anti-RNA Polymerase III.
- **D.** Anti-topoisomerase I.

QUESTIONS (27–32) REFER TO THE FOLLOWING INFORMATION

Match each of the following clinical scenarios with the autoantibody that it is most strongly associated with the following clinical scenario:

    A. Anti-Mi2.
    B. Anti-RNA polymerase III.
    C. Anti-Sm.
    D. Anti-SRP.
    E. Anti-SSA/Ro.
    F. Anti-centromere.
    G. Anti-topoisomerase I (Scl-70).
    H. Anti-U1 RNP.

27. Classic manifestations of dermatomyositis with good treatment response.

28. Necrotising autoimmune myositis with treatment resistant disease.

29. Myositis with Raynaud's phenomenon and swollen digits and synovitis of the hands.

30. Scleroderma renal crisis.

31. Subacute cutaneous lupus.

32. Systemic sclerosis with interstitial lung disease.

QUESTIONS (33–37) REFER TO THE FOLLOWING INFORMATION

Which of the following diagnosis best explains the constellation of clinical findings and radiological changes?

    A. Ankylosing spondylitis.
    B. Antiphospholipid syndrome.
    C. Behcet's syndrome.
    D. Kawasaki disease
    E. Polyarteritis nodosa (PAN).
    F. Systemic lupus erythematous.
    G. Granulomatosis with polyangiitis.
    H. Takayasu's arteritis.

33. A 35-year-old man presents with persistent low back pain and morning stiffness for seven months. Both the stiffness and the back pain improve with exercise but return again when he rests for any length of time. On examination, he has restriction of movements in his lumbar spine and flattening of his lumbar lordosis. Lateral compression of the pelvis reproduces pain in his lower back. A soft, 'blowing' early diastolic murmur can be heard at the left sternal edge. There are a few upper zone bilateral crepitations on lung auscultation.

34. A 31-year-old man presents with a two month history of weight loss, malaise, myalgias, and vague abdominal pain. On examination, he is hypertensive with BP 160/95 mmHg. There are several small skin lesions on the lower limbs, as shown in the picture below. He has mild renal impairment with serum creatinine 138 μmol/L [60–110]. His urine sediment is inactive and the urine albumin-to-creatinine ratio (ACR) is 10.5 mg/mmol/L [<2.5]. ANCA, ANA, and cryoglobulins are all negative. While investigating the cause of secondary hypertension, he undergoes a renal artery angiogram which demonstrates multiple microaneurysms involving the interlobar and arcuate arteries.

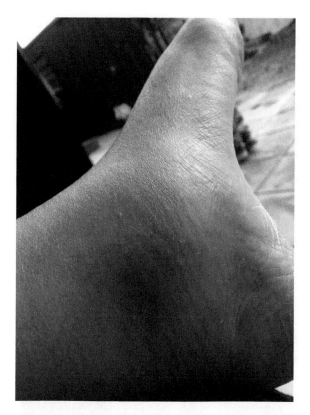

35. A 30-year-old woman presents with a sudden onset of left-sided weakness. An urgent MRI of the head confirms infarction of the right middle cerebral artery territory. She is a non-smoker and there are no other cardiovascular risk factors. She is not sexually active and has no children. She had one previous DVT after an injury to her calf whilst playing netball. She was on warfarin for six months and stopped two months ago. On examination, she is afebrile, BP is 130/80 mmHg, HR is 78 bpm and in sinus rhythm. There is bilateral fine reticular, dusky-coloured rash over the lower limbs. Neurological exam shows left hemiplegia.

36. A 52-year-old Japanese man has a purpuric rash over the lower limbs in the past four weeks. Duplex ultrasound revealed a left lower limb superficial vein thrombosis two weeks ago and he is taking apixaban. He also has a recurrent mouth ulcer despite taking large dose of multivitamin B. He presents to the emergency department today with bilateral acute painful red eyes with blurred vision and light sensitivity. He is diagnosed with uveitis.

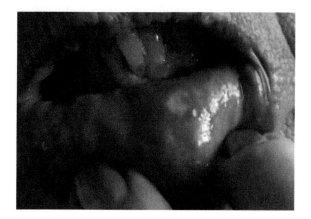

37. A 30-year-old woman is seen in the outpatient clinic because of gradual worsening of pain in the left arm and hand in the past three months. The pain is exacerbated by exercise and she has stopped going to gym. She also feels the left hand is cold and has a 'pins and needles' sensation. She has lost 4 kg of weight despite not going to the gym. On examination, there is no palpable pulse in either the left brachial or radial arteries. You measure the BP from the right arm which is 185/95 mmHg. There is a bruit over the right carotid artery. Her bilateral renal artery MR angiogram is shown below.

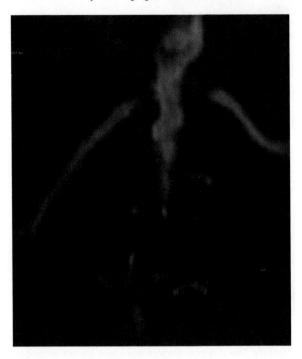

QUESTIONS (38–46) REFER TO THE FOLLOWING INFORMATION
Match the following adverse drug effects with disease-modifying antirheumatic drugs (DMARDs)
- **A.** Abnormal liver function tests, liver cirrhosis, pneumonitis, pulmonary fibrosis, mouth ulcers, alopecia.
- **B.** Rash, haemolytic anaemia, abnormal liver function tests, nausea, headache, oligospermia.
- **C.** Adrenal suppression, diabetes, hypertension, osteoporosis, psychosis, mania, delirium, depression, insomnia.
- **D.** Photosensitivity, haemolytic anaemia, blue–grey skin discolouration, corneal deposits, retinal toxicity.
- **E.** Alopecia, diarrhoea, gastrointestinal upset, hypertension, pneumonitis, peripheral neuropathy, hepatotoxicity.
- **F.** Abnormal liver function tests, myelosuppression, dyslipidaemia, reactivated tuberculosis, herpes zoster, venous thromboembolism.
- **G.** COPD exacerbation, hypertension, injection site reactions, anaphylaxis.
- **H.** Infusion reactions, anaphylaxis, myelosuppression.
- **I.** Injection site reactions, drug-induced lupus, demyelinating syndrome, malignancy, infection, reactivated tuberculosis, exacerbation of cardiac failure.
- **J.** Hypertension, myelosuppression, dyslipidaemia, gastrointestinal perforation, infection, abnormal liver function tests.
- **K.** Myelosuppression (neutropenia), injection site reactions, infection, anaphylaxis.

Questions:

38. Rituximab.

39. Methotrexate.

40. Tocilizumab.

41. TNF inhibitors.

42. Tofacitinib.

43. Hydroxychloroquine.

44. Prednisolone.

45. Sulfasalazine.

46. Leflunomide.

Answers

1. Answer: B

This woman has a likely diagnosis of antiphospholipid syndrome (APS) given her recurrent thromboembolic events involving both the arterial and venous systems. She also has a past medical history of obstetric complications such as frequent miscarriages without obvious explanation before 10 weeks' duration. Despite being on Warfarin with an INR level between 2 to 3, the patient has had another episode of arterial thromboembolism (i.e. an ischaemic stroke) and she has SLE.

Persistent antiphospholipid antibodies (aPL), including lupus-anticoagulant, anti-cardiolipin antibody, and anti-ß2-glycoprotein-1, tested more than three months apart with appropriate clinical features establish the diagnosis of APS. Activation of endothelial and complement systems are important factors in the pathogenesis of APS. Hydroxychloroquine is recommended in patients with a concurrent diagnosis of SLE and APS for primary and secondary prophylaxis. Rituximab has been used to treat non-thrombotic complications of APS. However, more studies are required to recommend the routine use of rituximab in APS.

Other clinical features, such as cognitive impairment (unrelated to stroke), mild to moderate thrombocytopenia, haemolytic anaemia, livedo reticularis, skin ulceration or necrosis, splinter haemorrhage, white matter lesions on brain imaging, valvular thickening or nodules, acute coronary syndrome, glomerular disease, thrombotic microangiopathy, thrombus in atypical sites, a prolonged APTT that fails to correct with mixing with normal plasma (due to the presence of a lupus anticoagulant) may be seen in patients with APS.

Testing for aPL should be considered in patients less than 50 years of age with high risk thrombotic or certain antenatal complications. This includes arterial, venous, microvascular thromboembolic events, or thrombosis at unusual sites. Pregnancy related complications in APS include foetal death after 10 weeks' gestation, premature birth due to severe preeclampsia or placental insufficiency, and recurrent miscarriages before 10 weeks' duration.

Warfarin is recommended for patients with a history of venous thromboembolism (VTE) in the context of APS. Anticoagulation should be continued long-term due to the risks of recurrence of VTE if it is stopped.

There is currently a lack of consensus for the best treatment for arterial thrombosis in patients with APS. A few treatment regimens are suggested by experts to prevent recurrent arterial thrombosis such as anticoagulation with warfarin (INR target of >3), or a combination of aspirin and warfarin with an INR target of 2–3. In patients with a past medical history of an ischaemic stroke and a positive aPL, aspirin and warfarin are equally effective in stroke prevention. Use of direct oral anticoagulants is not supported by current available evidence.

In the rare cases of 'catastrophic APS' where patients have multiple thrombi affecting three or more organ systems, systemic inflammatory response, and organ failure, the mortality rate is as high as 50%. Review of these cases has suggested that the combination treatment, including anticoagulation, high dose steroids, plasma exchange, and/or IVIG, achieved the highest rate of survival in patients with catastrophic APS.

Mezhov V, Segan J, Tran H, Cicuttini F. Antiphospholipid syndrome: a clinical review. Medical Journal of Australia. 2019;211(4): 184–188.
https://onlinelibrary.wiley.com/doi/abs/10.5694/mja2.50262

2. Answer: D

Different criteria have been proposed for the diagnosis of ankylosing spondylitis (AS). Common requirements include the presence of inflammatory back pain for at least 3 months in a patient younger than 45 years, limited lumbar spine motion, elevated inflammatory markers, and evidence of sacroiliitis on imaging. No additional tests are required to make the diagnosis of AS in this patient since there is already sacroiliac joint (SIJ) fusion on plain pelvic X-ray. This is reflective of longstanding sacroiliitis with subsequent end stage ankylosis. Earlier radiographic signs include SIJ space widening, sclerosis, and erosions. MRI showing sacroiliitis has increased the diagnostic sensitivity in the early stage of the disease.

This patient's clinical features are typical for AS with extra-articular manifestations. She has features of inflammatory back pain, which is the primary presenting complaint in the majority of cases. Inflammatory back pain features include her age (<45 years of age), insidious onset, improvement with exercise, worsening with rest and chronicity (> 3 months). The pain often makes patients wake during the second half of the night, with improvement on rising. Alternating buttock pain is also a clue to inflammation and reflects SIJ disease. Acute unilateral anterior uveitis is an important and serious extra-articular complication of AS.

There are no other clinical features to suggest a diagnosis of psoriatic arthritis (e.g. psoriatic plaques, onycholysis, dactylitis, telescoping of the digits) or reactive arthritis (e.g. preceding infections such as enteric of genitourinary infections). As a result, testing for sexually transmitted disease is not necessary.

ESR and CRP are likely to be positive in a patient with inflammatory arthritis and not specific. In most studies, HLA-B27 is present in 85 to 95% of Caucasian patients with AS but in only around 8% of the general population. HLA-B27 can be helpful to increase the confidence of a diagnosis of AS.

Taurog J, Chhabra A, Colbert R. Ankylosing Spondylitis and Axial Spondyloarthritis. New England Journal of Medicine. 2016;374(26): 2563–2574.
https://www.nejm.org/doi/full/10.1056/NEJMra1406182

3. Answer: A

Avascular necrosis (AVN), also known as osteonecrosis or aseptic necrosis, is a pathological process characterised by death of cellular components of bone secondary to an interruption of the subchondral blood supply. It typically affects the epiphysis of long bones at weight-bearing joints. AVN may be primary or idiopathic. Secondary AVN is associated with numerous conditions. Patients taking corticosteroids are particularly at risk of developing AVN. Causes of secondary AVN include:

- Systemic corticosteroid use
- Organ transplant recipients
- Trauma
- Alcohol abuse
- SLE, other connective-tissue diseases
- Sickle cell disease
- Haemophilia A or B
- Osteoporosis medications (i.e. bisphosphonates, denosumab)
- Bone disorders (slipped capital femoral epiphysis, congenital dysplasia of the hip)
- Radiation therapy
- Malignancy (marrow infiltration, malignant fibrous histiocytoma)
- Pregnancy
- Psoriasis
- Inflammatory bowel disease.

The overall incidence of AVN as a consequence of steroid therapy is approximately 4–25%. Patients treated with prolonged high doses of corticosteroids are at the greatest risk of developing AVN. A high index of suspicion is necessary for those with risk factors, particularly high-dose steroid use. MRI is far more sensitive than plain X-ray or bone scan in detecting AVN with a sensitivity approaching 100%. Therefore, MRI is effective in the evaluation of suspected AVN when plain X-ray or bone scintigraphy is negative or equivocal.

Buckley L, Humphrey M. Glucocorticoid-Induced Osteoporosis. New England Journal of Medicine. 2018;379(26): 2547–2556.
https://www.nejm.org/doi/full/10.1056/NEJMcp1800214

4. Answer: A

Approximately 95% of SLE patients are positive for ANA, but the specificity of the test is only 57% for the disease. The positive predictive value of the ANA test for SLE in the general population is poor at 7–11%. ANA titres cannot be used to monitor SLE and are not predictive of renal involvement. Change in titre is rarely clinically useful. Repeating ANA is also rarely clinically useful. ANA is NOT a marker of disease activity.

ANA is non-specific and laboratory dependent. The test is over-used. Do not order ANA testing without symptoms and/or signs suggestive of an autoimmune rheumatic disease (AIRD).

Pisetsky D. Antinuclear antibody testing — misunderstood or misbegotten? Nature Reviews Rheumatology. 2017;13(8): 495–502.
https://www.nature.com/articles/nrrheum.2017.74

5. Answer: A

Bone turnover markers (BTMs) are not used for diagnosis of osteoporosis and do not improve prediction of bone loss or fracture within a patient. Bone mineral density (BMD) test is used to diagnosis osteoporosis. Bone is constantly remodelled to cope with calcium metabolism and to repair microscopic damage in human body. There are two processes involved in bone turnover: resorption and formation which is a tightly coupled process. If there is disruption of the coupling process, there may be an underlying bone pathology. Due to the cost, local availability of BTMs and variation of BTMs assays in different laboratories, they are not recommended for routine clinical use. Blood should be collected fasting in the early morning to reduce variation.

Different BTMs may also be used based on local expertise and availability of the tests. The more commonly used are N-terminal propeptide of type I procollagen (P1NP), beta-C-terminal telopeptide (beta-CTx, also known as beta-CrossLaps) and bone specific alkaline phosphatase (ALP). P1NP is a bone formation marker whereas beta-CTx is released into the bloodstream during bone resorption and serves as a specific marker for the degradation of mature type I collagen. Elevated serum concentrations of beta-CTx have been reported in patients with increased bone resorption. Most of the BTMs are renally excreted, therefore increase in renal failure. ALP level is not affected by renal failure.

In patients taking bisphosphonates or hormone replacement therapy, a decrease of 25% or more from baseline beta-CTx levels 3 to 6 months after initiation of therapy indicates an adequate therapeutic response.

Serum concentrations of the C-terminal telopeptide of mature collagen are more useful in monitoring progress in osteoporosis and in bone resorption in multiple myeloma. A raised concentration has been associated with an increased risk of fractures independent of bone mineral density. Measurement may also be useful in monitoring the response to antiresorptive drugs such as bisphosphonates.

 Coates P. Bone turnover markers. Aust Fam Physician. 2013;42(5):285–287.https://www.racgp.org.au/afp/2013/may/bone-turnover-markers/

6. Answer: A

Acute calcium pyrophosphate (CPP) crystal arthritis, previously known as pseudogout, is an inflammatory arthritis produced by the deposition of CPP crystals in the synovium and periarticular soft tissues. Though acute crystal arthritis is a common finding, there is a spectrum of CPP related disease. According to the European League Against Rheumatism, calcium pyrophosphate dihydrate crystal deposition disease (CPPD) has been proposed as the key umbrella term to include several disease phenotypes that include: asymptomatic CPPD; acute CPP crystal arthritis; osteoarthritis (OA) with CPPD (previously, pseudo-OA); and the chronic CPP crystal inflammatory arthritis (previously, pseudorheumatoid arthritis).

Definitive diagnosis of CPPD is based on the demonstration of CPP crystals in the synovial fluid. Acute CPP crystal-induced synovitis, also called pseudogout is more common in the elderly. Any joint may be involved, but the knees and wrists are the commonest sites. As with gout, the attack is self-limiting. Several provoking factors are recognised, the most common being stress response to intercurrent illness or surgery, including lavage of the affected joint.

The knee X-ray reveals chondrocalcinosis (radiographic calcification in hyaline and/or fibrocartilage) as seen in this case. It is commonly present in patients with CPPD but is neither absolutely specific for CPPD nor universal among affected patients. Haemochromatosis is associated with the full spectrum of CPPD crystal-related joint disease (i.e. pseudogout, chondrocalcinosis, and chronic arthropathy). A variety of metabolic and endocrine disorders other than haemochromatosis are associated with CPPD. Clinical or radiographic evidence for CPPD crystal deposition disease, therefore, warrants exclusion of these disorders, particularly among younger individuals. The following have been associated with CPPD:

- Hyperparathyroidism
- Hypothyroidism
- Haemochromatosis
- Hypomagnesemia and hypophosphatasia
- Familial hypocalciuric hypercalcaemia.

 Rosenthal A, Ryan L. Calcium Pyrophosphate Deposition Disease. New England Journal of Medicine. 2016;374(26): 2575–2584.
https://www.nejm.org/doi/10.1056/NEJMra1511117

7. Answer: C

This patient may have co-existent crystal and septic arthritis. He has an acute monoarthritis of the knee on the background of chronic tophaceous gout and recent foot ulcer/infection. He has fever, neutrophilia, and a markedly elevated synovial fluid leucocyte count. This is highly suspicious of co-existence of crystal and septic arthritis. The presence of crystals on polarised microscope analysis of aspirated synovial fluid does not exclude a concomitant infection. Therefore, until culture result is available, empiric antibiotic treatment should be given.

Septic arthritis is a rare but serious complication of gout and presents a diagnostic difficulty. The injury to the joint from gout, paired with increased vascularity make the knee particularly susceptible to infection. Since both conditions may cause inflammation of the affected joint with redness and swelling, it is difficult to distinguish them from one another. Delay in diagnosis may cause destruction of the affected joint. It is thus important to diagnose these acute arthritides accurately in the initial management.

The diagnosis of septic arthritis in gout patients' rests on maintaining a high index of suspicion. An acutely inflamed joint in gout should also be worked up for septic arthritis. Synovial fluid WBC counts generally exceed 50,000/μL with more than 90% polymor- phonuclear cells (PMNs) in septic arthritis. Though this rule is not definitive, with particularly crystal arthritis able to produce cell counts well up to 100,000/μL. Other clinical information such as fever, recent skin, or soft tissue infection, immunocompromised, and high peripheral blood leucocyte count may be helpful.

Staphylococci or streptococci are the most common pathogens of septic arthritis in elderly patients. Hence, vancomycin is the empiric treatment of choice in immunocompetent patients with suspected septic arthritis whose Gram stain reveals gram-positive organism or Gram stain negative, but culture is pending. Vancomycin plus a third-generation cephalosporin such as ceftriaxone is recommended in immunosuppressed patients with suspected septic arthritis. Oral allopurinol 50 mg daily and reduction in azathioprine to 50 mg daily may be considered after septic arthritis has been excluded and the acute gout attack has settled. The other option, to avoid drug interaction, is to change azathioprine to mycophenolate.

Papanicolas L, Hakendorf P, Gordon D. Concomitant Septic Arthritis in Crystal Monoarthritis. The Journal of Rheumatology. 2011;39(1): 157-160.
http://www.jrheum.org/content/39/1/157

8. Answer: C

Idiopathic Inflammatory Myopathies (IIM) have many subtypes, distinguished by pattern of muscle weakness, CK level, EMG pat- tern, the presence of autoantibodies, interstitial lung disease, skin involvement, and muscle biopsy findings. MRI findings may show myoedema, muscle atrophy, or identify specific muscle involvement for further investigation with a muscle biopsy.

Patients with dermatomyositis may have a typical blue–purple (heliotrope) rash around the eyes, rashes around the face, back, and shoulders (a shawl sign), and a violaceous eruption (Gottron's rash) on the knuckles. These rashes are photosensitive and may be aggravated by ultraviolet light. Patients may also have dilated capillary loops at the nailfold, cracked palmar fingertips ('mechanic's hands'). In patients with the typical skin changes without myopathy, the condition is termed amyopathic dermatomyositis, although subclinical myositis is frequent. Muscle biopsy reveals perifascicular, perimysial or perivascular B cell infiltrates accompanied by CD4+ T helper cells. In patients over 45 years with dermatomyositis and positive anti-TIF-1 γ or anti-NXP-2 autoantibodies, there is an increased risk of malignancy such as ovarian cancer, breast cancer, colon cancer, melanoma, nasopharyngeal cancer (especially in Asians), and non-Hodgkin's lymphoma. Annual workup for malignancy is required in the first 3 years after disease onset due to dermatomyositis' association with malignancy. Sun light avoidance, topical steroids and calcineurin inhibitors may be helpful for skin manifestations.

Polymyositis is clinically and histopathologically distinct from dermatomyositis. Polymyositis has a subacute onset of proximal symmetrical muscle weakness, CK level can also be high and up to 50 times the upper limit of normal in early active disease, without skin involvement. EMG shows active and chronic myopathic units. Muscle biopsy reveals endomysial CD 8+ cells invading healthy fibrese; widespread expression of MHC class I antigen, no vacuoles.

Antisynthetase syndrome is another distinct IIM. The patients present with varying levels of interstitial lung disease, prominent arthritis, fever, and 'mechanic's hands'. Anti-Jo-1 antibodies are the most commonly detected antibody in this disease.

Necrotising autoimmune myositis is a severe IIM. It features acute or subacute onset of proximal weakness. CK level is also very high and can be up to 50 times the upper limit of normal in early active disease. EMG shows active myopathic units. Muscle histopathology demonstrates scatted necrotic fibers with macrophages, no CD8+ cells or vacuoles, deposits of complement on capillaries. Anti-signal recognition particle (anti-SRP) and anti-3-hydroxy-3-methylglutaryl-coenzyme A reductase (anti-HMGCR) autoantibodies are specific for necrotizing autoimmune myositis.

Patients with a diagnosis of inclusion-body myositis has a slow onset of proximal and distal muscle weakness, specific sites of muscle atrophy (i.e. quadriceps and forearms), frequent falls due to quadriceps atrophy, mild facial muscle weakness in people over 50 years of age. CK level can be up to 10 times the upper limit of normal and can also be normal or slightly elevated. EMG shows active and chronic myopathic units with some mixed large-size potentials. Muscle biopsy results reveals CD8+ cells invading healthy fibers, widespread expression of MHC class I antigen, autophagic vacuoles, ragged-red or ragged-blue fibers, congophilic amyloid deposits. Anti-cytosolic 5'-nucleotidase 1A (anti-cNIA) antibody is positive.

Dalakas M. Inflammatory Muscle Diseases. New England Journal of Medicine. 2015;372(18): 1734–1747.
https://www.nejm.org/doi/full/10.1056/NEJMra1402225

9. Answer: B

Gout is a common rheumatological condition associated with hyperuricaemia. It is often observed in patients with CKD, metabolic syndrome, diabetes, and has been associated with increased cardiovascular mortality in patients with coronary artery disease. The aim of gout treatment is to reduce the frequency of acute gout flares, reduce serum urate levels, improve quality of life, and reduce morbidity and mortality associated with gout. The target serum urate level is <0.36 mmol/L in patients with gout and <0.30 mmol/L in patients with gouty tophi. If chronic serum urate level is optimal, there may be reduction of acute gout flares, regression of crystal depositions in the joints and tophi.

Allopurinol remains the first-line medication for treatment of gout including patients with CKD. In patients with CKD, allopurinol should be started at a low dose and escalated to achieve target urate level according to tolerance rather than renal function. Probenecid, benzbromarone, or febuxostat can be used as second-line urate-lowering therapy according to clinical context.

The CARES study noted increased cardiovascular mortality and all-cause mortality with febuxostat when compared to allopurinol. This trial was conducted to help investigate the modestly higher rate of cardiovascular events with febuxostat in its initial development trials. However, the trial was not placebo-controlled, and it is unclear whether allopurinol had beneficial effects on mortality or whether febuxostat had adverse effects on cardiovascular and all-cause mortality.

Febuxostat should be reserved for use only in patients who have failed or do not tolerate allopurinol. Patients should seek medical advice on cardiovascular risks and seek medical attention immediately if there is a cardiovascular event. Febuxostat reduces metabolism of azathioprine and mercaptopurine, increasing the risk of severe bone marrow toxicity.

Allopurinol and its metabolites are structural analogues of both purine and pyrimidines and can affect enzymes in purine and pyrimidine metabolic pathways. They compete with hypoxanthine and xanthine for metabolism by xanthine oxidoreductase (XO), the enzyme responsible for the production of uric acid from purine metabolism. Febuxostat is a nonpurine inhibitor of XO and does not affect the activity of other enzymes involved in purine or pyrimidine synthesis or metabolism. When febuxostat is initiated, a prophylactic medication such as a NSAID, low-dose colchicine, or low-dose prednisolone may be used to reduce the increased risk of acute gout attacks, in much the same light as allopurinol.

White W, Saag K, Becker M, Borer J, Gorelick P, Whelton A et al. Cardiovascular Safety of Febuxostat or Allopurinol in Patients with Gout. New England Journal of Medicine. 2018;378(13): 1200–1210.
https://www.nejm.org/doi/full/10.1056/NEJMoa1710895

10. Answer: C

The patient has chronic and severe rheumatoid arthritis (RA), with neutropenia and splenomegaly. The presence of triad of these findings is suggestive of the diagnosis of Felty syndrome (FS), an uncommon extra-articular manifestation of seropositive RA. Anaemia of chronic disease is common in patients with RA. The mildly elevated CRP and ESR are likely a reflection of the underlying inflammatory condition in this clinical vignette.

Treatment of FS focuses on controlling the underlying RA and treatment of neutropenia to prevent severe infections. If neutropenia improves after treatment of RA with disease-modifying anti-rheumatic drugs (DMARDs) or biologics, this suggests FS. The presence of neutropenia is a necessary clinical feature to make the diagnosis of FS. FS is associated with risk factors such as seropositive RA, positive family history of RA, Caucasian background and HLA-DR4 allele.

Both cellular and humoral immune mechanisms have been implicated in the pathogenesis of FS. The presence of neutropenia is associated with bone marrow infiltration by cytotoxic lymphocytes and increased splenic sequestration.

Patients with neutropenia are prone to skin and respiratory infections. Maintaining oral hygiene and age-appropriate immunisation are important to prevent infections. If there are clinical features suggestive of febrile neutropenia, broad-spectrum antibiotics following a septic screen should be considered and appropriate neutropenic precautions taken. In asymptomatic patients with neutropenia, no treatment is required.

If patients are on a high dose of methotrexate, reduction of methotrexate dose may be necessary to minimise bone marrow suppression and neutropenic complications. In patients with severe neutropenia [Absolute neutrophil count (ANC) < 1 x 10^9/L] with severe and recurrent infections, G-CSF administration is likely to increase ANC within a week and reduce infection risks. In patients with FS who do not respond to medical treatment of neutropenia and have bleeding complications secondary to thrombocytopenia (due to splenomegaly), splenectomy could be considered. This is primarily to minimise the requirement for frequent blood transfusions. Currently there are no randomised control trials for management of FS, the recommendations are based on observational studies.

Patel R, Akhondi H. Felty Syndrome [Internet]. StatPearls. 2020 [cited 22 June 2020]. Available from: https://www.ncbi.nlm.nih.gov/books/NBK546693/

11. Answer: C

Fibromyalgia is a complex disorder characterised by widespread muscle pain, allodynia, and tenderness. Fibromyalgia also effects abnormal sleep rhythm with poorly refreshing sleep and increased fatigue. The disease process is underpinned by aberrant central nervous system processing of sensory input. The syndrome can have high levels of similarity and overlap with chronic fatigue syndrome and other central sensitisation conditions such as irritable bowel syndrome. However, myalgia is often the predominant complaint.

Given the long natural history of the disease, non-pharmacological measures are most appropriate in dealing with symptoms due to fibromyalgia. Non-pharmacological measures with some efficacy include acupuncture, cognitive behaviour therapy, graduated exercise, meditation, mindfulness, and multi-component therapy. In cases where non-pharmacologic measures have failed to improve symptoms, pharmacological management can be considered to improve quality of life. The agents with the most evidence for reducing symptoms of pain and sleep disorder are amitriptyline, pregabalin, cyclobenzaprine (a 5-HT2A receptor antagonist), and duloxetine. Potential therapeutic agents with little or no evidence to support use include growth hormone, monoamine oxidase inhibitors, NSAIDs, SSRIs, corticosteroids, opioids, and sodium oxybate.

Macfarlane G, Kronisch C, Dean L, Atzeni F, Häuser W, Fluß E et al. EULAR revised recommendations for the management of fibromyalgia. Annals of the Rheumatic Diseases. 2016;76(2): 318–328.
https://ard.bmj.com/content/76/2/318

12. Answer: D

Giant cell arteritis (GCA) is a clinical diagnosis that is supported by pathological findings rather than a clinical syndrome with a 'gold-standard' pathological test. The best clinical correlate to biopsy positivity is jaw claudication. In most settings, sensitivity of temporal artery biopsy is estimated to be around 60–70%, although in centres where optimal biopsy practices are used such as large segments sensitivity may be as high as 90%. Additionally, false-negative temporal artery biopsy may occur as a result of issues other than the specimen adequacy. For example, sectioning of the specimen may inadvertently skip the affected artery, or the temporal artery may not be involved by disease. Pathological interpretation can be difficult, particularly if the artery also has intimal hyperplasia due to atherosclerosis.

Diagnosis of GCA can be made on clinical grounds alone. For example, the American College of Rheumatology (ACR) guidelines for diagnosis of GCA require three of five criteria to be met out of age >50, new headache, temporal artery abnormality on examination, ESR > 50 mm/hr, and suggestive temporal artery biopsy. These criteria were revised in 2016 to include other discriminating clinical factors such as history of polymyalgia rheumatica, jaw claudication, unexplained fever, or anaemia. The receiver operator characteristics of the revised criteria could eliminate the need for biopsy in patients with a highly suggestive clinical picture, such as the case above.

The extreme morbidity associated with not treating GCA makes timely steroid treatment the most important. After prednisolone induction, Tocilizumab (an interleukin 6 receptor monoclonal antibody) is now used to maintain steroid free remission, in conjunction with prednisolone.

Banz Y, Stone J. Why do temporal arteries go wrong? Principles and pearls from a clinician and a pathologist. Rheumatology [Internet]. 2018 [cited 7 July 2020];57(suppl_2): ii3–ii10.
https://academic.oup.com/rheumatology/article/57/suppl_2/ii3/4898143

13. Answer: C

This patient has a diagnosis of inclusion body myositis (IBM). IBM is a rare, slowly progressive proximal and distal myopathy that occurs mostly in patients above the age of 50. It classically exhibits distal myopathy of the upper limb. T-cell–mediated cytotoxic effects and the enhancement of amyloid-related protein aggregates by pro-inflammatory cytokines are suggested to cause IBM. However, there is no effective immunosuppressive therapy for IBM, outside of intravenous immunoglobulin (IVIG) in patients with significant oropharyngeal dysphagia. Current recommended treatment is with non-pharmacologic interventions, such as physiotherapy, occupational therapy, and/or speech therapy.

IBM does not affect life expectancy of patients; however, patients with IBM may become wheelchair- or bed-bound and will require walking aids or wheelchair due to lower limb muscle weakness.

Dalakas M. Inflammatory Muscle Diseases. New England Journal of Medicine. 2015;372(18): 1734–1747.
https://www.nejm.org/doi/full/10.1056/NEJMra1402225

14. Answer: D

The X-ray findings are typical of changes of osteoarthritis (OA). In a small single-centre trial in 156 patients with a diagnosis of OA of the knee, patients were assigned to undergo physical therapy (e.g. manual physical therapy and home exercises) or to receive intraarticular glucocorticoid injections. Patients in the physical therapy group had less pain and functional disability at 1 year, compared to patients in the glucocorticoid injection group. It was also found that there were fewer patients that underwent knee replacement in the physical therapy group compared to patients who received intraarticular glucocorticoid injections. However, the results do not exclude the benefits of intraarticular glucocorticoid injections. The studies suggest that intraarticular glucocorticoids although convenient, should not be used in place of physical therapy or as the initial treatment for knee OA. The generalisability of the conclusions may be limited because of a small number of patients a single-centre format. The effect of NSAID treatment in OA decreases with time, there is no evidence to support NSAID therapy beyond three months in OA not to mention their side effects.

Deyle G, Allen C, Allison S, Gill N, Hando B, Petersen E et al. Physical Therapy versus Glucocorticoid Injection for Osteoarthritis of the Knee. New England Journal of Medicine. 2020;382(15): 1420–1429.
https://www.nejm.org/doi/full/10.1056/NEJMoa1905877

15. Answer: A

Osteoarthritis of the hip can be graded according to the features on plain X-ray.

- Grade 0: Normal
- Grade 1: Possible joint space narrowing and subtle osteophytes
- Grade 2: Definite joint space narrowing, defined osteophytes, and some sclerosis, especially in the acetabular region
- Grade 3: Marked joint space narrowing, small osteophytes, some sclerosis, cyst formation and deformity of femoral head and acetabulum. The above X-ray has these features.
- Grade 4: Gross loss of joint space with above features plus large osteophytes and increased deformity of the femoral head and acetabulum

The plain X-ray features of osteoporosis include decreased cortical thickness and loss of bony trabeculae. Vertebrae, proximal femur, calcaneum and tubular bones are examined for evidence of osteoporosis. Nevertheless, dual energy X-ray absorptiometry (DEXA) is the recommended imaging technique for diagnosing osteoporosis. The classical plain X-ray appearances of Paget's disease are expanded bone with a coarsened trabecular pattern. The pelvis, spine, skull, and proximal long bones are most frequently affected. There is no evidence of subcapital femoral neck fracture in this X-ray.

Hunter D, Bierma-Zeinstra S. Osteoarthritis. The Lancet. 2019;393(10182): 1745–1759.
https://www.thelancet.com/journals/lancet/article/PIIS0140-6736(19)30417-9/fulltext

16. Answer: A

This patient has extensive skeletal involvement secondary to Paget's disease, also known as osteitis deformans. Accelerated bone remodelling results in overgrowth of bone at selected sites and impaired integrity of affected bone. It is believed to be a disease of the osteoclasts. The patient's presenting symptoms are consistent with high output cardiac failure and low peripheral vascular resistance which can occur in patients with severe Paget's disease, current guidelines suggest treatment with a bisphosphonate. In patients with normal liver and biliary tract function, ALP can be used to monitor treatment effect. However, in patients with abnormal liver and biliary tract function, other bone turnover markers may be used to monitor treatment depending on the availability of the tests and cost.

Intravenous zoledronic acid is recommended as a first line treatment for patients with creatinine clearance > 30 mL/min and is usually very well tolerated. A single dose often induces a long-lasting remission. In patients who are intolerant of IV or oral bisphosphonate, calcitonin is recommended.

Singer F, Bone H, Hosking D, Lyles K, Murad M, Reid I et al. Paget's Disease of Bone: An Endocrine Society Clinical Practice Guideline. The Journal of Clinical Endocrinology & Metabolism. 2014;99(12): 4408–4422.
https://academic.oup.com/jcem/article/99/12/4408/2833929

17. Answer: C

This man has typical symptoms of polymyalgia rheumatica (PMR) with pain in the neck, both shoulders, bilateral upper arms, hips, and pelvic girdle that is worse in the morning. Serological tests suggest a diagnosis of rheumatoid arthritis is unlikely.

Up to 20% of patients with PMR develop giant cell arteritis (GCA). Conversely up to 50% of patients with GCA report PMR symptoms. The diagnosis of GCA should be confirmed with a temporal artery biopsy when possible and typical histologic findings include panarteritis with CD4+ and macrophage infiltration. Arteritic ischaemic optic neuropathy can cause irreversible vision loss in 10 – 15% of patients and should be treated as an emergency. Prompt temporal artery biopsy to confirm the diagnosis of GCA is imperative.

Current treatment recommendations are based on clinical experience. Steroids are the mainstay of treatment for GCA and PMR as they suppress IL-6. In patients with PMR, the recommended oral prednisolone dose is 15–20 mg daily for 1 to 2 months then tapers the dose down by 20% every month. In patients with GCA with unstable supply of blood to the eyes or the central nervous system, patients require IV methylprednisolone 1 g daily for three consecutive days to optimise immunosuppression and reduce tissue oedema. Once tissue necrosis occurs, the visual loss is irreversible. After IV methylprednisolone treatment is completed, commence oral prednisolone at 1 mg/kg daily for two to three weeks then taper the prednisolone dose down by 10–20% every month. When prednisolone dose is <10 mg/day for both GCA and PMR, prednisolone dose is tapered down slowly by 1 mg per month. Relapses of both diseases are common during the tapering of prednisolone and often respond to 10–20% increase in steroid dose. Currently there is not enough evidence to use steroid-sparing agents as induction therapy for both conditions.

Weyand C, Goronzy J. Giant-Cell Arteritis and Polymyalgia Rheumatica. New England Journal of Medicine. 2014;371(1): 50–57.
https://www.nejm.org/doi/pdf/10.1056/NEJMcp1214825

18. Answer: A

The presenting symptoms are suspicious of a diagnosis of Sjögren's syndrome, which is confirmed with positive anti-SSA (Ro) antibodies. Primary Sjögren's syndrome is associated with B-cell lymphoma (15–20 times higher compared to the general population). It is likely due to chronic activation of B-cells in Sjögren's syndrome. Lymphoma is commonly found in salivary glands or as primarily mucosa-associated lymphoid tissue (MALT) lymphomas. Hairy cell leukaemia (HCL) is recognised as a clonal B-cell malignancy, as identified by immunoglobulin gene rearrangements that result in a phenotype B-cell expression of surface antigens. These reflect the differentiation between the immature B-cell of chronic lymphocytic leukaemia and the plasma cell of multiple myeloma. HCL is associated with systemic immunologic disorders such as scleroderma, polymyositis, polyarteritis nodosa but there is no observed association between Sjögren's syndrome and HCL.

Factors are associated with increased risk of lymphoma in patients with primary Sjögren's syndrome include recurrent swelling of the parotid glands, splenomegaly, lymphadenopathy, purpura, score of > 5 on the EULAR Sjögren's Syndrome Disease Activity Index (ESSDAI), rheumatoid factor positivity, cyroglobulinaemia, low C4 level, CD4 T-cell lymphocytopenia, presence of ectopic germinal centres, focus score (the number of mononuclear-cell infiltrates containing at least 50 inflammatory cells per 4 mm^2 of labial salivary gland obtained on biopsy) and germinal mutations in TNFAIP3.

Surveillance blood tests are recommended every one to two years and every six months in patients with higher risks of developing lymphoma. This includes lymphocyte count, serum protein electrophoresis, rheumatoid factor, C3 and C4, and cryoglobulin. If lymphoma is suspected PET scan may be helpful to identify lymphoma. Tissue biopsy is required to confirm the diagnosis of lymphoma.

Mariette X, Criswell L. Primary Sjögren's Syndrome. New England Journal of Medicine. 2018;378(10): 931–939.
https://www.nejm.org/doi/10.1056/NEJMcp1702514

19. Answer: A

Psoriatic arthritis is a chronic seronegative inflammatory arthritis associated with psoriasis. Therefore, there are no serum markers can predict the occurrence of psoriatic arthritis or diagnose it; and thus, it is a clinical diagnosis. Psoriatic arthritis affects 20–35% of cutaneous psoriasis patients. The onset of psoriatic arthritis occurs after onset of psoriasis in about 60–85% of affected patients. There is no correlation between severity of psoriasis and severity of psoriatic arthritis; however, the incidence of psoriatic arthritis is higher in patients with severe psoriasis. This patient does have severe psoriasis as >10% of her skin has been affected (mild <3%, Moderate 3–10%).

Reference: Psoriatic Arthritis. Ritchlin CT, Colbert RA, Gladman DD. (2017) N Engl J Med 2017;376:957–70.

20. Answer: D

Raynaud's phenomenon is a condition resulting in discolouration of fingers and/or toes when a person is exposed to cold or emotional stress. At least biphasic (pallor or cyanosis) change in skin colour is required. Primary Raynaud's phenomenon is diagnosed when no underlying disease is found. Secondary Raynaud's phenomenon is associated with connective tissue diseases, such as scleroderma, SLE, dermatomyositis, Sjögren's syndrome, mixed connective tissue disease; cryoglobulins, paraneoplastic disorder, cold agglutinin, hypothyroidism, carpal tunnel syndrome, vibration exposure, frostbite, sympathomimetic disorder, interferon alfa-2b, ergotamine and chemotherapeutic agents.

Smoking, use of sympathomimetic medications, medications for migraine treatment and for attention deficit-hyperactivity disorder, should be avoided since they can worsen the symptoms of Raynaud's phenomenon.

Exposure to cold and stress causes the release of noradrenaline and can induce sympathetic vasoconstriction by acting on cold-sensitive α2-adrenoceptors. Endothelial dysfunction is present in patients with secondary Raynaud's phenomenon, but not in primary Raynaud's phenomenon. Endothelial dysfunction is associated with reduced activity of nitric oxide (NO) and increased expression and release of endothelin-1 (ET-1), leading to vasoconstriction.

The avoidance of cold is the most effective treatment for any cause of Raynaud's phenomenon. Systemic (with layered clothing, avoiding rapidly changing temperature and cold) and local warming (with gloves and rubbing the hands in warm water) can increase blood flow in the skin.

First-line pharmacotherapy includes low-dose sustained release dihydropyridine-class calcium-channel blocker (CCB) (nifedipine, amlodipine, felodipine) and titration of the dose up as required. If patients are unable to tolerate CCB, a phosphodiesterase type 5 (PDE-5), such as sildenafil or topical nitrate can be used. In patients with repeated digital ischaemic lesions, prostanoids (e.g. iloprost) or botulinum toxin injection, or both are treatment options. In patients with recurrent digital ulcers associated with scleroderma, ET-1 inhibitor (bosentan) can be added. Failing the medical treatment, patients may require amputation for severe digital ischaemia/gangrene.

Wigley F, Flavahan N. Raynaud's Phenomenon. New England Journal of Medicine. 2016;375(6): 556–565.
https://www.nejm.org/doi/full/10.1056/NEJMra1507638

21. Answer: C

This young male patient has a history of likely genitourinary infection around 4 weeks ago after he started a new relationship. His new onset of asymmetrical and monoarticular arthritis is the most likely due to reactive arthritis. Septic arthritis (particularly gonococcal) and crystal arthropathies are amongst possible differential diagnoses that are ruled out after the synovial fluid analysis showed low synovial WBC count and negative crystal findings, respectively.

Ruling out septic arthritis in a patient presenting with monoarticular arthritis is important to prevent joint destruction, disability, or death. Prompt evaluation of the joint, either by bedside arthrocentesis, open or arthroscopic drainage in the operating theatre, or imaging-guided drainage by a radiologist is mandatory.

Reactive arthritis is a subclass of seronegative spondyloarthropathies. A classic triad of symptoms of reactive arthritis include arthritis, urethritis, and conjunctivitis. However, not all patients present with the classic triad. Joint involvement in patients with reactive arthritis is oligoarticular, asymmetrical and affects the joints in the lower extremities, especially knees and ankles. Reactive arthritis is a clinical diagnosis.

American College of Rheumatology (ACR) provided diagnostic guidelines for reactive arthritis in 1999:

- Major criteria:
  o Asymmetric olio- or monoarthritis involving lower extremities
  o Either enteritis or urethritis symptoms preceding the onset of arthritis by a time interval of 3 days to 6 weeks
- Minor criteria:
  o Presence of a triggering infection as evidenced by culture positivity
  o Presence of persistent synovial involvement

Presence of genitourinary symptoms, metatarsophalangeal (MTP) joint involvement, elevated CRP and positive HLA-B27 gives 69% sensitivity and 93.5% specificity to the diagnosis of reactive arthritis.

Laboratory tests include stool culture for potential enteric pathogens, such as *Salmonella, Yersinia, Campylobacter, Shigella, C. difficile* and a urogenital swab/an early morning urine sample for *Chlamydia trachomatis* and *Neisseria Gonorrhoea*. Nucleic acid amplification test for *Mycoplasma genitalium* is also available and is relevant in men with urethritis. In areas where tuberculosis is endemic, patients need to have tuberculin skin test as well. Reactive arthritis is common in patients with HIV and in patients with new-onset symptoms suggestive of a diagnosis of reactive arthritis need to have HIV ruled out. A positive HLA-B27 correlated with disease severity but is not diagnostic. Sacroiliitis is more common in patients with a positive HLA-B27 test.

The initial treatment for reactive arthritis is with an NSAID in the acute phase. Intra-articular steroid for enthesitis or bursitis can be used in patients with mono-oligoarthritis. Systemic steroid is limited to severe polyarthritis. Disease-modifying antirheumatic drugs (DMARDs), sulphasalazine, is effective in treatment of both acute and chronic reactive arthritis. In patients with chronic arthritis, methotrexate and azathioprine have been shown to be helpful.

Diagnosis	Synovial fluid findings		
	Macroscopic appearance	WCC (10⁶/L)	% PMN
Normal	clear, viscous, pale yellow	0 to 200	<10%
Non-inflammatory	clear to slightly turbid	200 to 2,000	<20%
Non-infective inflammatory	slightly turbid	2,000 to 50,000	20 to 70%
Septic	turbid to purulent	> 50,000	>70%
		Note: Crystal arthropathy or severe rheumatoid arthritis may be associated with very high white cell counts that may be mistaken for infection.	

Cheeti A, Chakraborty R, Ramphul K. Reactive Arthritis (Reiter Syndrome) [Internet]. StatPearls. 2019 [cited 15 March 2020]. Available from: https://www.ncbi.nlm.nih.gov/books/NBK499831/

22. Answer: A

Tofacitinib is a janus kinase (JAK) inhibitor. JAKs are intracellular enzymes that transmit signals from cytokines binding to cell surface receptors signal transducers and activators of transcription (STATs). This process drives pro-inflammatory cellular responses.

Rituximab binds to the largely B cell molecule CD20 and depletes B-cells. Abatacept is a fusion protein of the Fc region of immunoglobulin IgG1 and extracellular domain of CTLA-4 and prevents antigen-presenting cells (APCs) from delivering the co-stimulatory signal, preventing T-cell activation. Etanercept is made from binding two human TNF receptors linked to an Fc portion of an IgG1. It reduces the effect of TNF by functioning as a decoy receptor that binds to TNF.

McInnes I, Schett G. Pathogenetic insights from the treatment of rheumatoid arthritis. The Lancet. 2017;389(10086): 2328–2337.
https://www.thelancet.com/journals/lancet/article/PIIS0140-6736(17)31472-1/fulltext

Guo Q, Wang Y, Xu D, Nossent J, Pavlos N, Xu J. Rheumatoid arthritis: pathological mechanisms and modern pharmacologic therapies. Bone Research. 2018;6(1).
https://www.ncbi.nlm.nih.gov/pmc/articles/PMC5920070/

23. Answer: C

Rheumatoid arthritis (RA) is a chronic, inflammatory polyarticular symmetric arthropathy that involves multiple joints bilaterally. The disease affects women 2 to 3 times more often than men and occurs at any age. The peak incidence is in the sixth decade. The pathophysiology of RA involves chronic inflammation of the synovial membrane, which can destroy articular cartilage and juxta-articular bone.

A patient with RA typically presents with pain and swelling in the joints of the hands and feet. The swelling is primarily in the wrists and metacarpophalangeal, metatarsophalangeal, and proximal interphalangeal joints. Predicting the course of an individual case of RA at the outset remains difficult, although the following all correlate with an unfavourable prognosis in terms of joint damage and disability:

- HLA-DRB1*04/04 genotype
- High serum titre of autoantibodies (e.g., rheumatoid factor, anti–CCP antibodies)
- Extra-articular manifestations
- Large number of involved joints
- Age younger than 30 years at onset
- Female sex
- Systemic symptoms
- Insidious onset.

This patient's bilateral hand X-ray shows multiple or large number of involved joints which confers a poor prognosis. Being a man aged 50 and the relatively acute onset may suggest a better prognosis for this patient.

Smolen J, Aletaha D, Barton A, Burmester G, Emery P, Firestein G et al. Rheumatoid arthritis. Nature Reviews Disease Primers. 2018;4(1).
https://www.nature.com/articles/nrdp20181

24. Answer: B

Systemic sclerosis (SSc), also called scleroderma, is a rare heterogenous autoimmune rheumatic disease, causing fibrosis of the skin, internal organs, and small arteries. There are two main subgroups of SSc, diffuse and limited. Limited SSc affects the areas below the elbows and the knees, with or without involvement of the face. Whereas diffuse SSc can extend above the elbows and the knees. Additionally, diffuse SSC can cause fibrosis of internal organs such as the heart, kidneys, gastrointestinal tract, lungs, and thyroid gland. CREST syndrome (calcinosis, Raynaud's phenomenon, oesophageal dysfunction, sclerodactyly, and telangiectasia) is associated with limited SSc. Other associated clinical features include pulmonary arterial hypertension, digital ulceration/gangrene/amputation, digital contractures, acro-osteolysis, Sjögren's syndrome, GORD, gastro antral vascular ectasia (GAVE), cardiac fibrosis, and scleroderma renal crisis. A small number of patients have clinical features and autoantibodies that are specific to SSc but without skin involvement, termed sine scleroderma. Systemic overlap syndrome can be found in patients in the subgroups, but it is most common in patients with limited cutaneous SSc.

SSc is associated with increased morbidity and mortality. Prognosis is determined by the organ involvement and death is often caused by heart, lung, or kidney involvement. Scleroderma is also associated with increased risks of cancer. Autoantibody profiles and ANA patterns are used as the classification criteria for SSc, target treatment and monitoring strategies for different internal organ complications.

ANA pattern/Autoantibody profiles	Associated subclass of SSc and clinical features
Anti-centromere ANA pattern	Limited SSc, pulmonary arterial hypertension
Anti-RNA polymerase III autoantibody	Diffuse SSc, scleroderma renal crisis, and hand disability
Anti-Scl-70 autoantibody	Diffuse SSc, progressive lung fibrosis, digital ulcers, and hand disability
Nucleolar ANA pattern	Progressive interstitial lung disease and pulmonary hypertension

Scleroderma renal crisis is a life-threatening, usually early complication of SSc. Episodes present with acute onset severe hypertension, rapidly progressive renal failure, hypertensive encephalopathy, CCF, and/or microangiopathic haemolytic anaemia. Factors predictive of scleroderma renal crisis include diffuse SSc, the presence of anti-RNA polymerase III antibodies, corticosteroid use in doses ≥ 15 mg of prednisolone or equivalent daily, tendon friction rubs, new onset anaemia, pericarditis, and CCF.

It is usual to begin treatment of severe hypertension associated with scleroderma renal crisis with short-acting ACE inhibitors, such as captopril to lower systolic BP by 20 mmHg in 24 hours. The aim is to reach the target BP of 120/70 mmHg within 72 hours. Once BP is stabilised, long-acting ACE inhibitor can be substituted in equivalent doses. If BP is not able to be controlled with maximum doses of ACE inhibitors, a dihydropyridine calcium channel blocker can be added. Corticosteroid doses ≥ 15 mg of prednisolone or equivalent per day should be avoided to reduce the risks of precipitating scleroderma renal crisis.

Denton, C. and Khanna, D. (2017). Systemic sclerosis. The Lancet, 390(10103), pp.1685–1699. https://www.thelancet.com/journals/lancet/article/PIIS0140-6736(17)30933-9/fulltext

25. Answer: C

SLE is a chronic autoimmune disease with an unpredictable disease course, which can affect multiple organs. It predominantly affects young females. A recent 2019 international reclassification has increased the specificity of diagnosing the disease while maintaining similar sensitivity in diagnosing the condition. ESR is a non-specific inflammatory marker that can be elevated in many different rheumatological conditions. ANA is a sensitive marker, and it is measured as a titre based on the presence of autoantibody titre after dilution. A titre of 1:160 is considered weakly positive. However, ANA is also positive in 10–15% of general population and it is a sensitive marker but not specific for the diagnosis of SLE.

If SLE is suspected based on the presenting symptoms and a positive ANA titre, further investigations with anti-dsDNA antibody and anti-Sm antibody should be ordered to confirm the diagnosis. Other investigations that may be helpful include complement levels (hypocomplementaemia is common in SLE), antiphospholipid antibodies (lupus anti-coagulant, cardiolipin antibody, beta-2-glycoprotein 1 antibody).

Early diagnosis and initiation of treatment is important for management of SLE. Due to its multi-system involvement, a coordinated approach among different specialists will be important to reduce morbidity and mortality. Currently, hydroxychloroquine is considered the anchor medication for SLE treatment. It is usually well tolerated and does not increase risks of infection. Patients who are on hydroxychloroquine need to have regular visual field checks as hydroxychloroquine-related retinopathy is a well-known complication of long-term therapy.

In moderate to severe disease, particularly lupus nephritis, immunosuppressants including pulse cyclophosphamide, and recently mycophenolate has been shown equivalent efficacy without gonadal toxicity as compared with cyclophosphamide. Cyclophosphamide remains an important treatment option for patients with relapsed SLE or lupus nephritis. Rituximab is used off-label currently to suppress B cell activity. However, further studies are required before more widely usage of Rituximab. Belimumab is the only biologic agent approved for SLE, though anifrolumab has shown promise in early trials. Abatacept is generally ineffective in SLE.

Ongoing research and guideline development is required to identify treatment options that are less toxic and reduce long term systemic glucocorticoid exposure. This is particularly important in reducing cardiovascular risks long-term. Patients with SLE have a 2-fold increase in cardiovascular mortality compared to sex and age-group matched cohorts. This make cardiovascular disease the leading cause of death in this cohort. Osteoporosis is also a debilitating complication of SLE associated with chronic inflammation, low vitamin D level, chronic corticosteroid use and low sun exposure due to the skin condition.

In patients presenting with symptoms and signs of arterial or venous thrombus, screening for antiphospholipid syndrome is important since the patient will require life-long anticoagulation to thromboembolic events.

Aringer M, Costenbader K, Daikh D, Brinks R, Mosca M, Ramsey-Goldman R et al. 2019 European League Against Rheumatism/American College of Rheumatology classification criteria for systemic lupus erythematosus. Annals of the Rheumatic Diseases. 2019;78(9): 1151–1159.
https://ard.bmj.com/content/78/9/1151

26. Answer: B

Systemic sclerosis (SSc) is a rare, chronic, debilitating, immune-mediated rheumatic disease that causes skin and internal organ fibrosis and vasculopathy. It is associated with a high morbidity and mortality rate, especially in patients with cardiopulmonary involvement.

Antisynthetase syndrome (ASSD) is a differential diagnosis in this case. It is a descriptive name for a constellation of clinical findings and suggestive serology in patients. The disease process is relatively acute in onset with constitutional symptoms (e.g. fever and weight loss), myositis, Raynaud's phenomenon, non-erosive arthritis, thickened skin of tips and margins of the fingers ('mechanic's hands') and interstitial lung disease. Whilst thought of as a myositis syndrome, patients do not necessarily need myopathy to satisfy the criteria. Anti Jo-1 antibodies are the main markers of the ASSD, though multiple other antibodies have been described.

SSc is a heterogenous disease with variable presenting symptoms and signs such as dyspnoea, fatigue, weight loss, swollen fingers, calcinosis, Raynaud's phenomenon, oesophageal dysmotility, sclerodactyly, telangiectasia (CREST syndrome) and digital contractures. Complications of SSc include digital ulceration, gangrene, autoamputation, acro-osteolysis, osteomyelitis, pulmonary fibrosis, interstitial lung disease, pulmonary hypertension, intestinal pseudo-obstruction, gastric antral vascular ectasia (GAVE), gastrointestinal tract bleeding, malnutrition, bacterial overgrowth, cardiac fibrosis and scleroderma renal crisis.

Traditionally, SSc is categorised based on the extent of skin involvement with 4 major subsets of systemic sclerosis, including limited cutaneous SSc (distal skin sclerosis below the knees and elbows), diffuse cutaneous SSc (proximal limb or trunk involvement, with skin sclerosis), sine scleroderma (no skin thickening) and SSc overlap syndrome (coexisting autoimmune/rheumatic disease). To make a diagnosis of SSc, patients' symptoms need to fulfil the 2013 European League Against Rheumatism (EULAR) and American College of Rheumatology (ACR) classification criteria. Scleroderma-like disease can be associated with L-tryptophan, gadolinium contrast usage in patients with CKD, vinyl chloride monomer exposure, organic solvents exposure, chemotherapy agents, such as taxanes or gemcitabine and radiotherapy.

ANA patterns are generally mutually exclusive and autoantibody profiles help to stratify the subgroups of SSc. The presence of anti-RNA polymerase III, anti-centromere, or anti-topoisomerase I antibodies are part of the criteria for diagnosis. Anti-RNA polymerase III antibody is associated with diffuse SSc, scleroderma renal crisis, hand disability, and malignancy; anti-centromere antibody is associated with limited SSc and pulmonary arterial hypertension, and anti-Scl-70 antibody is associated with diffuse SSc, progressive lung fibrosis, digital ulcers, and hand disability.

Because of their rare prevalence in autoimmune rheumatic disease (AIRD) patients, isolated anti-DFS70 antibodies are being increasingly considered as an important biomarker to exclude the diagnosis of AIRD.

Denton C, Khanna D. Systemic sclerosis. Lancet. 2017; 390: 1685–99.
https://www.ncbi.nlm.nih.gov/pubmed/28413064

27. Answer: A

28. Answer: D

29. Answer: H

30. Answer: B

31. Answer: E

32. Answer: G

In many autoimmune conditions, serum biomarkers can be useful in diagnosis, prognosis, sub-classification, monitoring and to inform therapeutic decisions. Consequently, an understanding of the clinical associations between antibodies and disease states can be extremely useful. In rheumatoid arthritis (RA), rheumatoid factor (RF) and anti-CCP antibodies are most clinically useful. RF is an antibody to immunoglobulin G isotopes, which predicts severity of disease and extra-articular manifestations. RF is found in 70–80% of patients with RA, but is also found in other systemic diseases and the healthy population; RF is incorporated into diagnostic criteria for RA. Anti-CCP antibodies are more specific for RA, and the combination of the two antibodies together is nearly 100% specific for the diagnosis of RA. Anti-CCP antibodies tend to develop early, often prior to the onset of symptoms and predict erosive joint disease.

SLE associated antibodies are wide-ranging but have particular associations with disease manifestations. Diagnosis of SLE includes both clinical and laboratory criteria, with anti-nuclear, anti-dsDNA, anti-Smith (Anti-Sm), antiphospholipid antibodies all forming part of diagnostic criteria. Antibodies are typically present in patients prior to the presentation of disease. However, as optimal treatment and monitoring for such patients is not established, testing for antibodies is usually only considered once a patient is symptomatic.

ANAs are considered as screening antibodies for SLE as a wide array of nuclear antibodies can cause a positive result. Specificity for SLE is low as infections, autoimmune disorders and even healthy aging can cause positive results. Among ANAs, anti-dsDNA is the most specific for a diagnosis of SLE, however sensitivity is low. Anti-Sm antibodies have even higher specificity than anti-dsDNA as well as low sensitivity. Anti-U1 RNP is strongly associated with mixed connective tissue disease – a disorder where features of SLE are mixed with those of other connective tissue disorders, most typically myositis and systemic sclerosis. Anti-SSA/Ro and Anti-SSB/La are typically described in Sjögren's syndrome, but they are commonly present in SLE. Anti-SSA/Ro is present in up to 30% of patients with SLE and is present in 70-90% of patients with subacute cutaneous lupus. Anti-SSA/Ro antibodies also correlate with photosensitivity, cutaneous vasculitis, and haematological complications. Anti-SSB/La is present in only 10% of patients with SLE, but in 30% of patients with subacute cutaneous lupus and 90% of patients with neonatal lupus and congenital heart block. Anti-SSB/La may also be predictive of fewer and less severe neurological and renal complications.

Antiphospholipid antibodies such as anti-cardiolipin antibodies and lupus anticoagulant are present in approximately one third of patients with SLE. Antiphospholipid antibodies are predictive of venous and arterial thromboembolic disease, focal neurological damage, haemolytic anaemia, and recurrent pregnancy loss. More recently, associations have been found between anti-ribosomal P antibodies and neuropsychiatric SLE, as well as between anti-C1q antibodies and renal SLE.

Systemic sclerosis is associated with autoantibodies that are usually mutually exclusive. Anti-centromere, anti-topoisomerase I (Scl-70) and anti-RNA polymerase III antibodies form part of diagnostic criteria. Part of the diagnostic sieve for systemic sclerosis is in differentiating diffuse from limited disease and antibody status often adds to this by further stratifying disease status. For example, anti-Scl-70 antibodies are associated with diffuse cutaneous involvement and require monitoring for interstitial lung disease. Anti-centromere antibodies are associated with limited cutaneous involvement, pulmonary arterial hypertension, and better survival. Anti-RNA polymerase III antibodies are associated with scleroderma renal crisis and gastric antral vascular ectasia. Anti-PM/Scl is associated with limited cutaneous involvement, polymyositis/dermatomyositis as well as better survival.

Idiopathic inflammatory myositis (IIM) encompasses a group of diagnoses with bilateral inflammatory muscle weakness as the core clinical feature. Dermatomyositis and polymyositis are the archetypal disease states in this group; however, the anti-synthetase syndrome is also an important diagnosis, due to the concomitant extramuscular manifestations. Many of the antibodies discussed above are present in IIM as well, for example anti-U1 RNP, anti-PM-Scl and anti SSA/Ro. Antibodies specific to IIM include the anti-synthetase antibodies, most commonly anti-Jo-1 but also anti-PL 12, PL 7, OJ and EJ. Common extramuscular manifestations of this syndrome include interstitial lung disease, arthritis, fever, Raynaud's phenomenon, and 'mechanic's hands'. Anti-Mi2 and anti-SRP are specific antibodies for IIM – these antibodies predict classic dermatomyositis with good response to treatment, and severe, treatment resistant disease, respectively.

Mohan C, Assassi S. Biomarkers in rhematic diseases: how can they facilitate diagnosis and assessment of disease activity? BMJ. 2015; 351: h5079.
https://www.bmj.com/content/351/bmj.h5079/rapid-responses

33. Answer: A

Spondyloarthropathy (SpA) is a heterogeneous group of rheumatic diseases which can be classified as peripheral or axial (axSpA) depended on what parts of the musculoskeletal system are predominantly affected. Ankylosing spondylitis (AS), a type of SpA, is an autoimmune disease that mainly involves spine joints, sacroiliac joints (SIJs) and their adjacent soft tissues, such as tendons. AS can be progressive and lead to fibrosis and calcification, resulting in the loss of flexibility and the fusion of the spine, resembling 'bamboo' with an immobile position. The main clinical features are back pain and progressive spinal rigidity as well as inflammation of the hips, shoulders, peripheral joints. The extra-articular manifestations include uveitis, inflammatory bowel disease (IBD), aortic incompetence as in this case, upper lobe pulmonary fibrosis, and renal disease secondary to amyloid deposition.

AS is associated with HLA-B27. In the HLA-B27-positive population, the prevalence rate of AS is 5–6%. Modified New York and European Spondyloarthropathy Study Group criteria are frequently used in clinical practice to help clinicians make diagnoses. A patient needs to meet at least one clinical and one radiological criterion for the diagnosis of AS.

AS should be managed by a multidisciplinary team. NSAIDs are the first-line treatment for AS. If needed, local intra-articular steroid injections into the sacroiliac and peripheral joints can offer relief. However, systemic glucocorticoid treatment has not been proven to be as efficacious for AS when compared to other inflammatory conditions. Long term steroid use can also contribute to osteoporosis. Disease-modifying anti-rheumatic drugs, such as methotrexate and leflunomide, are not routinely used in AS due to lack of evidence for efficacy. Sulphasalazine is useful for extra-axial joint involvement. If patients have persistently high disease activity despite the above therapeutic options, then the next step would be treatment with biologic agents which include TNF inhibitors. The agents currently recommended are adalimumab, certolizumab pegol, etanercept, golimumab, and infliximab, and their biosimilars. There is good evidence to support the use of biologics in AS. Spinal inflammation, as detected by MRI, has been shown to reduce after anti-TNF treatment. Up to 60% of patients have a good response to these agents.

Taurog J, Chhabra A, Colbert R. Ankylosing Spondylitis and Axial Spondyloarthritis. New England Journal of Medicine. 2016;374(26): 2563–2574.
https://www.nejm.org/doi/10.1056/NEJMra1406182

34. Answer: E

This patient has a typical presentation of polyarteritis nodosa (PAN) which includes constitutional, musculoskeletal symptoms, rash, subcutaneous nodules, and renal involvement. The renal artery angiogram is diagnostic in this case, demonstrating irregular stenoses in the larger vessels, multiple 1–5 mm peripheral aneurysms and arterial occlusions. For unknown reasons, PAN typically occurs at small and medium vessel bifurcations. Locations commonly involved include kidneys (70–80%), gastrointestinal tract, peripheral nerves, skin (50%), skeletal muscles, mesentery (30%), and central nervous system (10%). PAN is an acute multisystem disease. Patients with cutaneous-only PAN or other single-organ presentations of PAN must also be followed regularly for the possible development of disease in new organ systems.

Ozen S. The changing face of polyarteritis nodosa and necrotizing vasculitis. Nature Reviews Rheumatology. 2017;13(6): 381–386.
https://www.nature.com/articles/nrrheum.2017.68

35. Answer: B

Antiphospholipid syndrome (APS) is a systemic autoimmune disorder with a wide range of vascular and obstetric manifestations. These are associated with thrombotic and inflammatory mechanisms orchestrated by antiphospholipid (aPL) antibodies. Common APS clinical presentations include venous thromboembolism often in unusual sites such as upper limbs, hepatic vein, stroke, recurrent early miscarriages, late pregnancy losses and livedo reticularis as in this case. aPL antibodies can be one of three types: lupus anticoagulant, anticardiolipin antibodies or anti-β2 glycoprotein I antibodies. Definite APS, fulfilling at least one clinical and one laboratory criteria of the updated Sapporo classification criteria, can occur in association with other autoimmune diseases, such as SLE, Sjögren's syndrome, rheumatoid arthritis or in its primary form (primary APS). Rarely, a life-threatening form of multiorgan thrombosis, known as catastrophic APS, can occur.

Limper M, Scirè C, Talarico R, Amoura Z, Avcin T, Basile M et al. Antiphospholipid syndrome: state of the art on clinical practice guidelines. RMD Open. 2018;4(Suppl 1): e000785.
https://rmdopen.bmj.com/content/4/Suppl_1/e000785

36. Answer: C

Behçet's disease (BD) is a multi-systemic vasculitic disorder characterised by recurrent oral aphthous ulcers, genital ulcers, and uveitis. Painful oral lesions (aphthous or herpetiform) are one of the criteria for diagnosis and may be the first manifestation (70% of cases). Cutaneous manifestations can occur in up 75% of patients with BD and can range from acneiform lesions, to nodules and erythema nodosum. It usually affects young adults and the aetiology is likely autoimmune. BD is unique among vasculitides in that it can affect small, medium, and large vessels.

Diagnosis is based on clinical criteria from the International Study Group for Behçet's Disease, because specific diagnostic tests are lacking. The genetic susceptibility is the HLA allele HLA-B*51. The treatment approach depends on the individual patient, severity of disease, and major organ involvement.

Ocular presentations (anterior or posterior uveitis, hypopyon, retinal vasculitis, cystoid macular degeneration) represent the first manifestation of disease in 10% of patients with BD.

 Hatemi G, et al. 2018 update of the EULAR recommendations for the management of Behçet's syndrome. Ann Rheum Dis 2018; 0: 1–11.
https://pubmed.ncbi.nlm.nih.gov/29625968/

37. Answer: H

This patient's clinical features are consistent with Takayasu arteritis. Takayasu arteritis is an inflammatory disease of large- and medium-sized arteries, with a predilection for the aorta and its branches. The pathological inflammatory process leads to stenotic, occlusive, or aneurysmal vessels. The renal arteries are involved in 24% to 68% of Takayasu arteritis cases and it is often bilateral, causing hypertension, as seen in this case. Although conventional angiography is the gold standard for diagnosis and evaluation of the extent of disease, CT and MR angiogram is the initial choice of investigation.

The aetiology of Takayasu arteritis is unknown. The underlying pathologic process is likely autoimmune. Genetic susceptibility factors have been identified, particularly HLA-B*52 allele. Takayasu arteritis is a chronic relapsing and remitting disorder. The overall 10-year survival rate is approximately 90%. The overall morbidity in Takayasu arteritis depends on the severity of the lesions and organ involved. Complications of the disease include stroke, intracranial haemorrhage, ischemia, and organ failure.

The American College of Rheumatology has established classification criteria for Takayasu arteritis (3 of 6 criteria are necessary). The presence of any 3 or more criteria yields a sensitivity of 90.5% and a specificity of 97.8%. The criteria are as follows:

- Age of 40 years or younger at disease onset
- Claudication of the extremities
- Decreased pulsation of one or both brachial arteries
- Difference of at least 10 mmHg in systolic blood pressure between arms
- Bruit over one or both subclavian arteries or the abdominal aorta
- Arteriographic narrowing or occlusion of the entire aorta, its primary branches, or large arteries in the upper or lower extremities that is not due to arteriosclerosis, fibromuscular dysplasia, or other causes

Medical management of Takayasu arteritis focuses on controlling the inflammatory process and controlling hypertension. Glucocorticoids are the mainstay of therapy for active Takayasu arteritis. Some patients may also require other immunosuppressants to achieve remission and taper of long-term glucocorticoids treatment.

 Águeda AF, Monti S, Luqmani RA, *et al*. Management of Takayasu arteritis: a systematic literature review informing the 2018 update of the EULAR recommendation for the management of large vessel vasculitis. RMD Open 2019;**5**: e001020.
https://pubmed.ncbi.nlm.nih.gov/31673416/

38. Answer: H

39. Answer: A

40. Answer: J

41. Answer: I

42. Answer: F

43. Answer: D

44. Answer: C

45. Answer: B

46. Answer: E

Most disease-modifying anti-rheumatic drugs (DMARDs) have side effects that include myelosuppression, hepatotoxicity, malignancy, and infection but many also have important and specific adverse effects.

Wilsdon T, Hill C. Managing the drug treatment of rheumatoid arthritis. Australian Prescriber. 2017;40(2): 51–58. https://www.nps.org.au/australian-prescriber/articles/managing-the-drug-treatment-of-rheumatoid-arthritis

21 Basic Science

Questions

Answers can be found in the Basic Science Answers section at the end of this chapter.

1. A 68-year-old woman is admitted to ICU with hypotension and abdominal pain. Her lactate level is 5.8 mmol/L [0.5–1.0]. Which one of the following is correct?
   A. D-Lactate is the predominant isomer in humans.
   B. Elevated levels are associated with mortality only in critical illness due to sepsis.
   C. Lactate is generated from pyruvate.
   D. Type B lactic acidosis is due to inadequate oxygen delivery.

2. Which of one the following is **NOT** correct concerning the morphologic and biochemical changes in apoptosis?
   A. Apoptotic cells do not cause an inflammatory reaction.
   B. Apoptotic cells show cytoplasmic shrinking and increased eosinophilic staining.
   C. Apoptotic cells' mitochondria are enlarged and swollen.
   D. The apoptotic process requires gene expression, protein synthesis, and energy consumption.

3. Where is the primary auditory cortex located in the brain?
   A. Frontoparietal lobe.
   B. Occipital lobe.
   C. Parietal lobe.
   D. Temporal lobe.

4. A 56-year-old man presents with severe difficulty in controlling his hypertension. He is taking four antihypertensive medications. A CT angiogram reveals 50% stenosis of his proximal right renal artery. The blood flow to the right kidney will be reduced by
   A. 2-fold.
   B. 4-fold.
   C. 8-fold.
   D. 16-fold.

5. Cell-free DNA (cfDNA) analysis is emerging as an important and non-invasive adjunct to standard tumour biopsy. Which of the following is correct?
   A. cfDNA is more accurate in the diagnosis of cancer type than a tumour biopsy.
   B. cfDNA is not found in healthy patients.
   C. cfDNA is obtained from tumour biopsies.
   D. cfDNA levels reflect tumour progression and treatment response.

6. A 78-year-old man presents with ischaemic chest pain. He has a new left bundle branch block on his ECG and elevated troponin T. Which coronary artery is most likely to have significant disease during the coronary angiogram?
   A. Left anterior descending artery.
   B. Left circumflex artery.
   C. Obtuse marginal artery.
   D. Right coronary artery.

How to Pass the FRACP Written Examination, First Edition. Jonathan Gleadle, Jordan Li, Danielle Wu, and Paul Kleinig.
© 2022 John Wiley & Sons Ltd. Published 2022 by John Wiley & Sons Ltd.

7. In regarding COVID-19 infection, which one of the following is **NOT TRUE**?
   A. Both SARS-CoV-2 viral RNA and live virus have been detected in patient saliva and sputum.
   B. Nasopharyngeal viral load peaks 1 day prior to symptom onset, correlating to peak time of infectiousness.
   C. SARS-CoV-2 is a descending infection; in later disease, viral loads are higher in the lower respiratory tract, especially in ARDS.
   D. Severity of COVID-19 infection correlates with SARS-CoV-2 viral load in the blood.

8. Which one of the following statements regarding the health risks associated with climate change is **INCORRECT**?
   A. Climate change is associated with decreased cognitive performance.
   B. Climate change is associated with decreased risk of obesity.
   C. Climate change is associated with increased risk of lung cancer.
   D. Climate change is associated with increased risk of stroke.

9. Regarding human papilloma viruses (HPV), which one of the following statements is correct?
   A. HPV are double stranded RNA viruses.
   B. HPV integrate viral genome into cellular DNA to initiate cervical cancer.
   C. HPV types 1 to 180 are known to cause cervical cancer.
   D. HPV vaccine is a live virus vaccine attenuated by mutagenesis.

10. Which one of the following statements regarding hypoxia inducible factor (HIF) is correct?
   A. HIF causes the downregulation of production of erythropoietin.
   B. HIF causes upregulation of the VEGF gene.
   C. HIF promotes cell survival in hypoxia by switching metabolism from anaerobic to aerobic.
   D. Many tumours show suppression of HIF.

11. A 32-year-old GP registrar in Melbourne develops a cough, low grade-fever, and malaise after spending time in a crowded place. He receives a nasopharyngeal swab test for COVID-19 which is negative. He is feeling better 2 days later but still has cough and low-grade fever. He wants to return to work as there are many patients waiting to see him. What is your advice?
   A. Retest for COVID-19 and other respiratory viruses, and self-isolation.
   B. Return to work and do telehealth consults only.
   C. Return to work and see his patients.
   D. Self-isolate at home until all symptoms settle.

12. Which of the following effects is observed with acute severe metabolic acidosis?
   A. Decreased protein degradation.
   B. Decreased pulmonary vascular resistance.
   C. Increased adenosine triphosphate (ATP) generation.
   D. Increased resistance to catecholamines.

13. A 65-year-old homeless man is admitted to hospital complaining of chronic diarrhoea for a month. He has a poor appetite and eats one small meal a day. Past medical history includes rheumatoid arthritis, CKD stage 4, alcohol misuse, active smoker, hypertension, and occasional marijuana and recreational drug use. He does not take regular medications. On examination, his weight is 48 kg (baseline weight: 70 kg around 12 months ago), height is 175 cm, eyes appear sunken, there is loose skin and muscle atrophy around his arms, legs, and abdomen. Dietician reports reduced muscle mass by measuring the mid-arm muscle circumference and reduced hand-grip strength.
   What is your assessment of his nutritional status?
   A. No malnutrition.
   B. Mild malnutrition.
   C. Moderate malnutrition.
   D. Severe malnutrition.

14. Which of the following changes is not observed in patients with obesity hypoventilation syndrome (OHS)?
   A. Reduced total lung capacity.
   B. Reduced expiratory reserve volume (ERV).
   C. Increased tidal volume.
   D. Reduced functional residual capacity (FRC).

15. Which is the most common origin of idiopathic ventricular tachycardia in patients without structural heart disease?

A. Epicardium.

B. Great cardiac vein.

C. His-Purkinje system.

D. Ventricular outflow tract.

16. Routine use of MRI in patients with lower back pain has been shown to have no net clinical benefit. This practice is a typical example of:

A. Overdetection.

B. Overdiagnosis.

C. Overmedicalisation.

D. Overutilisation.

17. A 28-year-old Aboriginal and Torres Strait Islander presents with one-month history of cough, sputum, and weight loss. He has a recent TB contact history. You perform a polymerase chain reaction (PCR) sputum test to detect Mycobacterium tuberculosis. Which of the following is correct regarding this test?

A. 16 DNA duplexes are obtained from one DNA duplex after eight cycles of PCR.

B. PCR involves the synthesis of DNA from deoxynucleotide substrates on one stranded DNA template.

C. The primers used for the process of PCR are double stranded DNA oligonucleotides.

D. Taq polymerase is a heat sensitive DNA polymerase and DNA synthesis takes place at 37 °C.

18. The time interval between the entry of SARS-CoV-2 into a patient with systemic lupus erythematosus (SLE) on hydroxychloroquine and the onset of respiratory symptoms is termed:

A. Communicable period.

B. Decubation period.

C. Incubation period.

D. Pre-infectious period.

19. A 78-year-old woman is diagnosed with right rotator cuff syndrome. You explain to your medical student attached to your clinic what groups of muscles make up the rotator cuff.

A. Latissimus dorsi, levator scapulae, teres major, and supraspinatus.

B. Serratus anterior, teres minor, trapezius, and infraspinatus.

C. Supraspinatus, infraspinatus, teres minor, and subscapularis.

D. Teres major, teres minor, deltoid, and latissimus.

20. Regarding the Sodium/Glucose Cotransporter 2 (SGLT2), which of the following statements is correct?

A. Glucose can only be transported into human cells by SGLT2.

B. SGLT2 mediates 50% of glucose reabsorption in the proximal convoluted tubule.

C. SGLT2 inhibitors can cause hypoglycaemia by inhibiting glucose reabsorption in the small intestine.

D. SGLT2 is an active transporter whereas facilitated glucose transporters (GLUT) are passive transporters.

Answers

1. Answer: C

There is clear evidence that elevated levels of lactate in critically ill patients correlate with worse mortality and morbidity, regardless of cause. Serial blood lactate level measurements are a valuable tool to monitor progress in patients with circulatory shock. Targeting a reduction of blood lactate level of more than 20% in patients with a lactate level of > 3 mmol/L over 2 hours is associated with improved mortality rate in hospital. Lactic acidosis can occur due to: (i) excessive tissue lactate production and/or (ii) impaired hepatic metabolism of lactate. The causes of lactic acidosis are conventionally divided into those associated with obviously impaired tissue oxygenation (type A) and those in which systemic impairment in oxygenation does not exist or is not readily apparent (type B), in some critically ill patients there may be a combination. Plasma lactate level is found to be > 1.5 mmol/L in patients with acute circulatory failure. Lactic acidosis is generally defined as a plasma lactate concentration > 4 mmol/L. Lactic acid is >99% dissociated into lactate anions and protons (H+) at physiological pH. It has two optical isomers, L- and D-lactate. The latter can be produced by overgrowth of intestinal flora. L-lactate is produced from pyruvate by lactate dehydrogenase (LDH) during anaerobic metabolism.

Vincent J, De Backer D. Circulatory Shock. New England Journal of Medicine. 2013;369(18):1726–1734.https://www.nejm.org/doi/10.1056/NEJMra1208943

2. Answer: C

Apoptosis is the process of programmed cell death. It is characteriseds by distinct morphological and biochemical characteristics. It requires gene expression, protein synthesis and energy consumption. Apoptosis is a vital component of various processes such as healthy cell turnover, proper development and functioning of the immune system, hormone-dependent atrophy, and chemical-induced cell death. Inappropriate apoptosis is involved in the pathogenesis of many diseases including cancer, autoimmune disorders, and neurodegenerative diseases.

Morphological changes and features of apoptosis include:

- Involves single cell or small clusters of cells
- Cytoplasmic shrinking and increased eosinophilic staining
- Chromatin condensation and fragmentation
- Formation of apoptotic bodies, which consist of cytoplasm with tightly packed organelles with or without a nuclear fragment
- Pyknosis secondary to chromatin condensation which is the most characteristic feature of apoptosis
- All organelle integrity maintained during apoptotic process
- The mitochondria shrink or remains the same size

There is no inflammatory reaction associated with the process of apoptosis nor with the removal of apoptotic cells because: (i) apoptotic cells do not release their cellular constituents into the surrounding interstitial tissue, (ii) they are quickly phagocytosed by surrounding cells thus likely preventing secondary necrosis, and (iii) the engulfing cells do not produce inflammatory cytokines.

Nagata S. Apoptosis and Clearance of Apoptotic Cells. Annual Review of Immunology 2018 36:1, 489–517. https://www.annualreviews.org/doi/abs/10.1146/annurev-immunol-042617-053010

3. Answer: D

The auditory system and its function are complex. The system can localise, analyse, and interpret a sound that then extrapolates into useful information that the individual can respond to with simultaneous integration with other sensory stimuli. The auditory cortex plays a critical role in the perception of complex sounds. The auditory cortex has traditionally been subdivided into primary (A1), secondary (A2) and tertiary (A3) areas, this terminology has now been replaced by core, belt and parabelt, respectively. The primary auditory cortex (A1) is located on the superior temporal gyrus in the temporal lobe and receives point-to-point input from the ventral division of the medial geniculate complex.

Hackett T. Anatomic organization of the auditory cortex. The Human Auditory System – Fundamental Organization and Clinical Disorders. 2015; 129: 27–53.
https://pubmed.ncbi.nlm.nih.gov/25726261/

4. Answer: D

Blood flow in a vessel can be expressed as: $Q = \Delta P/R$, where Q is blood flow, ΔP is the pressure gradient between both ends of the vessel, and R is the resistance. Blood flow is inversely proportional to resistance. According to the equation, $R = 8nl/\pi r^4$, where R is resistance, n is viscosity of blood, l is the length of the blood vessel, and r^4 is the radius of the blood vessel wall to the fourth power, the resistance is inversely proportional to the fourth power of the radius (Poiseuille's law). In other words, if the radius is reduced by one half, the resistance is multiplied by 16. Therefore, when the resistance is increased by 16-fold, blood flow decreases by 16-fold.

5. Answer: D

Liquid biopsies, particularly those involving cell-free DNA (cfDNA) from plasma, are rapidly emerging as an important and minimally invasive adjunct to standard tumour biopsies and, in some cases, even a potential alternative approach. Blood is not the only bodily fluid that can be used for liquid-biopsy approaches. Urine, stool, CSF, saliva, pleural fluid, and ascites are all potential sources of tumour-derived cfDNA.

cfDNA is released into the bloodstream through apoptosis or necrosis, and cfDNA is typically found as double-stranded fragments of approximately 150 to 200 base pairs in length, corresponding to nucleosome-associated DNA. Molecules of cfDNA are rapidly cleared from the circulation, with a half-life of an hour or less.

The cfDNA from normal cells is found in plasma at low levels in healthy persons, and the cfDNA level can increase under conditions of tissue stress, including ischaemia, sepsis, inflammation, surgery, and trauma. Patients with cancer have higher overall levels of cfDNA than persons without cancer because cancer release cfDNA into blood. The fraction of tumour cfDNA in total cfDNA in patients with cancer can vary greatly, from less than 0.1% to more than 90%. The fraction of tumour cfDNA tends to parallel tumour burden within an individual patient, substantial variability has been observed among patients with the same cancer type.

Corcoran R, Chabner B. Application of Cell-free DNA Analysis to Cancer Treatment. New England Journal of Medicine. 2018;379(18):1754–1765.
https://www.ncbi.nlm.nih.gov/pubmed/30380390

6. Answer: A

Blood supply to cardiac conduction system:
- Blood Supply to the Sinoatrial (SA) Node
  - *Right Coronary Artery*: 60% of patients
  - *Left Circumflex Artery*: 40% of patients
- Blood Supply to the Atrioventricular (AV) Node
  - *Right Coronary Artery*: 90% of patients
  - *Left Circumflex Artery*: 10% of patients
- Blood Supply to the His Bundle
  - *Right Coronary Artery*: main blood supply
  - *Septal Perforators of the Left Anterior Descending Coronary Artery*: minor contribution
- Main/Proximal Left Bundle Branch
  - *Left Anterior Descending Artery*: main blood supply
  - *Right Coronary Artery*: collateral flow
  - *Left Circumflex Artery*: collateral flow
- Right Bundle Branch
  - *Septal Perforators of the Left Anterior Descending Artery*: main blood supply
  - *Right Coronary Artery*: some collateral flow (depending on dominance of the system)
  - *Left Circumflex Artery*: some collateral flow (depending on dominance of the system)

Villa A, Sammut E, Nair A, Rajani R, Bonamini R, Chiribiri A. Coronary artery anomalies overview: The normal and the abnormal. World Journal of Radiology. 2016;8(6): 537.
https://www.wjgnet.com/1949-8470/full/v8/i6/537.htm

7. Answer: D

COVID-19 infection is caused by SARS-CoV-2 RNA virus. Nasopharyngeal viral load peaks around 1 day prior to symptom onset, correlating to peak time of infectiousness. SARS-CoV-2 is a descending infection; in later disease, viral loads are higher in the lower respiratory tract especially in severe/critical illness. In mild cases, live virus is isolated up to day 8 after symptom onset. There can be prolonged shedding of viral RNA lasting many weeks, particularly after critical illness. Correlation with infectiousness is unknown. Studies differ on whether severity of illness correlates with viral load.

The following table summarises the samples that can be used to detect SARS-CoV-2 RNA or live virus and the mode of transmission. The saliva may become an important and convenient sampling site for diagnosis.

Sample source	SARS-CoV-2 RNA PCR	Live SARS-CoV-2 virus	Mode of transmission
Blood	Uncertain	No	No confirmed bloodborne transmissions to date
Cat	Yes	Yes	Cats can transmit SARS-CoV-2 between each other. Not certain about cat to human transmission
Conjunctiva	Yes	Yes	Direct contact
Nasopharynx	Yes	Yes	Droplet and direct contact transmission
Saliva	Yes	Yes	Direct contact transmission
Sputum	Yes	Yes	Airborne is possible in some circumstances
Stool	Yes	Yes	No evidence faecal-oral to date
Urine	Yes	Yes	Unknown

Watson J, Whiting P, Brush J. Interpreting a covid-19 test result [Internet]. The BMJ. 2020 [cited 7 July 2020]. Available from: https://www.bmj.com/content/369/bmj.m1808

8. Answer: B

Climate change is expected to alter the geographic range and burden of a variety of climate-sensitive health outcomes and to affect the health care systems. Extreme weather-related events and disasters can cause four Ds: damage, distress, disease, and death. Climate change is associated with ***increased risk*** of:

1. Respiratory diseases such as allergies, asthma, chronic lung diseases, and lung cancer. Changes in CO_2 concentrations, air temperatures, and precipitation can lead to more ozone, pollen, mould spores, fine particles, and chemicals in the air that causing above respiratory illness.
2. Insect-borne infectious diseases. Changes in temperature, rainfall, humidity, and other weather patterns can facilitate the spread, persistence, and behaviour of mosquitoes, ticks, and other insects that can carry such diseases as malaria, dengue, Zika, Ross River fever, Hendra virus infection, and Lyme disease.
3. Foodborne diseases. Changes in temperatures and sea levels, as well as extreme weather events can create conditions ripe for the spread of disease-causing microbes which can then contaminate food, such as campylobacter infection, cholera, cryptosporidiosis.
4. Malnourishment or obesity. Climate change can affect food production by adversely affecting both plants and animals, leading to decreased availability of more natural, healthy foods, such as fruits and vegetables. All of these may lead to increased reliance on highly processed, unhealthy foods.
5. Cardiovascular diseases and stroke. More extreme temperatures along with poorer air quality as well as psychological stress from extreme weather events can increase stress and other cardiovascular risk factors.
6. Skin cancer and cataracts. Destruction of the ozone layer allows the passage of more ultraviolet radiation, which can then lead to increased risk of skin cancers and cataracts.
7. Heat exhaustion or heat stroke and related admission.
8. Mental health and stress-related issues. Extreme weather events, such as flooding, wildfires, and tornadoes can exacerbate stress, anxiety, and depression.
9. Cognitive performance. Elevated CO_2 levels in occupied buildings are a well-known indoor air quality concern, with studies reporting associations with declines in cognitive performance and increased risk of sick building syndrome in office workers and school children. As outdoor CO_2 levels rise, background indoor levels rise too. Current guidelines recommend keeping indoor CO_2 levels below 1000–1500 ppm.

Haines A, Ebi K. The Imperative for Climate Action to Protect Health. New England Journal of Medicine. 2019;380(3): 263–273.
https://www.ncbi.nlm.nih.gov/pubmed/30650330

9. Answer: B

HPV are non-enveloped viruses. The viral particles consist of a circular double-stranded DNA genome, encompassing eight open reading frames (ORF), as well as a non-enveloped icosahedral capsid. HPV infections are sexually transmitted diseases in both sexes and are strongly implicated in the pathogenesis of different types of cancer, especially cervical cancer. 'High-risk' mucosal HPV types, predominantly types 16, 18, 31, 33 and 35, are associated with most cervical, penile, vulvar, vaginal, anal, and oropharyngeal cancers as well as pre-cancers. HPV cause cancer by integrating viral genome into cellular DNA. The highly effective HPV vaccine is a whole virus, chemically inactivated vaccine.

 Crosbie E, Einstein M, Franceschi S, Kitchener H. Human papillomavirus and cervical cancer. The Lancet. 2013;382(9895):889–899.
https://pubmed.ncbi.nlm.nih.gov/23618600/

10. Answer: B

Hypoxia-inducible-factors (HIFs) are transcriptional regulators that are induced by hypoxia and bind to specific DNA sequences, thus controlling the rate of gene transcription. HIF-1 is a dimer consisting of HIF-1α and HIF-1β subunits. HIF-1β is constitutively present, but HIF-1α is present at very low levels under normoxic conditions. The degradation of HIF in normoxic conditions is mediated by oxygen dependent prolyl hydroxylation by the PHD enzymes of the HIF protein, recognition, and binding by the von Hippel Lindau (VHL) tumour suppressor and subsequent proteasomal degradation. In hypoxic conditions prolyl hydroxylation and VHL recognition and destruction is reduced. VHL is commonly mutated in renal cell carcinoma leading to unrestrained HIF activation.

HIF is known to induce transcription of more than 60 target genes, including vascular endothelial growth factor (VEGF) and erythropoietin that are involved in angiogenesis and erythropoiesis contributing to the adaptation to chronic hypoxia. In addition, some genes are downregulated, such as PDK1, leading to decreased mitochondrial oxygen consumption. HIF-1α promotes cell survival under hypoxic conditions by switching metabolism from aerobic to anaerobic or glycolytic by enhancing expression of glycolytic genes.

One important HIF-1 function is to promote angiogenesis. This is done via HIF-1 regulation of angiogenic growth factors such as VEGF. VEGF is a major regulator of angiogenesis, which promotes endothelial cell migration toward a hypoxic area. Such endothelial cells help to form new blood vessels. HIF-1 plays a critical part in tumour proliferation. As a tumour develops and grows, a hypoxic environment is created because of the extreme energy demands of the numerous, rapidly dividing cells.

 West J. Physiological Effects of Chronic Hypoxia. New England Journal of Medicine. 2017;376(20):1965–1971.
https://www.ncbi.nlm.nih.gov/pubmed/28514605

11. Answer: A

Interpreting the result of a test for COVID-19 depends on two things: the accuracy of the test, and the pre-test probability or estimated risk of disease before testing. A positive RT-PCR test for COVID-19 test has more weight than a negative test because of the test's high specificity but moderate sensitivity. A single negative COVID-19 test should not be used to rule-out patients with strongly suggestive symptoms and high pre-test probability, as seen in this case. If this GP returns to work and subsequently the test is confirmed as a false negative, this will have significant consequences for his patients, colleagues, and everyone with whom he came into contact. It is therefore safest for this GP with suggestive symptoms to retest and self-isolate.

The accuracy of COVID-19 PCR test has a false negative rate of between 2% and 29% (equating to sensitivity of 71–98%), based on negative PCR tests which were positive on repeat testing. The sensitivity of viral PCR test in clinical practice is dependent on the swab site and quality of sampling. It is about 93% for bronchoalveolar lavage, 72% for sputum, 63% for nasal swabs, and only 32% for throat swabs. Accuracy is also likely to vary depending on stage of disease and degree of viral multiplication or clearance. Higher sensitivities are reported depending on which gene targets are used, and whether multiple gene tests are used in combination.

 Good C, Hernandez I, Smith K. Interpreting COVID-19 Test Results: a Bayesian Approach. Journal of General Internal Medicine. 2020.
https://link.springer.com/article/10.1007/s11606-020-05918-8

12. Answer: D

Acute metabolic acidosis is common in seriously ill patients and when severe, is associated with increased mortality and poor clinical outcomes. Therefore, rapid recognition and effective treatment are essential. The main adverse and beneficial effects of metabolic acidosis are listed below:

Adverse effects

- Decreased cardiac contractility and cardiac output
- Arteriolar dilatation and venoconstriction
- Decreased tissue oxygen delivery
- Hypotension, decreased hepatic, renal and cerebral blood flow
- Predisposition to cardiac arrhythmias
- Resistance to catecholamines
- Pulmonary arterial vasoconstriction, causing pulmonary hypertension and right heart failure
- Decreased adenosine triphosphate (ATP) generation
- Increased insulin resistance
- Stimulation of inflammatory mediators
- Impairment of the immune response
- Impaired phagocytosis
- Increased apoptosis
- Increased protein degradation

Beneficial effects

- Decreased affinity of haemoglobin for oxygen leading to favourable haemoglobin-oxygen dissociation for tissue extraction of oxygen. The reduction in 2,3-diphosphoglycerate (2,3-DPG) counteracts this rightward shift. A severe rightward shift may result in poor haemoglobin saturation when passing through pulmonary capillaries
- Vasodilatation of vessels with increased blood flow to tissues
- Increased ionised calcium with augmented myocardial contractility

Jung B, Martinez M, Claessens Y, Darmon M, Klouche K, Lautrette A et al. Diagnosis and management of metabolic acidosis: guidelines from a French expert panel. Annals of Intensive Care. 2019;9(1). https://annalsofintensivecare.springeropen.com/articles/10.1186/s13613-019-0563-2#citeas

13. Answer: D

The Global Leadership Initiative on Malnutrition (GLIM) recommended in 2016 a two-step approach for diagnosis of malnutrition. The first step is to identify 'at risk' status by using any validated nutritional risk screening tools, and the second step is to assess the severity of malnutrition. The diagnosis of malnutrition is made if patients fitting at least one of the agreed phenotypic criterion (e.g. weight loss, low BMI, and reduced muscle mass) and one aetiologic criterion, such as reduced food intake or assimilation, and inflammation or disease burden.

Phenotypic criteria for the diagnosis of malnutrition as listed in the table below:

Table 21.1:

Phenotypic criteria			Aetiology Criteria	
Weight loss (%)	Low BMI (kg/m²)	Reduced muscle mass	Reduced food intake or assimilation	Inflammation
>5% within past 6 months, or >10% beyond 6 months	<20 if < 70 years, or <22, if ≥70 years Asians: <18.5 if <70 years, or <20 if ≥70 years	Reduced by validated body composition measuring techniques[a]	≤50% or energy requirements > 1 week, or any reduction for >2 weeks, or any chronic gastrointestinal condition that adversely impacts food assimilation or absorption	Acute disease/injury or chronic disease-related

[a]For example appendicular lean mass index (kg/m²) by dual-energy absorptiometry or corresponding standard using other body composition methods like bioelectrical impedance analysis, CT, or MRI. When not available or by regional preference, physical examination or standard anthropometric measures like mid-arm muscle or calf circumferences may be used. Functional assessment like hand-grip strength may be used as a supportive measure.

Table 21.2: Grading of malnutrition severity.

Phenotypic criteria			
	Weight loss (%)	**Low BMI (kg/m²)**	**Reduced muscle mass (see the footnote in Table 21.1)**
Stage 1/Moderate malnutrition (Requires 1 phenotypic criterion that meets this grade)	5 – 10% within the past 6 months, or 10–20% beyond 6 months	<20 if <70 years, <22 if ≥70 years	Mild to moderate deficit (per validated assessment methods)
Stage 2/Severe malnutrition (Requires 1 phenotypic criterion that meets this grade)	>10% within the past 6 months, or >20% beyond 6 months	< 18.5 if < 70 years, <20 if ≥70 years	Severe deficit (per validated assessment methods)

His calculated BMI is 15.7 kg/m². He has a significant weight loss: of 31% beyond 6 months. Weight loss %: (70 – 48)/70 x 100% = 31%.

This man fits the diagnostic criteria of malnutrition (all three of the phenotypic criteria and both of the aetiology criteria (i.e. chronic diarrhoea, rheumatoid arthritis, and CKD), furthermore, he fits all three criteria for severe malnutrition.

The patient is also at risk of refeeding syndrome. It is recommended to have careful monitoring of electrolytes, such as potassium, calcium, magnesium, phosphate levels and replacement of these electrolytes to maintain normal levels. Thiamine should be commenced immediately for a total of at least 10 days to prevent Wernicke's encephalopathy or Korsakoff's syndrome. Refeeding should be started at a low level of energy replacement in consultation with a dietician.

Cederholm T, Jensen G, Correia M, et al. GLIM criteria for the diagnosis of malnutrition – A consensus report from the global clinical nutrition community. Journal of Cachexia, Sarcopenia and Muscle. 2019;10(1):207–217. https://onlinelibrary.wiley.com/doi/full/10.1002/jcsm.12383

14. Answer: C

Obesity hypoventilation syndrome (OHS) is defined by obesity (BMI ⩾30 kg/m²), sleep disordered breathing and daytime hypercapnia (PaCO2 ⩾45 mmHg) during wakefulness occurring in the absence of an alternative neuromuscular, mechanical, or metabolic explanation for hypoventilation.

The excess of adipose tissue in the abdomen and chest wall reduces total lung capacity, reduced lung volumes, functional residual capacity (FRC) and expiratory reserve volume (ERV). Fat deposits impede diaphragm motion, decrease lung compliance, and increase lower airway resistance. Gas trapped due to premature airway closure generates intrinsic positive end-expiratory pressure and favours ventilation/perfusion mismatches. There is also development of atelectasis of the lower lobes of the lungs. OHS patients show a greater impairment in respiratory mechanics than the morbidly obese without OHS, with associated weakness in respiratory muscles. Overall, there is an increase in the work required for breathing that needs to be compensated by elevated drive from the respiratory centres to the respiratory muscles.

Masa J, Pépin J, Borel J, et al. Obesity hypoventilation syndrome. European Respiratory Review. 2019;28(151):180097.https://err.ersjournals.com/content/errev/28/151/180097.full.pdf

15. Answer: D

Idiopathic ventricular arrhythmias (VAs) are comprised of ventricular premature depolarisations, non-sustained VT and rarely sustained VT, and these typically occur in the absence of structural heart disease. The mechanism of these arrhythmias is usually triggered activity or abnormal automaticity, and this usually manifests as a focal source. Idiopathic VAs tend to have a benign prognosis. Sudden cardiac death is uncommon.

Idiopathic VAs originate most commonly from the ventricular outflow tract (OT) region, but they can also arise from the His-Purkinje system, the papillary muscles, and other perivalvular locations. OT VAs can originate from the right and left ventricular outflow tracts (RVOT or LVOT), either above or below the pulmonic and aortic valves. They can also originate in the vicinity of the great cardiac vein and/or the anterior inter-ventricular vein, and the left ventricular summit region.

Structural diseases such as arrhythmogenic right ventricular cardiomyopathy and sarcoidosis need to be excluded before a diagnosis can be made. VT with structural heart disease has poor prognosis and warrants an implantable cardioverter defibrillator (ICD). Beta-blockers, calcium-channel blockers, or catheter ablation are effective in treating idiopathic VAs.

Killu AM, Stevenson WG. Ventricular tachycardia in the absence of structural heart disease. Heart 2018; 0:1–12. https://heart.bmj.com/content/105/8/645

16. Answer: D

Overdiagnosis is defined as the diagnosis of a condition that, if unrecognised, would not cause symptoms or harm a patient during his or her lifetime. In other words, the diagnosis does not produce a net benefit for that patient. Overdiagnosis is increasingly recognised because of screening for cancer and other conditions. It is problematic for patients, clinicians, and health care policymakers.

Overdetection is defined as the detection of a clinical finding in an asymptomatic person, usually by an investigation. This clinical finding does not produce a net benefit for that patient. In fact, it may produce harm due to further investigation or subsequent treatment. A typical example is the incidentaloma found on a CT scan or PSA testing in an asymptomatic elderly man who has significant comorbidities.

Overutilisation refers to the establishment of a standard practice that does not provide net benefit to patients. Routine MRI lumbar spine for patients presenting with lower back pain without 'red flag' symptoms is a typical example.

Overmedicalisation is altering the meaning or understanding of experiences in such a way that non-medical problems are re-interpreted as medical problems requiring medical treatment without net benefit to patients. Harm to health can be caused by undue treatment and undesirable side effects of the medication administered.

The above concepts are interrelated. Overdetection and overdiagnosis cause overtreatment and overutilisation.

Kale M, Korenstein D. Overdiagnosis in primary care: framing the problem and finding solutions. BMJ. 2018; k2820. https://www.bmj.com/content/362/bmj.k2820

17. Answer: B

PCR allows for specific detection and production of large amounts of DNA. PCR is widely used by clinicians to diagnose diseases, detect pathogens, clone, and sequence genes, as well as carry out sophisticated quantitative and genomic studies in a rapid and very sensitive manner. PCR can be performed using source DNA from a variety of tissues and organisms, including microbes, peripheral blood, skin, hair, saliva, and sputum such as in this case. Only trace amounts of DNA are needed for PCR to generate enough copies to be analysed using conventional laboratory methods. Therefore, PCR can be a highly sensitive assay and contamination can cause false positive results.

Each PCR assay requires the presence of template DNA, primers, nucleotides, and heat resistant DNA polymerase. The primers are short DNA fragments with a defined sequence complementary to the target DNA that is to be detected and amplified. These serve as an extension point for the DNA polymerase to build on. The reaction solution is first heated to 94 °C, which allows two complementary DNA strands of the target DNA to separate, which is called denaturation. The temperature is then lowered to 74 °C to allow the specific primers to bind to the target DNA segments, a process known as hybridisation or annealing. Annealing between primers and the target DNA occurs only if they are complementary in sequence (e.g. A binding to G). The temperature is raised again, at which time the heat resistant DNA polymerase is able to extend the primers by adding nucleotides to the developing DNA strand. DNA polymerase synthesizes DNA in a 5'→3' direction and can add nucleotides in the 3' end of a custom-designed oligonucleotide. With each repetition of these three steps, the number of copied DNA molecules doubles and exponentially increases.

There are two main methods of visualising the PCR products: (i) staining of the amplified DNA product with a chemical dye such as ethidium bromide, which intercalates between the two strands of the duplex, or (ii) labelling the PCR primers or nucleotides with fluorescent dyes (fluorophores) prior to PCR amplification.

When PCR is used to detect the presence or absence of a specific DNA product, it is called qualitative PCR. Qualitative PCR is a good technique to use when PCR is performed for cloning purposes or to identify a pathogen.

Quantitative real-time or qRT-PCR provides information beyond mere detection of DNA. It indicates how much of a specific DNA or gene is present in the sample. qRT-PCR allows for both detection and quantification of the PCR product in real-time, while it is being synthesised. Real-time PCR can be combined with reverse transcription, which allows messenger RNA to be converted into cDNA (i.e., reverse transcription), after which quantification of the cDNA is performed with qPCR.

PCR uses the enzyme DNA polymerase that directs the synthesis of DNA from deoxynucleotide substrates on one stranded DNA template. After each cycle, the number of duplexes doubles itself thus after the first cycle there are two DNA duplexes. A duplex has two DNA strands thus after second cycle there will be four duplexes, after third cycle there will be eight DNA duplexes. Lastly, after the fourth cycle there will be 16 duplexes.

Ghannam M, Varacallo M. Biochemistry, Polymerase Chain Reaction (PCR) [Internet]. Statpearls.com. 2018 [cited 18 February 2020]. Available from: https://www.statpearls.com/kb/viewarticle/27414/

18. Answer: C

The incubation period of an infectious disease is the time between exposure/entry an infectious organism and the first symptom of the disease. Knowledge of the incubation period is essential in the investigation and control of infectious disease. Decubation period is the time from the disappearance of symptoms until the recovery and the absence of infectious organism. Communicable period is the time during which an infectious agent may be transferred directly or indirectly from an infected person to another person. Latent period or the pre-infectious period is the time interval between when an individual or host is infected by an organism and when he or she becomes infectious.

COVID-19 is caused by severe acute respiratory syndrome coronavirus (SARS-CoV-2), a novel coronavirus belonging to the family of β-coronaviruses. It mainly spreads through the respiratory tract. Human-to-human transmission is the main source of contagion, which occurs mainly through contaminated droplets, hands, or surfaces. Virus particles, which are present in secretions from an infected person's respiratory system, infect others through direct contact with mucous membranes with an incubation period of between 2 and 14 days (median 5.1 days).

Virus transmission by asymptomatic patients during the incubation period (pre-symptomatic transmission) has been documented through contact tracing and enhanced investigation of clusters of confirmed cases. This is supported by data that some people can test positive for COVID-19 from one to three days before they develop symptoms. Thus, patients infected with COVID-19 could transmit the virus before symptoms develop. An asymptomatic laboratory-confirmed case is a person infected with COVID-19 who does not develop symptoms. Asymptomatic transmission refers to transmission of SARS-CoV-2 from a person, who does not develop symptoms. Asymptomatic cases have been reported as part of contact tracing efforts. There is no evidence that hydroxychloroquine can prevent COVID-19 or reduce a patient's infectious status.

McAloon C, Collins Á, Hunt K, Barber A, Byrne A, Butler F et al. Incubation period of COVID-19: a rapid systematic review and meta-analysis of observational research. BMJ Open. 2020;10(8):e039652. https://bmjopen.bmj.com/content/10/8/e039652

19. Answer: C

The rotator cuff (RC) is an anatomic coalescence of the muscles and tendons of supraspinatus, infraspinatus, teres minor, and subscapularis. Rotator cuff syndrome (RCS) constitutes a spectrum of disease across a wide range of pathologies associated with injury or degenerative conditions affecting the RC.

RCS includes subacromial impingement syndrome, subacromial bursitis, RC tendonitis, partial- versus full-thickness RC tears and, chronically, can influence the development of glenohumeral degenerative disease and rotator cuff arthropathy. Detailed history and examination enable early diagnosis even in the asymptomatic RC tear. Ultrasonography and MRI are the mainstay of investigations. While conservative measures are successful in elderly patients with minimal lesions and demands, early surgery should be considered in younger, healthier, active, and symptomatic patients.

Sambandam S. Rotator cuff tears: An evidence based approach. World Journal of Orthopedics. 2015;6(11):902. https://www.wjgnet.com/2218-5836/full/v6/i11/902.htm

20. Answer: D

Healthy people are able to maintain tight glucose homeostasis by closely regulating glucose production, reabsorption, and utilisation. Glucose is transported into human cells by facilitated diffusion and secondary active transport via the glucose transporters (GLUTs) and SGLT transporters, respectively. Approximately 180 g of glucose is filtered daily by the renal glomeruli and is then reabsorbed in the proximal convoluted tubule (PCT). This is achieved by GLUTs and SGLTs. There are two main SGLTs, SGLT1 in the small intestine, and SGLT2 in the PCT which contributes to 90% of glucose reabsorption. SGLT2 inhibitors work by inhibiting SGLT2 in the PCT to prevent reabsorption of glucose and facilitate its excretion in urine leading to an improvement in glycaemic control in patients with type 2 diabetes. However, SGLT2 inhibitors inhibit only 30–50% of the filtered glucose load.

Liu J, Lee T, DeFronzo R. Why Do SGLT2 Inhibitors Inhibit Only 30–50% of Renal Glucose Reabsorption in Humans? Diabetes. 2012;61(9):2199–2204.
https://www.ncbi.nlm.nih.gov/pmc/articles/PMC3425428/

Index

AA *see* aplastic anaemia
AAA *see* abdominal aortic aneurysm
AATD *see* α1-antitrypsin deficiency
abatacept 436, **451**
abdominal aortic aneurysm (AAA) 1, **13**
ABG *see* arterial blood gas
ABMR *see* antibody-mediated rejection
ABPA *see* allergic bronchopulmonary aspergillosis
ACD *see* angioedema of chronic disease
ACE inhibitors, angioedema 223, **228**
acetylcholine receptor antibodies 337, **351**
acid-base homeostasis, kidney function 307, **325**
acromegaly 71, **79**
ACS *see* acute coronary syndrome
ACTH *see* adrenocorticotropic hormone
activated protein C 193, **219**
acute coronary syndrome (ACS) **215**
acute eosinophilic pneumonia (AEP) 394–395, **415**
acute generalised exanthematous pustulosis 62, **69**
acute HIV infections 238–239, **248–249**
acute intermittent porphyria **66**
acute interstitial nephritis (AIN) 302–303, **313–314**
acute kidney injury (AKI) 37, **49–50**, 303, **314**
acute metabolic acidosis 459, **465**
acute myeloid leukaemia (AML) 197, **221**, 270, **276–277**
acute myocardial infarction (AMI) 142, **154**
acute myocarditis 145, **162**
acute necrotising pancreatitis (ANP) 107–108, **119**
acute pancreatitis 107–108, **118–119**
acute post-streptococcal glomerulonephritis (APSGN) 302, **312**
acute pulmonary oedema (APO) 404, **425**
acute red eye 141, **151**
acute respiratory distress syndrome (ARDS) 34, **43**
acute rheumatic fever (ARF) 7, **26**
acute severe asthma 42, **55**
acute vertebral osteomyelitis 241, **256**
acyclovir 369, **381**
AD *see* Alzheimer's disease
ADA *see* adenosine deaminase
adaptive immunity, antibody production 223, **229**
ADB *see* adynamic bone disease
addiction medicine 368–392
    cocaine overdose 375, **392**
    opioid use disorder 371–372, **384–385**
    see also pharmacology
Addison's disease 369, **380**
adenoma, pituitary 75–76, **90–91**

adenosine deaminase (ADA) **423**
adipocytes 73, **82**
ADPKD *see* autosomal dominant polycystic kidney disease
adrenal crisis 72, **80**
adrenal incidentaloma 72, **80**
adrenaline autoinjectors 223, **228**
adrenocorticotropic hormone (ACTH) 73, **82–83**
adult T-cell lymphoma (ATL) 239, **249**
advance care planning 36, **47**, 361, **365**
advanced adenocarcinoma of the lung 271, **279–280**
adverse effects
    antidepressant cessation 291, **298**
    chemotherapy 272–273, **285–286**
    lithium 292, **301**, 305, **320**
    psychotropic medications 292, **301**
    vancomycin 374, **392**
    see also polypharmacy; toxicology
adynamic bone disease (ADB) 302, **313**
AEP *see* acute eosinophilic pneumonia
AF *see* atrial fibrillation
ageing
    normal physiological changes 141, **151–152**
    pharmacology 368, **376**
age-related macular degeneration (AMD) 141, **152**
AIH *see* amiodarone-induced hypothyroidism
AIHA *see* autoimmune haemolytic anaemia
AIN *see* acute interstitial nephritis
AKI *see* acute kidney injury
AL *see* light chain amyloidosis
alcohol
    oxidative metabolism 141, **153**
    withdrawal syndrome 141–142, **153**
Alirocumab 6, **23**
allergic bronchopulmonary aspergillosis (ABPA) 394–395, 401,
        407, **415**, **424**, **427**
allergies 223–236
    adrenaline autoinjectors 223, **228**
    amoxicillin 223, **228–229**
    anaphylaxis 223, 224, 225, **228**, **231**, **233–234**
    hereditary angioedema 224, **231**
    penicillin 225, **228**, **232**
    systemic mastocytosis 225, **233**
allopurinol 369, **381**
alpha 1-antitrypsin deficiency 173, **182**
alpha methyldopa 369, **381**
Alport's syndrome 309, **330–331**
alveolar proteinosis (AP) 407, **428**

How to Pass the FRACP Written Examination, First Edition. Jonathan Gleadle, Jordan Li, Danielle Wu, and Paul Kleinig.
© 2022 John Wiley & Sons Ltd. Published 2022 by John Wiley & Sons Ltd.

Alzheimer's disease (AD), pharmacologic therapies   369, **379**
AMD *see* age-related macular degeneration
amiodarone, pulmonary side effects   393, **409–410**
amiodarone-induced hypothyroidism (AIH)   72, **81**
AML *see* acute myeloid leukaemia
amlodipine   369, **381**
amoebiasis   148, **167**
amoxicillin, allergies   223, **228–229**
ampicillin elimination   368, **376**
amyloidosis, cardiac   3, **16–17**
amyotrophic lateral sclerosis (ALS)   337, **350**
ANA *see* antinuclear antibodies
anaemia
    aplastic   185, **200–201**
    autoimmune haemolytic   184, **199–200**
    microcytic   194, **220–221**
    pernicious   189–190, **212**
anaemia of chronic disease (ACD)   187, **206**
anaphylaxis
    adrenaline autoinjectors   223, **228**
    food-dependent, exercise-induced   224, **231**
    systemic mastocytosis   225, **233**
    tryptase levels   225, **233–234**
    vancomycin   **392**
aneurysm, abdominal aortic   1, **13**
Angelman syndrome   171, **178–179**
angina, nitrate tolerance   371, **383**
angiogenesis, cancer   269, **274**
angioedema, ACE inhibitors   223, **228**
ankylosing spondylitis (AS)   430, **442–443**
ANP *see* acute necrotising pancreatitis
anthracycline cardiomyopathy   2, **14**
antibacterial agents
    mechanisms of action   242, **258–259**
    see also individual drugs...
antibody-mediated rejection (ABMR)   223, **229**, 303,
    314–315
antibody production   223, **229**
anticholinergic medicines
    elderly patients   368, 371, **376–377, 384**
    toxicity   371, **384**
anticonvulsant medications   340, **357**
antidepressants
    adverse events on cessation   291, **298**
    mechanisms of action   292, **300–301**
antifungal agents   237, **245**
anti-GBM disease *see* anti-glomerular basement membrane
    disease
anti-glomerular basement membrane (anti-GBM)
    disease   303–304, **315**
anti-microbial resistance mechanisms   242–243, **259–260**
antinuclear antibodies (ANA)   430, **443**
antiphospholipid syndrome (APS)   **204**, 262, **264**, 430, **442**
antisynthetase syndrome (ASSD)   **453**
antithrombotic therapy   2, **15**
α1-antitrypsin deficiency (AATD)   393, **409**
antivirals, mechanisms of action   243, **260**
aortic stenosis (AS)   2, 8, **14–15, 28**

aortic valve area (AVA), stenosis   2, **15**
AP *see* alveolar proteinosis
aplastic anaemia (AA)   185, **200–201**
apoptosis
    BCL-2 family proteins   185, **201**
    morphologic/biochemical changes   458, **461**
    programmed death ligand 1 (PD-L1)   271, **281**
APS *see* antiphospholipid syndrome; autoimmune polyendocrine
    syndrome
APSGN *see* acute post-streptococcal glomerulonephritis
ARDS *see* acute respiratory distress syndrome
ARF *see* acute rheumatic fever
arithmetic mean   97, **100**
artemisinin-based combination therapy (ACT)   **251**
arterial blood gas (ABG)   401–402, **424–425**
arteries, transposition   12, **32–33**
artesunate   239–240, **251**
arthritis
    crystal   431, **444–445**
    psoriatic   436, **450**
    reactive   436, **450–451**
    rheumatoid   433, 436–437, **446, 451–452**
    septic   431–432, **444–445**
AS *see* ankylosing spondylitis; aortic stenosis
ASB *see* asymptomatic bacteriuria
asbestos exposure   397, **421–422**
ascertainment bias   97, **101–102**
ascites   108, **119–120**
ASCT *see* autologous stem-cell transplantation
ASD *see* atrial septal defect
aspiration pneumonia   403, **425**
aspirin, preeclampsia   263, **266–267**
ASSD *see* antisynthetase syndrome
asthma
    monoclonal antibodies   393, **410–411**
    omalizumab   393, **410–411**
    pregnancy   262, **264**
    severe   38, 42, **50–51, 55**
    treatment measures   393, **410**
asymptomatic bacteriuria (ASB)   146, **165**
ATL *see* adult T-cell lymphoma
atrial fibrillation (AF)   1, 2, **13–14, 15**
atrial septal defect (ASD)   12, **32**
attack rate   98, **105**
ATTR *see* transthyretin amyloidosis
atypical haemolytic uraemic syndrome (aHUS)   196, **221**
auditory cortex   458, **461**
autoantibodies
    associated conditions   438–440, **454–455**
    neurological effects   227, **236**
autoimmune haemolytic anaemia (AIHA)   184, **199–200**
autoimmune (Hashimoto's) thyroiditis   76, **92–93**
autoimmune hepatitis (AIH)   108, **120**
autoimmune polyendocrine syndrome (APS)   72, **81–82**
autoinfection, strongyloidiasis   241, **254–255**
autologous stem-cell transplantation (ASCT)   **206**
autosomal dominant arteriopathy with subcortical infarcts and
    leukoencephalopathy (CADASIL)   341–342, **358**

autosomal dominant polycystic kidney disease (ADPKD)   302, **312–313**
AVA *see* aortic valve area
avascular necrosis (AVN)   430, **443**
averages   97, **100**
AVN *see* avascular necrosis
azathioprine   107, **119**
azithromycin   **53**, 368, 374, **377, 391**
azoles   237, **245**

Bacillus Calmete-Guerin (BCG) vaccine   226, **235**
back pain   144–145, **161**
   metastatic compression   271, **278–279**
bacterial overgrowth, small bowel   116, **138**
BAE *see* bronchial artery embolism
bariatric surgery, metabolic/nutritional complications   77–78, **95–96**
Barrett's oesophagus (BO)   108–109, **121**
basal cell carcinoma (BCC)   61, **68**
BCC *see* basal cell carcinoma
B cell lymphoma 2 (BCL-2) proteins   185, **201**
B cells   226, **234**
BCG *see* Bacillus Calmete-Guerin
BCL-2 *see* B cell lymphoma 2 proteins
BD *see* Behçet's disease
Becker muscular dystrophy   **176–177**
Beers criteria   **163–164**
Behçet's disease (BD)   439, **456**
Bell's palsy   334, **342**
benign paroxysmal positional vertigo (BPPV)   334, **342–343**
benralizumab   **411**
benzodiazepines   145–146, **163**
β-blockers   2, 11, **15–16, 31**, 374, **392**
beta-thalassemia   170, **175**
bevacizumab   269, **274**
bias   98–99, **104–106, 105–106**
   ascertainment   97, **101–102**
   information   98–99, **105–106**
   publication   98, **104**
   randomisation   97, **101–102**
   recall   97, **101–102**
   selection   97, 98–99, **101–102, 105–106**
bifascicular block   39, **51–52**
biliopancreatic diversion (BPD)   **95**
bioavailability   371, **384**
biosimilar medications   368, **377–378**
bipolar disorder, pregnancy   289, **293**
Birt–Hogg–Dube syndrome   **181**
bisphosphonates   369, **378**
bite wounds, human   239, **249**
biventricular pacemaker and defibrillator   4–5, **20**
BK virus nephropathy (BKVN)   306, **323–324**
BKVN *see* BK virus nephropathy
blood pressure, critical care medications   41, **54**
BMD *see* bone mineral density
bone-kidney endocrine axis   307, **324**
bone mineral density (BMD)   431, **444**
bones

Paget's disease   75, **87–88**
   radioisotope scans   143, **154**
   see also *rheumatology*
bone turnover markers (BTMs)   431, **444**
BPD *see* biliopancreatic diversion
BRCA1/BRCA2 mutations   269, **275**
breast cancer, *BRCA1/BRCA2* mutations   269, **275**
brentuximab vedotin (BV)   **206**
brigatinib   273, **287**
Broca's area   341, **359**
bronchial artery embolism (BAE)   395, **416**
bronchiectasis   394, **411**
brown fat   73, **82**
Brugada syndrome (BS)   2–3, **16**
brush border microvilli   109, **121**
BS *see* Brugada syndrome
BTMs *see* bone turnover markers
Budd–Chiari syndrome   189, **211**
bullous pemphigoid   57, 60, **63, 66–67**
Burkholderia pseudomallei   240, **251–252**
BV *see* brentuximab vedotin

C2-3 facet joint injuries   145, **162**
C3 glomerulopathy   304, **316**
CA *see* cardiac amyloidosis
CABG *see* coronary artery bypass graft surgery
CAD *see* coronary artery disease
CADASIL *see* autosomal dominant arteriopathy with subcortical infarcts and leukoencephalopathy
calciphylaxis, risk factors   304, **316–317**
calcium oxalate dihydrate crystals   109, **121–122**
calcium pyrophosphate (CPP) crystal arthritis   431, **444**
calcium pyrophosphate dihydrate (CPPD) crystal arthritis   431, **444**
cancer
   acute myeloid leukaemia   197, **221**, 270, **276–277**
   angiogenesis   269, **274**
   autoimmunity   227, **236**
   basal cell carcinoma   61, **68**
   breast   269, **275**
   cervical screening program   269, **275–276**
   chronic myeloid leukaemia   189, 197–198, **211–212, 221–222**
   colon   110, **124**
   cytogenic abnormalities   193–194, **219–220**
   disseminated intravascular coagulation   186, **204**
   gastric   112, **126–127**
   HIV-associated   243, **261**
   Hodgkin's lymphoma   187, **206–207**
   lenalidomide   188, **208**
   leptomeningeal carcinomatosis   270, **277**
   Lynch syndrome   270, **278**
   malignant mesothelioma   395, **416–417**
   melanoma   59, **65–66**
   metastatic cord compression   271, **278–279**
   metastatic renal cell cancer   269, **274**
   multiple endocrine neoplasia   74, **86–87**
   multiple myeloma   188–189, **208–210**
   non-Hodgkin lymphoma   189, **211**

cancer (*Contd.*)
  non-small cell lung   270, 271, **276**, **279–280**
  obesity   271, **280**
  opioid rotation   361, **364–365**
  ovarian   272, **283**
  palliative medicine   361–362, **364–366**
  post-transplant   307, 308, **326**, **328**
  premature ovarian failure   74, **85**
  programmed death ligand 1 (PD-L1) 271, **281**
  prostate   271–272, **279**, **281–282**
  small cell lung   227, **236**, 338, **353**, 399, **423**
  sunscreen usage   61, **68**
  thyroid   76–77, **93–94**
  see also chemotherapy; oncology
cancer of unknown primary (CUP)   270, **278**
Candida auris   237, **244**
cannabinoids   334, **343**
CAP see community acquired pneumonia
Captopril   11, **31**
carbamazepine   292, **301**
carbapenemase-producing Enterobacterales (CPE)   238, **246**
carbon monoxide (CO) poisoning   34, **44**
carcinoid heart disease   143, **154**
carcinoma
  basal cell   61, **68**
  hepatocellular   113, **130–131**
  thyroid   76–77, **93–94**
cardiac amyloidosis (CA)   3, **16–17**
cardiac arrest   40, **53**
cardiac catheterisation   35–36, **45**
cardiac output, increasing   3, **17–18**
cardiac syncope   3, **18**
cardiac tamponade   34, **43–44**
cardiology
  abdominal aortic aneurysm   1, **13**
  acute rheumatic fever   7, **26**
  amiodarone-induced hypothyroidism   72, **81**
  amyloidosis   3, **16–17**
  anthracycline cardiomyopathy   2, **14**
  antithrombotic therapy   2, **15–16**
  aortic stenosis   2, 8, **14–15**, **28**
  atrial fibrillation   1, 2, **13–14**, **15**
  atrial septal defect   12, **32**
  β-blockers   2, 11, **15–16**, **31**
  bifascicular block   39, **51–52**
  Brugada syndrome   2–3, **16**
  carcinoid heart disease   143, **154**
  cardiac output   3, **17–18**
  cholesterol embolisation   3–4, **18–19**
  computed tomography coronary angiography (CTCA)   4, **19–20**
  congenital conditions   12, **32–33**
  coronary artery disease   2, 9, **15–16**, **28**
  Eisenmenger's syndrome   12, **32**
  heart block   35, 39, 40, **45**, **51–52**
  heart failure with preserved ejection fraction (HFpEF)   5, **21**
  Holter monitoring   6, **23**
  hyperkalaemia   35–36, **45**
  hypertensive retinopathy   6, **22**

hypertrophic obstructive cardiomyopathy   5, **22**
implantable cardioverter-defibrillators (ICDs)   2, 4–5, 6, **15**, **16**, **20**, **22–23**
infective endocarditits   4, **20**
intra-aortic balloon pump   36, **47**
left bundle branch block (LBBB)   35, 39, **45**, **51–52**, 458, **462**
lipid-lowering agents   6, **23**
long QT syndrome   7, **23–24**
Marfan's syndrome   12, **32**
medications   11, **31**
mitral stenosis   7, **24**
Mobitz type I heart block   40, **51–52**
Mobitz type II 2:1 heart block   39, **51–52**
multivessel coronary artery disease   9, **28**
myocardial infarction (MI)   8, 9–10, **26–27**, **29–30**, 35–36, 38–40, **45**, **51–52**, 142, **154**
pacemakers   4–5, **20**
patent ductus arteriosus   12, **33**
pericarditis   35–36, **45**
polyunsaturated fatty acids   7, **24–25**
restrictive cardiomyopathy   7, **25**
rheumatic fever   7, **24**, **26**
right ventricular myocardial infarction   8, **26–27**
sinus node dysfunction   8, **27**
ST elevation acute myocardial infarction (STEMI)   35–36, **45**
syncope   3, **18**
Takotsubo cardiomyopathy   8, **27–28**
temporary pacing   38–40, **51–52**
Tetralogy of Fallot   12, **32**
torsade de pointes   42, **56**
transcatheter aortic valve implantation   8, **28**
transposition of the great arteries   12, **32–33**
treatment-resistant hypertension   7, **25**
troponins   9, **29**
type 2 diabetes   5, **21**
ventricular septal defects   12, **32**
Wolff–Parkinson–White syndrome   10–11, **30–31**
cardiomyopathy
  anthracycline   2, **14**
  hypertrophic   5, **22**
  restrictive   7, **25**
  Takotsubo-type   8, **27–28**
Carotid artery stenosis   339, **356**
CAR T see chimeric antigen receptor T-cells
carvedilol   374, **392**
case-control studies   99, **103**
case fatality   98, **105**
catecholamines, phaeochromocytoma   75, **89–90**
CCRT see concurrent chemoradiotherapy
CD see conversion disorder; Crohn's disease
CDI see *Clostridium difficile* infection
cell-free DNA (cfDNA)   458, **462**
cellulitis, acute interstitial nephritis   302–303, **313–314**
central tendency   97, **100**
central venous sinus thrombosis (CVST)   335, **344**
cephalosporin resistance   239, **250–251**
cerebrospinal fluid (CSF), components   335, **345**
cervical screening program   269, **275–276**

cervicogenic headaches   145, **162**
cessation
    antidepressant   291, **298**
    dialysis   360, **363–364**
CF *see* cystic fibrosis
cfDNA *see* cell-free DNA
CFS *see* chronic fatigue syndrome
CGM *see* continuous glucose monitoring
Charcot-Marie-Tooth (CMT) disease   340–341, **358**
chemotherapy
    adverse events   272–273, **285–286**
    concurrent radiotherapy   272, **282**
    premature ovarian failure   74, **85**
    targeted molecular agents   273, **287–288**
    tumor lysis syndrome   272, **283–284**
chemotherapy-induced nausea and vomiting (CINV)   269, **276**
Cheyne-Stokes respirations   362, **366**
chiasma   341, **359**
chimeric antigen receptor T-cells (CAR T)   269, **275**
Chi-squared test   98, 98, **102–103**, **104**
Chlamydia trachomatis   237, **245**
chloroquine   239–240, **251**
cholesterol embolisation   3–4, **18–19**
cholinesterase inhibitors, Alzheimer's disease   **379**
chromaffin cells   75, **89–90**
chronic fatigue syndrome (CFS)   143, **155**
chronic idiopathic constipation   111, **125**
chronic inflammatory demyelinating polyradiculoneuropathy
    (CIDP)   335, **344–345**
chronic kidney disease (CKD)
    adynamic bone disease   302, **313**
    ampicillin elimination   368, **376**
    bone-kidney endocrine axis   307, **324**
    darbepoetin   307, **324**
    diabetic nephropathy   73, **83**, 310, **331–332**
    secondary hyperparathyroidism   74, **86**
    see also nephrology
chronic kidney disease–mineral and bone disorders
    (CKD-MBD)   302, 304, **313**, **317**
chronic liver disease   108, **119–122**
    encephalopathy   112, **128**
chronic lymphocytic leukaemia (CLL)   185, **203**
chronic mesenteric iscaemia   114, **134**
chronic myeloid leukaemia (CML)   189, 197–198, **211–212**, **221–222**
chronic obstructive pulmonary disease (COPD)   394, 396, **414**,
    417, **420**
chronic thromboembolic pulmonary hypertension (CTEPH)   394,
    412–413
CIDP *see* chronic inflammatory demyelinating
    polyradiculoneuropathy
CIN *see* contrast-induced nephropathy
CINV *see* chemotherapy-induced nausea and vomiting
circulatory shock   34, **44–45**
cirrhosis   108, 110, 112, 115, **119–120**, **122–123**, **127–128**, **137**
cisplatin   273, **286**
citalopram   292, **301**
citrate   74, **86**
CKD *see* chronic kidney disease

CKD-MBD *see* chronic kidney disease–mineral and bone disorders
classifications
    adipocytes   73, **82**
    myocardial infarction   9–10, **29–30**
climate change   459, **462**
clinical trials   99, **103**
    see also research
CLL *see* chronic lymphocytic leukaemia
clopidogrel   369, **379**
Clostridium difficile infection (CDI)   38, **49**, **51**, 237, **244**
clozapine   289, 292, **294**, **301**
CML *see* chronic myeloid leukaemia
CMT *see* Charcott-Marie-Tooth disease
CO *see* carbon monoxide
CoA *see* coarctation of the aorta
coagulopathies, cirrhosis-related   110, **122–123**
coal workers' pneumoconiosis   396, **419**
coarctation of the aorta (CoA)   12, **32**
cocaine overdose   375, **392**
Cockcroft–Gault formula   370, **381**
coeliac disease   57, **63**, 110, **123–124**
colon cancer   110, **124**
colorectal cancer, Lynch syndrome   270, **278**
commencement, dialysis   304–305, **318**
common variable immunodeficiency (CVID)   224, **230**
community acquired pneumonia (CAP)   394, **411**, **413**
competitive inhibition   369, **381**
components of cerebrospinal fluid   335, **345**
computed tomography coronary angiography (CTCA)   4, **19–20**
concurrent chemoradiotherapy (CCRT)   272, **282**
confidentiality, mental health   291, **298–299**
confounding   98–99, **105–106**
congenital heart disease   12, **32–33**
conjugate vaccines   226, **235**
Conn's syndrome   149, **168**
consent
    mental health   291, **298–299**
    research   98, **103–104**
constipation   111, **125**
continuous glucose monitoring (CGM)   76, **91–92**
continuous positive airway pressure (CPAP)   396, **418–419**
contraindications, extracorporeal membrane oxygenation   **46**
contrast-induced nephropathy (CIN)   308, **326–327**
conversion disorder (CD)   289, **295**
COP *see* cryptogenic organizing pneumonia
COPD *see* chronic obstructive pulmonary disease
coronary artery bypass graft surgery (CABG)   9, **28**
coronary artery disease (CAD)   2, **15–16**
    multivessel   9, **28**
corpus callosum   341, **359**
correlation   98, **102–103**
corticosteroids, palliative medicine   361–362, **366**
Covid-19   225, **232–233**, 237, **245–246**, 459, 460, **462–463**,
    464, **468**
Coxiella burnetii   241, **254**
CPAP *see* continuous positive airway pressure
CPE *see* carbapenemase-producing Enterobacterales
CPP *see* calcium pyrophosphate

CPPD *see* calcium pyrophosphate dihydrate
cranial nerve palsy 341, **359**
critical care 34–56
  acute kidney injury 37, **49–50**
  acute respiratory distress syndrome 34, **43**
  advance care planning 36, **47**
  bifascicular block 39, **51–52**
  carbon monoxide poisoning 34, **44**
  cardiac arrest 40, **53**
  cardiac tamponade 34, **43–44**
  circulatory shock 34, **44–45**
  dialysis 37, **49–50**
  disseminated intravascular coagulation 34, **44**
  early goal-directed therapy 38, **50**
  encephalopathy 36, **46**
  extracorporeal membrane oxygenation 36, **46**
  gastrointestinal bleeding 37, **49**
  head injuries 40, **52**
  hyperkalaemia 35–36, 42, **45**, **55–56**
  intra-aortic balloon pump 36, **47**
  left bundle branch block 35, 39, **45**, **51–52**
  Mobitz type I heart block 40, **51–52**
  Mobitz type II 2:1 heart block 39, **51–52**
  myocardial infarction 35–36, 38–40, **45**, **51–52**
  necrotising fasciitis 36, **47–48**
  opiate toxicity 42, **56**
  paracetamol overdose management 37, **48**
  pericarditis 35–36, **45**
  pulseless electrical activity 37, **48–49**
  septic shock 37–38, 40–41, **49–50**, **51**, **53–54**
  severe asthma 38, 42, **50–51**, **55**
  ST elevation acute myocardial infarction 35–36, **45**
  temporary pacing 38–40, **51–52**
  torsade de pointes 42, **56**
  tranexamic acid 40, **52**
  venous blood gas (VBG) 40, **52**
Crohn's disease (CD) 109, **122**
crossover studies 369, **379–380**
cross-sectional studies 99, **103**
crude rates 98, **105**
cryoglobulinaemia 224, **230**
cryptogenic organizing pneumonia (COP) 407, **427**
crystal arthritis 431, **444–445**
CSF *see* cerebrospinal fluid
CTCA *see* computed tomography coronary angiography
CTEPH *see* chronic thromboembolic pulmonary hypertension
CUP *see* cancer of unknown primary
Cushing's syndrome 72, 73, **80**, **82–83**
CVID *see* common variable immunodeficiency
CVST *see* central venous sinus thrombosis
CYP446 enzymes, pharmacology 372, **386**
cyproterone acetate 77, **94**
cystine crystals 109, **121–122**
cystic fibrosis (CF) 170, **175**, 394, **412**
cytogenic abnormalities, malignancies 193–194, **219–220**

DAA *see* direct-acting antiviral therapy
dafrafenib 273, **287**

dapagliflozin 76, **92**
darbepoetin 307, **324**
dasatinib 273, **287**
D-dimer degradation product of fibrin 394, **414**
deep vein thrombosis (DVT) 192, **217**
degradation, fibrin 394, **414**
dementia 143, 150, **155–156**, **168**
dendritic cells 226, **235**
  metabolism 74, **86**
dengue haemorrhagic fever 238, **246–247**
denosumab **378**
depression 290–291, 291, **295–296**, **298**
dermatitis herpetiformis (DH) 57, **63**
dermatology 57–70
  acute generalised exanthematous pustulosis 62, **69**
  basal cell carcinoma 61, **68**
  bullous pemphigoid 57, 60, **63**, **66–67**
  coeliac disease 57, **63**
  dermatitis herpetiformis 57, **63**
  drug rash with eosinophilia and systemic symptoms 61, **69**
  erythema nodosum 58–59, **63–64**
  Henoch-Schönlein purpura 59, **64–65**
  melanoma 59, **65–66**
  porphyria cutanea tarda 60, **66–67**
  rosacea 60, **67**
  scabies 61, **67**
  skin layers 61, **68**
  Staphylococcal scalded skin syndrome 62, **69**
  Stevens Johnson Syndrome 61, 62, **68–69**
  sunscreen usage 61, **68**
  toxic epidermal necrolysis 61, 62, **68–69**
dermatomyositis **445**
descriptors of mental health 291–292, **299–300**
DH *see* dermatitis herpetiformis
diabetes
  continuous glucose monitoring 76, **91–92**
  dapagliflozin treatment 76, **92**
  maturity-onset of the young (MODY) 74, **87**, 170–171, **177–178**
diabetic gastroparesis 75, **88–89**
diabetic ketoacidosis (DKA) 73, **83–84**
diabetic nephropathy (DN) 73, **83**, 310, **331–332**
diabetic neuropathy, painful 75, **88**
dialysis 37, **49–50**
  commencement 304–305, **318**
  peritoneal 307, **325**
  withdrawal at end-of-life 360, **363–364**
digoxin 145–146, **163**
direct-acting antiviral (DAA) therapy 113, **129**
disease-modifying antirheumatic drugs (DMARDs) 440–441, **457**
dispersion measures 98, **103**
disseminated intravascular coagulation (DIC) 34, **44**, 186, **204**
  D-dimer degradation product of fibrin 394, **414**
distribution-free tests 97, **100–101**
Dix–Hallpike manoeuvre 334, **342–343**
DKA *see* diabetic ketoacidosis
DMARDs *see* disease-modifying antirheumatic drugs

DMD *see* Duchenne muscular dystrophy
DMEs *see* drug metabolising enzymes
DN *see* diabetic nephropathy
DNA
  cell-free 458, **462**
  mitochondrial 172, **180**
  see also epigenetics; genetics; mutations
dobutamine 41, **54**
Dobutamine Stress Echocardiography (DSE) 2, **14–15**
Down's syndrome 170, **176**
doxorubicin 273, **286–287**
  anthracycline cardiomyopathy 2, **14**
dropouts, as source of bias 97, **101–102**
drug allergies
  amoxicillin 223, **228–229**
  penicillin 225, **228**, **232**
drug-induced acute interstitial nephritis 302–303, **313–314**
drug-induced Parkinsonism 292, **301**
drug metabolising enzymes (DMEs), variation 372, **386**
drug rash with eosinophilia and systemic symptoms 61, **69**
dry mouth, palliative medicine 360, **363**
Dubin–Johnson syndrome 112, **127**
Duchenne muscular dystrophy (DMD) 170, **176–177**
duloxetine 292, **300–301**
DVT *see* deep vein thrombosis
dyskinesias, levodopa-induced 338, **354**
dysphagia, oesophageal 115, **135–136**
dyspnoea, chronic thromboembolic pulmonary hypertension 394, **412–413**

early goal-directed therapy (EGDT) 38, **50**
echinocandins 237, **245**
ECMO *see* extracorporeal membrane oxygenation
ECT *see* electroconvulsive therapy
eculizumab 184, **199**
EGDT *see* early goal-directed therapy
eGFR *see* estimated glomerular filtration rates
EGPA *see* eosinophilic granulomatosis with polyangiitis
Eisenmenger's syndrome 12, **32**
elder abuse 143, **156–157**
elderly patients
  anticholinergic medicines 368, **376–377**
  polypharmacy 372–373, **387**
  see also geriatric medicine
electroconvulsive therapy (ECT) 290, 296
electromechanical dissociation *see* pulseless electrical activity
electronic cigarettes 143, **157**
embolisation, cholesterol 3–4, **18–19**
EMD (electromechanical dissociation) *see* pulseless electrical activity
emphysema 394, **414**
encephalopathy, critical care 36, **46**
encephalitis
  herpes simplex viruses 336, **347–348**
  small cell lung cancer 338, **353**
endocarditis, infective 4, **20**
endocrinology 71–96
  acromegaly 71, **79**

adipocytes 73, **82**
adrenal crisis 72, **80**
adrenal incidentaloma 72, **80**
amiodarone-induced hypothyroidism 72, **81**
autoimmune polyendocrine syndrome 72, **81–82**
bariatric surgery 77–78, **95–96**
bariatric surgery complications 77–78, **95–96**
Cushing's syndrome 72, 73, **80**, **82–83**
dapagliflozin effects 76, **92**
dendritic cell metabolism 74, **86**
diabetic gastroparesis 75, **88–89**
diabetic ketoacidosis 73, **83–84**
diabetic nephropathy 73, **83**
erectile dysfunction 74, **84–85**
gastrointestinal 117, **137–143**
gender-affirmation treatment 77, **94–95**
HbA1c levels 75, **90**
hypogonadism 74, **85**
hypothyroidism 76, 78, **92–93**, **96**
macrophage metabolites 74, **86**
maturity-onset diabetes of the young 74, **87**
multiple endocrine neoplasia 74, **86–87**
Paget's disease of bone 75, **87–88**
painful diabetic neuropathy 75, **88**
phaeochromocytoma 75, **89–90**
pituitary tumours 75–76, **90–91**
polycystic ovarian syndrome 75, **89**
premature ovarian failure 74, **85**
secondary hyperparathyroidism 74, **86**
testosterone treatment 74, **84–85**
thyroid carcinomas 76–77, **93–94**
thyroid nodules 77, **94**
end-of-life care *see* palliative medicine
endovascular thrombectomy 336, **348–349**
end-stage kidney disease (ESKD)
  secondary hyperparathyroidism 74, **86**
  see also nephrology
eosinophilic esophagitis (EoE) 111, **125**
eosinophilic granulomatosis with polyangiitis (EGPA) 401, 408, **424**, **429**
eosinophilic/Th2 asthma 393, **410–411**
epidemiology 97–106
  attack rate 98, **105**
  case fatality 98, **105**
  confounding 98–99, **105–106**
  crude rates 98, **105**
  forest plots 98–99, **103–103**
  incidence rate 98, **105**
  odds ratio 97, **101**
  population attributable risk 98, **105**
  prevalence 98, 98, **102**, **104**
  risk 98, **104–105**
epigenetics 170, **177**
epilepsy
  cannabinoids 334, **343**
  lamotrigine dosage 335, **345–346**
EpiPens 223, **228**
EPO *see* erythropoietin

erectile dysfunction (ED)   74, **84–85**
erythema nodosum   58–59, **63–64**
erythropoiesis, roxadustat   306, **322–323**
erythropoietin (EPO)   307, **324**
Escherichia coli   **256**
ESGYS *see* Evaluation of Guidelines in SYncope study
ESKD *see* end-stage kidney disease
essential thrombocythaemia (ET)   186, **204–205**
estimated glomerular filtration rates (eGFR)   370, **381**
ET *see* essential thrombocythaemia
etanercept   436, **451**
ethosuximide   340, **357**
ethylene glycol poisoning   370, **381**
Evaluation of Guidelines in SYncope study (ESGYS) scores   **18**
evolocumab   6, **23**
exhaustion, heat   144, **159**
extracorporeal membrane oxygenation (ECMO)   36, **46**
exudates, pleural   397, **421**
ezetimibe   6, **23**

factor deficiencies   185–186, 192–193, **203–204**, **218**
faecal calprotectin (FC)   111, **126**
FC *see* faecal calprotectin
FDEIA *see* food-dependent, exercise-induced anaphylaxis
febrile neutropaenia (FN)   186, **205**
febuxostat   433, **446**
feminising hormone therapy   77, **94–95**
fertility, transplant recipients   263, **267–268**
fertility preservation
   chemotherapy   74, **85**
   gender-affirmation treatment   **95**
FGF-23   307, **324**
fibrillation, atrial   1, 2, **13–14**, **15**
fibrin, degradation   394, **414**
fibromyalgia   433, **447**
first-pass metabolism   368, 370, **376**, **382**
Fisher's exact test   98, **103**
fluorouracil   273, **285**
FN *see* febrile neutropaenia
food-dependent, exercise-induced anaphylaxis (FDEIA)   224, **231**
forest plots   98–99, **103–103**
frontotemporal dementia   150, **168**
FSGS *see* focal segmental glomerulosclerosis
funnel plots   98, **104**

gabapentin   340, **357**
ganciclovir   370, **381**
Gardner syndrome   173, **182**
gastric bypass, metabolic/nutritional complications   77–78, **95–96**
gastric cancer (GC)   112, **126–127**
gastrin   117, **137**
gastroenterology   107–143
   ascites   108, **119–120**
   autoimmune hepatitis   108, **120**
   Barrett's oesophagus   108–109, **121**
   brush border microvilli   109, **121**
   cirrhosis   108, 110, 112, 115, **119–120**, **122–123**, **127–128**, **137**

coeliac disease   110, **123–124**
colon cancer   110, **124**
constipation   111, **125**
Crohn's disease   109, **122**
endocrinology   117, **137–143**
eosinophilic esophagitis   111, **125**
gastric cancer   112, **126–127**
HBsAg positivity   112, **129**
Helicobacter pylori   112, **128**
hepatic encephalopathy   112, **128**
hepatic steatosis   114, **134–135**
hepatitis viruses   112–113, **129–130**
hepatocellular carcinoma   113, **130–131**
hepatorenal syndrome   116, **139**
hereditary haemochromatosis   113, **131**
high-resolution manometry   115, **135**
hypergastrinemia   117, **137**
inflammatory bowel disease   111, **126**
irritable bowel syndrome   113, **131–132**
lactose intolerance   113, **132–133**
liver transplants   114, 116, **133**, **138–139**
lower GI bleeding   114, **133–134**
mesenteric iscaemia   107, 114, **118**, **134**
oesophageal dysphagia   115, **135–136**
Ogilvie's syndrome   116–117, **137–138**
pancreatitis   107–108, **118–119**
primary biliary cirrhosis   112, 115, **127–128**, **137**
proton-pump inhibitors   115, **136–137**
renal calculi   109, **121–122**
small bowel bacterial overgrowth   116, **138**
unconjugated hyperbilirubinemia   112, **127–128**
upper gastrointestinal bleeding   116–117, **139–137**
gastrointestinal bleeding   37, **49**
gastroparesis, diabetic   75, **88–89**
gating, radiotherapy   272, **283**
GBM *see* glioblastoma multiforme
GBS *see* Guillain–Barré syndrome
GC *see* gastric cancer
GCA *see* giant cell arteritis
gender-affirmation treatment   77, **94–95**
general medicine   141–169
genetic medicine   170–183
   Angelman syndrome   171, **178–179**
   autoimmune polyendocrine syndrome   **81–82**
   beta-thalassemia   170, **175**
   cystic fibrosis   170, **175**
   Down's syndrome   170, **176**
   Duchenne muscular dystrophy   170, **176–177**
   epigenetics   170, **177**
   Gardner syndrome   173, **182**
   Huntington's disease   171, **178**
   inheritance patterns   173–174, **182–185**
   Klinefelter syndrome   171, **179**
   maternal inheritance   171–172, **179–180**
   melanoma   59, **65**
   mitochondrial DNA mutations   172, **180**
   multiple endocrine neoplasia   74, **86–87**
   Paget's disease of bone   75, **87–88**
   Prader–Willi syndrome   **182**

small interfering RNA 172, **180–181**
spina bifida 173, **182**
spinocerebellar ataxia 172, **181**
thyroid carcinomas 76–77, **93–94**
tuberous sclerosis complex 172, **181–182**
variants of uncertain significance 170–171, **177–178**
Von Hippel–Lindau syndrome **87**, **181**
Wilson's disease 173, **182**
geometric mean 97, **100**
geriatric medicine 141–169
  anticholinergic medicines 368, 371, **376–377**, **384**
  pharmacokinetics 368, **376**
  polypharmacy 372–373, **387**
GH *see* growth hormone
giant cell arteritis (GCA) 433, **447**
Gilbert syndrome (GS) 112, **127**
GLIM *see* Global Leadership Initiative on Malnutrition
glioblastoma multiforme (GBM) 338–339, **355**
Global Leadership Initiative on Malnutrition (GLIM) 459,
  465–466
glomerulonephritis
  IgA nephropathy 305, 307, **319–320**, **325**
  membranoproliferative 309–310, **331**
  synpharyngitic 150, **168**
glyceryl trinitrate 11, **31**
gonadotrophin-releasing hormone analogues 77, **94**
Goodpasture's syndrome 310–311, **332**
gout 431–432, 433, **444–445**, **446**
graft-versus-host disease (GVHD) 191, **214**, **215**
granulotomatosis with polyangiitis (GPA) 401, 405, **424**, **426**
great arteries, transpositions 12, **32–33**
growth hormone (GH), acromegaly 71, **79**
GS *see* Gilbert syndrome
Guillain–Barré syndrome (GBS) 335–336, 337, **346**, **349–350**
GVHD *see* graft-versus-host disease
gynaecomastia 143, **158**

HAART *see* highly active antiretroviral therapy
HAE *see* hereditary angioedema
haematology 184–222
  acute myeloid leukaemia 197, **221**
  anaemia of chronic disease 187, **206**
  aplastic anaemia 185, **200–201**
  apoptosis 185, **201**
  atypical haemolytic uraemic syndrome 196, **221**
  autoimmune haemolytic anaemia 184, **199–200**
  BCL-2 family proteins 185, **201**
  chronic lymphocytic leukaemia 185, **203**
  chronic myeloid leukaemia 189, 197–198, **211–212**, **221–222**
  cytogenetics of malignancies 193–194, **219–220**
  deep vein thrombosis 192, **217**
  disseminated intravascular coagulation 186, **204**
  essential thrombocythaemia 186, **204–205**
  factor deficiencies 185–186, 192–193, **203–204**, **218**
  febrile neutropaenia 186, **205**
  graft-versus-host disease 191, **214**, **215**
  haemolytic anaemia 184, **199–200**
  haemolytic uraemic syndrome 184, **199**

heparin-induced thrombocytopenia 186, **205–206**
hereditary spherocytosis 194, **220**
Hodgkin's lymphoma 187, **206–207**
idiopathic thrombocytopenic purpura 187–188, **207–208**
inherited thrombophilia 191, **216**
iron metabolism 187, **207**
lenalidomide 188, **208**
leukaemia 185, **203**
malignancy-related venous thromboembolism 184, **200**
microcytic anaemia 194, **220–221**
monoclonal gammopathy of undetermined significance 188,
  208
multiple myeloma 188–189, **208–210**
myeloproliferative neoplasms 189, 191, **211**, **213–214**
non-Hodgkin lymphoma 189, **211**
peripheral blood film examination 194–198, **220–222**
peripheral blood stem cell transplants 191, **215**
pernicious anaemia 189–190, **212**
platelet counts in pregnancy 263, **268**
polycythaemia vera 189, 191, **211**, **213–214**
progressive multifocal leukoencephalopathy 190, **213**
prolonged prothrombin time 185–186, **203–204**
protein C 193, **219**
sickle cell disease 191, **214–215**
transfusion-related acute lung injury 191–192, **216–217**
venous thromboembolism 184, **200**
von Willebrand disease 192–193, **218**
Waldenström macroglobulinaemia 193, **218–219**
warfarin 185, **201–203**
haematopoietic cell transplantation (HCT), graft-versus-host
  disease 191, **214**, **215**
haemochromatosis, hereditary 113, **131**
haemolytic anaemia, autoimmune 184, **199–200**
haemolytic uraemic syndrome (HUS) 184, **199**
haemoptysis 395, **416**
Hashimoto thyroiditis 76, **92–93**
HbA1c levels 75, **90**
HBS *see* Hungry bone syndrome
HBsAg positivity 112, **129**
HBV *see* hepatitis B
HCAIs *see* healthcare-associated infections
HCC *see* hepatocellular carcinoma
HCV *see* hepatitis C
HD *see* Huntington's disease
headaches
  cervicogenic 145, **162**
  medication overuse 337, **349**
  neuroimaging needs 336, **346–347**
head cancer, concurrent chemoradiotherapy 272, **282**
head injuries
  subdural haematoma 339, **356**
  tranexamic acid 40, **52**
healthcare-associated infections (HCAIs) 239, **250**
heart block
  bifascicular 39, **51–52**
  left bundle branch 35, 39, **45**, **51–52**, 458, **462**
  Mobitz type I 40, **51–52**
  Mobitz type II 2:1 39, **51–52**
heart failure with preserved ejection fraction (HFpEF) 5, **21**

heat exhaustion   144, **159**

Helicobacter pylori   112, **128**

helper T lymphocytes   226, **234**

hemiballismus   341, **358**

Henoch-Schönlein purpura (HSP)   59, **64–65**

heparin-induced thrombocytopenia (HIT)   186, **205–206**,
   370–371, **382–383**

hepatic steatosis   114, **134–135**

hepatitis
   ascites   108, **119–120**
   autoimmune   108, **120**
   cirrhosis   108, 110, 112, 115, **119–120**, **122–123**, **127–128**,
      137
   coagulopathies   110, **122–123**
   encephalopathies   112, **128**
   liver transplants   114, 116, **133**, **138–139**
   primary biliary cirrhosis   112, 115, **127–128**, **137**

hepatitis B (HBV) infection   112, **129**

hepatitis C (HCV) infection   113, **129**, 224, **230**

hepatitis E (HEV) infection   113, **130**

hepatocellular carcinoma (HCC)   113, **130–131**

hepatorenal syndrome, terlipressin   116, **139**

hepatotoxicity, paracetamol   115, **136**

hepcidin   187, **206**

hereditary nonpolyposis colorectal cancer (HNPCC)   270, **278**

hereditary spherocytosis   194, **220**

hereditary angioedema (HAE)   224, **231**

hereditary haemochromatosis (HH)   113, **131**

herpes simplex viruses (HSV)   242, **257**, 336, **347–348**

HEV *see* hepatitis E

HFpEF *see* heart failure with preserved ejection fraction

HG *see* hyperemesis gravidarum

HH *see* hereditary haemochromatosis

highly active antiretroviral therapy (HAART), immune reconstitution
   inflammatory syndrome   238, **247–248**

high-resolution manometry (HRM)   115, **135**

Hiprex *see* methenamine hippurate

HIT *see* heparin-induced thrombocytopenia

HIV infections   238–239, **247–249**
   acute   238–239, **248–249**
   associated cancers   243, **261**
   immune reconstitution inflammatory syndrome   238, **247–248**
   pre-exposure prophylaxis   238, **248**

HNPCC *see* hereditary nonpolyposis colorectal cancer

HOCM *see* hypertrophic obstructive cardiomyopathy

Hodgkin's lymphoma   187, **206–207**

Holter monitoring   6, **23**

hormone replacement therapy (HRT)   145, **161–162**

hormones, gastrointestinal   117, **137–143**

hormone therapy
   feminising   77, **94–95**
   masculinising   **94**

Horner's syndrome   334, **343**

HRT *see* hormone replacement therapy

HSP *see* Henoch-Schönlein purpura

HTLV-1 *see* Human T-cell lymphotropic virus type 1

human bite wounds   239, **249**

human papilloma viruses (HPV)   269, **275–276**, 459, **464**

Human T-cell lymphotropic virus type 1 (HTLV-1)   239, **249**

Hungry bone syndrome (HBS)   **86**

Huntington's disease (HD)   171, **178**

HUS *see* haemolytic uraemic syndrome

hydralazine   11, **31**

hydrocephalus   150, **168–169**

hydroxychloroquine   441, **457**

hyperammonaemia, valproic acid-induced   146–147, **166**

hyperbilirubinemia   112, **127–128**

hypercarbia   36, **46**

hyperemesis gravidarum (HG)   262, **265**

hypergastrinemia   117, **137**

hyperkalaemia   35–36, 42, **45**, **55–56**, 305, **318–319**, **321**

hyperparathyroidism   107, **118–119**
   secondary   74, **86**

hypertension
   chronic thromboembolic pulmonary   394, **412–413**
   clinical features   148–150, **167–168**
   pregnancy   262, 263, **265**, **266–267**
   treatment-resistant   7, **25**

hypertensive retinopathy   6, **22**

hypertrophic cardiomyopathy (HOCM)   5, **22**

hypocalcaemia   74, **86**

hypoglycaemia   144, **159**

hypogonadism   74, **85**

hypokalaemia   74, **86**

hypomagnesaemia   74, **86**

hyponatraemia   306, **323**

hypophosphataemia   74, **86**

hypotension, postural   146, **164**

hypothyroidism   76, 78, **92–93**, **96**
   amiodarone-induced   72, **81**
   pregnancy   262, **266**

hypoxia   36, **46**

hypoxia-inducible factors (HIF)   306, **322–323**, 459, **464**

IABP *see* intra-aortic balloon pump

IBD *see* inflammatory bowel disease

IBM *see* inclusion body myositis

IBS *see* irritable bowel syndrome

ICD *see* implantable cardioverter-defibrillator

ICO *see* internal carotid artery

idarubicin, anthracycline cardiomyopathy   2, **14**

IDH *see* isocitrate dehydrogenase

idiopathic inflammatory myopathies (IIM)   432, **445**

idiopathic pulmonary fibrosis (IPF)   398–399, 407, **422–423**,
   428

idiopathic thrombocytopenic purpura (ITP)   187–188, **207–208**

idiopathic ventricular arrhythmias   460, **466–467**

IE *see* infective endocarditis

ifosfamide   272–273, **285**

IgAN *see* IgA nephropathy

IgA nephropathy (IgAN)   305, 307, **319–320**, **325**

IGF-1 *see* insulin like growth factor 1

IgG4-related disease (IgG4-RD)   107, **119**, 225, **232**

IIM *see* idiopathic inflammatory myopathies

IMiD *see* immunomodulatory imide drugs

immune reconstitution inflammatory syndrome (IRIS) 238,
  247–248
immunology 223–236
  anaphylaxis 223, 224, 225, **228**, **231**, **233–234**
  antibody-mediated rejection 223, **229**, 303, **314–315**
  antibody production 223, **229**
  cell types and functions 226, **234–235**
  common variable immunodeficiency 224, **230**
  cryoglobulinaemia 224, **230**
  hereditary angioedema 224, **231**
  IgG4-related disease 107, **119**, 225, **232**
  neurological autoantibody effects 227, **236**
  RNA vaccines 225, **232–233**
  systemic mastocytosis 225, **233**
  toll-like receptors 226, **234**
  vaccinations 225, 226, **232–233**, **235–236**
immunomodulatory imide drugs (IMiD)
  lenalidomide 188, **208**
  multiple myeloma 188, 189, **208**, **210**
immunosuppressants, mechanisms of action 308–309, **329–330**
implantable cardioverter-defibrillator (ICD) 2, 4–5, 6, **15**, **16**, **20**,
  22–23
incidence rate 98, **105**
inclusion body myositis (IBM) 433–434, **445**, **447**
incubation periods 460, **468**
indapamide 371, **383**
indications
  extracorporeal membrane oxygenation **46**
  high-resolution manometry 115, **135**
  intra-aortic balloon pump **47**
  liver transplants 114, **133**
  non-invasive positive pressure ventilation 396, **418**
Indigenous Australians, acute kidney injury 303, **314**
infarct-related artery (IRA) revascularisation 9, **28**
infectious diseases 237–261
  acute vertebral osteomyelitis 241, **256**
  antibacterial agents 242, **258–259**
  antifungal agents 237, **245**
  antimicrobial resistance 242–243, **259–260**
  antivirals 243, **260**
  Burkholderia pseudomallei 240, **251–252**
  Candida auris 237, **244**
  carbapenemase-producing Enterobacterales 238, **246**
  cephalosporin resistance 239, **250–251**
  Chlamydia trachomatis 237, **245**
  Clostridium difficile 38, **49**, **51**, 237, **244**
  community acquired pneumonia 394, **411–412**, **413**
  dengue haemorrhagic fever 238, **246–247**
  Escherichia coli **256**
  healthcare-associated 239, **250**
  Helicobacter pylori 112, **128**
  hepatitis B 112, **129**
  hepatitis C 113, **129**, 224, **230**
  hepatitis E 113, **130**
  herpes zoster 242, **257**
  HIV 238–239, 243, **247–249**, **261**
  human bite wounds 239, **249**
  human papilloma viruses 269, **275–276**, 459, **464**

Human T-cell lymphotropic virus type 1 239, **249**
immune reconstitution inflammatory syndrome 238, **247–248**
incubation periods 460, **468**
influenza vaccinations 239, **250**
JC virus 190, **213**
Legionella 395, **415**
Listeria monocytogenes 239, **250–251**
meningococcal follow-up 242, **257–258**
methenamine hippurate treatment 240, **252**
necrotising fasciitis 36, **47–48**
Norovirus 241, **253**
Plasmodium falciparum 239, **251**
Pseudomonas aeruginosa **256**, 371, **383–384**
pulmonary tuberculosis 241, **255**
pyrexia of unknown origin 241, **253–254**
Q fever 241, **254**
SARS-CoV-2 225, **232–233**, 237, **245–246**, 459, 460,
  462–463, **464**, **468**
Staphylococcus aureus 241, **255**, **256**
Streptococcus pneumoniae 394, **411–412**, **413**
Streptococcus pyogenes **256**
strongyloidiasis 148, **166–167**, 241, **254–255**
syphilis 240, **252–253**
vaccinations 225, 226, **232–233**, **235–236**
varicella-zoster virus 242, **257**
Zika virus 242, **257**
infective endocarditis (IE) 4, **20**
inflammatory bowel disease (IBD) 111, **126**
influenza vaccinations 239, **250**
information bias 98–99, **105–106**
informed consent
  mental health 291, **298–299**
  research 98, **103–104**
inheritance patterns 173–174, **182–185**
inherited thrombophilia 191, **216**
inhibition
  competitive/non-competitive 369, **381**
  low-density lipoprotein receptors 6, **23**
  P-glycoprotein 372, **385**
  SGLT2 5, **21**, 76, **83**, **92**, 308, **327**
insomnia 144, **160**
insulin like growth factor 1 (IGF-1), acromegaly 71, **79**
intermittently scanned continuous glucose monitoring 76, **91–92**
internal carotid artery (ICO) 336, **348**
International Society of Thrombosis and Haemostasis (ISTH)
  scores 34, **44**
interquartile range (IQR) 98, **103**
interstitial lung disease (ILD) 400–401, **424**
intolerances, lactose 113, **132–133**
intra-aortic balloon pump (IABP) 36, **47**
intracranial parenchymal haemorrhage 336, **348**
ionotropes, critical care 41, **54**
IPF *see* idiopathic pulmonary fibrosis
IQR *see* interquartile range
IRA *see* infarct-related artery revascularisation
IRIS *see* immune reconstitution inflammatory syndrome
iron deficiency anaemia 75, **90**
iron metabolism 187, **207**

irritable bowel syndrome (IBS)   113, **131–132**
ischaemic stroke   336–337, 339, **348–349**, **356**
   pharmacological treatment   373–384, **389**
isocitrate dehydrogenase (IDH), cancerous mutations   270,
   276–277
ISTH *see* International Society of Thrombosis and Haemostasis
I² test   98, **104**
ITP *see* idiopathic thrombocytopenic purpura
ixazomib   189, **210**

JC virus   190, **213**
juvenile epilepsy syndrome   334, **343**

ketoacidosis, diabetic   73, **83–84**
kidneys
   diabetic nephropathy   73, **83**
   transplantation   263, **267–268**
   see also acute kidney injury; chronic kidney disease; end-stage
      kidney disease; nephrology
Klinefelter syndrome (KS)   171, **179**
Krebs cycle   74, **86**
kyphoscoliosis   397, **420**

L5 radiculopathy   339, **355**
lactate levels   458, **461**
lactose intolerance   113, **132–133**
lacunar stroke syndromes   336, **348**
LAM *see* lymphangioleiomyomatosis
lamotrigine   335, **345–346**
laparoscopic sleeve gastrectomy (LSG)   77, **95**
lapatinib   273, **288**
large vessel occlusions (LVO)   336, **348**
lateral medullary syndrome   338, **355**
layers of the skin   61, **68**
LBBB *see* left bundle branch block
LCSD *see* left cardiac sympathetic denervation
leflunomide   441, **457**
left bundle branch block (LBBB)   35, 39, **45**, **51–52**, 458, **462**
left cardiac sympathetic denervation (LCSD)   7, **23–24**
left ventricular hypertrophy (LVH)   35–36, **45**
Legionella Sp.   395, **415**
leg ulcers, venous   144, **160–161**
lenalidomide   188, **208**
leptomeningeal carcinomatosis   270, **277**
lesions, neurological   341, **358–359**
leukaemia
   acute myeloid   197, **221**, 270, **276–277**
   chronic lymphocytic   185, **203**
   chronic myeloid   189, 197–198, **211–212**, **221–222**
levodopa-induced dyskinesias   338, **354**
levosimendan   41, **54**
Lewy bodies   143, **156**
LGIB *see* lower gastrointestinal bleeding
light chain amyloidosis (AL)   3, **16–17**
Light's criteria   397, **421**, **423**
linezolid   371, **383–384**

lipodermatosclerosis   302–303, **313–314**
liquid biopsies   458, **462**
Listeria monocytogenes   239, **250–251**
lithium   78, **96**
   adverse effects   292, **301**, 305, **320**
   pregnancy   289, **293**
liver transplants   114, 116, **133**, **138–139**
Löfgren syndrome   406, **426–427**
long QT syndrome (LQT)   7, **23–24**, 42, **56**
   psychotropic medications   292, **301**
low back pain   144–145, **161**
low-density lipoprotein (LDL) receptors, inhibition   6, **23**
lower gastrointestinal bleeding (LGIB)   114, **134**
LQT *see* long QT syndrome
LS *see* Lynch syndrome
LSG *see* laparoscopic sleeve gastrectomy
lung cancer
   management   270, 271, **276**, **279–280**
   metastatic   402–403, **425**
   mutations   271, **279–280**
   small cell   227, **236**, 338, **353**, 399, **423**
lungs, transfusion-related acute injury (TRALI)   191–192, **216–217**
lupus nephritis   305, **320–321**
LVH *see* left ventricular hypertrophy
LVO *see* large vessel occlusions
lymphangioleiomyomatosis (LAM)   408–409, **428**
lymphocytes
   antibody production   223, **229**
   cell types and functions   226, **234–235**
lymphoproliferative disorder, post-transplant (PTLD)   307, 308,
   326, **328**
Lynch syndrome (LS)   270, **278**

MACE *see* major adverse cardiac events
macrocytic anaemia   189–190, **212**
macrophages   226, **234**
   metabolism   74, **86**
magnesium sulphate, preeclampsia   263, **267**
major adverse cardiac events (MACE), perioperative
   management   145, **163**
malaria   239, **251**
malignancy-related venous thromboembolism   184, **200**
malignant bowel obstruction   360, **363**
malignant mesothelioma   395, **416–417**
malignant transformation, melanoma   59, **65**
malnutrition   459, **465–466**
manometry, high-resolution   115, **135**
MAPK *see* mitogen-activated protein kinase
Marfan's syndrome   12, **32**
masculinising hormone therapy   **94**
maternal inheritance   171–172, **179–180**
maternally inherited diabetes and deafness (MIDD)   171–172,
   179–180
maturity-onset diabetes of the young (MODY)   74, **87**, 170–171,
   177–178
mean   97, **100**
measures of central tendency   97, **100**
mechanisms of action

antibacterial agents   242, **258–259**
antidepressants   292, **300–301**
antivirals   243, **260**
bisphosphonates   369, **378**
immunosuppressants   308–309, **329–330**
opioids   372, **386–387**
risperidone   373, **389**
SGLT2   460, **469**
median   97, **100**
Medical Emergency Response Teams   42, **55–56**
medical obstetrics   262–268
   see also obstetrics
medical oncology   269–288
   see also oncology
medication overuse headaches   337, **349**
medications
   calciphylaxis risk   304, **316–317**
   cardiology   11, **31**
   hyperkalaemia   305, **318–319**
   multiple myeloma   **210**
melanoma
   gene mutations   59, **65**
   surgical interventions   59, **65–66**
meliodosis   240, **251–252**
memantine   **379**
membranoproliferative glomerulonephritis (MPGN)   309–310, **331**
membranous nephropathy (MN)   306, **321–322**
MEN see multiple endocrine neoplasia
meningococcal disease   242, **257–258**
menopause   145, **161–162**
mental health   289–301
   adverse psychotropic effects   292, **301**
   antidepressant cessation   291, **298**
   antidepressant mechanisms   292, **300–301**
   bipolar disorder   289, **293**
   clozapine   289, **294**
   confidentiality   291, **298–299**
   conversion disorder   289, **295**
   depression   290–291, 291, **295–296, 298**
   descriptors   291–292, **299–300**
   electroconvulsive therapy   290, 296
   neuroleptic malignant syndrome   290, **297**
   schizophrenia   289, 290, **294, 297–298**
   self-harm   290, 291, **296–297, 298**
   serotonin syndrome   290, **297**
   suicide   289, 290, **293, 296–297**
mepolizumab   **51, 410–411**
mesenteric ischaemia   107, 114, **118, 134**
metabolic complications, bariatric surgery   77–78, **95–96**
metabolic encephalopathy   36, **46**
metabolism
   dendritic cells   74, **86**
   iron metabolism   187, **207**
   macrophages   74, **86**
metanephrines   75, **89–90**
metaraminol   41, **54**
metastatic cord compression   271, **278–279**
metastatic lung cancer   402–403, **425**

metastatic renal cell cancer (mRCC)   269, **274**
methenamine hippurate (Hiprex)   240, **252**
methotrexate   273, **286**, 440, **457**
MFS see Miller Fisher syndrome
MG see myasthenia gravis
MGUS see monoclonal gammopathy of undetermined significance
MI see myocardial infarction
microcytic anaemia   194, **220–221**
MIDD see maternally inherited diabetes and deafness
Miller Fisher syndrome (MFS)   **349–350**
milrinone   41, **54**
mineralocorticoid receptor agonists (MRA)   7, **25**
minoxidil   11, **31**
mipomersen   6, **23**
mirtazapine   292, **300–301**
mitochondrial DNA (mtDNA)   172, **180**
mitogen-activated protein kinase (MAPK) pathway, thyroid carcinomas   77, **94**
mitral stenosis   7, **24**
mitral valve disease   7, **24**
mitral-valve infective endocarditits   4, **20**
MM see multiple myeloma
MN see membranous nephropathy
MND see motor neurone disease
Mobitz type II 2:1 heart block   39, **51–52**
Mobitz type I (Wenckebach) heart block   40, **51–52**
mode   97, **100**
MODY see maturity-onset diabetes of the young
monoclonal antibodies, asthma   393, **410–411**
monoclonal gammopathy of undetermined significance (MGUS)   188, **208**
MOR see μ-opioid receptor
mosaic Down's syndrome   170, **176**
motor neurone disease (MND)   337, **350**, 361, **364**
moxonidine   11, **31**
MPGN see membranoproliferative glomerulonephritis
MPNs see myeloproliferative neoplasms
MRA see mineralocorticoid receptor agonists
mRCC see metastatic renal cell cancer
MS see multiple sclerosis
mtDNA see mitochondrial DNA
multiple endocrine neoplasia (MEN)   74, **86–87**
multiple myeloma (MM)   188–189, **208–210**
   diagnosis   188–189, **208–209**
   lenalidomide   188, **208**
   treatment options   189, **209–210**
multiple sclerosis (MS), optic neuritis   337, **351–352**
multivessel coronary disease   9, **28**
muscular dystrophy   170, **176–177**
mutations
   advanced adenocarcinoma of the lung   271, **279–280**
   Angelman syndrome   171, **178–179**
   autoimmune polyendocrine syndrome   **81–82**
   beta-thalassemia   170, **175**
   BRCA1/BRCA2   269, **275**
   chronic myeloid leukaemia   **211–212**
   CYP2D6 gene   372, **386**
   cystic fibrosis   170, **175**

mutations (*Contd.*)
  Down's syndrome   170, **176**
  essential thrombocythaemia   **204–205**
  hereditary angioedema   **231**
  Huntington's disease   171, **178**
  inheritance patterns   173–174, **182–185**
  isocitrate dehydrogenase   270, **276–277**
  Klinefelter syndrome   171, **179**
  maternal inheritance   171–172, **179–180**
  melanoma   59, **65**
  mitochondrial DNA   172, **180**
  multiple endocrine neoplasia   74, **86–87**
  muscular dystrophy   **176–177**
  neurological conditions   340–341, **357–358**
  Paget's disease of bone   75, **87–88**
  Prader–Willi syndrome   **182**
  spinocerebellar ataxia   172, **181**
  systemic mastocytosis   225, **233**
  thyroid carcinomas   76–77, **93–94**
  tuberous sclerosis complex   172, **181–182**
  variants of uncertain significance   170–171, **177–178**
  Von Hippel–Lindau syndrome   **87, 181**
myasthenia gravis (MG)   337, **351**
Mycobacterium tuberculosis   241, **255**
myeloproliferative neoplasms (MPNs)   189, 191, **211, 213–214**
myocardial infarction (MI)   142, **154**
  classifications   9–10, **29–30**
  intra-aortic balloon pump   36, **47**
  right ventricular   8, **26–27**
  ST elevation   35–36, **45**
  temporary pacing   38–40, **51–52**
myocarditis, acute   145, **162**

NAFLD *see* non-alcoholic fatty liver disease
naive mature B cells   226, **234**
narcolepsy   396, **417**
nausea and vomiting, chemotherapy-induced   269, **276**
nausea and vomiting in pregnancy (NVP)   262, **265**
nebivolol   11, **31**
neck cancer, concurrent chemoradiotherapy   272, **282**
neck pain   145, **162**
necrotising fasciitis   36, **47–48**
necrotising immune myositis   **445**
nephrology   302–333
  acid-base homeostasis   307, **325**
  acute interstitial nephritis   302–303, **313–314**
  acute kidney injury   303, **314**
  acute post-streptococcal glomerulonephritis   302, **312**
  adynamic bone disease   302, **313**
  allograft rejection   308, **328**
  Alport's syndrome   309, **330–331**
  antibody-mediated rejection   303, **314–315**
  anti-glomerular basement membrane disease   303–304, **315**
  autosomal dominant polycystic kidney disease   302, **312–313**
  BK virus nephropathy   306, **323–324**
  bone-kidney endocrine axis   307, **324**
  C3 glomerulopathy   304, **316**
  calciphylaxis risk of medications   304, **316–317**
  contrast-induced nephropathy   308, **326–327**
  dapagliflozin   308, **327**
  darbepoetin   307, **324**
  diabetic nephropathy   310, **331–332**
  dialysis commencement   304–305, **318**
  differential diagnoses   309–311, **330–333**
  estimated glomerular filtration rates   370, **381**
  Goodpasture's syndrome   310–311, **332**
  hyperkalaemia   305, **318–319, 321**
  hyponatraemia   306, **323**
  IgA nephropathy   305, 307, **319–320, 325**
  immunosuppressant activity mechanisms   308–309, **329–330**
  Indigenous Australians   303, **314**
  lithium risks   305, **320**
  membranoproliferative glomerulonephritis   309–310, **331**
  membranous nephropathy   306, **321–322**
  nephrotic syndrome   308, 311, **327, 332–333**
  podocytes   307, **325–326**
  post-transplant lymphoproliferative disorders   307, 308, **326, 328**
  primary focal segmental glomerulosclerosis   309, 311, **330, 333**
  rhabdomyolysis   306, **322**
  roxadustat   306, **322–323**
  SGLT2 inhibitors   308, **327**
  systemic lupus erythematosus   305, **320–321**
  thin basement membrane nephropathy   309, **331**
  trimethoprim   308, **328**
nephrotic syndrome   308, 311, **327, 332–333**
nerve compression   339, **355**
neurofibromatosis   173, **182**, 340, **357–358**
neurogenic orthostatic hypotension   338, **352**
neuroimaging, headaches   336, **346–347**
neuroleptic malignant syndrome (NMS)   290, **297**
neurological effects, autoantibodies   227, **236**
neurology   334–359
  anticonvulsant medications   340, **357**
  Bell's palsy   334, **342**
  benign paroxysmal positional vertigo   334, **342–343**
  cannabinoids   334, **343**
  central venous sinus thrombosis   335, **344**
  cerebrospinal fluid components   335, **345**
  chronic inflammatory demyelinating polyradiculoneuropathy   335, **344–345**
  encephalitis   336, 338, **347–348, 353**
  endovascular thrombectomy   336, **348–349**
  genetic mutations   340–341, **357–358**
  Guillain–Barré syndrome   335–336, 337, **346, 349–350**
  headaches   336, 337, **346–347, 349**
  herpes simplex virus encephalitis   336, **347–348**
  Horner's syndrome   334, **343**
  intracranial parenchymal haemorrhage   336, **348**
  juvenile epilepsy syndrome   334, **343**
  lacunar stroke syndromes   336, **348**
  lamotrigine in pregnancy   335, **345–346**
  lesion presentations   341, **358–359**
  levodopa-induced dyskinesias   338, **354**
  motor neuron disease   337, **350**
  myasthenia gravis   337, **351**

nerve compression 339, **355**
nitrous oxide abuse 338, **354–355**
optic neuritis 337, **351–352**
orthostatic hypotension 338, **352**
Parkinson's disease 338, 341, **352, 353–354, 358**
paroxysmal nocturnal haemoglobinuria 335, **344**
primary central nervous system tumours 338–339, **355**
radiculopathies 339, **355**
stroke 336–337, 338, 339, **348–349, 355, 356**
subacute combined degeneration 338, **354–355**
subdural haematoma 339, **356**
trigeminal neuralgia 340, **357**
neuromyelitis optica (NMO) 337, **351–352**
neurosyphilis 240, **252–253**
neutropaenia
  febrile 186, **205**
  rheumatoid arthritis 433, **446**
NHL see non-Hodgkin lymphoma
nilotinib 189, **211–212**
nitrate tolerance 371, **383**
nitrous oxide abuse 338, **354–355**
nivolumab 271, **280**–281
NMO see neuromyelitis optica
NMS see neuroleptic malignant syndrome
NNT see number needed to treat
noisy breathing, palliative medicine 362, **366**
non-alcoholic fatty liver disease (NAFLD) 114, **134–135**
non-communicating hydrocephalus 341, **359**
non-competitive inhibition 369, **381**
non-Hodgkin lymphoma (NHL) 189, **211**
non-invasive positive pressure ventilation (NPPV) 396, **418**
non-parametric tests 97, **100–101**
non-small cell lung cancer (NSCLC)
  management 270, **276**
  mutations 271, **279–280**
noradrenaline 41, **54**
normal physiological changes, ageing 141, **151–152**
normal pressure hydrocephalus 150, **168–169**
Norovirus 241, **253**
NPPV see non-invasive positive pressure ventilation
NSCLC see non-small cell lung cancer
number needed to treat (NNT) 97, **101**
nutritional complications, bariatric surgery 77–78, **95–96**
NVP see nausea and vomiting in pregnancy

OA see osteoarthritis
obesity
  cancer risk 271, **280**
  drug dosing 372, **386**
obesity hypoventilation syndrome (OHS) 466
obstetrics 262–268
  antiphospholipid syndrome 262, **264**
  asthma 262, **264**
  bipolar disorder 289, **293**
  hypertension 262, 263, **265, 266–267**
  hypothyroidism 262, **266**
  lamotrigine dosage 335, **345–346**

lithium 289, **293**
  nausea and vomiting 262, **265**
  platelet counts 263, **268**
  pre-eclampsia 263, **266–267**
  transplant recipients 263, **267–268**
obstructive sleep apnoea (OSA) 150, **168**, 396, **418–420**
OCPs see oral contraceptive pills
ODC see oxygen dissociation curve
odds ratio (OR) 97, **101**
oesophageal dysphagia 115, **135–136**
Ogilvie's syndrome 116–117, **137–138**
OHS see obesity hyperventilation syndrome
olanzapine 292, **301**
omalizumab 393, **410–411**
omecamtiv 41, **54**
omega-3 fatty acids 7, **24–25**
oncology 269–288
  adverse events of chemotherapeutics 272–273, **285–286**
  bevacizumab 269, **274**
  BRCA1/BRCA2 mutations 269, **275**
  cancer of unknown primary 270, **278**
  cervical screening program 269, **275–276**
  chemotherapy-induced nausea and vomiting 269, **276**
  chimeric antigen receptor T-cells 269, **275**
  concurrent chemoradiotherapy 272, **282**
  head and neck cancer 272, **282**
  isocitrate dehydrogenase mutations 270, **276–277**
  leptomeningeal carcinomatosis 270, **277**
  Lynch syndrome 270, **278**
  metastatic cord compression 271, **278–279**
  nivolumab 271, **280**–281
  non small cell lung cancer 270, 271, **276, 279–280**
  obesity risks 271, **280**
  ovarian cancer 272, **283**
  programmed death ligand 1 (PD-L1) 271, **281**
  prostate cancer 271–272, **279, 281–282**
  radiotherapy 272, **282–283**
  sunitinib 269, **274**
  targeted chemotherapeutic agents 273, **287–288**
  tumour lysis syndrome 272, **283–284**
  tumour markers 272, **284–285**
one compartment models 369, **378–379**
μ-opioid receptor (MOR) 372, **386–387**
opioids
  mechanisms of action 372, **386–387**
  rotation 361, **364–365**
  toxicity 42, **56**, 361, **365**
  use disorder 371–372, **384–385**
optic chiasm 341, **359**
optic neuritis 337, **351–352**
OR see odds ratio
oral contraceptive pills (OCPs), side effects 112, **127**
organ transplant recipients, suncreen usage 61, **68**
orthostatic hypotension, Parkinson's disease 338, **352**
OSA see obstructive sleep apnoea
osimertinib 273, **287**
osteitis deformans 434–435, **448**
osteoarthritis (OA) 434, **448**

osteoporosis, bone turnover markers   431, **444**
ovarian cancer   272, **283**
ovarian failure, premature   74, **85**
ovaries, polycystic syndrome   75, **89**
overanticoagulation   374, **391**
overdetection   460, **467**
overdiagnosis   460, **467**
overdose management
   cocaine   375, **392**
   paracetamol   37, **48**
overmedicalisation   460, **467**
oxaliplatin   273, **285–286**
oxidative metabolism, alcohol   141, **153**
oxybutynin   145–146, **163**, 371, **384**
oxycodone   145–146, **163**
oxygen dissociation curve (ODC)   396, **420**

pacemakers   4–5, **20**
   implantable cardioverter-defibrillators   6, **22–23**
Paget's disease of bone (PDB)   75, **87–88**, 434–435, **448–449**
painful diabetic neuropathy (PDN)   75, **88**
palliative medicine   360–367
   advance care planning   361, **365**
   cancer   361–362, **364–366**
   corticosteroids   361–362, **366**
   haemodialysis withdrawal   360, **363–364**
   malignant bowel obstruction   360, **363**
   motor neurone disease   361, **364**
   noisy breathing   362, **366**
   opioid rotation   361, **364–365**
   thirst and dry mouth   360, **363**
   tube feeding withdrawal   362, **367**
PAN see polyarteritis nodosa
pancreatitis   107–108, **118–119**
   IgG4-related autoimmune   225, **232**
panniculitis, erythema nodosum   58–59, **63–64**
PAP see pulmonary alveolar proteinosis
papillary thyroid carcinoma (PTC)   76–77, **93**
paracetamol
   hepatotoxicity risk   115, **136**
   overdose management   37, **48**
paraneoplastic autoimmune conditions   227, **236**
paraneoplastic neurological syndromes (PNS)   338, **353**
Parkinson's disease
   clinical features   338, 341, **353–354, 358**
   levodopa-induced dyskinesias   338, **354**
   orthostatic hypotension   338, **352**
paroxysmal nocturnal haemoglobinuria (PNH)   335, **344**
patent ductus arteriosus (PDA)   12, **33**
patiromer   305, **321**
pazopanib   273, **288**
PBC see primary biliary cirrhosis
PBSCT see peripheral blood stem cell transplant
PCI see percutaneous coronary intervention
PCOS see polycystic ovarian syndrome
PCR see polymerase chain reaction
PCT see porphyria cutanea tarda

PD see peritoneal dialysis
PDA see patent ductus arteriosus
PDB see Paget's disease of bone
PD-L1 see programmed death ligand 1
PDN see painful diabetic neuropathy
PEA see pulseless electrical activity
penicillin, allergies   225, **228, 232**
percutaneous coronary intervention (PCI)   9, **28**
pericarditis   35–36, **45**
perioperative management   145, **163**
   warfarin   **201–203**
peripheral blood film examination   194–198, **220–222**
peripheral blood stem cell transplant (PBSCT)   191, **215**
peritoneal dialysis (PD)   307, **325**
pernicious anaemia   189–190, **212**
peroneal nerve compression   339, **355**
P-glycoprotein (P-gp) inhibitors   372, **385**
phaeochromocytoma   75, **89–90**
pharmacodynamics   372, **385**
pharmacokinetics, ageing   368, **376**
pharmacology   368–392
   Addison's disease   369, **380**
   ageing   368, **376**
   Alzheimer's disease   369, **379**
   ampicillin elimination   368, **376**
   anticholinergic medicines   368, 371, **376–377, 384**
   azithromycin   368, 374, **377, 391**
   β-blockers   374, **392**
   bioavailability   371, **384**
   biosimilar medications   368, **377–378**
   bisphosphonates   369, **378**
   BMI considerations   372, **386**
   clopidogrel   369, **379**
   cocaine overdose   375, **392**
   competitive/non-competitive inhibition   369, **381**
   crossover studies   369, **379–380**
   drug metabolising enzymes   372, **386**
   estimated glomerular filtration rates   370, **381**
   first-pass metabolism   368, 370, **376, 382**
   heparin-induced thrombocytopenia   370–371, **382–383**
   indapamide   371, **383**
   ischaemic stroke treatments   373–384, **389**
   nitrate tolerance   371, **383**
   μ-opioid receptor   372, **386–387**
   opioid use disorder   371–372, **384–385**
   pharmacodynamics   372, **385**
   polypharmacy   372–373, **387**
   pramipexole   373, **388**
   prodrugs   373, **388**
   Pseudomonas aeruginosa treatment   371, **383–384**
   risperidone   373, **389**
   steady-state concentrations   369, **378–379**
   vancomycin   374, **390–391, 392**
   warfarin interactions   374, **391**
phenelzine   292, **300–301**
phenylephrine   41, **54**
phenytoin   340, **357**
pituitary tumours   75–76, **90–91**

Plasmodium falciparum 239, **251**

platelet counts, pregnancy 263, **268**

pleural effusion 397, 399–400, **421**, **423**

pleural effusion transudates 397, **421**

PML *see* progressive multifocal leukoencephalopathy

PMR *see* polymyalgia rheumatica

pneumonia
aspiration 403, **425**
cryptogenic organizing 407, **427**
silicosis 396, **419**
urinary antigen tests 394, **411–412**

pneumothorax 398, 402, **422**, **425**

PNH *see* paroxysmal nocturnal haemoglobinuria

PNS *see* paraneoplastic neurological syndromes

podocytes 307, **325–326**

poisoning
carbon monoxide 34, **44**
ethylene glycol 370, **381**

polyarteritis nodosa (PAN) 438, **456**

polycystic ovarian syndrome (PCOS) 75, **89**

polycythaemia vera (PV) 189, 191, **211**, **213–214**

polyenes 237, **245**

polymerase chain reaction (PCR) tests 460, **467–468**

polymorphic ventricular tachycardia (PVTs) 2–3, **16**

polymyalgia rheumatica (PMR) 435, **449**

polymyositis **445**

polypharmacy 372–373, **387**, **389**
statins 373, **389**
warfarin 374, **391**

polysaccharide vaccines 226, **235**

polyunsaturated fatty acids (PUFAs) 7, **24–25**

population attributable risk 98, **105**

porphyria cutanea tarda (PCT) 60, **66–67**

posterior tibial nerve compression 339, **355**

post-transplant lymphoproliferative disorders (PTLD) 307, 308, **326**, **328**

postural hypotension 146, **164**

PPI *see* proton-pump inhibitors

Prader–Willi syndrome (PWS) **182**

pramipexole 373, **388**

prednisolone 441, **457**

preeclampsia 263, **266–267**

pre-excitation Wolff–Parkinson–White syndrome 10–11, **30–31**

pre-exposure prophylaxis (PrEP) 238, **248**

pregnancy *see* obstetrics

premature ovarian failure 74, **85**

PrEP *see* pre-exposure prophylaxis

prevalence 98, 98, **102**, **104**

primary aldosteronism 149, **168**

primary biliary cirrhosis (PBC) 112, 115, **127–128**, **137**

primary central nervous system tumours 338–339, **355**

primary focal segmental glomerulosclerosis (FSGS) 309, 311, **330**, **333**

primary membranous nephropathy 306, **321–322**

primary spontaneous pneumothorax (PSP) 398, **422**

procalcitonin **254**

prodrugs 373, **388**

progestins, gender-affirmation treatment 77, **94**

programmed death ligand 1 (PD-L1) 271, **281**

progressive multifocal leukoencephalopathy (PML) 190, **213**

prolactin levels 75–76, **90–91**

prolonged prothrombin time (PT) 185–186, **203–204**

prospective cohort studies 99, **103**

prostate cancer
biopsy 271–272, **279**, **282**
risk factors 271, **281**

protein C 193, **219**

prothrombin time (PT) 185–186, **203–204**

proton-pump inhibitors (PPIs) 115, **136–137**

protoporphyria 60, **66–67**

proximal Roux-en-Y gastric bypass (RYGB) 77, **95**

PSA values *see* prostate specific antigen 271–272, **282**

pseudogout 431, **444**

Pseudomonas aeruginosa **256**, 371, **383–384**

psoriatic arthritis 436, **450**

PSP *see* primary spontaneous pneumothorax

PT *see* prothrombin time (PT)

PTC *see* papillary thyroid carcinoma

PTLD *see* post-transplant lymphoproliferative disorders

puberty blockers 77, **94**

publication bias 98, **104**

public health measures, meningococcal disease 242, **257–258**

pulmonary alveolar proteinosis (PAP) 407, **428**

pulmonary embolism (PE) 394, 403–404, **412–413**, **425**

pulmonary tuberculosis 241, **255**

pulseless electrical activity (PEA) 37, **48–49**

PUO *see* pyrexia of unknown origin

PV *see* polycythaemia vera

PVTs *see* polymorphic ventricular tachycardia

PWS *see* Prader–Willi syndrome

pyrexia of unknown origin (PUO) 241, **253–254**

pyrimidine analogues 237, **245**

Q fever 241, **254**

RAAS blockade *see* renin–angiotensin–aldosterone system blockade

radioisotope bone scans 143, **154**

radiotherapy
concurrent chemotherapy 272, **282**
gating 272, **283**

randomisation, bias 97, **101–102**

range 98, **103**

RCM *see* restrictive cardiomyopathy

reactive arthritis 436, **450–451**

real-time continuous glucose monitoring (RTCGM) 76, **91–92**

recall bias 97, **101–102**

recombinant vaccines 226, **235**

red eye, acute 141, **151**

red person syndrome **392**

refeeding syndrome (RFS) 146, **164–165**

regorafenib 273, **288**

regulatory T cells (Tregs) 226, **234**

renal calculi 109, **121–122**

renal transplants, antibody-mediated rejection 223, **229**
renin–angiotensin–aldosterone system (RAAS) blockade **83**
research 97–106
  confounding 98–99, **105–106**
  correlation 98, **102–103**
  crossover studies 369, **379–380**
  dispersion measures 98, **103**
  forest plots 98–99, **103–103**
  informed consent 98, **103–104**
  non-parametric tests 97, **100–101**
  number needed to treat 97, **101**
  odds ratio 97, **101**
  prevalence 98, 98, **102, 104**
  publication bias 98, **104**
  randomisation 97, **101–102**
  study types 99, **103**
resistance, antimicrobials 242–243, **259–260**
respiratory medicine 393–429
  acute eosinophilic pneumonia 394–395, **415**
  acute pulmonary oedema 404, **425**
  allergic bronchopulmonary aspergillosis
      394–395, 401, 407, **415, 424, 427**
  amiodarone 393, **409–410**
  α1-antitrypsin deficiency 393, **409**
  arterial blood gas measurement 401–402, **424–425**
  asbestos exposure 397, **421–422**
  aspiration pneumonia 403, **425**
  asthma 393–394, **410–411**
  bronchiectasis 394, **411**
  chronic thromboembolic pulmonary
      hypertension 394, **412–413**
  community acquired pneumonia 394, **411–412, 413**
  continuous positive airway pressure 396, **418–419**
  COPD 394, 396, **414, 417, 420**
  cryptogenic organizing pneumonia 407, **427**
  cystic fibrosis 394, **412**
  D-dimer degradation product of fibrin 394, **414**
  eosinophilic granulomatosis with polyangiitis
      401, 408, **424, 429**
  granulomatosis with polyangiitis 405, **426**
  haemoptysis 395, **416**
  idiopathic pulmonary fibrosis 398–399, 407, **422–423, 428**
  interstitial lung disease 400–401, **424**
  kyphoscoliosis 397, **420**
  Legionella Sp. 395, **415**
  Löfgren syndrome 406, **426–427**
  lymphangioleiomyomatosis 408–409, **428**
  malignant mesothelioma 395, **416–417**
  metastatic lung cancer 402–403, **425**
  non-invasive positive pressure ventilation 396, **418**
  obstructive sleep apnoea 396, **418–420**
  pleural effusion 397, 399–400, **421, 423**
  pneumothorax 398, 402, **422, 425**
  pulmonary alveolar proteinosis 407, **428**
  pulmonary embolism 394, 403–404, **412–413, 425**
  silicosis 396, **419**
  small cell lung cancer 399, **423**
    tension pneumothorax 398, **422**
    urinary antigen tests 394, **411–412**
restrictive cardiomyopathy (RCM) 7, **25**
retinopathy, hypertensive 6, **22**
RFS *see* refeeding syndrome
rhabdomyolysis 306, **322**
rheumatic fever 7, **24, 26**
rheumatoid arthritis (RA) 433, 436–437, **446, 451–452**
rheumatology 430–457
  ankylosing spondylitis 430, **442–443**
  antinuclear antibodies 430, **443**
  antiphospholipid syndrome 430, **442**
  arthritis 431–432, 436, **444–445, 450–451**
  autoimmune biomarkers 438–440, **454–455**
  avascular necrosis 430, **443**
  Behçet's disease 439, **456**
  bone turnover markers 431, **444**
  disease-modifying antirheumatic drugs 440–441, **457**
  giant cell arteritis 433, **447**
  gout 431–432, 433, **444–445, 446**
  idiopathic inflammatory myopathies 432, **445**
  inclusion body myositis 433–434, **445, 447**
  neutropaenia 433, **446**
  osteoarthritis 434, **448**
  osteoporosis 431, **444**
  Paget's disease of bone 434–435, **448–449**
  polyarteritis nodosa 438, **456**
  polymyalgia rheumatica 435, **449**
  psoriatic arthritis 436, **450**
  reactive arthritis 436, **450–451**
  rheumatoid arthritis 433, 436–437, **446, 451–452**
  Sjögren's syndrome 435–436, **449–450**
  spondyloarthropathy 438, **455**
  systemic lupus erythematosus 430, 437, **443, 453**
  systemic sclerosis 437, **452–453**
  Takayasu arteritis 440, **456–457**
RIFLE criteria *see* risk, injury, failure, loss, and end-stage kidney
    disease
right ventricular myocardial infarction (RVMI) 8, **26–27**
risk 98, **104–105**
risk factors
  contrast-induced nephropathy 308, **326–327**
  prostate cancer 271, **281**
risk, injury, failure, loss, and end-stage kidney disease (RIFLE)
    criteria **49–50**
risperidone 373, **389**
rituximab 436, 440, **451, 457**
rivaroxaban 2, **15**
RNA
  small interfering 172, **180–181**
  vaccines 225, **232–233**
Romberg's sign 240, **252–253**, 338
rosacea 60, **67**
rosuvastatin 6, **23**
rotator cuff (RC) 460, **468**
Roux-en-Y gastric bypass (RYGB) 77, **95**
roxadustat 306, **322–323**

RTCGM *see* real-time continuous glucose monitoring
RVMI *see* right ventricular myocardial infarction
RYGB *see* Roux-en-Y gastric bypass

S1 radiculopathy 339, **355**
sacubitril 11, **31**
"saddleback" ST segment elevation 36, **45**
sarcopenia 146, **165**
SARS-CoV-2 225, **232–233**, 237, **245–246**, 459, 460, **462–463**, **464**, **468**
SAVE trial 396, **418–419**
SAVR *see* surgical aortic valve replacement
SCA *see* spinocerebellar ataxia
scabies 61, **67**
scalded skin syndrome, Staphylococcal 62, **69**
SCD *see* sickle cell disease; subacute combined degeneration
schizophrenia 289, 290, **294**, **297–298**
sciatica 144–145, **161**
SCLC *see* small cell lung cancer
scleroderma 437, **452–453**
Screening Tool of Older Persons' Potentially inappropriate Prescriptions (STOPP) **163–164**
Screening Tool to Alert Doctors to Right Treatment (START) criteria **163**
scurvy 147–148, **166**
SD *see* standard deviation
SDH *see* subdural haematoma
secondary hyperparathyroidism 74, **86**
selection bias 97, 98–99, **101–102**, **105–106**
self-harm 290, 291, **296–297**, **298**
sentinel lymph node biopsy (SLNB) 59, **65–66**
sepsis 38, 40–41, **51**, **53–54**
septic arthritis 431–432, **444–445**
septic shock 34, 37–38, 40–41, **44–45**, **49–50**, **51**, **53–54**
serotonin syndrome (SS) 290, **297**
serum biomarkers, autoimmune conditions 438–440, **454–455**
severe aortic stenosis 2, 8, **14–15**, **28**
severe asthma 38, 42, **50–51**, **55**
severe back pain 144–145, **161**
severe mitral stenosis 7, **24**
SGLT2, mechanism of action 460, **469**
SGLT2 inhibitors (SGLT2i) 5, **21**, **83**
  nephropathies 308, **327**
  side effects 76, **92**
sickle cell disease (SCD) 191, **214–215**
silicosis 396, **419**
sinus node dysfunction 8, **27**
siRNA *see* small interfering RNA
Sjögren's syndrome 435–436, **449–450**
SJS *see* Stevens Johnson Syndrome
skin, layers 61, **68**
sleep medicine 393–429
  narcolepsy 396, **417**
  obstructive sleep apnoea 396, **418–419**
SLNB *see* sentinel lymph node biopsy
small bowel bacterial overgrowth 116, **138**

small cell lung cancer (SCLC) 227, **236**, 338, **353**, 399, **423**
small interfering RNA (siRNA) 172, **180–181**
smoking, electronic cigarettes 143, **157**
SpA *see* spondyloarthropathy
Spearman's rank correlation 98, **102**
spina bifida 173, **182**
spinal cord, metastatic compression 271, **278–279**
spinocerebellar ataxia (SCA) 172, **181**
splenectomies, vaccine requirements 226, **235–236**
spondyloarthropathy (SpA) 438, **455**
SS *see* serotonin syndrome
SSc *see* systemic sclerosis
SSC *see* Surviving Sepsis Campaign
standard deviation (SD) 98, **103**
Staphylococcal scalded skin syndrome 62, **69**
Staphylococcus aureus 241, **255**, **256**
START criteria *see* Screening Tool to Alert Doctors to Right Treatment criteria
statins 6, **23**, 373, **389**
statistics 97–106
  attack rate 98, **105**
  bias 98–99, **104–106**
  case fatality 98, **105**
  central tendency 97, **100**
  confounding 98–99, **105–106**
  correlation 98, **102–103**
  crude rates 98, **105**
  dispersion measures 98, **103**
  forest plots 98–99, **103–103**
  incidence rate 98, **105**
  non-parametric tests 97, **100–101**
  number needed to treat 97, **101**
  odds ratio 97, **101**
  population attributable risk 98, **105**
  prevalence 98, 98, **102**, **104**
  randomisation 97, **101–102**
  risk 98, **104–105**
steady-state concentrations 369, **378–379**
ST elevation acute myocardial infarction (STEMI) 35–36, **45**
stem-cell transplants
  graft-versus-host disease 191, **214**, **215**
  peripheral blood stem cells 191, **215**
STEMI *see* ST elevation acute myocardial infarction
stenoses
  aortic 2, 8, **14–15**, **28**
  mitral 7, **24**
Stevens Johnson Syndrome (SJS) 61, 62, **68–69**, 292, **301**
STOPP *see* Screening Tool of Older Persons' Potentially inappropriate Prescriptions
Streptococcus pneumoniae 394, **411–412**, 413
Streptococcus pyogenes **256**
stress, Takotsubo cardiomyopathy 8, **27–28**
stroke 336–337, 338, 339, **348–349**, **355**, **356**
  pharmacological treatment 373–384, **389**
strongyloidiasis 148, **166–167**, 241, **254–255**
Students t-test 98, **103**
subacute combined degeneration (SCD) 338, **354–355**

subclinical hypothyroidism   76, **92–93**
subdural haematoma (SDH)   339, **356**
suicide   289, 290, **293**, **296–297**
sulfasalazine   441, **457**
sunscreen usage   61, **68**
sunitinib   269, **274**
surgical aortic valve replacement (SAVR)   2, **15**
surgical interventions, melanoma   59, **65–66**
Surviving Sepsis Campaign (SSC)   **51**, **54**
switching antidepressants   291, **298**
syncope   3, **18**
   Holter monitoring   6, **23**
synpharyngitic glomerulonephritis   150, **168**
syphilis   240, **252–253**
systemic lupus erythematosus (SLE)
   antinuclear antibodies   430, **443**
   laboratory testing   437, **453**
   nephrology   305, **320–321**
systemic mastocytosis   225, **233**
systemic sclerosis (SSc)   437, **452–453**

tacrolimus   116, **138–139**
Takayasu arteritis   440, **456–457**
Takotsubo cardiomyopathy   8, **27–28**
targeted chemotherapeutic agents   273, **287–288**
TAVI *see* transcatheter aortic valve implantation
TB *see* tuberculosis
TBMN *see* thin basement membrane nephropathy
TCA *see* tricarboxylic acid cycle
T cells   226, **234**
   Staphylococcus aureus   241, **255**
TE *see* thromboembolism
temazepam   145–146, **163**
temporary pacing   38–40, **51–52**
TEN *see* Toxic epidermal necrolysis
tension pneumothorax   398, **422**
"tented" T waves   35, **45**
teriparatide   **378**
terlipressin   116, **139**
testosterone replacement therapy (TRT)   74, **84–85**
Tetralogy of Fallot   12, **32**
TGA *see* transient global amnesia
TGD *see* transgender persons
thermogenic beige adipocytes   **82**
thin basement membrane nephropathy (TBMN)   309, **331**
thirst, palliative medicine   360, **363**
thrombocytopenia
   heparin-induced   186, **205–206**, 370–371, **382–383**
   idiopathic purpura   187–188, **207–208**
thromboembolism (TE), warfarin treatment   185, **201–203**
thrombophilia, inherited   191, **216**
thyroid carcinomas   76–77, **93–94**
thyroid function tests (TFTs)   78, **96**
thyroid nodules   77, **94**
thyroxine, pregnancy   262, **266**
TLRs *see* toll-like receptors
TLS *see* tumour lysis syndrome

TNF inhibitors   441, **457**
toclizumab   440, **457**
tofacitinib   436, 441, **451**, **457**
tolerance, nitrates   371, **383**
toll-like receptors (TLRs)   226, **234**
topiramate   340, **357**
topoisomerase (Top) 2α inhibition   2, **14**
torsade de pointes   42, **56**
Toxic epidermal necrolysis (TEN)   61, 62, **68–69**, **69**,
   292, **301**
toxicology   368–392
   ampicillin   368, **376**
   azithromycin   368, **377**
   cocaine overdose   375, **392**
   ethylene glycol   370, **381**
   indapamide   371, **383**
   P-glycoprotein inhibition   372, **385**
   P-glycoprotein inhibitors   372, **385**
   polypharmacy   372–373, **387**, **389**
   vancomycin   374, **392**
   see also pharmacology
toxoid vaccines   226, **235**
TRALI *see* transfusion-related acute lung injury
tranexamic acid   40, **52**
transcatheter aortic valve implantation (TAVI)   2, 8, **15**, **28**
transfusion-related acute lung injury (TRALI)   191–192, **216–217**
transgender (TGD) persons, hormone therapy   77
transient global amnesia (TGA)   374, **390**
transplant indicators, liver   114, **133**
transplant recipients
   antibody-mediated rejection   223, **229**, 303, **314–315**
   BK virus nephropathy   306, **323–324**
   failure to adhere   308, **328**
   graft-versus-host disease   191, **214**, **215**
   lymphoproliferative disorders   307, 308, **326**, **328**
   peripheral blood stem cells   191, **215**
   pregnancy   263, **267–268**
   sunscreen usage   61, **68**
   vaccination recommendations   241, **256**
transposition of the great arteries   12, **32–33**
transrectal ultrasound (TRUS)   271, **279**
transthyretin amyloidosis (ATTR)   3, **16–17**
transudates, pleural   397, **421**
treatment-resistant hypertension   7, **25**
treatment-resistant schizophrenia, clozapine   289, **294**
Tregs *see* regulatory T cells
tricarboxylic acid cycle (TCA)   74, **86**
trigeminal neuralgia   340, **357**
trimethoprim   308, **328**
trisomy 21   170, **176**
troponins   9, **29**
TRT *see* testosterone replacement therapy
TRUS *see* transrectal ultrasound
tryptase levels, anaphylaxis   225, **233–234**
TSC *see* tuberous sclerosis complex
tube feeding withdrawal   362, **367**
tuberculosis (TB), pulmonary   241, **255**
tuberous sclerosis complex (TSC)   172, **181–182**

tumour lysis syndrome (TLS)   272, **283–284**
tumour markers   272, **284–285**
tumours
  adrenal incidentaloma   72, **80**
  central nervous system   338–339, **355**
  multiple endocrine neoplasia   74, **86–87**
  pituitary   75–76, **90–91**
  see also cancer
type 2 diabetes, with cardiovascular disease   5, **21**

UAT *see* urinary antigen tests
UGIB *see* upper gastrointestinal bleeding
unconjugated hyperbilirubinemia   112, **127–128**
uncoupling protein-1   **82**
unilateral neglect   341, **359**
unpaired t-test   98, **103**
upper gastrointestinal bleeding (UGIB)   116–117, **139–137**
uric acid crystals   109, **121–122**
urinary antigen tests (UAT), pneumonia   394, **411–412**
urosepsis, septic shock   40–41, **53**

VA *see* ventricular arrhythmias
vaccinations   226, **235–236**
  influenza   239, **250**
  RNA-based   225, **232–233**
  splenectomies   226, **235–236**
  transplant recipients   241, **256**
valproic acid (VPA)-induced hyperammonaemia   146–147, **166**
vancomycin   374, **390–391**, **392**
vaping   143, **157**
variants of uncertain significance (VUS)   170–171, **177–178**
varicella-zoster virus (VZV)   242, **257**, 336, **347–348**
vascular dementia   150, **168**
vasopressin   41, **54**
vasopressin analogues, terlipressin   116, **139**
vasopressors, critical care   41, **54**
VBG *see* venous blood gas
venous blood gas (VBG)   40, **52**
venous disease   144, **160–161**

venous thromboembolism (VTE)
  D-dimer degradation product of fibrin   394, **414**
  inherited thrombophilia   191, **216**
  malignancy-related   184, **200**
ventricular arrhythmias (VA)   460, **466–467**
ventricular septal defect (VSD)   12, **32**
ventricular tachycardia (VT)   40, **53**
VHL *see* Von Hippel–Lindau mutations
vitamin A deficiency   77, **95**
vitamin B1 deficiency   77, **95**
vitamin B12 deficiency   77, **95**, 189–190, **212**, 338, **354–355**
vitamin C deficiency   147–148, **166**
vitamin deficiencies, gastric bypass surgery   77–78, **95–96**
Von Hippel–Lindau (VHL) mutations   **87**, **181**
von Willebrand disease (VWD)   192–193, **218**
VPA *see* valproic acid
VSD *see* ventricular septal defect
VT *see* ventricular tachycardia
VTE *see* venous thromboembolism
VUS *see* variants of uncertain significance
VWD *see* von Willebrand disease
VZV *see* varicella-zoster virus

Waldenström macroglobulinaemia (WM)   193, **218–219**
warfarin   185, **201–203**, 304, **316–317**
  polypharmacy   374, **391**
water deprivation test   78, **96**
Wenckebach (Mobitz type I) heart block   40, **51–52**
Whipple's disease   107, **118–119**
white adipocytes   **82**
Wilson's disease   173, **182**
withdrawal syndromes, alcohol   141–142, **153**
WM *see* Waldenström macroglobulinaemia
Wolff–Parkinson–White (WPW) syndrome   10–11, **30–31**
WPW syndrome *see* Wolff–Parkinson–White syndrome

Zika virus   242, **257**
zinc deficiency   77–78, **95–96**
Zollinger–Ellison syndrome   117, **137**

Printed and bound by CPI Group (UK) Ltd, Croydon, CR0 4YY

21/10/2024

14576965-0001

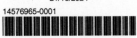